Atlas of
Osteopathic
Techniques

Third Edition

Atlas of
Osteopathic
Techniques

Third Edition

Alexander S. Nicholas, DO, FAAO

Professor and Chairman
Department of Osteopathic Manipulative Medicine
Philadelphia College of Osteopathic Medicine
Philadelphia, Pennsylvania

Evan A. Nicholas, DO

Associate Professor
Department of Osteopathic Manipulative Medicine
Philadelphia College of Osteopathic Medicine
Philadelphia, Pennsylvania

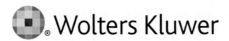 Wolters Kluwer

Philadelphia • Baltimore • New York • London
Buenos Aires • Hong Kong • Sydney • Tokyo

Acquisitions Editor: Tari Broderick
Product Development Editor: Greg Nicholl
Marketing Manager: Joy Fisher Williams
Production Project Manager: David Orzechowski
Design Coordinator: Elaine Kasmer
Art Director: Jennifer Clements
Manufacturing Coordinator: Margie Orzech
Prepress Vendor: SPi Global

3rd edition

Library of Congress Cataloging-in-Publication Data
Nicholas, Alexander S., author.
Atlas of osteopathic techniques / Alexander S. Nicholas, Evan A. Nicholas. — Third edition.
   p. ; cm.
  Osteopathic techniques
  Includes bibliographical references and index.
  ISBN 978-1-4511-9341-1
 I. Nicholas, Evan A., author. II. Title. III. Title: Osteopathic techniques.
  [DNLM: 1. Manipulation, Osteopathic—Atlases. WB 17]
  RZ342
  615.5'33—dc23

                                                              2015011291

LWW.com

CCS0915

Dedication

"Dr. Nick"

In 1974, the authors' father, Nicholas S. Nicholas, DO, FAAO, chairman of the Osteopathic Principles and Practice Department at Philadelphia College of Osteopathic Medicine (PCOM) published the first edition of *Atlas of Osteopathic Techniques*. His goal was to put into print a number of the commonly used osteopathic manipulative techniques of that time. They were to be used by medical students to reference the techniques being taught in the classroom and to standardize the techniques so that in the oral examination, the evaluation of their work could be more objectively evaluated.

Nicholas S. Nicholas, DO, a 1939 graduate of Kirksville College of Osteopathy, was a general practitioner who also specialized in industrial and sports medicine. He used osteopathic techniques routinely in his practice, and because of the clinical results, he was very excited to teach these techniques to medical students. Affectionately known as Dr. Nick to his students, he began teaching at PCOM in 1946 and in 1974 became the chairman of the Osteopathic Principles and Practice Department. In 1974, he enlisted PCOM faculty members to develop a list of techniques to include in the original edition of his atlas. These faculty members included David Heilig, DO, FAAO; Robert England, DO, FAAO; Marvin Blumberg, DO, FAAO; Jerome Sulman, DO; and Katherine England, DO.

The students benefited, and their attempts to learn the techniques were improved, as was seen during PCOM examinations. As word of this text spread, PCOM alumni and other osteopathic physicians also saw a need for this text as a review and/or reference of standard techniques for their practices. Because of illness, Dr. Nick was able to produce only two editions of his work.

Over the years, the atlas gave way to videotape demonstrations of techniques and further edited and expanded versions of the written techniques. From the time of the inception of the atlas, the number of named styles of osteopathic techniques being taught in osteopathic medical schools has grown from approximately 3 to 12 distinctly named styles. Many of the styles have similarities that can lead to confusion, which is why we have decided to expand the original version and update it to the present level of practice.

We dedicate this book to our father, who would most likely have wanted to dedicate it to all of his former students and to all the future osteopathic physicians he thought would appreciate a comprehensive work on osteopathic manipulative techniques.

Preface to the Third Edition

The third edition of the *Atlas of Osteopathic Techniques* continues to build on the osteopathic armamentarium of safe and effective manipulative treatment by adding and modifying a number of techniques, better defining techniques in a number of chapters, and by moving some techniques to chapters that better follow their principles. We continue to illustrate and describe these techniques in the most visually effective manner, so that the photos relate most closely to the proximal text. Again, we have attempted as much as possible, to keep each technique on the same or, whenever necessary, on the adjacent page.

In this third edition, we have continued to modify and expand the counterstrain and muscle energy chapters, as well as modify the principles and descriptions within the "Osteopathic Cranial Manipulative Medicine" chapter (formerly "Osteopathy in the Cranial Field") in order to follow the recommended curriculum and terminology of the Education Council on Osteopathic Principles (ECOP) of the American Association of Colleges of Osteopathic Medicine (AACOM).

Videos

For this updated third edition, we have also added video callouts to various technique headings. These references make it easier for those using the text to view dynamically illustrated videos associated with the particular technique in the book. In addition, several new videos have been added to the lineup offering even more footage. Hopefully, this improved method of referencing the videos creates a more productive and pleasing experience for everyone who uses the book.

A.S. Nicholas
E.A. Nicholas

Preface to the First Edition

Osteopathic medicine as taught and practiced in the United States at the end of the 19th century through the beginning of the 21st century has undergone many changes. The evolution of scientific findings and understanding of biologic processes by which the body functions and attempts to maintain health has had a direct effect on the way osteopathic medical curricula are developed.

During our osteopathic medical school matriculation, we were taught only three or four separate styles of osteopathic technique. Since that time, many new diagnostic and therapeutic procedures have been added to the armamentarium of osteopathic treatment, and there are now over a dozen individual styles. Some of these styles are very similar, and as described in the chapters of this atlas, they have developed by nuance into distinct, individually named categories of technique.

Because of these additions and changes, both osteopathic medical students and practitioners have had a much more difficult time trying to learn and remember these techniques, and practitioners have faced an increasingly complex process in deciding which technique is clinically indicated for a particular patient. To aid the study and practice, we have gradually developed a compilation of techniques that are commonly used by osteopathic physicians and that are clinically effective. The result of this effort is the *Atlas of Osteopathic Techniques*.

At Philadelphia College of Osteopathic Medicine, a tradition of technique atlas goes back to at least 1949 with the publication of *Osteopathic Techniques*, by Samuel Rubinstein, DO. It was dedicated to two highly respected physicians, Otterbein Dressler, DO, and John Eimerbrink, DO. In his preface, Dr. Rubinstein noted, "The necessity for this type of textbook has become increasingly apparent with time" because of the need to have a visual record of the various physician and patient positions and force vectors at play. Yet no other example was readily reproduced until N. S. Nicholas, DO, FAAO, published his *Atlas of Osteopathic Technique* in 1974.

Throughout our years of teaching, many practicing physicians have asked us why there were no new editions of the *Atlas of Osteopathic Technique*. Our initial answer was that other texts had been published. However, these reference textbooks focus on the philosophy and principles of osteopathic medical practice and include only a few useful techniques. The need for an updated, comprehensive atlas of techniques became increasingly clear, and we have responded with a textbook that includes a straightforward, highly organized, and easily navigable compendium of osteopathic techniques along with the philosophy and principles that support them. This material is intended to help students and practitioners understand the reasoning behind the procedures and the ramifications of their use in the clinical setting.

One of the major improvements in the *Atlas of Osteopathic Techniques* is the presentation of more than 1,000 color photos of every procedural step involved in each technique. The photos for each technique are placed together on the same or adjacent pages, along with descriptive text, to make the book easy to use in the clinical setting. The new photos were created specifically for this atlas under the direction of the authors and a professional photographer. Arrows and other annotations directly on the photos guide the reader through the techniques. The clarity of these photos and their annotations, combined with their organization into an easy-to-use format, make this atlas an extremely useful tool in both the laboratory and the clinic.

Also included in the atlas are the various diagnostic procedures common to osteopathic medicine. The descriptions for these include the musculoskeletal structural examination, regional range of motion assessment, layer-by-layer palpatory examination, and the intersegmental examination of the spinal and pelvic regions. Diagnosis is included so the reader can relate the specific treatment to the diagnostic criteria that govern its use. This is important, as the physician must understand the nature of the dysfunction and the technique best suited to treat it successfully.

We have organized this atlas into two sections: Part 1, Osteopathic Principles in Diagnosis, and Part 2, Osteopathic Manipulative Techniques. The order of Part 1 is similar to how we present the material to osteopathic medical students and is in keeping with what we believe is the most appropriate and safe method of performing the osteopathic musculoskeletal examination.

We have arranged Part 2 in what we consider the classical format, by technique style, as the reader should first decide on a style and then proceed to the appropriate chapter and to the specific anatomic region within that chapter.

We hope that the reader will find this useful in all stages of osteopathic education: undergraduate, postgraduate residency, and continuing medical education. We hope use of this text will instill more confidence in performing these techniques and thereby help readers to better help patients. As physicians, we are trained to use our minds and hands, and as osteopathic physicians, we are frequently reminded that it is inherent to our practice to do so, as the seal of Philadelphia College of Osteopathic Medicine states, "Mens et Manus."

A.S. Nicholas
E.A. Nicholas

Acknowledgments

As stated in the acknowledgments section of the first edition of this work, it was our goal to "maintain a historical continuum of the many variations of osteopathic manipulative techniques." In this third edition, we have tried our best to continue this endeavor by seeking input from our colleagues on the Educational Council on Osteopathic Principles, members of the American Academy of Osteopathy, colleagues from many departments of Osteopathic Manipulative Medicine (OMM) of the colleges of Osteopathic Medicine, as well as our associates in the PCOM department of OMM.

We have of course enlisted the feedback of our medical students at PCOM, as well as from osteopathic medical students across the country. In addition, through our contacts with physicians in Germany through the German-American Academy of Osteopathy and the courses that we teach there, we have gained a fresh viewpoint in our approach to the development of this text. A number of techniques that we taught for years have been modified slightly to better suit a wide variety of medical practitioners and their patients.

We must also thank some individuals personally for going that extra step in helping edit the text, finding errors, and giving their expertise so that those reading this work may better and more easily understand the techniques. First, we want to thank Abraham Zellis, DO, our long-time friend and colleague for his editorial expertise in recommending changes and corrections. David Fuller, DO, FAAO, has been extremely valuable as a set of new eyes in corroborating the veracity of the work. He was very helpful in recommending better explanations and descriptions in the "Techniques of Still" chapter. We also wish to thank Donna Mueller, DO, for her assistance in editing of the "Osteopathic Cranial Manipulative Medicine" chapter.

As we did in the second edition, would like to thank our friend and colleague Bruce Fairfield for his photographic expertise for the added and edited techniques. Lastly, thanks to our undergraduate fellows Christopher Mulholland and Philip Koehler for their editing and overall student feedback. Philip Koehler (again) for his help as a patient model for the added techniques.

We would especially like to extend our gratitude to Greg Nicholl at Wolters Kluwer for his tireless efforts in guiding us to the completion of this work.

Contents

PART 1 | OSTEOPATHIC PRINCIPLES IN DIAGNOSIS

PART 2 | OSTEOPATHIC MANIPULATIVE TECHNIQUES

List of Techniques

Chapter 11

PART 1

Osteopathic Principles in Diagnosis

Osteopathic diagnosis involves all classical methods of physical examination (e.g., observation, palpation, auscultation). In addition, some distinct techniques are most common to osteopathic medicine and are less commonly used in allopathic medicine. These techniques have to do with fine methods of tissue texture evaluation and epicritic intersegmental evaluation of the cardinal axes (x-, y-, and z-axes) of spinal motion. Evaluating the patient using both observation and palpation of specific landmarks in these axes to assess symmetry, asymmetry, and so on may be referred to as *three-plane motion* diagnosis in later chapters.

Principles of the Osteopathic Examination

Osteopathic Principles (Philosophy)

The primary goal of the Educational Council on Osteopathic Principles (ECOP) of the American Association of Colleges of Osteopathic Medicine is to evaluate the most current knowledge base in the fields of biomechanics, neuroscience, and osteopathic principles and practice. By constantly studying the most current trends in osteopathic principles and practice, as well as the basic science database, this committee produces a glossary of osteopathic terminology that is the language standard for teaching this subject. It was originally created to develop a single, unified osteopathic terminology to be used in all American osteopathic medical schools. One of the reasons Nicholas S. Nicholas, DO, FAAO, published his original *Atlas of Osteopathic Techniques* was to help in this endeavor. He and his associate, David Heilig, DO, FAAO, were two of the original members of this committee as representatives of one of the original sponsors, the Philadelphia College of Osteopathic Medicine. Over time, with its glossary review committee, the ECOP has produced frequent updates of the *Glossary of Osteopathic Terminology*, issued each year in the *American Osteopathic Association Yearbook and Directory of Osteopathic Physicians* (1). It was previously printed in the first two editions of *Foundations for Osteopathic Medicine* and most recently is now printed in *Foundations of Osteopathic Medicine* (2).

The ECOP glossary defines osteopathic philosophy as "a concept of health care supported by expanding scientific knowledge that embraces the concept of the unity of the living organism's structure (anatomy) and function (physiology). Osteopathic philosophy emphasizes the following principles: (a) The human being is a dynamic unit of function. (b) The body possesses self-regulatory mechanisms that are self-healing in nature. (c) Structure and function are interrelated at all levels. (d) Rational treatment is based on these principles" (1). The diagnostic and therapeutic applications illustrated in this atlas are all based upon these principles.

Structural Components

Structure and Function

Structure and function concepts of the myofascial and articular portions of the musculoskeletal system are inherent to understanding osteopathic diagnostic and therapeutic techniques. For example, knowledge of the origin and insertion of muscles (functional anatomy) is imperative in the performance of muscle energy technique. Understanding the structure of the spinal joints helps in the evaluation of spinal mechanics and in the direction of applied forces in techniques such as high-velocity, low-amplitude (HVLA) manipulations, such as when it is necessary to consider oblique cervical facets and coupled joint motion.

Barrier Concepts

Barriers are also an important concept in the understanding and application of osteopathic techniques. In osteopathic medicine, various barriers to motion have been classically described within the framework of normal physiologic motion.

The greatest range of motion (ROM) in a specified region is the *anatomic* range, and its passive limit is described as the *anatomic barrier* (1). This barrier may be the most important to understand, as movement beyond this point can disrupt the tissues and may result in subluxation or dislocation. Osteopathic techniques should never involve movement past this barrier.

The *physiologic* ROM is the limit of active motion given normal anatomic structures and the articular, myofascial, and osseous components (1). The point at which the physiologic motion ends is the *physiologic barrier*. The term *elastic barrier* is used to describe the motion between the physiologic and anatomic barriers, which is available secondary to passive myofascial and ligamentous stretching (1).

When a dysfunctional state exists, reduced motion or function occurs, and a *restrictive barrier* between the physiologic barriers may be demonstrated (1). The restrictive barrier, the major aspect of the overall dysfunctional pattern, can be eliminated or minimized with osteopathic treatment. Manipulative techniques incorporate activating forces in an attempt to remove the restrictive barrier, but these forces should be kept within the bounds of the physiologic barriers whenever possible. A *pathologic barrier* is more permanent; it may be related to contractures within the soft tissues, osteophytic development, and other degenerative changes (e.g., osteoarthritis).

To avoid further injuring the patient with diagnostic or therapeutic techniques, the practitioner must understand the normal compliance of tissues and the limits they maintain. These different barriers must be understood completely, as they may cause the physician to alter the technique chosen (i.e., indirect vs. direct) or may limit the motion directed into the tissues and/or joints during treatment.

In osteopathic principles, the present system of describing the cardinal motion dynamics in spinal mechanics is based on the positional and/or motion asymmetry related to the freedom of motion (1). Previously, there have been other ways to describe these asymmetries. The direction in which the motion was restricted was the most common early method. Other past descriptions included whether the joint was open or closed. These were also based on the mechanical findings revealed on palpation. Today, the governing system in use names the biomechanical findings based on motion restriction and/or asymmetry and the directions in which motion is most free. This motion freedom is also called ease, free, and loose. In myofascial diagnostic findings, it is common to see both the freedom and the limitation used (i.e., loose, tight; ease, bind; and free, restricted). Yet the use of these descriptions does not allow for problems in which motion is symmetrically and/or universally restricted, as seen in some patients.

One of the most important principles in diagnosis and treatment is to control the tissue, joint, or other structure within its normally adaptive motion limits. Thus, the motion in a treatment technique should be within normal physiologic limits. Certainly, the motion used should always be within anatomic limits. It is our philosophy that controlling motion within the physiologic limits ensures greater safety and efficacy, whereas moving closer to the anatomic limits increases risk with little increase in efficacy.

For example, in an HVLA technique, the restrictive barrier should be engaged if engagement is tolerated. The movement necessary to affect this barrier, however, should be only 1 to 2 degrees of motion (still within the physiologic limits), whereas the actual physiologic barrier of normal motion may be 5 to 6 degrees further.

Somatic Dysfunction

Somatic dysfunction is the diagnostic criterion for which osteopathic manipulation is indicated. The ECOP definition of somatic dysfunction is as follows:

Impaired or altered function of related components of the somatic (body framework) system: skeletal, arthrodial, and myofascial structures and related vascular, lymphatic, and neural elements. Somatic dysfunction is treatable using osteopathic manipulative treatment. The positional and motion aspects of somatic dysfunction are best described using at least one of three parameters: (a) the position of a body part as determined by palpation and referenced to its adjacent defined structure; (b) the directions in which motion is freer; and (c) the directions in which motion is restricted (1).

Associated criteria for somatic dysfunction are related to *tissue texture abnormality*, *asymmetry*, *restriction of motion*, and *tenderness* (acronym *TART*). The glossary of osteopathic terminology states that any one of these must be present for the diagnosis. The primary findings we use for the diagnosis of somatic dysfunction are motion restriction (and related motion asymmetry, if present) and tissue texture changes. Tenderness (some prefer sensitivity) can be one of the great pretenders in the clinical presentation of a problem. Tenderness may be elicited on palpation due to pressure or because the patient wants the physician to believe there is pain. Pain may be present in one area but the primary dysfunction or problem distant. Therefore, we believe tenderness (sensitivity or pain) to be the weakest of the aforementioned criteria, and in our practice, it is used in a limited fashion, mostly when implementing counterstrain techniques.

Certain qualities of these criteria are particularly common in specific types of dysfunctions arising from acute and chronic states. Increased heat, moisture, hypertonicity, and so on are common with acute processes. Decreased heat, dryness, atrophy, and stringiness of tissues are more common with chronic problems.

Myofascial-Articular Components

As the presence of somatic dysfunction by definition may include myofascial and articular components, the palpatory examination is an important part of the evaluation. Palpation will determine whether there is a primary myofascial or articular component or both and lead to the development of the most appropriate treatment plan. Specific types of dysfunctions are best treated by certain techniques. For example, a primary tissue texture abnormality in the fascia is best treated by a technique that most affects change at that level (e.g., myofascial release), whereas another technique may have no real effect on the specific tissue involved (e.g., HVLA). Articular dysfunctions, on the other hand, are best treated with an articular technique, such as HVLA, and myofascial release would be less appropriate.

Visceral-Autonomic Components

Some dysfunctions may directly affect an area (e.g., small intestines with adhesions), while other dysfunctions may be more reflexively important (i.e., cardiac arrhythmia–somatovisceral reflex). Somatic dysfunction may cause reactions within the autonomic nervous system and result in many clinical presentations, or visceral disorders present with a number of somatic components (3).

Order of Examination

The order of the osteopathic physical examination is best based on the patient's history and clinical presentation. In general, it is best to begin the examination by performing the steps that have the least impact on the patient physically and that lead to the least tissue reactivity and least secondary reflex stimulation.

General Observation

It is recommended that the physician begins with general observation of the static posture and then the dynamic posture (gait and regional ROM). For safety, it is best to begin by observing function and ROM with active regional motion testing. After examining the patient in this manner, the physician may decide to observe the patient's limits by passive ROM testing. The passive ranges should typically be slightly greater than those elicited during active motion assessment. After identifying any asymmetries or abnormalities at this point, it is reasonable to proceed to the palpatory examination.

Layer-by-Layer Palpation

The palpatory examination is also best started by observing the area of interest for any vasomotor, dermatologic, or developmental abnormalities. The examination may then proceed to temperature evaluation. The physician may now make contact with the patient following a layer-by-layer approach to the examination to evaluate the tissue texture. This approach permits the examiner to distinctly monitor each anatomic layer from a superficial to deep perspective to best determine the magnitude of and specific tissues involved in the dysfunctional state. The tissues are progressively evaluated through each ensuing layer and depth by adding a slightly greater pressure with the palpating fingers or hand. The physician should also attempt to monitor the tissue texture quality and any dynamic fluid movement or change in tissue compliance. During palpation over a viscera, the mobility of that organ may be evaluated along with any inherent motility present within that organ.

Another method that we commonly use is a screening evaluation using percussion over the paraspinal musculature, with patient seated or prone, to determine differences in muscle tone at various spinal levels. In the thoracic and lumbar areas, a hypertympanic reaction to percussion appears to be associated with the side of the rotational component.

These steps in the examination evaluate the postural and regional movement ramifications involved in the patient's problem, in addition to eliciting any gross and fine tissue texture changes. The final step in the examination is to determine whether there is a related articular component to the patient's problem. This involves controlling a joint and putting it through very fine small motion arcs in all phases of its normal capabilities (intersegmental motion testing). The physician attempts with a three-plane motion examination to determine whether the motion is normal and symmetric or whether pathology is restricting motion, with or without asymmetry in the cardinal axes. For example, the C1 segment may be restricted within its normal physiologic range of rotation and exhibit either a bilaterally symmetric restriction in rotation (e.g., 30 degrees right and left) or an asymmetry of motion with greater freedom in one direction than in the other (e.g., 30 degrees right, 40 degrees left). As stated previously, most descriptions of somatic dysfunction relate to the asymmetric restrictions, but symmetric restrictions are seen clinically.

In performing the stepwise layer-by-layer palpatory examination and finishing with the intersegmental motion evaluation, the physician can determine the specific tissues involved in the dysfunction (e.g., muscle, ligament, capsular), the extent to which it is present (e.g., single segment, regional), and whether the process is acute, subacute, or chronic. These determinations prepare the physician to develop the most appropriate treatment plan for the somatic dysfunction or dysfunctions.

References

1. Glossary Review Committee, Educational Council on Osteopathic Principles of the American Association of Colleges of Osteopathic Medicine. Glossary of Osteopathic Terminology. http://www.aacom.org
2. Chila AG, exec.ed. Foundations of Osteopathic Medicine. 3rd ed. Baltimore, MD: Lippincott Williams & Wilkins, 2011.
3. Nicholas AS, DeBias DA, Ehrenfeuchter W, et al. A somatic component to myocardial infarction. Br Med J 1985;291:13–17.

Osteopathic Static Musculoskeletal Examination

The osteopathic structural examination has both static and dynamic components. The physician will normally use static examination as a method to discern obvious structural asymmetries of osseous and myofascial origin and extrapolate from that information to determine etiologies that affect function. Therefore, on visual examination alone, a physician can postulate what the subsequent specific dynamic examination will elicit.

Observance of gait may preface the static examination, as the patient can be observed walking into the examination room. A number of conditions produce obvious antalgic and asymmetric tendencies, such as osteoarthritis of the hips and knee, degenerative discogenic spondylosis of the lumbar spine, and acute problems, including strains and sprains. The visual observance of gait and the associated static examination (which may be performed either before or after gait evaluation) will help the physician understand the patient's medical and psychological status and also help avoid portions of the examination that may be painful or in other ways detrimental to the patient. These types of scrutiny affect the patient less than do dynamic examinations with physical contact and therefore are less likely to cause pain or damage to the patient.

As an example, a patient with the asymmetric findings illustrated in Figure 2.1 (see p. 7) could be reasonably expected to exhibit motion restriction and motion asymmetry in the thoracic and lumbar spine with restrictions in lumbar side bending to the left and midthoracic side bending to the right. These findings would also cause the physician to be concerned with right and left latissimus dorsi, psoas, and erector spinae tension asymmetries affecting range of motion of the hip, pelvis, and shoulder girdle **(Fig. 2.1)**.

Therefore, the physician should observe the patient in posterior, anterior, and lateral (sagittal and coronal plane) views to develop the most complete understanding of the patient's physical makeup before performing the remainder of the examination. These views may be started at the feet or at the head. We generally recommend starting at the feet, as that is the gravitational contact point.

The static musculoskeletal (structural) examination uses superficial anatomic landmarks that help the physician "see the forest for the trees." Sometimes, slight asymmetries are missed, but aligning two or three landmarks makes the asymmetry obvious. Some anatomic landmarks are important for finding the spinal vertebral levels. The spine of the scapula is typically at the level of T3, and the inferior angle of the scapula is typically at the level of the spinous process of T7 and transverse processes of T8 **(Fig. 2.2)**. Some landmarks assist in locating a more clinically important landmark. The mastoid process and the angle of the mandible are commonly used to help the novice palpate the C1 transverse process **(Fig. 2.3)**. Other landmarks, such as the coracoid process, bicipital groove of the humerus, and greater and lesser tuberosities of the humerus, help distinguish one tendon from another, hence differentiating between a rotator cuff syndrome and another somatic problem **(Fig. 2.4)**. The most commonly used landmarks tend to be the ones that determine horizontal symmetry or asymmetry **(Figs. 2.5 to 2.10)**. Landmarks such as the tibial tuberosities, anterior superior iliac spines, posterior superior iliac spines, iliac crests, nipples, shoulders at the acromioclavicular joint, earlobes, and eyes as horizontal levels plane are often used for this purpose.

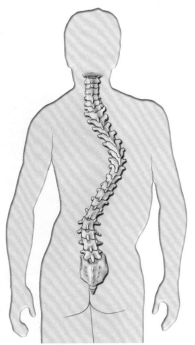

Figure 2.1. Asymmetry in scoliosis. (Anatomical Chart Company. Human Spine Disorders Anatomical Chart. 2nd ed. Baltimore, MD: Lippincott Williams & Wilkins, 2004.)

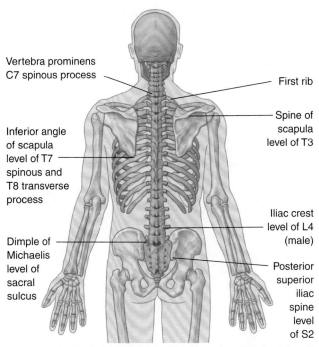

Vertebra prominens C7 spinous process

First rib

Spine of scapula level of T3

Inferior angle of scapula level of T7 spinous and T8 transverse process

Iliac crest level of L4 (male)

Dimple of Michaelis level of sacral sulcus

Posterior superior iliac spine level of S2

Figure 2.2. Relating scapular landmarks to spinal level. (Moore KL, Agur AMR, Dalley AF. Essential Clinical Anatomy. 5th ed. Baltimore, MD: Lippincott Williams & Wilkins, 2015.)

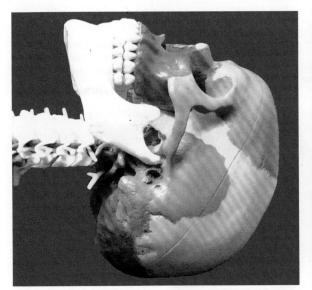

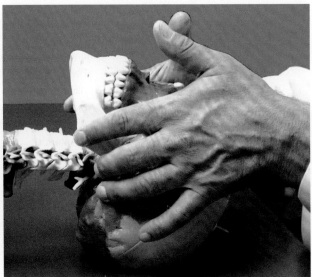

A

B

Figure 2.3. A and B. Landmarks to locate the C1 transverse process.

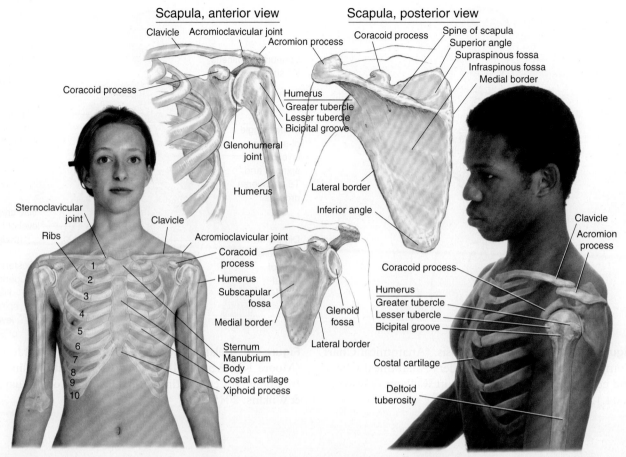

Figure 2.4. Important landmarks of the shoulder girdle. (Clay JH, Pounds DM. Basic Clinical Massage Therapy: Integrating Anatomy and Treatment. 2nd ed. Baltimore, MD: Lippincott Williams & Wilkins, 2003.)

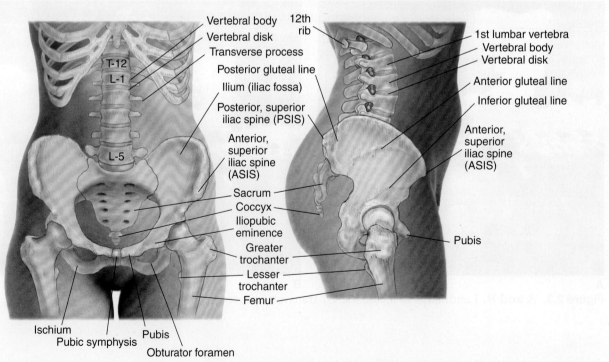

Figure 2.5. Important landmarks of the lumbar spine and pelvis. (Clay JH, Pounds DM. Basic Clinical Massage Therapy: Integrating Anatomy and Treatment. 2nd ed. Baltimore, MD: Lippincott Williams & Wilkins, 2008.)

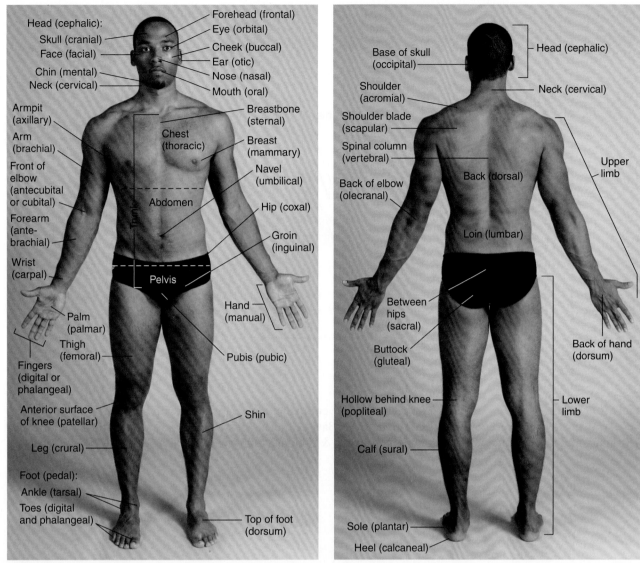

Figure 2.6. Landmarks to help determine horizontal levelness. (Premakur K. Anatomy and Physiology. 2nd ed. Baltimore, MD: Lippincott Williams & Wilkins, 2004.)

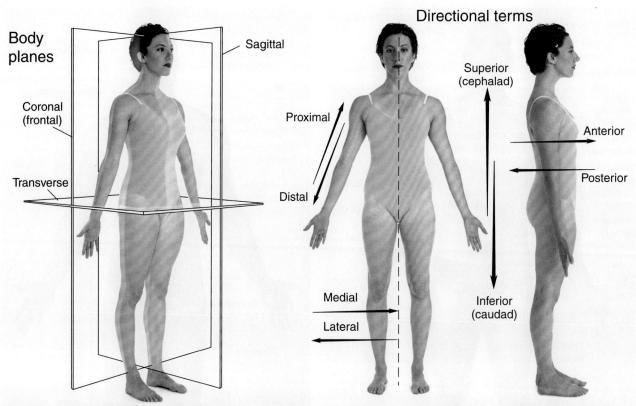

Figure 2.7. Planes of the body and directional terms. The coronal plane is associated with both the ventral (anterior) and dorsal (posterior) aspects. (Clay JH, Pounds DM. Basic Clinical Massage Therapy: Integrating Anatomy and Treatment. 2nd ed. Baltimore, MD: Lippincott Williams & Wilkins, 2008.)

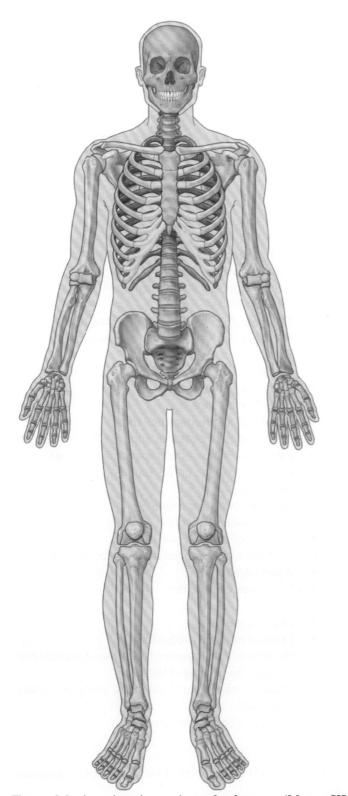

On examination note:
- Midgravitational line
- Lateral body line
- Position of feet
  - Pronation
  - Supination
  - Levelness of tibial tuberosities
- Levelness of patellae
- Anterior superior iliac spines
  - Level?
  - Anteroposterior: rotational prominence
- Prominence of hips
- Iliac crests, levelness
- Fullness over iliac crest
- Relation of forearms to iliac crests
  - One longer
  - Anteroposterior relation
  - Nearness to body
- Prominence of costal arches
- Thoracic symmetry or asymmetry
- Prominence of sternal angle
- Position of shoulders
  - Level or unlevel
  - Anteroposterior relations
- Prominence of sternal end of clavicle
- Prominence of sternocleidomastoid muscles
- Direction of symphysis menti
- Symmetry of face (any scoliosis capitis)
- Nasal deviation
- Angles of mouth
- Level of eyes
- Level of supraciliary arches (eyebrows)
- Head position relative to shoulders and body

Figure 2.8. Anterior view points of reference. (Moore KL, Agur AMR, Dalley AF. Essential Clinical Anatomy. 5th ed. Baltimore, MD: Lippincott Williams & Wilkins, 2015.)

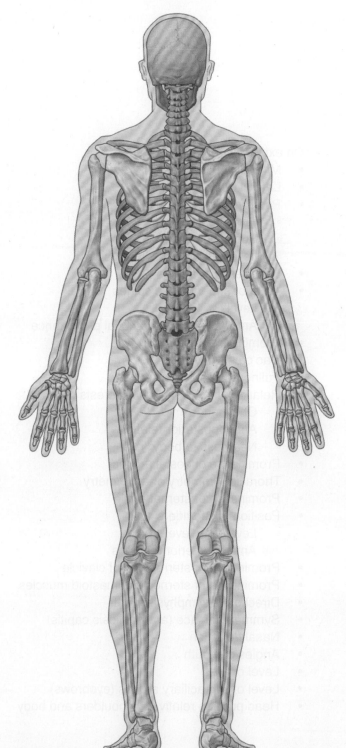

On examination note:
- Midgravitational line
- Achilles tendon: straight, curved?
- Position of feet
- Relation of spine to midline (curves, etc.)
- Prominence of sacrospinalis muscle mass
- Symmetry of calves
- Symmetry of thighs (including any folds)
- Symmetry of buttocks
- Lateral body lines
- Levelness of greater trochanters
- Prominence of posterior superior iliac spines
- Levelness of posterior superior iliac spines
- Levelness of iliac crests (supine, prone, sitting, standing)
- Fullness over iliac crests
- Prominence of scapula
- Position of scapula and its parts
- Levelness and relation of fingertips to body
- Arms (relations)
- Levelness of shoulder
- Neck-shoulder angles
- Level of earlobes
- Level of mastoid processes
- Position of body relative to a straight vertical line through the midspinal line
- Posterior cervical muscle mass (more prominent, equal, etc.)
- Head position: lateral inclination

Figure 2.9. Posterior view points of reference. (Moore KL, Agur AMR, Dalley AF. Essential Clinical Anatomy. 5th ed. Baltimore, MD: Lippincott Williams & Wilkins, 2015.)

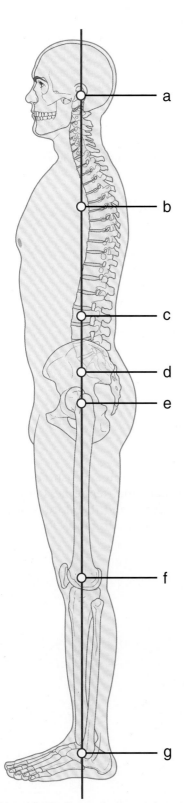

On examination note:
- Lateral midgravitational line
  - a   External auditory canal
  - b   Lateral head of the humerus
  - c   Third lumbar vertebra
  - d   Anterior third of the sacrum
  - e   Greater trochanter of the femur
  - f   Lateral condyle of the knee
  - g   Lateral malleolus
- Anterior and posterior body line
- Feet: degree of arching or flatness
- Knees: degree of flexion or extension
- Spinal curves: increase, decreased, or normal
  - Cervical lordosis: posterior concavity
  - Thoracic kyphosis: posterior convexity
  - Lumbar lordosis: posterior concavity
  - Sacrum, lumbosacral angle
- Arms: position relative to body
- Abdomen: prominence or flatness
- Sternal angle
- Thorax: prominence or flatness
- Head: relation to shoulder and body

Figure 2.10. Lateral view points of reference and midgravity line. (Nelson KE, Glonek T. Somatic Dysfunction in Osteopathic Family Medicine. 2nd ed. Baltimore, MD: Wolters Kluwer Health, 2015.)

See Video 2.1
(Anterior Skull)

 See Video 2.2
(Lateral Skull)

 See Video 2.3
(Posterior Skull)

 See Video 2.4
(Joints of Luschka)

 See Video 2.5
(Anterior Shoulder)

 See Video 2.6
(Posterior Shoulder)

 See Video 2.7
(Anterior Rib Cage)

 See Video 2.8
(Posterior Rib Cage)

 See Video 2.9
(Anterior Pelvis)

 See Video 2.10
(Posterior Pelvis)

See Video 2.11
(Elbow)

 See Video 2.12
(Wrist)

 See Video 2.13
(Knee, Anterior/Posterior View)

 See Video 2.14
(Foot/Ankle, Anterior/Posterior View)

 See Video 2.15
(Foot/Ankle, Lateral View)

 See Video 2.16
(Foot/Ankle, Medial View)

 See Video 2.17
(Foot/Ankle, Dorsal View)

 See Video 2.18
(Anterior View)

 See Video 2.19
(Posterior View)

 See Video 2.20
(Lateral View)

Asymmetry is one of the three measurable components of somatic dysfunction (tenderness or sensitivity being more subjective) and therefore is one of the basic steps to develop the diagnosis for somatic dysfunction.

Spinal Regional Range of Motion

3

Regional motion testing evaluates patients' ability to move through the cardinal axes of motion and reflects their ability to move normally or with pain, degenerative joint disease, muscle hypertonicity, strain or sprain, and so on. The static structural/postural examination will give clues of motion patterns to expect on intersegmental motion testing to be performed later in the exam process. The ranges that are accepted as normal depend upon the patient's somatotype, as well as the condition causing them dysfunction. As such, they may vary from one type of patient to another, hence the term *ranges*. Mesomorphic patients should be midrange, ectomorphic (long-linear) patients at the high range and endomorphic patients (brevilinear) at the lower ranges of motion expectation. Realizing that patients exhibit different body types with the potential of having varied preference to muscle type, elasticity, etc., the physician can have a better idea of the overall dysfunctional state with which the patient presents. This can be important in the choice of osteopathic technique for the treatment of the patient's dysfunction or in prevention, such as the exercise and training methods an athlete should use. For example, some people may never be able to bend and touch their toes, while others are hypermobile and may have joint instabilities.

This type of motion testing evaluates a group of segments that make up a specific region of the spine (e.g., cervical region—occiput through C7). Therefore, during the examination process, it is important to monitor the *transition zone* where the lowest segment of the region being evaluated articulates with the most superior segment of the region immediately below (e.g., C7–T1) and measure only the motion of the region being tested; otherwise, an incorrect increased motion may be elicited. As the following techniques demonstrate, the physician palpates the two segments of the transition zone while the motion being tested is performed and stops that motion at the point where further motion would cause movement of the lower (inferior) segment.

During this process, the physician has the option of having the patient demonstrate the motions (*active*) and/or, with the patient relaxed without muscle contraction, the physician may move the patient's anatomic region through the various cardinal axes *(passive)*. After eliciting the medical history and finding no contraindications (severe trauma, loss of consciousness, etc.) for this type of examination, it is best to start with *active* motion testing; as with active movement, patients will typically stop or resist further movement before exacerbating their symptoms and/or condition. Passive motion testing will typically produce a greater regional range as compared to active motion testing. By evaluating with both methods, the physician may gain a clearer picture of the patient's condition (e.g., degree of severity, fracture, dislocation, somatization disorder, symptom magnification, etc.) affecting the degree of range seen on exam.

By evaluating the patient's regional range of motion, the physician is able to assess both the *asymmetry* and *restriction* of motion criteria for somatic dysfunction. It is, also, the most objective and reproducible method of testing, as it can be measured in degrees with a goniometer, protractor, or other measuring device from visit to visit, allowing the physician to better determine the patient's functional response to treatment. Therefore, it may be the most important method used for the evaluation and diagnosis of the patient's condition (i.e., somatic dysfunction) and, more important, the salient factor in determining the effectiveness of osteopathic treatment and prognosis for recovery.

 See Video 3.1
(Spinal Regional Range of Motion)

 See Video 3.2
(Cervical Regional Range of Motion)

 See Video 3.3
(Thoracic Regional Range of Motion)

Table 3.1 Normal Spinal Ranges of Motion for Active and Passive Testing

	Guides to Evaluation of Permanent Impairment (AMA)*	Angus Cathie, D.O.†			Revised PCOM‡		
NORMAL DEGREES OF MOTION—CERVICAL SPINE							
Flexion	50	90			45–90		
Extension	60	45			45–90		
Side bending R/L	45	30–40			30–45		
Rotation R/L	80	90			70–90		
NORMAL DEGREES OF MOTION—THORACIC SPINE							
		T1–T3	T4–T8	T8–L1	T1–T4	T5–T8	T9–T12
Flexion	45						
Extension	0						
Side bending R/L	45	35	45		5–25	10–30	20–40
Rotation R/L	30			90			30–45
NORMAL DEGREES OF MOTION—LUMBAR SPINE							
Flexion	60+				70–90		
Extension	25				30–45		
Side bending R/L	25	25			25–30		
Rotation R/L							

Flexion, forward bending; extension, backward bending; R/L, right and left.
*Rondinelli RD. Guides to the Evaluation of Permanent Impairment. 6th ed. New York, NY: American Medical Association, 2009.
†Cathie A; Philadelphia College of Osteopathy. From Dr. Cathie's PCOM (OPP) notebook, published in THE D.O., June 1969 and reprinted in the 1974 Yearbook of the American Academy of Osteopathy. Colorado Springs, CO: American Academy of Osteopathy, 1974:72.
‡Nicholas A. Osteopathic Manipulative Medicine Manual. Philadelphia, PA: Philadelphia College of Osteopathic Medicine, 2014.

Cervical Spine

Forward/Backward Bending (Flexion/Extension), Active

 See Video 3.4

1. The patient is seated.

2. The physician stands at the side of the patient.

3. The physician palpates the C7–T1 spinous process interspace **(Fig. 3.1)** or the spinous processes **(Figs. 3.2 and 3.3)**.

4. The patient is instructed to bend the head and neck forward to the functional and pain-free limitation of motion **(Fig. 3.4)**.

5. The degree of forward bending (flexion) is noted. *Normal forward bending of the cervical spine is 45 to 90 degrees.*

6. The patient is instructed to bend the head and neck backward as far as possible within the physiologic and pain-free range of motion **(Fig. 3.5)**.

7. The degree of backward bending (extension) is noted. *Normal backward bending of the cervical spine is 45 to 90 degrees.*

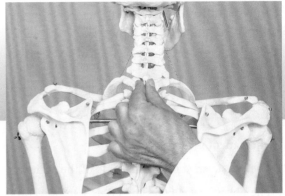

Figure 3.1. Step 3.

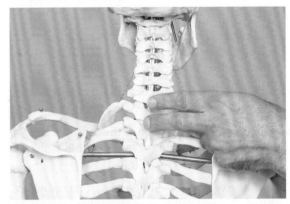

Figure 3.2. Step 3.

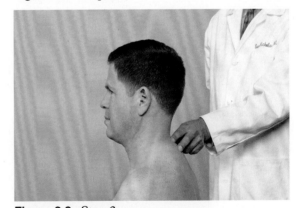

Figure 3.3. Step 3.

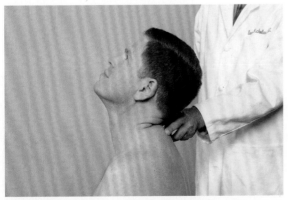

Figure 3.5. Step 6, active backward bending.

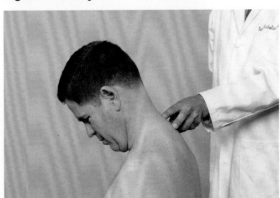

Figure 3.4. Step 4, active forward bending.

Cervical Spine

Forward/Backward Bending (Flexion/Extension), Passive

1. The patient is seated.

2. The physician stands at the side of the patient.

3. The physician palpates the C7–T1 spinous process interspace **(Fig. 3.6)** or the spinous processes **(Figs. 3.7 and 3.8)**.

4. The physician bends the patient's head and neck forward while monitoring C7 and T1 and stops when motion is detected at T1 **(Fig. 3.9)**.

5. The degree of forward bending (flexion) is noted. *Normal flexion of the cervical spine is 45 to 90 degrees.*

6. The physician then extends the patient's head and neck while monitoring C7 and T1 and stops when motion is detected at T1 **(Fig. 3.10)**.

7. The degree of backward bending (extension) is noted. *Normal extension of the cervical spine is 45 to 90 degrees.*

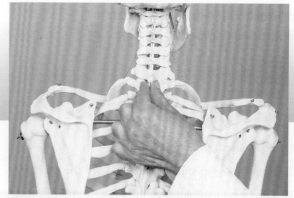

Figure 3.6. Step 3.

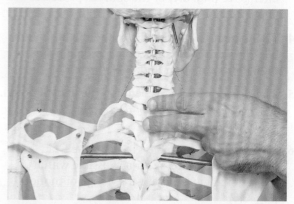

Figure 3.7. Step 3.

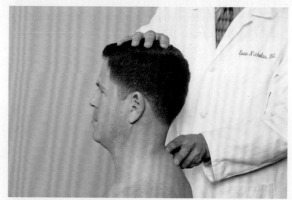

Figure 3.8. Step 3.

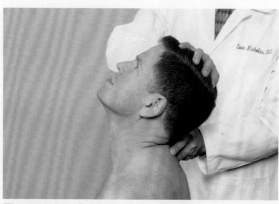

Figure 3.10. Step 6, passive backward bending.

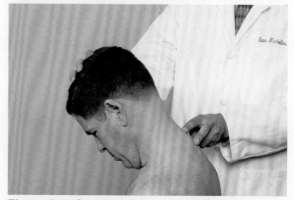

Figure 3.9. Step 4, passive forward bending.

Cervical Spine

Side Bending, Active/Passive

 See Video 3.5

1. The patient is seated.

2. The physician stands at the side of the patient.

3. The physician palpates the transverse processes of C7 and T1 **(Fig. 3.11)**.

4. The patient is instructed to side bend the head and neck to the right to the functional and pain-free limitation of motion **(Fig. 3.12)**. This is repeated to the left **(Fig. 3.13)**.

5. The physician side bends the patient's head and neck to the right while monitoring C7 and T1 and stops when motion is detected at T1 **(Fig. 3.14)**. This is repeated to the left **(Fig. 3.15)**.

6. The degree of both active and passive side bending is noted. *Normal side bending in the cervical spine is 30 to 45 degrees.*

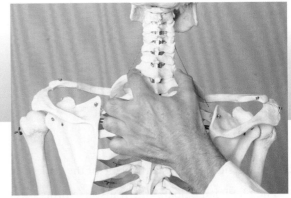

Figure 3.11. Step 3.

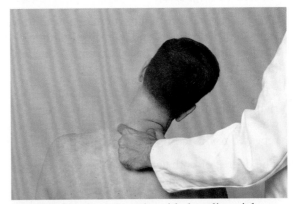

Figure 3.12. Step 3, active side bending right.

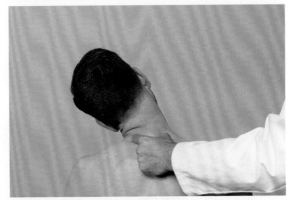

Figure 3.13. Step 4, active side bending left.

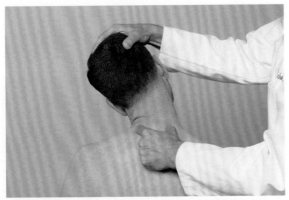

Figure 3.15. Step 5, passive side bending left.

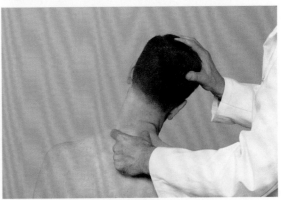

Figure 3.14. Step 5, passive side bending right.

Cervical Spine

Rotation, Active/Passive

 See Video 3.2

1. The patient is seated.

2. The physician stands at the side of the patient.

3. The physician palpates the transverse processes of C7 and T1 **(Fig. 3.16)**.

4. The patient is instructed to rotate the head to the right to the functional and pain-free limitation of motion **(Fig. 3.17)**. This is repeated to the left **(Fig. 3.18)**.

5. The physician rotates the patient's head to the right while monitoring C7 and T1 and stops when motion is detected at T1 **(Fig. 3.19)**. This is repeated to the left **(Fig. 3.20)**.

6. The degree of both active and passive rotation is noted. *Normal rotation in the cervical spine is 30 to 45 degrees.*

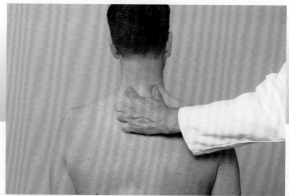

Figure 3.16. Step 3.

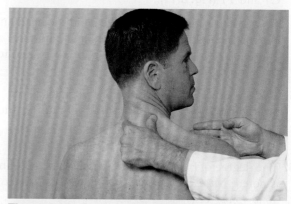

Figure 3.17. Step 4, active rotation right.

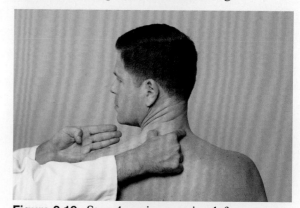

Figure 3.18. Step 4, active rotation left.

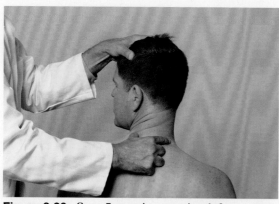

Figure 3.20. Step 5, passive rotation left.

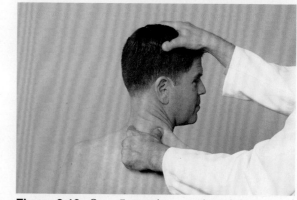

Figure 3.19. Step 5, passive rotation right.

Thoracic Spine

T1–T4, Side Bending, Passive

1. The patient is seated.

2. The physician stands behind the patient.

3. The physician's left index finger or thumb may palpate the transverse processes of T4 and T5 or the interspace between them to monitor motion. The webbing between the physician's right index finger and thumb is placed on the patient's right shoulder closest to midline at the level of T1 **(Fig. 3.21)**.

4. A gentle springing force is directed toward the vertebral body of T4 until the physician feels motion of T4 on T5. This is done by creating a vector with the forearm that is directly in line with the vertebral body of T4 **(Fig. 3.22)**. This is repeated to the opposite side **(Figs. 3.23 and 3.24)**.

5. The degree of passive side bending on each side is noted. *Normal side bending for T1–T4 is 5 to 25 degrees.*

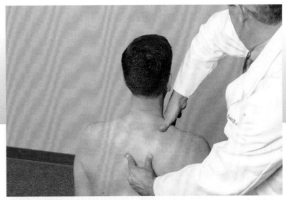

Figure 3.21. Step 3.

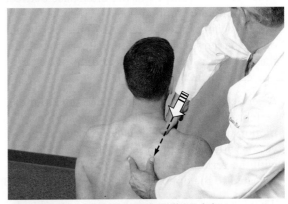

Figure 3.22. Step 4, side heading right.

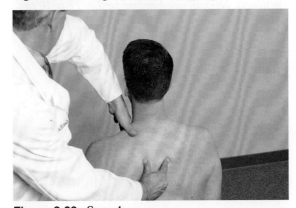

Figure 3.23. Step 4.

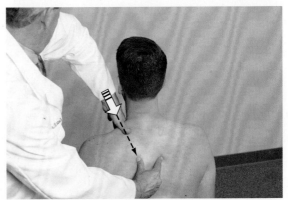

Figure 3.24. Step 4, side bending left.

Thoracic Spine

T5–T8, Side Bending, Passive

1. The patient is seated.

2. The physician stands behind the patient.

3. The physician's left hand palpates the transverse processes of T8 and T9 or the interspace between them to monitor motion. The webbing between the physician's index finger and thumb is placed on the patient's right shoulder halfway between the base of the patient's neck and the acromion process **(Fig. 3.25)**.

4. A gentle springing force is directed toward the vertebral body of T8 until the physician feels motion of T8 on T9. This is done by creating a vector with the forearm that is directly in line with the vertebral body of T8 **(Fig. 3.26)**. This is repeated to the opposite side **(Figs. 3.27 and 3.28)**.

5. The degree of passive side bending on each side is noted. *Normal side bending for T5–T8 is 10 to 30 degrees.*

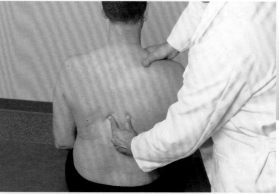

Figure 3.25. Step 3.

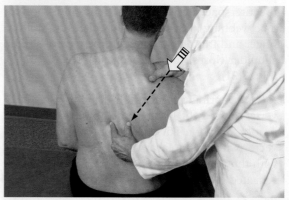

Figure 3.26. Step 4, side bending right.

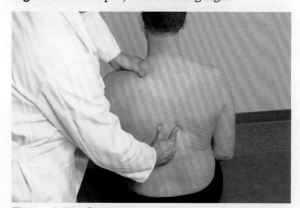

Figure 3.27. Step 4.

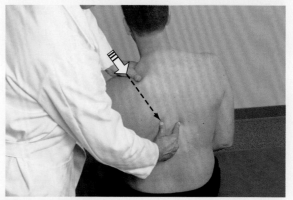

Figure 3.28. Step 4, side bending left.

Thoracic Spine

T9–T12, Side Bending, Passive

1. The patient is seated.

2. The physician stands behind the patient.

3. The physician's left hand may palpate the transverse processes of T12 and L1 or the interspace between them to monitor motion. The space (webbed skin) between the physician's index finger and thumb is placed on the patient's right shoulder at the acromioclavicular region **(Fig. 3.29)**.

4. A gentle springing force is directed toward the vertebral body of T12 until the physician feels motion of T12 on L1. This is done by creating a vector with the forearm that is directly in line with the vertebral body of T12 **(Fig. 3.30)**. This is repeated to the opposite side **(Figs. 3.31 and 3.32)**.

5. The degree of passive side bending is noted on each side. *Normal side bending for T9–T12 is 20 to 40 degrees.*

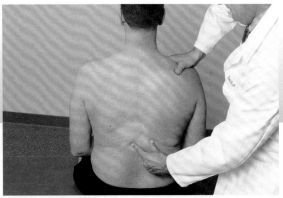

Figure 3.29. Step 3.

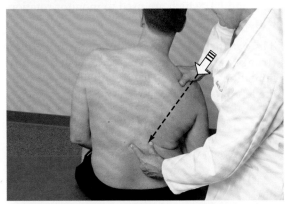

Figure 3.30. Step 4, side bending right.

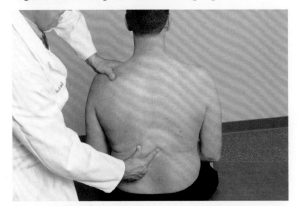

Figure 3.31. Step 4.

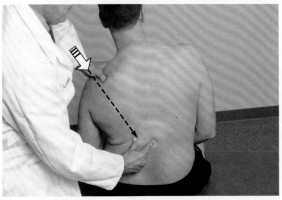

Figure 3.32. Step 4, side bending left.

Thoracic Spine

T9–T12, Rotation, Active

1. The patient is seated with the arms crossed so that the elbows make a V formation.

2. The physician stands at the side of the patient and palpates the patient's transverse processes of T12 and L1, which are used to monitor rotation **(Fig. 3.33)**.

3. The patient is instructed to rotate the upper body (trunk) to the right to the functional and pain-free limitation of motion **(Fig. 3.34)**. This is repeated to the left **(Fig. 3.35)**.

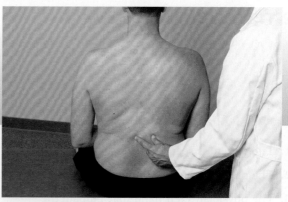

Figure 3.33. Step 2.

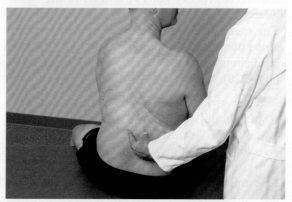

Figure 3.34. Step 3, active rotation right.

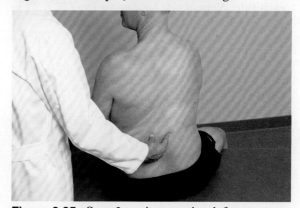

Figure 3.35. Step 3, active rotation left.

Thoracic Spine

T9–T12, Rotation, Passive

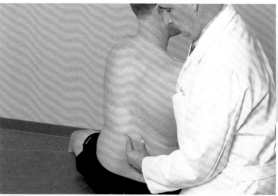

Figure 3.36. Step 3, passive rotation right.

1. The patient is seated with the arms crossed so that the elbows make a V formation.

2. The physician stands at the side of the patient and palpates the patient's transverse processes of T12 and L1, which are used to monitor rotation **(Fig. 3.33)**.

3. To test passive right rotation, the physician's right hand is placed on the patient's elbows or opposing left shoulder. The physician rotates the patient toward the right while monitoring motion at T12 and L1 **(Fig. 3.36)**. This is repeated to the opposite side **(Fig. 3.37)**.

4. The degree of active and passive rotation is noted. *Normal rotation for T9–T12 is 30 to 45 degrees.*

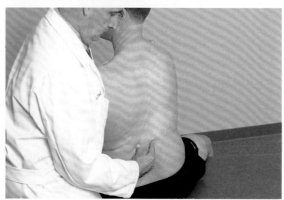

Figure 3.37. Step 3, passive rotation left.

Lumbar Spine

Forward/Backward Bending (Flexion/Extension), Active

 See Video 3.6

1. The patient stands in a neutral position with feet shoulder's width apart.

2. The physician stands to the side of the patient so as to view the patient in a sagittal plane **(Fig. 3.38)**.

3. The patient is instructed to bend forward and attempt to touch the toes without bending the knees to the functional and pain-free limitation of motion **(Fig. 3.39)**.

4. The degree of active forward bending (flexion) is noted. *Normal flexion for the lumbar spine is 70 to 90 degrees.*

5. Motion is then tested for backward bending in the lumbar region. The patient stands in a neutral position with feet a shoulder width apart. The patient is instructed to bend backward to the functional and pain-free limitation of motion, while the physician supports the patient's upper body **(Fig. 3.40)**.

6. The degree of active backward bending (extension) is noted. *Normal extension for the lumbar spine is 30 to 45 degrees.*

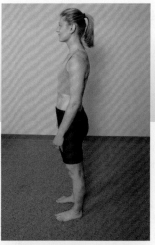

Figure 3.38. Step 2.

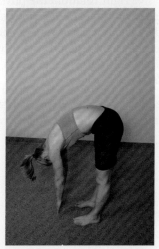

Figure 3.39. Step 3, active forward bending.

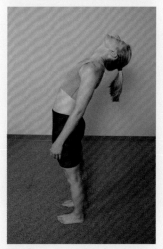

Figure 3.40. Step 5, active backward bending.

Lumbar Spine

Side Bending, Active

 See Video 3.7

1. The patient stands in a neutral position with feet shoulder's width apart.

2. The physician stands behind the patient so as to view the patient in a coronal plane **(Fig. 3.41)**.

3. The patient is instructed to reach down with the right hand toward the knee to the functional and pain-free limitation of motion **(Fig. 3.42)**. This is repeated to the opposite side **(Fig. 3.43)**.

4. The degree of active side bending is noted. *Normal side bending in the lumbar spine is 25 to 30 degrees.*

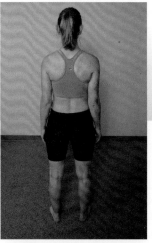

Figure 3.41. Step 2.

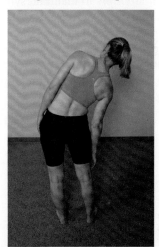

Figure 3.42. Step 3, active side bending right.

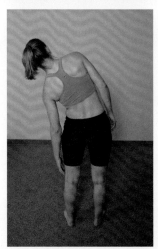

Figure 3.43. Step 3, active side bending left.

Lumbar Spine

Side Bending, *Passive* with Active "Hip Drop" Test

 See Video 3.8

1. The patient stands in a neutral position with feet shoulder's width apart.

2. The physician stands behind the patient so as to view the patient in a coronal plane. The physician's eyes should be level with the lumbar spine **(Fig. 3.44)**.

3. The patient attempts to maintain symmetric weight bearing on both legs and then quickly flexes the right knee, causing a right sacral base declination, hence causing the pelvis to compensate with a lateral translation to the left **(Fig. 3.45)**. This is repeated on the opposite side **(Fig. 3.46)**.

4. The degree of left lumbar side bending is noted. *Normal side bending in the lumbar spine is 25 to 30 degrees.*

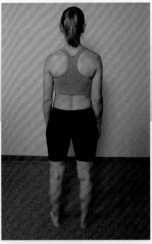

Figure 3.44. Step 2.

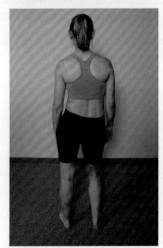

Figure 3.45. Step 3, passive side bending left with right sacral base unleveling.

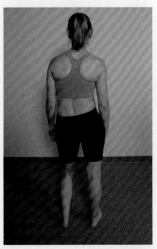

Figure 3.46. Step 3, passive side bending right with left sacral base unleveling.

4

Osteopathic Layer-by-Layer Palpation

Principles of Palpation

Palpation is the most important aspect of osteopathic physical diagnosis. The criteria that we use to determine the presence of somatic dysfunction, other than observation, are all based on those revealed during some form of palpation. These would include tissue texture changes associated with acute and chronic conditions, as well as those associated with autonomic and visceral disturbances. The relative health of the tissues including temperature, relative humidity, tone, trophicity, turgor, and elastic properties can all be manually sensed during the palpation process, giving various clues to the patient's state of health (1).

The palpatory exam is best performed by using specific locations of the palmar surfaces of the pads of the second and third digits and/or thumbs, depending on what body region and/or depth of tissue the physician is examining. At times, the olecranon process of the elbow can even be used to palpate very deep tissues, especially tendons (e.g., piriformis) of muscles, as the physician's joint and capsular mechanoreceptors will be stimulated, thereby guiding the palpation. The manner in which the exam is carried out depends on the history of the patient and the area to be palpated. As the patient and physician may alternately and continuously respond to touch (*cybernetic loop*, Korr), the exam is typically begun with observation and then temperature evaluation, as these cause the least reaction by the patient and the tissues to be later palpated (2). As we make physical contact with the patient and penetrate through the various layers of somatic tissues, it is important to understand what sensory receptors we use for palpation and where they are located (i.e., *mechanoreceptors* and *thermoreceptors*), as these are located in various locations, depth, and magnitudes in the finger pads, palm of hands, and thenar or hypothenar eminences. The act of palpating a patient to gather information uses a complicated set of somatic senses that allow the physician to interpret tissue texture changes from hypertonicity of muscle to edema of the interstitial spaces. These include the following commonly referenced tactile receptors that enable us to determine the depth of a mass, its size, its resistance to pressure, and whether it is mobile or fixed, pulsatile, warm, cold, etc. (3):

1. Free nerve endings
2. Meissner corpuscles
3. Merkel disks
4. Ruffini organs
5. Pacinian corpuscles
6. Krause corpuscles

Therefore, during the osteopathic palpatory exam, the physician may use the pads of the fingertips for tissue and depth quality but use the volar surface of the wrist or the dorsal hypothenar eminence of the hand to determine temperature levels. As the physician continues to palpate from superficial to deep levels and move from segment to segment (spinal) or throughout a larger geographic area, a three-dimensional palpatory "visualization" is generated. Over time, practicing this kinesthetic skill can be improved upon, not only making examination of the musculoskeletal system more sophisticated but also helping in the examination of the abdomen and other body regions.

 See Video 4.1
(Introduction: Layer-by-Layer Palpation)

 See Video 4.2
(Examination: Layer-by-Layer Palpation)

Examination Sequence

1. Observation
2. Temperature
3. Skin topography and texture
4. Fascia
5. Muscle
6. Tendon
7. Ligament
8. Erythema friction rub

Observation

Prior to touching the patient, the physician should visualize the area to be examined for evidence of trauma, infection, anomalies, gross asymmetries, skin lesions,

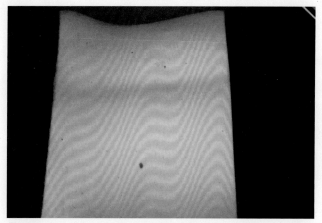

Figure 4.1. Visual observation of the patient.

Skin Topography and Texture

A very light touch will be used. Gentle palpation with the palmar surface of the tips of the fingers will provide the necessary pressure. The pressure will permit the finger pads to glide gently over the skin without drag (friction). There should be no change in the color of the physician's nail beds. When the physician is touching the patient, it is important to explain the nature of the examination and receive the patient's acceptance before continuing. Therefore, it is important to be prepared mentally to apply the hand as confidently and professionally as possible.

Skin topography and texture are evaluated for increased or decreased humidity, oiliness, thickening, roughness, and so on.

and/or anatomic variations. The patient should be positioned comfortably so that the most complete examination can be performed. At this point, the primary interest is in changes associated with somatic dysfunction and any autonomic related effects. The physician should visually inspect the area for clues that somatic dysfunction may be present (e.g., hyperemia, abnormal hair patterns, nevi, follicular eruptions) **(Fig. 4.1)**.

Fascia

The physician adds enough pressure to move the skin with the hand to evaluate the fascia. This pressure will cause slight reddening of the nail bed. The physician moves the hand very gently in cephalad, caudad, left, right, clockwise, and counterclockwise directions to elicit motion and tension quality barriers of ease and bind **(Fig. 4.3)**. Minimal changes in pressure to evaluate the different levels of fascia are helpful.

Temperature

Temperature is evaluated by using the volar aspect of the wrist or the dorsal hypothenar eminence of the hand. The physician does this by placing the wrists or hands a few inches above the area to be tested and using both hands to evaluate the paravertebral areas bilaterally and simultaneously **(Fig. 4.2)**. Changes in heat distribution may be palpated paraspinally as secondary effects of metabolic processes, trauma, and so on (acute inflammatory vs. chronic fibrotic effects). Heat radiation may also be palpated in other areas of the body (e.g., extremities, abdomen). If unable to determine the thermal status of the region in question, the physician may at this point make slight physical contact with the appropriate area of the palpating hand.

Muscle

Muscle is deeper tissue; therefore, the next degree of palpatory pressure is applied. The physician adds slightly more pressure to evaluate the muscle's consistency and determines whether there is ropiness, resistance to pressure, stringiness, and so on. This pressure will cause blanching of the physician's nail beds **(Fig. 4.4)**.

Tendons

Tendons should be traced to their bony attachments as well as to their continuity with muscle. Any fibrous thickening, change in elasticity, and so on should be noted.

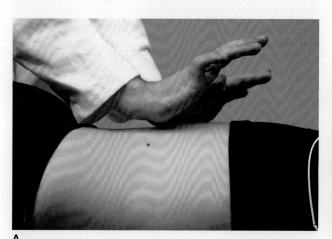
A

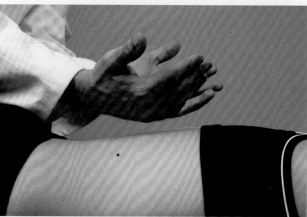
B

Figure 4.2. A and B. Evaluation for thermal asymmetry.

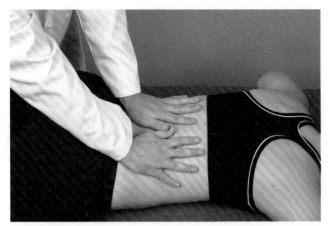

Figure 4.3. Fascial evaluation for ease-bind asymmetry.

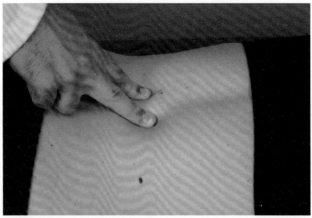

Figure 4.4. Blanching of the nail bed with muscle depth palpation.

Ligaments

Ligaments must be considered when restriction of joint motion, hypermobility (joint laxity), pain, and so on are present. Obviously, ligaments vary in type and are more or less palpable depending on their anatomic placement.

Erythema Friction Rub

The final step is to perform the erythema friction rub, in which the pads of the physician's second and third digits are placed just paraspinally and then in two to three quick

strokes are drawn down the spine cephalad to caudad. Pallor or reddening is evaluated per spinal segment for vasomotor changes that may be secondary to dysfunction. This is not typically done on the extremities, as the purpose of this test is to identify central spinal areas of autonomic change related to segmental dysfunction **(Fig. 4.5)**.

Percussion

Percussion is a quick and easy palpatory technique that does not require adept palpatory skills. Commonly

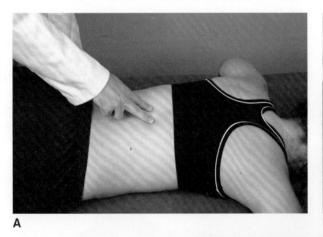

A

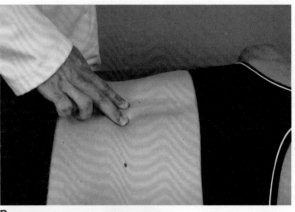

B

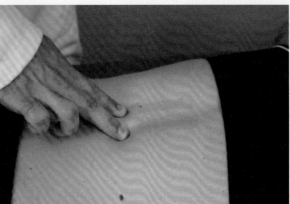

C

Figure 4.5. A–C. Erythema friction rub.

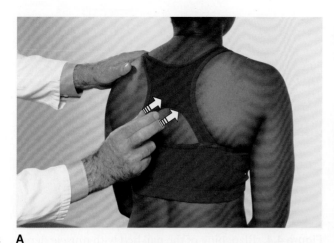 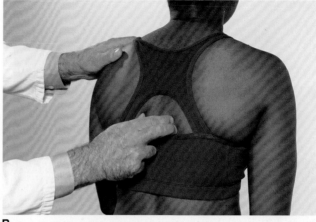

A   **B**

Figure 4.6. A. Bilateral percussion using whipping motion of wrist/fingers. **B.** Contact sensing tissue texture changes in tension.

described in physical examination texts for examining the chest cage for cardiac and pulmonary involvement, as well as in the abdominal examination, this technique can be used in the osteopathic structural examination as a variation of the layer-by-layer palpatory approach for changes in tissue texture and myofascial changes including hypertonicity and flaccidity. William Johnston, D.O. (*Personal Communication May 2000*), frequently used this method to quickly identify areas of greatest tension in the posterior thoracic and lumbar paraspinal region. He used this as a diagnostic technique for his "functional oriented techniques" and would monitor changes there as he positioned the patient indirectly, as pertained to the dysfunctional hypertonic tissue (4). The patient can stand, sit, or lie prone for this evaluation. The physician, using the index and third fingers, can percuss the tissues with a snapping or whipping motion of the fingers and wrist, as if to elicit a deep tendon response. The physician may do this unilaterally or, using a fast method to determine

laterality of the problem, tap bilaterally and simultaneously over the paraspinal tissues by joining the index and third fingers of the hand on one paraspinal myofascial area while using the thumb on the other side at the same level **(Fig. 4.6A and B)**. For example, the physician will start percussing bilaterally at T1 and with each percussion descend inferiorly one segment at a time, eventually reaching the L5 level. If percussion reveals that one side feels harder or more dense, the physician can move to that side and tap with the fingers of one hand to determine the extent of this change (i.e., T2–T7 on the left) **(Fig. 4.7A and B)**. If the tissue's texture is difficult to distinguish, or if the physician prefers, listening to the pitch of the sound the percussive tap elicits can easily distinguish between an area of hypertonicity (like a drum which is taut—higher pitched) compared to an area of normal tonicity or flaccidity (like a drum which is loose—lower pitched). This is similar to percussion over the chest wall to determine air, mass, or fluid presence by the acoustic tone of the percussion.

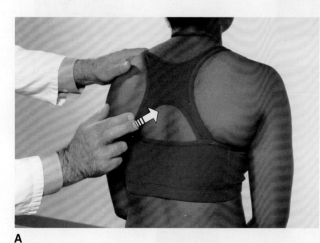 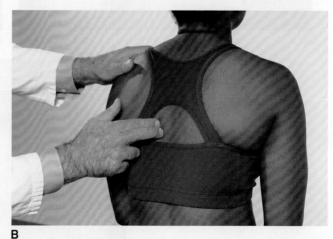

A   **B**

Figure 4.7. A. Unilateral percussion using whipping motion of wrist/fingers. **B.** Contact sensing tissue texture changes in tension.

Thoracic Region Cross Section

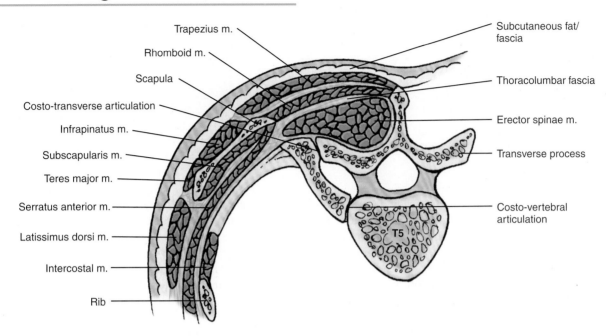

Lumbar Region Cross Section

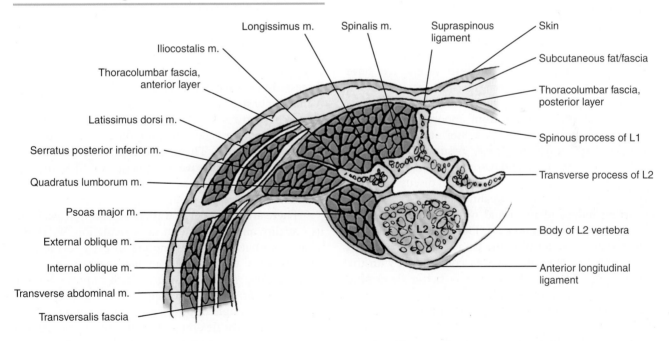

References

1. Nicholas A. Palpation in osteopathic medicine. Osteopath Ann 1978;6(7):36–42.
2. Korr IM. Osteopathic research: the needed paradigm shift. J Am Osteopath Assoc 1991;91(2):156.
3. Guyton A, Hall J. Textbook of Medical Physiology. 12th ed. Philadelphia, PA: Saunders, 2011.
4. Johnston WL, Friedman HD. Functional Methods: A Manual for Palpatory Skill Development in Osteopathic Examination and Manipulation of Motor Function. Indianapolis, IN: American Academy of Osteopathy, 1994.

5

Intersegmental Motion Testing

Intersegmental motion testing is classically described as an evaluation of spinal articulatory (facet) motion. In this chapter, it is also considered as a technique to elicit any motion at a joint (articulation), whether spinal, pelvic, costal, or extremity. Depending on the joint, the motions evaluated may include flexion and extension; rotation; side bending and rotation coupling; translational motions anteriorly, posteriorly, or laterally; separation or approximation of joint surfaces; and torsional movements. An important aspect of this type of palpation is to determine not only the symmetry/asymmetry and quantity of motion present at the segment(s) being examined but also the quality of the motion throughout the range. The quality of motion as the anatomic, physiologic, or restrictive barrier is approached is referred to as *end feel* (1–3). Various qualities of end feel have been described as *capsular, bone on bone, ligamentous and soft tissue approximation, springy, empty*, etc., attempting to differentiate normal from abnormal (4). Those originally described by Cyriax as normal include bone to bone (hard, unyielding), soft tissue approximation (yielding compression), and tissue stretch (hard or firm/springy) with a slight give (4). Mennell discussed "joint play" as it related to these qualities and described it as occurring independent of and not introduced by voluntary muscle contraction (3). This has clinical impact when trying to determine the veracity of the patient's complaint. In examining such, in conjunction with the patient's history, the physician may better determine the cause of the articular motion disturbance so that the safest and most effective treatment protocol can be developed.

In spinal motion testing, the physician attempts to discern the *three-plane motion* and the relation between side bending and rotation (coupling). The physician can determine the coupling status and whether the articular somatic dysfunction is exhibiting a Type I (opposite side) or Type II (same side) pattern **(Figs. 5.1 and 5.2)**. In the thoracic or lumbar region, if the dysfunctional pattern is found to be Type I, the examination is complete, as the segment has a neutral relation with the coupling.

If the dysfunction exhibits a Type II coupling pattern, the physician must typically continue the examination to determine whether a flexion or extension component is associated with the coupled motions of the dysfunction. In the cervical spine, these coupling relations follow a different set of biomechanical rules from those of the thoracic and lumbar regions. In the cervical spine, flexion, extension, and neutral components may be found with Type I or Type II coupling, or in the case of C1–C2 motion, there may be no coupling at all.

Some physicians prefer to start with the flexion and extension portion of the examination and then follow with rotation and/or side bending to determine the coupling components for determination of a Type I or Type II dysfunction. Because of the biomechanical patterns inherent to specific regions, the motion most easily tested may vary. For example, in the C2–C7 region, it may be best to test side bending first. However, it is always best to test the coupled segments together and test the flexion or extension components before or after the coupled testing. This is also true when performing osteopathic manipulative treatment (OMT), such as muscle energy technique, when all three axes are to be treated. The coupling should always be kept unified.

There are a number of ways to test motion availability (quality and quantity) at an articulation. We prefer a method that introduces motion directly to the joint using physical contact on bony landmarks (e.g., cervical articular processes) using a quick impulse. We use the term *positive* when referring to this form of motion testing. An example of positive motion testing is a lumbar spring test for flexion and extension components of dysfunction. Motion availability can be instantly ascertained in whichever direction the impulse was vectored, and the physician has a high degree of certainty that the motion palpated is occurring at this location.

Another common method is use of visual clues. In this method, the physician looks for a change in relation (symmetry or asymmetry) of superficial anatomic landmarks as the patient actively moves through a range of motion. We use the term *presumptive* when referring

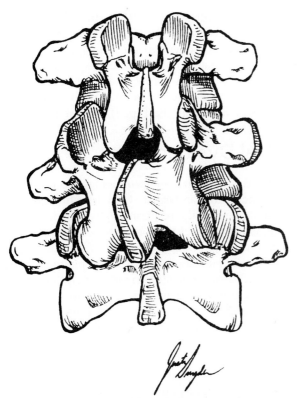

Figure 5.1. Type I spinal coupled pattern.

to this form of motion testing. Examples of presumptive motion testing are the standing and seated flexion (forward bending) tests for sacroiliac region dysfunction. In this form of motion testing, the physician has a lower

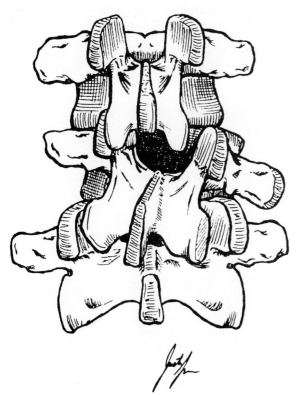

Figure 5.2. Type II spinal coupled pattern.

degree of certainty that the designated joint has motion reduction or asymmetry (dysfunction). Many postural factors (e.g., sacral base unleveling, tight hamstring muscles) other than motion disturbance at the joint can cause false positives in this type of testing, and therefore, we limit its use.

When documenting the motion preferences revealed on intersegmental motion testing, it is understood that the following abbreviations are accepted and used consistently within the osteopathic profession to denote the *x*, *y*, and *z* components in the *three-plane* diagnosis and will be used in the following chapters to describe the dysfunction's free motion characteristics: Flexion = F; Extension = E; Neutral = N; Side bending right = SR; Side bending left = SL; Rotation right = RR; and Rotation left = RL.

After determining what motion restriction(s) and ease-bind asymmetries are present, the articular dysfunction must be documented. When the osteopathic profession decided to change its terminology describing musculoskeletal problems from *osteopathic lesion* to *somatic dysfunction*, it also changed the manner in which we describe the dysfunction. Previously, osteopathic physicians described the lesion (dysfunction) by the direction of motion restriction that typically caused pain. When the term somatic dysfunction was adopted, a three-dimensional (*x*-, *y*-, and *z-cardinal axis*) type description based on the *positional* relationship of the superior segment of the coupled dysfunctional vertebral unit became the standard. In addition, it was found that the positional diagnosis correlated with the motion parameters that were most free. In doing so, it led to describing somatic dysfunction by its *least* dysfunctional parameter. This has led to some confusion for the novice student or other manual medicine physician groups (e.g., European manual medicine physician specialists) who better understand the older "restriction" referencing, which is based on the *loss of function and/or pain*.

In developing ways to document the dysfunctional findings by the present American osteopathic method, osteopathic physicians have used a number of abridgments as described previously, for example, NSRRL. Originally, because of the motion parameters involved at different spinal levels associated with Type I (opposite-sided coupling) or Type II (same-sided coupling), it was common to describe the Type I, neutral dysfunctions by writing the side-bending component first and following with the rotational component of the dysfunction, for example, T5, NSLRR. Whereas in a Type II dysfunction, the rotational component followed the flexion or extension component, followed last by the side-bending component, for example, T5, FRRSR, or ERRSR. Presently, this has been continued by purists who want students to remember that in various cases, rotation or side bending should be the first barrier engaged with osteopathic technique (e.g., muscle energy) after the flexion, extension, or neutral component, respectively.

Trying to palpate these coupled motions and seeing how rotation and side bending relate differently in neutral and nonneutral biomechanics is a useful practice in understanding how fulcrums and pivot points are developed. Some osteopathic physicians prefer a more abbreviated variation by noting the nonneutral component followed by the motion freedom/direction associated with the last letter of the abbreviation; examples being ERS_R (ESR_R) for extended, rotated right, side bent right and FRS_L (FSR_L) for flexed, rotated left, side bent left. In neutral dysfunctions, this can be used as NSR_L for neutral, side bent right, rotated left; however, the practitioner must understand completely the coupling relationship in neutral biomechanics to abridge this correctly! In national testing situations, it may be common to have no abbreviations, and the entire dysfunction may be seen as written out completely, that is, neutral, side bent right, and rotated left.

Group and Single Segment Dysfunctions

As a patient suffering from spinal somatic dysfunction may have either a Type I or Type II dysfunction, it is important to know that there are subtle differences that may be presented in these two types. Classically, Type I dysfunctions have been described as a collective or "group curve" dysfunction (thoracic and lumbar) involving more than one segment (1). These dysfunctions may follow common postural movements, common compensatory fascial patterns, or mild-to-moderate physical stresses. Type II dysfunctions are classically described as presenting as single segment dysfunctions and less

commonly as a group. Type II dysfunctions (thoracic and lumbar) follow movements that added a flexion or extension component to the coupled motions and, therefore, generated increased forces through greater long levering than those developed in neutral posturing. This may, at times, cause a more symptomatic or more painful presentation in the Type II dysfunction.

Costal Dysfunctions

In costal dysfunctions, the terminology has been somewhat difficult to standardize. Costal dysfunctions have been described by the respiratory/physiologic and non-physiologic/positional motion patterns. Some prefer to describe the dysfunction in terms of motion freedom related to the inhalation or exhalation phase of respiration (e.g., 1st rib, inhalation right), which follows more closely the way in which dysfunctions are described in other areas of the body, while others prefer to describe the same problem by the way the rib is being held (e.g., 1st rib right, held/caught in inhalation) (1). Some clinicians describe costal dysfunctions by their altered positions: elevated or depressed, anterior or posterior.

Because costal dysfunctions may typically follow a vertebral dysfunction, single segment or group dysfunctions may be possible in this region. Also, when both vertebral and costal dysfunctions occur at the same level, it can be frequently effective to treat only the vertebral dysfunction, as the costal dysfunction may have been secondary to the vertebral somatic component. However, in our clinical experience, we believe that 1st rib and 12th (floating) rib are commonly dysfunctional without the vertebral relationship.

Lumbar Intersegmental Motion Testing

L1–L5, Rotation
Prone, Short-Lever Method
Ex: L4

 See Videos 5.1 and 5.2

1. The patient lies prone on the treatment table with the head in neutral (if a face hole is present) or rotated to the more comfortable side. *Remember, the side to which the head is rotated will passively increase the rotational effect to that side.*

2. The physician stands at either side of the table and palpates the L4 transverse processes (level of the iliac crest) with the pads of the thumbs **(Figs. 5.3 and 5.4)**.

3. The physician alternately presses on the left and right transverse processes of L4 with firm ventrally directed impulses to evaluate for ease (freedom) of left and right rotation **(Figs. 5.5 and 5.6)**.

4. If the right transverse process moves anteriorly (inward) (*white arrow*) more easily and the left transverse process is resistant, the segment is rotating left more freely (rotated left) **(Fig. 5.7)**.

5. If the *left* transverse process moves anteriorly (*white arrow*) more easily and the right transverse process is resistant, the segment is rotating right more freely (rotated right) **(Fig. 5.8)**.

6. The left transverse process of L4 in this example may present more prominently (posteriorly) on static (layer-by-layer) palpation in a rotated left dysfunction.

7. The physician performs these steps at each segment of the lumbar spine and documents the rotational freedom of movement.

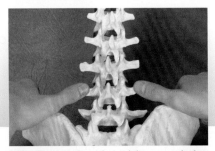
Figure 5.3. Step 2, hand position on skeleton.

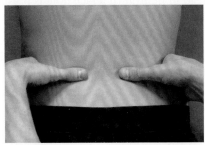
Figure 5.4. Step 2, hand position on the patient.

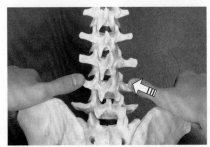
Figure 5.5. Step 3, skeleton, rotation left.

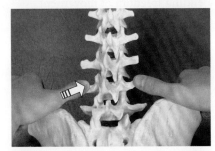
Figure 5.6. Step 3, skeleton, rotation right.

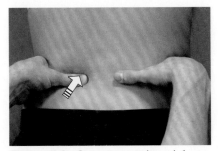
Figure 5.8. Step 5, rotation right.

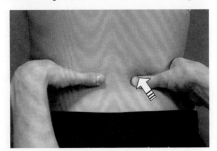
Figure 5.7. Step 4, rotation left.

Lumbar Intersegmental Motion Testing

L1–L5, Side Bending
Prone, Short-Lever Translatory Method
Ex: L4

 See Videos 5.3 and 5.4

1. The patient lies prone on the treatment table with the head in neutral (if a face hole is present) or rotated to the more comfortable side.

2. The physician's thumbs rest on the posterolateral aspect of the transverse processes **(Figs. 5.9 and 5.10)**.

3. The physician introduces an alternating translatory glide, left and right, to evaluate for ease of left and right side bending.

4. If the thumb translates the segment more easily from left to right, the segment has its ease in left side bending and is termed *side bent left* **(Figs. 5.11 and 5.12)**.

5. If the thumb translates the segment more easily from right to left, the segment has its ease in right side bending and is termed *side bent right* **(Figs. 5.13 and 5.14)**.

6. The physician performs these steps at each segment of the lumbar spine and documents the side-bending freedom of movement.

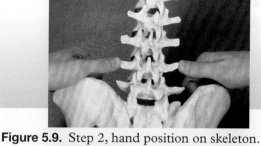
Figure 5.9. Step 2, hand position on skeleton.

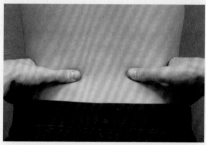
Figure 5.10. Step 2, hand position on the patient.

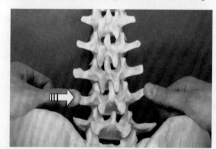
Figure 5.11. Step 4, side bending left on skeleton.

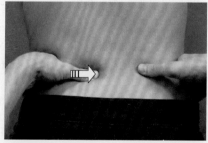
Figure 5.12. Step 4, side bending left on the patient.

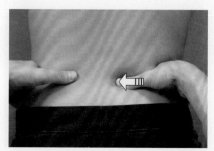
Figure 5.14. Step 5, side bending right on the patient.

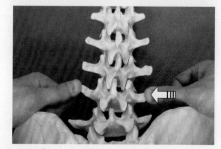
Figure 5.13. Step 5, side bending right on skeleton.

Lumbar Intersegmental Motion Testing

L1–L5, Extension/Flexion
Prone Sphinx Position/Seated Flexion
Ex: L1, Type II (Nonneutral Dysfunction)

1. After determining that the rotational and side-bending components are coupled in a Type II pattern (same-side pattern of ease), the physician's thumbs are placed on the posterolateral aspect of the transverse processes **(Fig. 5.15)** of the prone patient.

2. The patient is instructed to extend the thoracolumbar region by elevating the chest off the table with the support of the elbows and resting the head on the supporting hands, to relax the paraspinal musculature **(Fig. 5.16)**.

3. The physician retests the rotational and/or side-bending components in this position. If the static and dynamic components of the dysfunction improve, the dysfunction is *extended* **(Fig. 5.17)**. If the static and dynamic components of the dysfunction become more asymmetric, the dysfunction is *flexed* (or neutral). A more patient active test can be performed by asking the seated patient to extend backward (as if looking up toward the ceiling) and similarly reevaluating the dysfunctional components.

4. Using a flexion-oriented evaluation, the patient sits on the table and the physician stands or sits behind the patient. The physician's thumbs or index fingers are placed over the transverse processes of the dysfunctional segment. The patient is asked to slowly forward bend, and the physician notes whether an improvement or exacerbation of the dysfunctional components occurred. If the dysfunctional components appear more symmetric in this position, the dysfunction is termed *flexed*. If they are more asymmetric in this position, it is termed *extended* **(Fig. 5.18)**. Some prefer to have the patient curl up in a knees-to-chest position to promote relative flexion and retest the dysfunctional rotation and side-bending components; however, we feel that this is difficult for a large percent of our patients.

5. The physician must perform only one of these as long as there is a known Type II coupling pattern; perform the most comfortable test.

6. The physician will document the findings in the progress note according to the position or freedom of movement elicited.

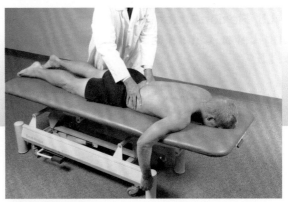

Figure 5.15. Step 1.

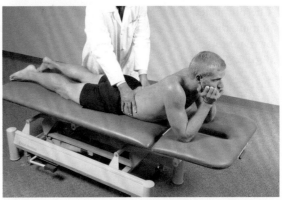

Figure 5.16. Step 2, lumbar sphinx position.

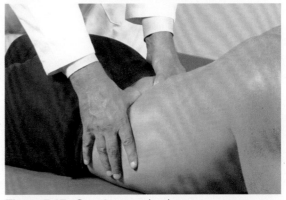

Figure 5.17. Step 3, extension improves asymmetry.

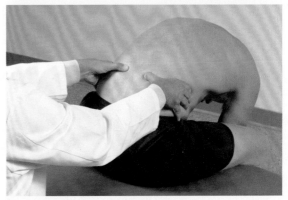

Figure 5.18. Step 4, flexion.

Lumbar Intersegmental Motion Testing

L1–L5, Flexion/Extension
Long-Lever, Lateral Recumbent Method
Ex: L5

 See Video 5.5

1. The patient lies in the lateral recumbent (side-lying) position.

2. The physician stands at the side of the treatment table facing the front of the patient.

3. The physician's finger pads of the cephalad hand palpate the spinous processes of L5–S1 **(Fig. 5.19)** or the interspinous space between L5 and S1 **(Fig. 5.20)**.

4. The physician's caudad hand controls the patient's flexed lower extremities, and the physician's thigh may be placed against the patient's tibial tuberosities for greater balance and control during positioning **(Fig. 5.21)**.

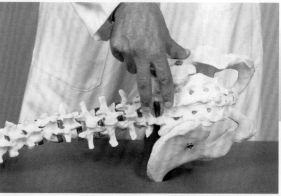

Figure 5.19. Step 3, palpation of spinous processes.

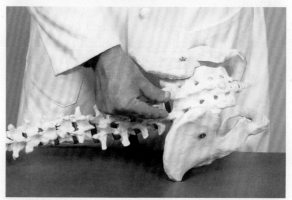

Figure 5.20. Step 3, palpation of L5–S1 interspace.

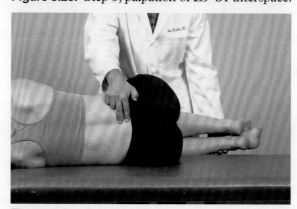

Figure 5.21. Step 4.

5. The physician slowly flexes and extends the patient's hips with the caudad hand and thigh while the cephalad hand constantly monitors the spinous processes to determine the relative freedom of lumbar flexion and extension of L5 on S1 **(Figs. 5.22 and 5.23)**.

6. The physician assesses the ability of the upper of the two segments to flex and extend on the lower. If L5 flexes and extends equally (symmetrically) on S1, then L5 is termed neutral. If there is asymmetry of motion between the two segments, the dysfunction is named for the direction of ease of motion of the upper of the two segments (e.g., if L5 moves more easily in flexion, L5 is *flexed*; if the segment moves more freely into extension, L5 is *extended*).

7. The physician performs these steps at each segmental level of the lumbar spine.

8. The physician will document the findings in the progress note according to the position or freedom of movement elicited.

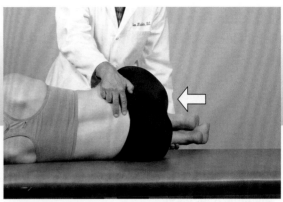

Figure 5.22. Step 5, flexion, spinous process separate.

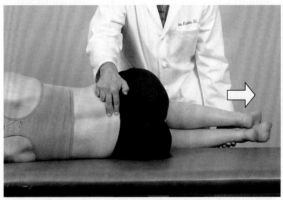

Figure 5.23. Step 5, extension, spinous process approximate.

Lumbar Intersegmental Motion Testing

L1–L5, Side Bending
Lateral Recumbent, Long-Lever Method
Ex: L5

 See Video 5.6

1. The physician flexes the patient's hips to approximately 90 degrees and gently moves the patient's lower extremities slightly off the edge of the table (**Fig. 5.24**).

2. The physician slowly flexes and extends the patient's hips until L5 is neutral relative to S1.

3. The finger pads of the physician's cephalad hand palpate the left and right transverse processes of L5 (**Fig. 5.25**) *or* the interspace between their transverse processes.

4. The physician's caudad hand slowly raises the patient's feet and ankles upward as the cephalad hand monitors the approximation of the transverse processes on the side to which the feet are raised (or the separation of the transverse processes on the side to which the patient is lying) (**Fig. 5.26**).

5. The physician then lowers the patient's feet and ankles while the cephalad hand monitors the approximation of the transverse processes on the side to which the feet are lowered (or the separation of the transverse processes on the side opposite to which the patient is lying) (**Fig. 5.27**).

6. The physician assesses the ability of the upper of the two segments (L5) to side bend left and side bend right. In this test, side bending occurs on the side to which the feet and ankles are moved.

7. The physician performs these steps at each segmental level of the lumbar spine.

8. The physician will document the findings in the progress note according to the position or freedom of movement elicited.

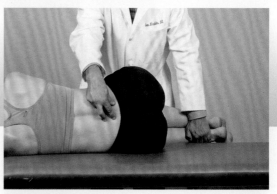
Figure 5.24. Step 1.

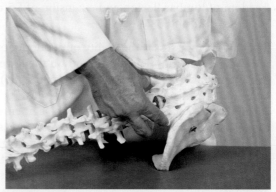
Figure 5.25. Step 3, palpation of L5 transverse processes.

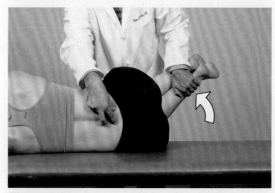
Figure 5.26. Step 4, side bending right.

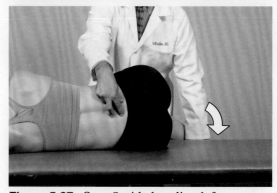
Figure 5.27. Step 5, side bending left.

Lumbar Intersegmental Motion Testing

L1–L5, Flexion/Extension
Prone, Spring Test Method
Ex: L4 (May Be Used in Thoracic Spine)

1. After determining that the rotational and side-bending components are coupled in a Type II pattern (same-side pattern of ease), the physician's thumb and index finger of one hand are placed immediately paraspinal and between the spinous processes of the dysfunctional vertebral unit (upper and lower segments) of the prone patient, or the physician may use the thumbs placed bilaterally between the spinous processes of the dysfunctional vertebral unit (upper and lower segments) **(Fig. 5.28A and B)**.

2. The physician imparts a quick, springing impulse that is vectored ventrally (toward the table) **(Fig. 5.29)**. This is similar to the *lumbosacral spring test* used to determine anterior (forward) or posterior (backward) sacral dysfunctions.

3. If increased resistance is met and the segments do not move easily into an extension relationship, the dysfunctional component related to the Type II coupling is flexion.

4. If less or no resistance is met and the segments move easily into extension, the dysfunctional component related to the Type II coupling is extension.

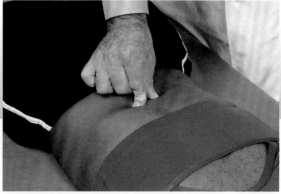

Figure 5.28. A. Step 1, springing with the thumb and index finger.

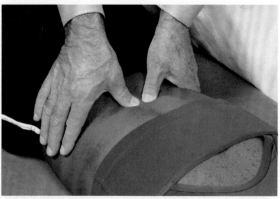

Figure 5.28. B. Step 1, springing with the thumbs bilaterally.

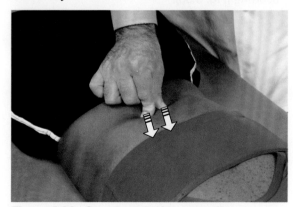

Figure 5.29. Step 2, springing ventrally.

Thoracic Intersegmental Motion Testing

T1–T4, Flexion/Extension
T1–T4, Side Bending/Rotation
Seated, Long-Lever Method

 See Video 5.7

1. The patient is seated with the physician standing behind the patient.

2. The physician controls the patient's head with one hand and palpates the spinous processes of T1 and T2 with the index and third finger of the other hand.

3. The physician slowly moves the patient's head forward and backward while constantly monitoring the ability of the upper of the segments to move in the respective direction tested **(Figs. 5.30 and 5.31).**

4. The physician, while controlling the patient's head, palpates the left transverse processes of T1 and T2 and moves the patient's head to the left shoulder, assessing the ability of the left T1 transverse process to approximate the left T2 transverse process. This elicits left side bending **(Fig. 5.32).** This is repeated on the right to elicit right side bending **(Fig. 5.33).**

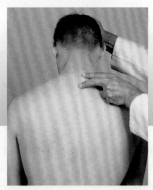

Figure 5.30. Step 3, flexion-spinous processes separate.

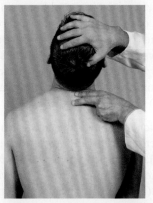

Figure 5.31. Step 3, extension-spinous processes approximate.

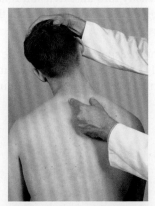

Figure 5.32. Step 4, side bending left.

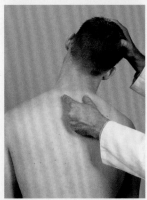

Figure 5.33. Step 4, side bending right.

5. While monitoring the left transverse processes, the physician slowly rotates the patient's head to the left. This evaluates left rotation; it is sensed by a simultaneous posterior movement of the transverse process on that side **(Fig. 5.34)**. This is repeated on the right to elicit right rotation **(Fig. 5.35)**.

6. The physician performs these steps at each segmental level T2–T3, T3–T4, and T4–T5.

7. The physician will document the findings in the progress note according to the position or freedom of motion elicited.

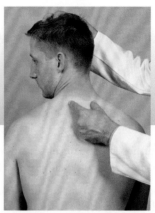

Figure 5.34. Step 5, rotation left.

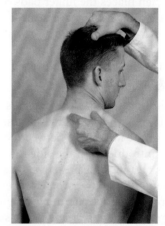

Figure 5.35. Step 5, rotation right.

Thoracic Intersegmental Motion Testing

T1–T4, Side Bending
Lateral Recumbent, Long-Lever Method
Ex: T2

 See Video 5.8

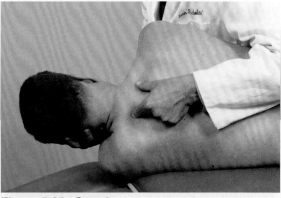

Figure 5.36. Step 3.

1. The patient lies in the lateral recumbent position with the back close to the side of the table.

2. The physician sits in front of the patient at the side of the table, facing the patient's head.

3. The physician places the finger pads of the caudad hand over the transverse processes of the dysfunctional segment or the interspace between them while the cephalad hand reaches under the patient's head and carefully lifts it off the table **(Fig. 5.36)**.

4. The physician gently lifts the patient's head while monitoring the involved segment's transverse processes or the interspace between them. Side bending is introduced on the side to which the head is moved. This presents as a sense of approximation of the transverse processes on the upward side and separation of the transverse processes on the opposite side (table side) **(Fig. 5.37)**.

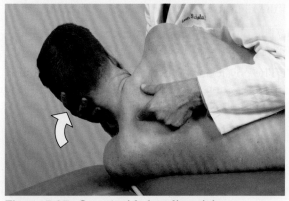

Figure 5.37. Step 4, side bending right.

5. The physician reverses the movement by gently lowering the head toward the table **(Fig. 5.38)** while monitoring the approximation of the transverse processes on the lower side (table side) and/or separation on the opposite side. *Again, the side to which the head moves is the side on which side bending occurs.*

6. The physician repeats this sequence throughout the T1–T4 region to determine side-bending preference or ease of motion and then documents the findings in the progress note.

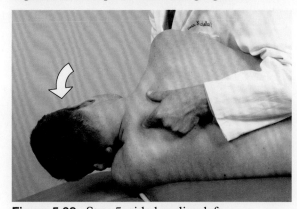

Figure 5.38. Step 5, side bending left.

Thoracic Intersegmental Motion Testing

T1–T12, Flexion/Extension
Seated, Short-Lever/Translatory Method
Ex: T6

 See Video 5.9

1. The patient is seated with the physician standing behind and to the side.

2. The physician places the thumb and index finger of one hand between the spinous processes of T6 and T7 or the index and third finger palpate the spinous processes of T6 and T7, respectively **(Fig. 5.39)**.

3. The patient's arms are crossed, anteriorly, in a V formation. The physician's right arm and hand are placed under the patient's crossed elbows while the left hand remains on the T6–T7 interspace **(Fig. 5.40)**.

4. The physician instructs the patient to completely relax forward, resting the forehead on the forearm as the left hand monitors flexion of T6 on T7 (separation of the spinous processes). The patient must be completely relaxed and not guarding **(Fig. 5.41)**.

5. The physician's posterior hand gently pushes or glides the spinous process or interspace anteriorly as the other hand lifts the patient's elbows slightly to evaluate extension of T6 on T7. This is noted by the approximation of the spinous processes **(Fig. 5.42)**. The patient must be completely relaxed and not guarding. Care must be taken to avoid hyperextension.

6. Steps 4 and 5 are performed at each thoracic segmental level.

7. The physician will document the findings in the progress notes according to the position or freedom of motion elicited.

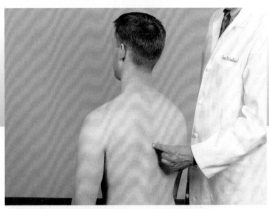

Figure 5.39. Step 2.

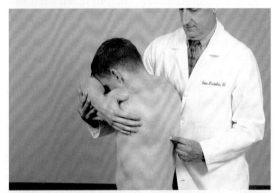

Figure 5.40. Step 3.

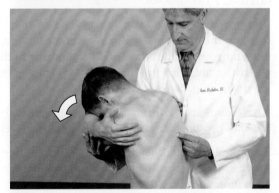

Figure 5.41. Step 4, flexion-spinous processes separate.

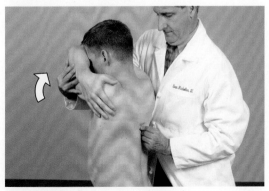

Figure 5.42. Step 5, extension-spinous processes approximate.

Thoracic Intersegmental Motion Testing

T1–T12, Side Bending
Seated, Short-Lever/Translatory Method
Ex: T6

 See Video 5.10

1. The patient is seated and the physician stands behind and to the side.

2. The physician places the left thumb and index finger between the spinous processes of T6 and T7 **(Fig. 5.43)**. Alternatively, the physician's left thumb and index finger palpate the spinous process of T6.

3. The physician reaches across the front of the patient's chest with the right arm and places the right hand on the patient's left shoulder with the physician's right axilla resting on the patient's right shoulder **(Fig. 5.44)**.

4. The physician's right axilla applies a downward force on the patient's right shoulder as the left hand simultaneously glides or pushes the T6–T7 interspace to the patient's left. This causes a left translatory effect that produces right side bending of T6 on T7 **(Fig. 5.45)**.

5. The physician's right hand applies a downward force on the patient's left shoulder as the left hand simultaneously glides the T6–T7 interspace to the patient's right. This produces left side bending of T6 on T7 **(Fig. 5.46)**.

6. These steps are performed to evaluate right and left side bending at each thoracic segmental level.

7. The physician will document the findings in the progress note according to the position or freedom of motion elicited.

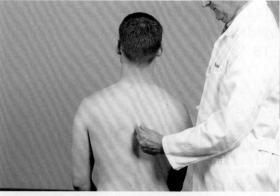

Figure 5.43. Step 2.

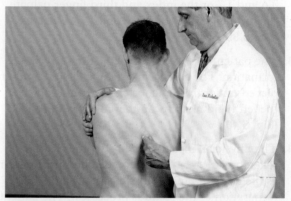

Figure 5.44. Step 3.

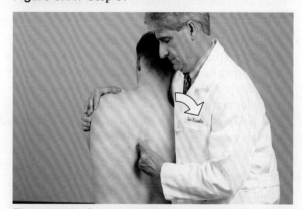

Figure 5.45. Step 4, translatory side bending right.

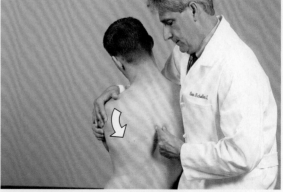

Figure 5.46. Step 5, translatory side bending left.

Thoracic Intersegmental Motion Testing

T1–T12, Rotation/Side Bending
Prone, Short-Lever Method
Ex: T7

1. The patient lies prone with the head in neutral. If this is not possible, the patient should turn the head to the more comfortable side. Note any change below.

2. The physician stands at either side of the table and palpates the T7 transverse process with the pads of the thumbs or index fingers.

3. The physician alternately presses on the left and right transverse processes of T7, evaluating for ease of movement.

4. If the right transverse process moves anteriorly (inward) more easily, the segment is rotating left more freely and vice versa **(Figs. 5.47 and 5.48)**.

5. In the step 4 scenario, the left transverse process may be palpated more prominently (posteriorly) on layer-by-layer palpation.

6. Next, with the thumbs palpating over the most lateral aspect of the transverse processes, an alternating translatory glide to the left and right is introduced to test side bending.

7. If the thumb translates the segment more easily from left to right, left side bending is occurring and vice versa **(Figs. 5.49 and 5.50)**.

8. These steps are performed to evaluate right and left rotation and side bending at each segmental level (T1–T2, T2–T3, T3–T4, and so on to T12–L1).

9. The physician will document these findings in the progress note according to the position or freedom of motion palpated.

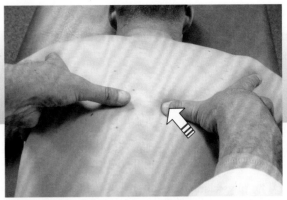

Figure 5.47. Step 4, rotation left.

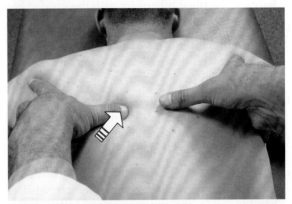

Figure 5.48. Step 4, rotation right.

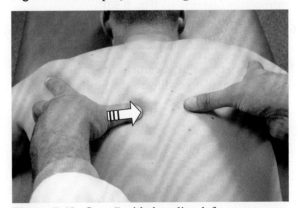

Figure 5.49. Step 7, side bending left.

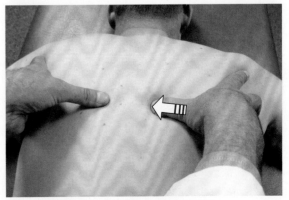

Figure 5.50. Step 7, side bending right.

Thoracic Intersegmental Motion Testing

T8–T12, Flexion/Extension
Long-Lever, Lateral Recumbent Method
Ex: T12

 See Video 5.11

1. The patient lies in the lateral recumbent position with the hips and knees flexed (fetal position).

2. The physician stands on the side of the table facing the front of the patient and controls the patient's knees at the tibial tuberosity with the caudad hand.

3. The physician's cephalad hand palpates the spinous processes of T12 and L1 or their interspace with the index and/or long finger **(Fig. 5.51)**.

4. The physician slowly flexes the hips by bringing the knees to the chest as the physician's cephalad hand monitors the separation of the spinous processes (flexion) **(Fig. 5.52)**.

5. The physician then extends the hips by bringing the knees away from the chest as the cephalad hand monitors the approximation of the spinous processes (extension) **(Fig. 5.53)**.

6. These steps are performed to evaluate flexion and extension at each thoracic segmental level.

7. The physician will document the findings in the progress note according to the position or freedom of motion elicited.

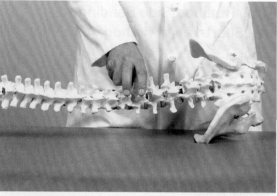

Figure 5.51. Step 3, spinous processes of T12–L1.

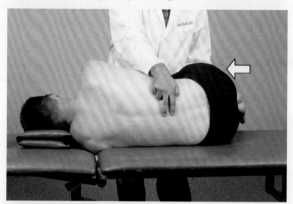

Figure 5.52. Step 4, flexion.

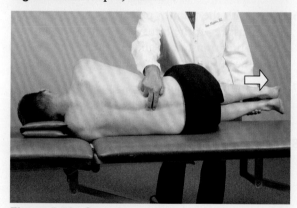

Figure 5.53. Step 5, extension.

Thoracic Intersegmental Motion Testing

T8–T12, Side Bending
Long-Lever, Lateral Recumbent Method
Ex: T12

 See Video 5.12

1. The patient lies in the lateral recumbent position with the hips and knees flexed (fetal position).

2. The physician stands on the side of the table facing the front of the patient and controls the patient's knees at the tibial tuberosity with the caudad hand.

3. The physician moves the patient's lower legs off the edge of the table, and while monitoring the transverse processes, the physician slowly raises the patient's feet toward the ceiling and then draws them toward the floor **(Fig. 5.54)**.

4. Side bending is evaluated by monitoring the approximation of the transverse processes on the side to which the feet are drawn (e.g., feet toward the right, side bending right) **(Figs. 5.55 and 5.56)**.

5. These steps are performed to evaluate left and right side bending at each thoracic segmental level.

6. The physician will document the findings in the progress note according to the position or freedom of motion elicited.

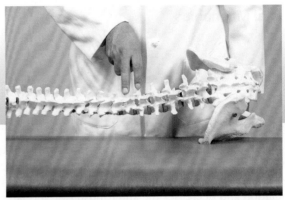

Figure 5.54. Step 3.

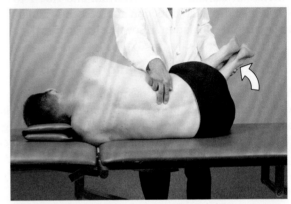

Figure 5.55. Step 4, side bending right.

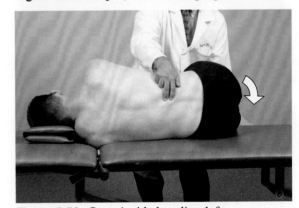

Figure 5.56. Step 4, side bending left.

Costal Motion Testing

Costal Mechanics

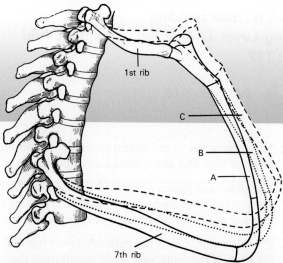

In respiration, the sternum and ribs move in a simultaneous and combined pattern that expands the chest in the anteroposterior and lateral diameters during inhalation and decreases the anteroposterior and lateral diameters in exhalation. The sternum and ribs 1 to 10 also rise in a cephalad direction and descend caudally in inhalation and exhalation, respectively **(Fig. 5.57)**.

Rib Excursion with Inhalation

The vertebral and sternal attachments combine to promote specific vectors of motion during normal inhalation, expanding the chest. This expansion moves through two major vector paths. These patterns are described as occurring through pump-handle and bucket-handle axes in both vertebrosternal ribs 1 to 6 and vertebrochondral ribs 7 to 10 **(Figs. 5.58 and 5.59)**.

Figure 5.57. Lateral view of the 1st and 7th ribs in position, showing the movements of the sternum and ribs in (*A*) ordinary expiration, (*B*) quiet inspiration, and (*C*) deep inspiration. (From Clemente CD. Gray's Anatomy. 13th ed. Baltimore, MD: Lippincott Williams & Wilkins, 1985, with permission.)

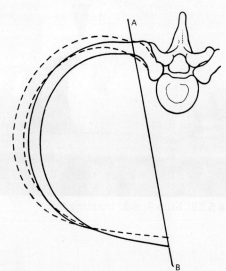

Figure 5.59. Axis of movement (*A–B*) of a vertebrochondral rib. The interrupted lines indicate the position of the rib in inhalation. (Used with permission of the AACOM. ©1983–2006. All rights reserved.)

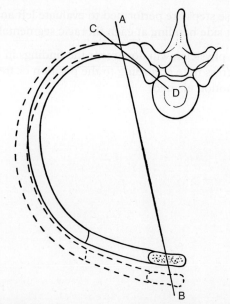

Figure 5.58. Axes of movement (*A–B* and *C–D*) of a vertebrosternal rib. Interrupted lines indicate the position of the rib in inhalation. (Used with permission of the AACOM. ©1983–2006. All rights reserved.)

Angle of Inclination of the Axes of Rib 1 and Rib 6

The costotransverse articulations combine with the costovertebral articulations at each vertebral level to develop angles through which axis of rotation a rib may move. Thus, the rib moves within this specific axis of rotation, and the angle changes from superior to inferior ribs. The angle, as it relates to the anteroposterior planes and the lateral body line, determines whether the rib motion produced through normal respiration is greatest at the anterior midclavicular line or the lateral clavicular-midaxillary line. Ribs 1 to 10 have some shared motion parameters in each of the axes of rotation. However, the motion pattern of the upper ribs is related to a predominant anterior or frontal plane axis, whereas in the lower ribs, a less frontal, more sagittal axis predominates. These differences produce the patterns of pump-handle motion preference of the upper ribs and the bucket-handle preference of the lower ribs (**Figs. 5.60 and 5.61**).

Pump-Handle Rib Motion

The term *pump-handle rib motion* describes the movement of a rib that can be compared to the motion of the handle of a water pump. Its motion is produced by one end being fixed in space and rotating around an axis that permits the opposite end to move through space (**Fig. 5.62**).

Bucket-Handle Rib Motion

The term *bucket-handle rib motion* describes the movement of a rib that can be best compared to the movement of the handle of a bucket as it is lifted up and off the rim of the bucket and then laid down on the same side. The motion is produced by both ends of the

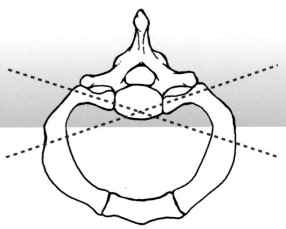

Figure 5.60. Rib 1: most frontal in plane, allowing a more purely "pump-handle" rib excursion.

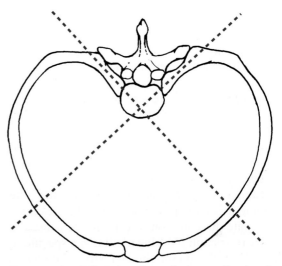

Figure 5.61. Rib 6: less frontal plane, allowing for greater ability to move in a "bucket-handle" type motion than can rib 1.

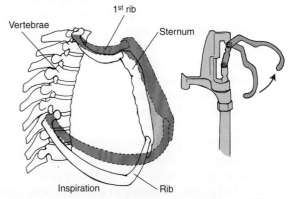

Figure 5.62. Pump-handle rib motion. (From Clay JH, Pounds DM. Basic Clinical Massage Therapy: Integrating Anatomy and Treatment. Baltimore, MD: Lippincott Williams & Wilkins, 2003, with permission.)

Costal Motion Testing

Costal Mechanics (Continued)

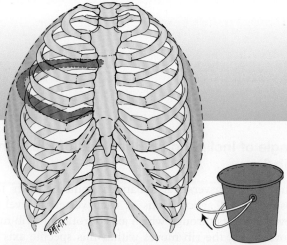

Figure 5.63. Bucket-handle rib motion. (From Clay JH, Pounds DM. Basic Clinical Massage Therapy: Integrating Anatomy and Treatment. Baltimore, MD: Lippincott Williams & Wilkins, 2003, with permission.)

handle being fixed at a rotational axis permitting only the area between the two points to move through space **(Fig. 5.63)**.

The "Key Rib" Dysfunction

The term *key lesion* (dysfunction) is defined as "the somatic dysfunction that maintains a total dysfunction pattern including other secondary dysfunctions" (2). In expanding this principle, the term *"key rib"* was introduced in muscle energy technique seminars to help determine which rib should be treated first when a group costal dysfunction was evident (5). This principle may or may not always be true, as somatic dysfunctions may be caused by a number of conditions including: a myofascial tug/pull that restricts motion opposite the pulling direction, a blockage of motion secondary to a joint restriction, or tissue that is indurated, edematous, etc., acting as a barrier to movement toward it. For example, a myofascial etiology may "tug" the rib by pulling it back in one direction and restricting it in the opposite direction, but it can also be caused by an articular restriction blocking motion in a specific direction, as if a wall is present in the restricted direction.

An example of the key rib postulate is the idea that with a group inhalation dysfunction treated by a direct technique (i.e., muscle energy), the corrective forces must be vectored toward the restriction; as in this case, exhalation. Therefore, if the motion we are improving is vectored toward exhalation, the most inferior rib must be treated first so that those superior can then move more easily in sequential procession; whereas in an exhalation dysfunction, the motion we are trying to improve is toward inhalation; treating the most superior rib first and permitting those inferior to follow in sequential procession. Therefore, the key ribs in *group inhalation and exhalation* costal dysfunctions are the most inferior in inhalation and the most superior in exhalation dysfunctions (5). Another way to picture this is a line of people marching in a straight line, where the leader of the march can be compared to the key rib. The leader (key rib) moves first toward the determined direction of the march and the others follow. An incorrect example would be a group of dominos falling one into the next one and so on.

Costal Motion Testing

Rib 1 and Rib 2, Physiologic Model
Supine, Respiratory Excursion Method
Ex: Pump-Handle Motion

1. The patient lies supine, and the physician sits or stands at the head of the table. (Or the patient may sit.)

2. The physician palpates the 1st ribs at their infraclavicular position at the sternoclavicular articulation (the supraclavicular position can also be used) **(Fig. 5.64)**.

3. The physician monitors the relative superior (cephalad) and inferior (caudad) relation of the pair and, on the symptomatic side, determines whether that rib is prominent or not and positioned superiorly or inferiorly.

4. The patient is instructed to inhale and exhale deeply through the mouth as the physician monitors the ability of the pair of 1st ribs to move superiorly and inferiorly.

5. If the rib on the symptomatic side is statically cephalad and on inhalation has greater cephalad (on exhalation, less caudad) movement, it is classified as an *inhalation rib dysfunction* **(Fig. 5.65)**.

6. If the rib on the symptomatic side is statically caudad and on inhalation has less cephalad (on exhalation, greater caudad) movement, it is classified as an *exhalation rib dysfunction* **(Fig. 5.66)**.

7. The physician next palpates the 2nd ribs approximately one finger's breadth below and one finger's breadth lateral to where the 1st rib was palpated and repeats steps 3 to 6 **(Fig. 5.67)**.

8. The movement of the rib on the symptomatic side that was freest is documented in the progress note (inhalation or exhalation based on the respiratory [physiologic] model).

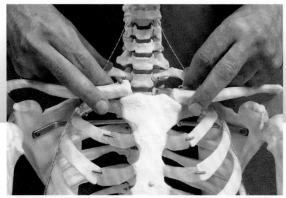

Figure 5.64. Step 2, palpation of the 1st rib.

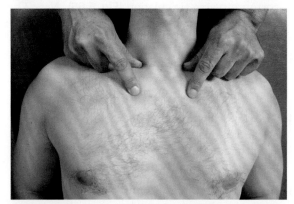

Figure 5.65. Step 5, inhalation rib dysfunction.

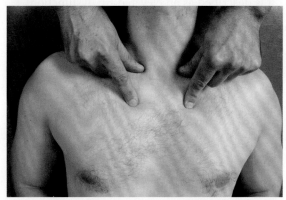

Figure 5.66. Step 6, exhalation rib dysfunction.

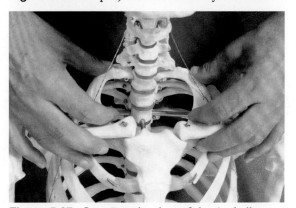

Figure 5.67. Step 7, palpation of the 2nd rib.

Costal Motion Testing

Rib 1, Nonrespiratory Model
Seated, Short-Lever Method
Ex: Rib 1, Elevated (Nonphysiologic)

 See Video 5.13

1. The patient is seated, and the physician stands behind the patient.

2. The physician palpates the posterolateral shaft of each 1st rib immediately lateral to the costotransverse articulation **(Fig. 5.68)**. *Note*: The trapezius borders may have to be pulled posteriorly **(Fig. 5.69)**.

3. With firm pressure of the thumbs or finger pads, the physician directs a downward (caudad) force alternately on each rib **(Figs. 5.70 and 5.71)**.

4. The physician monitors the relative cephalad or caudad relation of the pair and on the symptomatic side determines whether that rib is prominent superiorly as compared to its mate.

5. If a rib is prominent, painful, and has less spring (movement) on downward pressure than its mate, it is described as an elevated rib dysfunction.

6. This finding is documented in the progress note as an *elevated* 1st rib dysfunction. This is a nonrespiratory model of dysfunction.

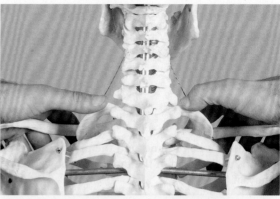

Figure 5.68. Step 2, palpation of the 1st rib.

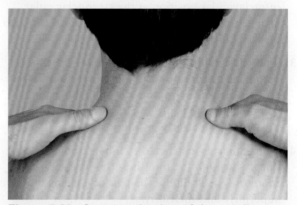

Figure 5.69. Step 2, palpation of the 1st rib.

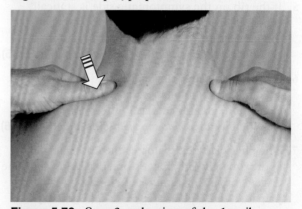

Figure 5.70. Step 3, palpation of the 1st rib.

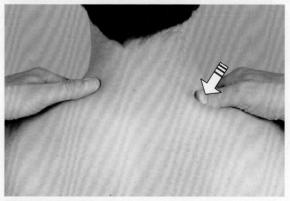

Figure 5.71. Step 3.

Costal Motion Testing

Rib 3–Rib 6, Physiologic Model
Supine, Respiratory Excursion Method
Ex: Pump/Bucket-Handle Motions

 See Video 5.14

1. The patient lies supine, and the physician stands on one side of the patient.

2. The physician's thumbs palpate the 3rd ribs bilaterally at their costochondral articulations for pump-handle motion and at the midaxillary line with the second or third fingertips for bucket-handle motion **(Fig. 5.72)**.

3. The physician monitors the relative cephalad or caudad relation of the pair and, on the symptomatic side, determines whether that rib is more or less prominent or superiorly or inferiorly positioned.

4. The patient is instructed to inhale and exhale deeply through the mouth as the physician monitors the relative cephalad and caudad movements of each rib with the palpating thumbs and fingertips **(Fig. 5.73)**.

5. If the rib on the symptomatic side is statically more cephalad and on inhalation has greater cephalad movement (on exhalation, less caudad movement), it is termed an *inhalation rib* (dysfunction) **(Fig. 5.74)**.

6. If the rib on the symptomatic side is statically more caudad and on inhalation has less cephalad movement (on exhalation, greater caudad movement), it is termed an *exhalation rib* (dysfunction) **(Fig. 5.75)**.

7. The physician next palpates ribs 4 to 6 at their costochondral ends with the thumbs and at their midaxillary lines with the fingertips and repeats steps 3 to 6.

8. The freest movement of the rib on the symptomatic side is then documented in the progress note (inhalation or exhalation based on the respiratory model).

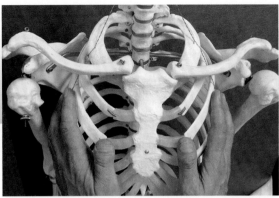

Figure 5.72. Step 2.

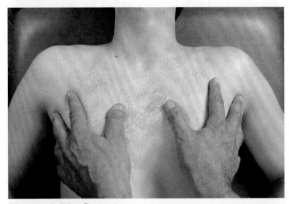

Figure 5.73. Step 4.

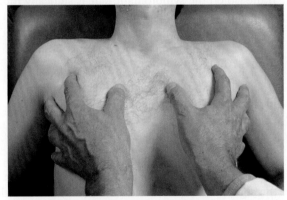

Figure 5.74. Step 5, inhalation rib.

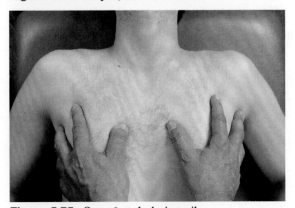

Figure 5.75. Step 6, exhalation rib.

Costal Motion Testing

Rib 7–Rib 10, Physiologic Model
Supine, Respiratory Excursion Method
Ex: Pump/Bucket-Handle Motions

 See Video 5.15

1. The patient is supine, and the physician stands on one side of the patient.

2. The physician's thumbs palpate the 7th ribs bilaterally at their costochondral articulations for pump-handle motion and at the midaxillary line with the second or third fingertips for bucket-handle motion **(Figs. 5.76 and 5.77)**.

3. The physician monitors the relative cephalad or caudad relation of the pair and determines on the symptomatic side whether that rib is more or less prominent or superiorly or inferiorly positioned.

4. The patient is instructed to inhale and exhale deeply through the mouth as the physician monitors the relative cephalad and caudad movements of each rib with the palpating thumbs and fingertips.

5. If the rib on the symptomatic side is statically more cephalad and on inhalation has greater cephalad movement (on exhalation, less caudad movement), it is termed an *inhalation rib* (dysfunction) **(Fig. 5.78)**.

6. If the rib on the symptomatic side is statically more caudad and on inhalation has less cephalad movement (on exhalation, greater caudad movement), it is termed an *exhalation rib* (dysfunction) **(Fig. 5.79)**.

7. The physician next palpates, sequentially, the 8th through 10th ribs at their costochondral ends with the thumbs and at their midaxillary lines with the fingertips and repeats steps 3 to 6.

8. The movement of the freest rib on the symptomatic side is then documented in the progress note (inhalation or exhalation based on the respiratory model).

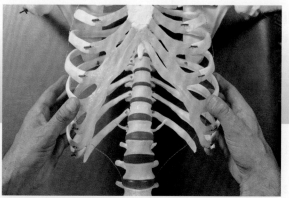

Figure 5.76. Step 2.

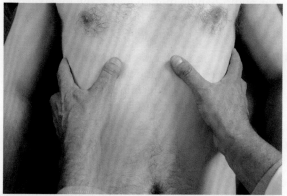

Figure 5.77. Step 2.

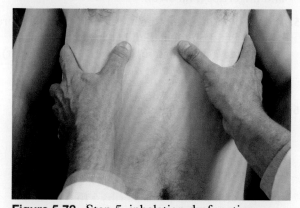

Figure 5.78. Step 5, inhalation dysfunction.

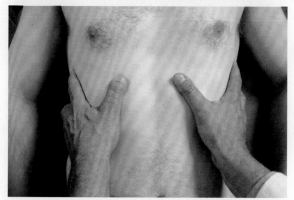

Figure 5.79. Step 6, exhalation dysfunction.

Costal Motion Testing

Rib 11 and Rib 12, Physiologic Model
Prone, Respiratory Excursion Method
Ex: Rib 11, Caliper Motion

 See Video 5.16

1. The patient lies prone, and the physician stands on either side of the patient.

2. The physician's thumb and thenar eminence palpate the shaft of each 11th rib **(Figs. 5.80 and 5.81)**.

3. The patient is instructed to inhale and exhale deeply through the mouth.

4. The physician notes any asymmetric motion at each rib.

5. If, on the symptomatic side, the patient's rib moves more posteriorly and inferiorly with inhalation and less anteriorly and superiorly with exhalation than its mate, it is classified as an *inhalation rib* (dysfunction) **(Fig. 5.82)**.

6. If, on the symptomatic side, the patient's rib moves more anteriorly and superiorly with exhalation and less posteriorly and inferiorly with inhalation than its mate, it is classified as an *exhalation rib* (dysfunction) **(Fig. 5.83)**.

7. These findings are documented in the progress note.

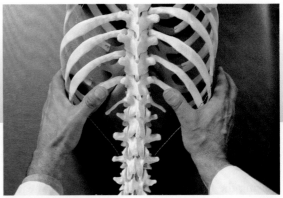

Figure 5.80. Step 2.

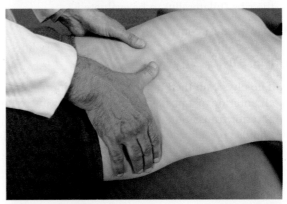

Figure 5.81. Step 2.

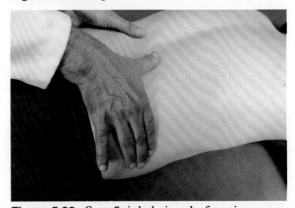

Figure 5.82. Step 5, inhalation dysfunction.

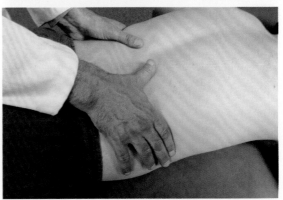

Figure 5.83. Step 6, exhalation dysfunction.

Costal Motion Testing

Rib 3–Rib 6, Nonphysiologic Model
Supine/Prone, Short-Lever Method
Anterior/Posterior/Lateral Translation

1. The patient lies supine, and the physician stands at the side of the table.

2. Using the thumbs and the index fingers of each hand, the physician attempts to contour them over the ribs (bilaterally) to be evaluated.

3. The greatest contact/pressure should occur between the midclavicular and midaxillary lines **(Fig. 5.84)**.

4. The physician then imparts a gentle impulse from an anterior to a posterior direction to evaluate for anterior translation of the rib. Resistance to the impulse reveals an anterior translation **(Fig. 5.85)**.

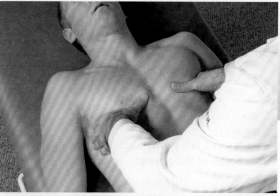

Figure 5.84. A. Steps 1 to 3, hand position.

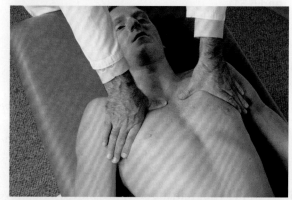

Figure 5.84. B. Steps 1 to 3, hand position variation.

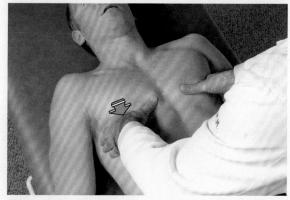

Figure 5.85. Step 4, anterior-to-posterior impulse.

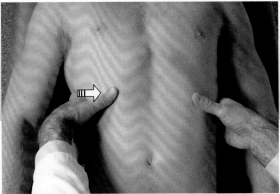

Figure 5.86. Step 5, lateral-to-medial impulse.

5. Next, the physician imparts a gentle impulse from a lateral to medial direction to evaluate for a lateral translation of the rib. Resistance to the impulse reveals a lateral translation **(Fig. 5.86)**.

6. The patient is then positioned in the prone position, and the physician stands at the side of the table.

7. Using the thumbs and the index fingers of each hand, the physician attempts to contour them over the ribs (bilaterally) to be evaluated.

8. The contact should be between the angle of the rib and the midaxillary line.

9. The physician then imparts a gentle impulse from a posterior to an anterior direction to evaluate for posterior translation of the rib. Resistance to the impulse reveals a posterior translation **(Fig. 5.87)**.

10. In the above steps, the freedom or ease of motion determines the type of dysfunction, but the resistance is generally the easiest to palpate. Therefore, the categorization of rib dysfunction would be named opposite the restriction.

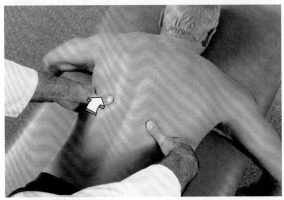

Figure 5.87. Step 9, posterior-to-anterior impulse.

Cervical Intersegmental Motion Testing

Occipitoatlantal (OA, C0–C1) Flexion/Extension, Side Bending/Rotation Translatory, Type I Motion Emphasis

 See Videos 5.17 and 5.18

1. The patient lies supine on the treatment table.

2. The physician sits at the head of the table.

3. The physician's index or third finger pad palpates the transverse processes of C1 **(Fig. 5.88)**.

4. The physician gently flexes and extends the patient's occiput in a "rocking-chair" motion, without moving the segments below the occiput **(Fig. 5.89)**.

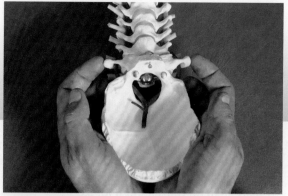

Figure 5.88. Step 3, C1 transverse process.

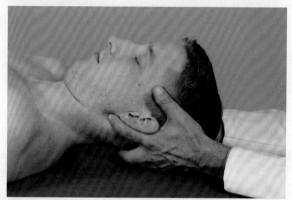

Figure 5.89. A. Step 4, flexion.

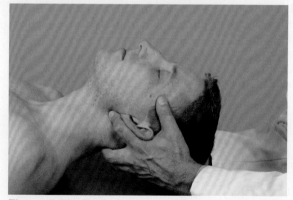

Figure 5.89. B. Step 4, extension.

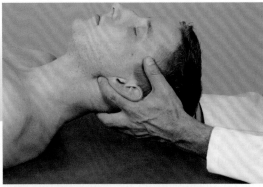

Figure 5.90. A. Step 5, extension.

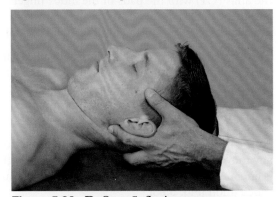

Figure 5.90. B. Step 5, flexion.

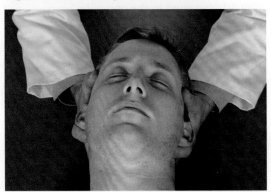

Figure 5.91. Step 6, left side bending/rotation coupling.

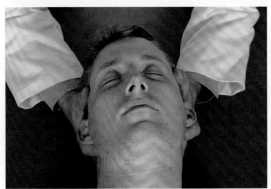

Figure 5.92. Step 6, right side bending/rotation coupling.

5. The physician may also gently move the occiput up off the table (extension) and down toward the table (flexion) in a translatory-type movement, without moving the segments below the occiput. This may also determine a motion preference **(Fig. 5.90)**.

6. To evaluate side bending and rotation, the physician minimally translates the patient's occiput alternately to the left and right over C1 (atlas) without inducing any movement of C1–C7 **(Figs. 5.91 and 5.92)**.

7. These steps are evaluated for asymmetric movement patterns that exhibit more side bending in one direction and more rotation in the other and should be repeated in a flexed, neutral, and extended position. This is to determine which of these components is involved with the coupled motions of the dysfunction (the position that elicits the least motion asymmetry is that component of the dysfunction).

8. The physician will document the findings in the progress note according to the position or freedom of motion elicited.

Cervical Intersegmental Motion Testing

Atlantoaxial (AA, C1–C2) Axial Rotation Emphasis

 See Video 5.19

1. The patient lies supine, and the physician sits at the head of the table.

2. The physician palpates the transverse processes of the atlas (C1) with the pads of the index fingers and the articular processes of the axis (C2) with the pads of the third or fourth fingers **(Fig. 5.93)**.

3. The physician slowly rotates the patient's head in one direction, careful not to add any side bending or flexion **(Fig. 5.94)**. (This eliminates any lower cervical movements and keeps motion vectored to this level.)

4. As the head is rotated, the physician monitors for any movement of the axis (C2) and *stops* when this is encountered. This is the limit of motion for this articulation **(Fig. 5.95)**.

5. Step 4 is repeated in the opposite direction **(Fig. 5.96)**.

6. The physician will document the findings in the progress note according to the position or freedom of motion elicited.

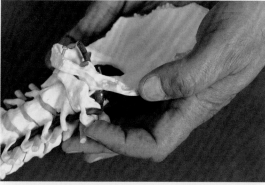

Figure 5.93. Step 2, transverse process of atlas and C2 articular process.

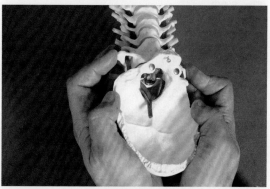

Figure 5.94. Step 3, rotation right.

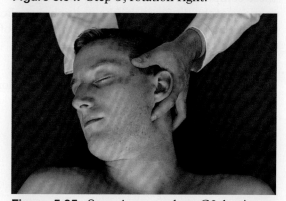

Figure 5.95. Step 4, stop when C2 begins to move.

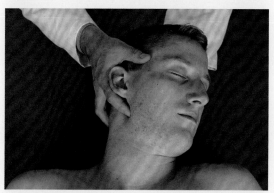

Figure 5.96. Step 5, rotation to opposite side.

Cervical Intersegmental Motion Testing

Atlantoaxial (AA, C1–C2)
Supine, Flexion Alternative
Axial Rotation Emphasis

 See Video 5.20

1. The patient lies supine on the treatment table.

2. The physician sits at the head of the table.

3. The physician slowly flexes (forward bends) the patient's head and neck to the comfortable passive motion limit to segmentally restrict the free coupled motions of the occipitoatlantal and C2–C7 segments **(Fig. 5.97)**.

4. The physician slowly and alternately rotates the patient's head to the comfortable right and left passive motion limits **(Figs. 5.98 and 5.99)**.

5. The physician is alert for any restricted and/or asymmetric rotation.

6. The physician then notes the asymmetric motion preference if present (C1-RR or C1-RL).

7. *Note*: Never do this type of motion test with the head and neck extended. We do not recommend this test, as it is presumptive, whereas the aforementioned C1 rotation test with the head in neutral positioning is a positive test and better tolerated by most patients.

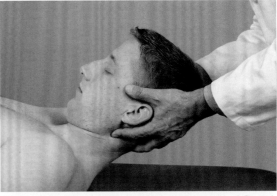

Figure 5.97. Step 3, C1 rotation with the head flexed.

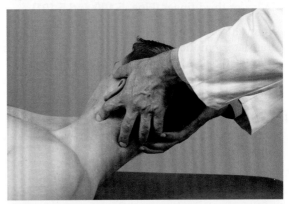

Figure 5.98. Step 4, C1 rotation right with the head flexed.

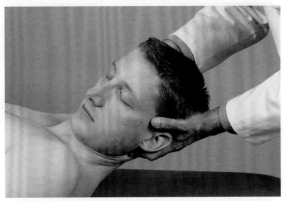

Figure 5.99. Step 4, C1 rotation left with the head flexed.

Cervical Intersegmental Motion Testing

C2–C7, Type II Motion
Short-Lever, Translatory Method
Ex: C4, Side Bending/Rotation Emphasis

 See Video 5.21

1. The patient lies supine on the treatment table, and the physician sits at the head of the table.

2. The physician palpates the articular processes of the segment to be evaluated with the pads of the index or third finger (**Figs. 5.100 and 5.101**).

3. To evaluate asymmetry in side bending, a translatory motion is introduced from left to right (**Fig. 5.102A and B**, left side bending) and then right to left (**Fig. 5.103A and B**, right side bending) through the articular processes.

4. Each cervical segment is evaluated in flexion, extension, and neutral to determine which position improves the asymmetry.

5. The physician will document the findings in the progress note according to the position or freedom of motion elicited.

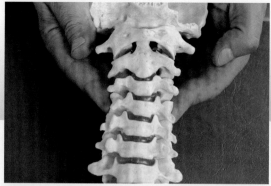
Figure 5.100. Step 2, cervical articular pillars on skeleton.

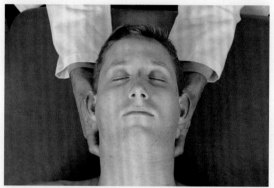
Figure 5.101. Step 2, cervical articular pillars on the patient.

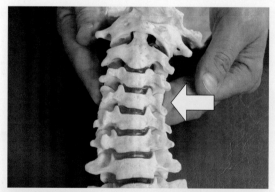
Figure 5.102. A. Step 3, side bending left.

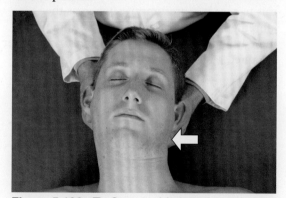
Figure 5.102. B. Step 3, side bending left.

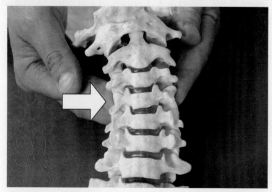
Figure 5.103. A. Step 3, side bending right.

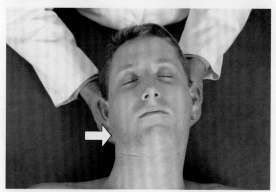
Figure 5.103. B. Step 3, side bending right.

Cervical Intersegmental Motion Testing

C2–C7, Type II Motion
Long-Lever Method
Ex: C3, Side Bending/Rotation Emphasis

1. Cervical intersegmental motion may be evaluated by long-lever method. Move the head in an ear-to-shoulder, arclike movement to the level of the dysfunctional segment for its side-bending ability **(Fig. 5.104)**.

2. At the end of the limit of side bending, a slight rotation is added to the direction of the side bending **(Fig. 5.105)**.

3. With the head in neutral for C2, flexion is increased approximately 5 to 7 degrees for each descending segment to be evaluated. The articular processes are positioned in side bending/rotation to the right and then the left until their limit is elicited **(Figs. 5.106 and 5.107)**.

4. Since C2–C7 side bend and rotate to the same side regardless of the sagittal plane, the physician must also assess flexion and extension motion preference or which position (flexion, extension, or neutral) improves the asymmetry at each segmental level (C2–C7).

5. The physician will document the findings in the progress note by recording the position or freedom of motion elicited in all three planes (F, E, or N—if there is no preference for flexion or extension preference, SRRR or SLRL).

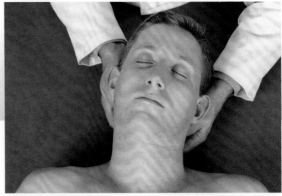

Figure 5.104. Step 1, "ear-to-shoulder" method.

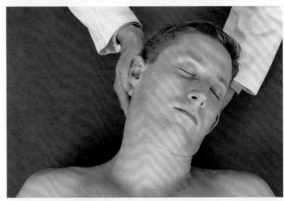

Figure 5.105. Step 2, rotation added.

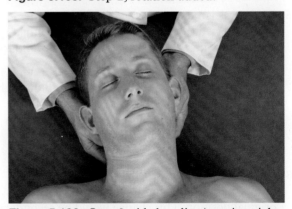

Figure 5.106. Step 3, side bending/rotation right.

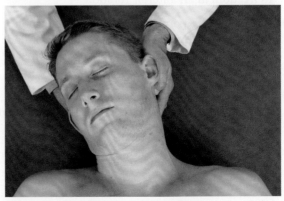

Figure 5.107. Step 3, side bending/rotation left.

Sacroiliac Joint Motion Testing

**Iliosacral, Anterior/Posterior Rotation
Supine, Long-Lever Method
Effect of Motion Testing on ASIS**

1. The patient lies supine on the treatment table.

2. The physician stands at the side of the table at the patient's hip.

3. The physician palpates the patient's anterior superior iliac spines (ASISs) and medial malleoli and notes the relation of the pair (cephalad or caudad, symmetric or asymmetric pattern) **(Fig. 5.108)**.

4. The physician instructs the patient to flex the hip and knee on one side. The physician's hands then control the patient's knee and ankle **(Fig. 5.109)**.

5. The physician takes the patient's hip through a range of motion starting with 130 degrees of flexion and progresses through external rotation and finally extension, bringing the patient to the neutral starting position **(Fig. 5.110)**.

6. The physician notes whether the ASIS on the motion-tested side appears more cephalad than its original position. This change would be secondary to freedom in posterior rotation.

7. The physician then takes the patient's hip through a range of motion starting with 90 degrees of flexion and progressing through internal rotation and finally extension, bringing the patient to the neutral starting position **(Fig. 5.111)**.

8. The physician notes whether the ASIS on the motion-tested side appears more caudad than its original position. This change would be secondary to freedom in an anterior rotation.

9. This is repeated on the other side to determine whether each joint has freedom in posterior and anterior rotation and if not, which joint is free or restricted in only one direction.

10. The physician will document the findings in the progress note according to the position or freedom of motion elicited.

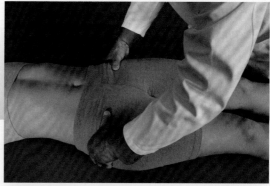

Figure 5.108. Step 3, palpating the "ASIS."

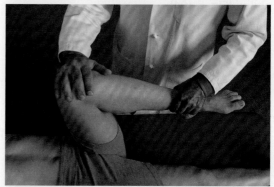

Figure 5.109. Step 4.

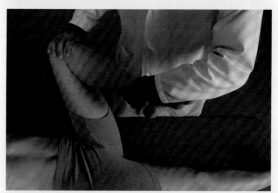

Figure 5.110. Step 5, flexion, external rotation, and extension.

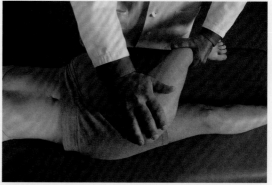

Figure 5.111. Step 7, flexion, internal rotation, and extension.

Sacroiliac Joint Motion Testing

Iliosacral (Innominate) Dysfunctions
Standing Flexion Test Method
Ex: Right, Positive Standing Flexion Test

1. The patient stands erect with the feet shoulder's width apart.

2. The physician stands or kneels behind the patient with the eyes at the level of the patient's posterior superior iliac spines (PSISs).

3. The physician's thumbs are placed on the inferior aspect of the patient's PSIS. Maintain firm pressure on the PSISs, *not* skin or fascial drag, to follow bony landmark motion **(Fig. 5.112)**.

4. The patient is instructed to actively forward bend and try to touch the toes within a pain-free range **(Fig. 5.113)**.

5. The test is positive on the side where the thumb (PSIS) moves more cephalad at the end range of motion **(Fig. 5.114)**. A positive standing flexion test identifies the side on which the sacroiliac joint is dysfunctional, not the specific type of dysfunction. A positive standing flexion test indicates that a pelvic (iliosacral) dysfunction (innominate on the sacrum) may be present. This is usually compared to the results of the seated flexion test to rule out a sacral dysfunction (sacrum on innominate).

6. This is a presumptive test reflecting asymmetry, which may be related to dysfunctions at the sacroiliac joint. It should not replace more objective motion testing specific to the sacroiliac joint that actually elicits motion availability.

7. The physician will document the findings in the progress note according to the position or freedom of motion elicited.

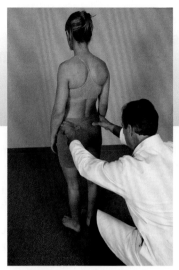

Figure 5.112. Step 3.

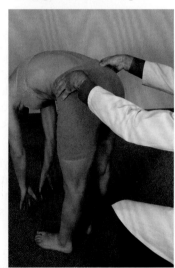

Figure 5.113. Step 4, forward bending.

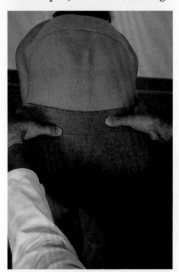

Figure 5.114. Step 5, positive standing flexion test right.

Sacroiliac Joint Motion Testing

Sacral Dysfunctions
Seated Flexion Test Method
Ex: Right, Positive Seated Flexion Test

1. The patient is seated on a stool or treatment table with both feet flat on the floor.

2. The physician stands or kneels behind the patient with the eyes at the level of the patient's PSISs.

3. The physician's thumbs are placed on the inferior aspect of the patient's PSISs, and a firm pressure is directed on the PSISs, *not* skin or fascial drag, to follow bony landmark motion **(Fig. 5.115)**.

4. The patient is instructed to forward bend as far as possible within a pain-free range **(Fig. 5.116)**.

5. The test is positive on the side where the thumb (PSIS) moves more cephalad at the end range of motion **(Fig. 5.117)**. A positive seated flexion test identifies the side of sacroiliac dysfunction (motion of the sacrum on the ilium), not the specific type of dysfunction.

6. This is a presumptive test reflecting asymmetry, which may be related to dysfunctions at the sacroiliac joint. It should not replace more objective motion testing specific to the sacroiliac joint.

7. The physician will document the findings in the progress note according to the position or freedom of motion elicited.

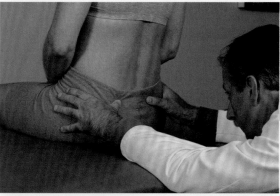

Figure 5.115. Step 3.

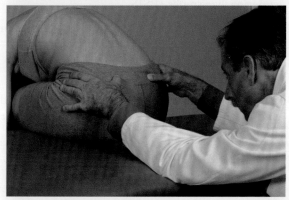

Figure 5.116. Step 4, forward bending.

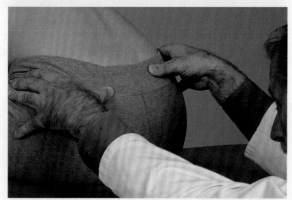

Figure 5.117. Step 5, positive seated flexion test, right.

Sacroiliac Joint Motion Testing

Iliosacral (Innominate) Dysfunctions
Prone, Long-Lever Method
Ex: Left, Iliosacral Motion Testing

1. The patient lies prone on the treatment table.

2. The physician stands to one side of the patient at the level of the hip.

3. The physician places the cephalad hand over the patient's sacroiliac joint with the finger pads of the index and third digits contacting the sacrum and PSIS, or the index finger contacts the PSIS while the thumb contacts the sacrum **(Fig. 5.118)**. If palpating the opposite sacroiliac joint, the finger pads will contact the landmark on the other side.

4. The physician's other hand grasps the patient's fully extended (straight) lower leg at the level of the tibial tuberosity **(Fig. 5.119)**.

5. The physician gently lifts the extended leg and then slowly and minimally lowers it while palpating the movement of the PSIS as it relates to the *sacrum* **(Fig. 5.120)**. The physician may also carry the leg across the midline **(Fig. 5.121)** and then laterally **(Fig. 5.122)**. Quality and quantity of motion, as well as ease-bind relations, are monitored.

6. The physician repeats this on the opposite side.

7. This motion test may determine joint motion restriction and/or motion asymmetry (e.g., sacroiliac restricted, free posteriorly).

8. This is a positive test, as compared to the standing and seated flexion tests, which are more presumptive.

9. The physician will document the findings in the progress note according to the position or freedom of motion elicited.

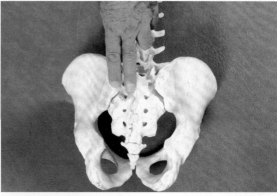

Figure 5.118. Step 3.

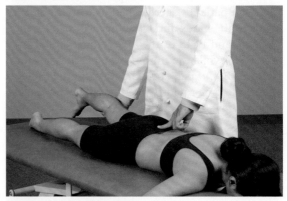

Figure 5.119. Step 4.

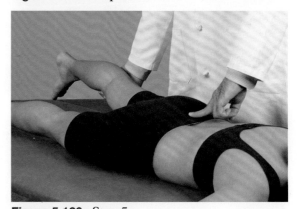

Figure 5.120. Step 5.

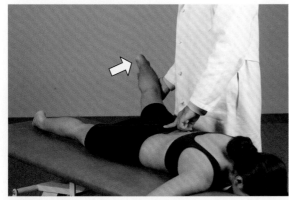

Figure 5.122. Step 5.

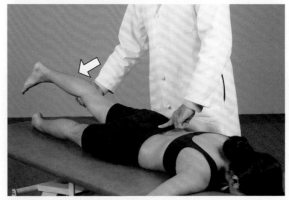

Figure 5.121. Step 5.

Sacroiliac Joint Motion Testing

Iliosacral (Innominate) Dysfunction
Prone, Long-Lever Method
Inflare/Outflare Emphasis

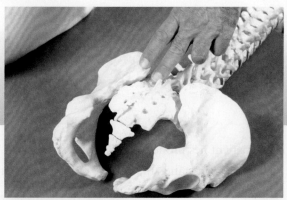

Figure 5.123. Step 3.

1. The patient lies prone on the treatment table.

2. The physician stands to one side of the patient at the level of the hip.

3. The physician places the cephalad-oriented hand over the patient's sacroiliac joint with the finger pads of the index and third digit contacting the sacrum and PSIS or the index finger contacts the PSIS while the thumb contacts the sacrum **(Fig. 5.123)**. If palpating the opposite sacroiliac joint, the finger pads will contact the landmark opposite what is noted above.

4. The physician instructs the patient to flex the lower leg (knee) approximately 90 degrees and then grasps the ankle **(Fig. 5.124)**.

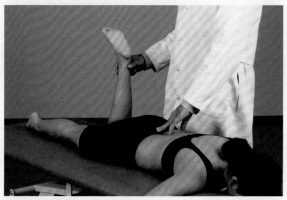

Figure 5.124. Step 4.

5. The physician then externally and internally rotates the patient's hip by moving the ankle medially and laterally, respectively **(Figs. 5.125 and 5.126)**. This approximates (outflare) and separates (inflare) the sacroiliac joint.

6. The physician then repeats this on the opposite side.

7. The above motion test may determine joint motion restriction and/or motion asymmetry (e.g., sacroiliac joint restricted, free inflare).

8. The physician will document the findings in the progress note according to the position or freedom of motion elicited.

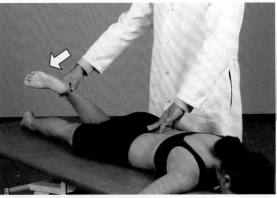

Figure 5.125. Step 5.

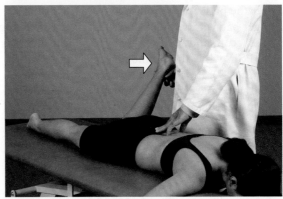

Figure 5.126. Step 5.

Sacroiliac Joint Motion Testing

**Iliosacral (Innominate) Dysfunction
Prone, Long-Lever Method
Anterior/Posterior Rotation Emphasis**

1. The patient lies prone on the treatment table.

2. The physician stands to one side of the patient at the level of the hip.

3. The physician places the cephalad-oriented hand over the patient's sacroiliac joint (SIJ) with the finger pads of the index and third digit contacting the sacrum and PSIS or the index finger contacts the PSIS while the thumb contacts the sacrum **(Fig. 5.127)**. If palpating the opposite sacroiliac joint, the finger pads will contact the landmark opposite what is noted above.

4. The physician instructs the patient to flex the lower leg (knee) approximately 90 degrees and then grasps the ankle **(Fig. 5.128)**.

5. The physician then quickly, with short up and down oscillations **(Fig. 5.129)** of the ankle, attempts to palpate (with the PSIS contacting finger) the quality and quantity of anterior/posterior innominate motion at the sacroiliac joint.

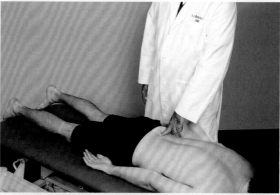

Figure 5.127. Step 3, identifying the SIJ.

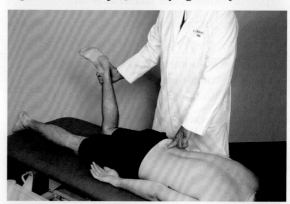

Figure 5.128. Step 4.

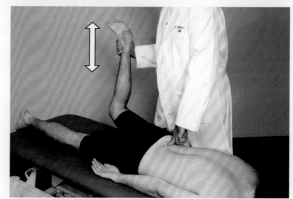

Figure 5.129. Step 5, lifting and lowering leg; anterior/posterior rotation effect.

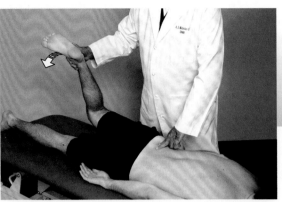

Figure 5.130. Step 6, SIJ approximation with external rotation of the hip.

6. This may then be repeated by quickly oscillating the ankle medially (external rotation of the hip) and laterally (internal rotation of the hip), causing a whiplike effect **(Figs. 5.130 and 5.131)** through the leg and innominate at the sacroiliac joint and assessing the quality and quality of motion at the sacroiliac joint.

7. The physician then repeats this on the opposite side.

8. If it is determined that there is motion dysfunction at the sacroiliac joint, the physician will then use observation of the pelvic landmarks to determine the type of dysfunction present (rotation, shear, etc.) based on the asymmetries observed.

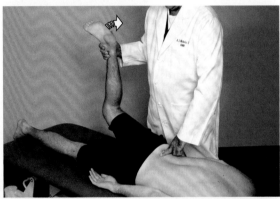

Figure 5.131. Step 6, SIJ separation (gapping) with internal rotation of the hip.

Sacroiliac Joint Motion Testing

Iliosacral (Innominate) Dysfunction
Prone, Short-Lever Method
Lateralization Emphasis

1. The patient lies prone on the treatment table.

2. The physician stands to one side of the patient at the level of the hip.

3. The physician places the thenar eminences over the patient's PSISs **(Fig. 5.132)**.

4. The physician alternately introduces a mild-to-moderate impulse through the PSISs with the thenar eminences **(Fig. 5.133)**.

5. The physician notes the quality (end feel) and quantity of motion on each side.

6. This is a positive test that will determine which sacroiliac joint is most restricted but will not determine the nature of the dysfunction.

7. The physician will document the findings in the progress note according to the position or freedom of motion elicited.

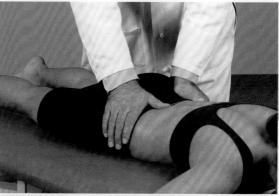

Figure 5.132. Step 3.

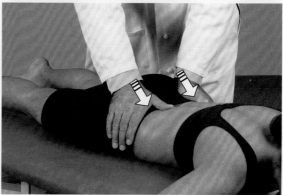

Figure 5.133. Step 4, prone short lever with alternating thenar impulse.

Sacroiliac Joint Motion Testing

Iliosacral (Innominate) Dysfunctions
Supine, Short-Lever Method
ASIS Compression/Lateralization Emphasis

1. The patient lies supine on the treatment table.

2. The physician stands at the level of the patient's hip.

3. The physician's palms or thenar eminences are placed inferior to the patient's ASISs **(Fig. 5.134)**.

4. The physician alternately introduces a mild-to-moderate impulse through the ASISs (may direct it posteriorly or slightly cephalad) **(Fig. 5.135A and B)**.

5. The physician notes quality (end feel) and quantity of motion on each side.

6. This will determine which sacroiliac joint is most restricted and may determine which motion preference is present (anterior or posterior rotation).

7. If a posterior innominate dysfunction is present, the symptomatic and restricted side will have a preference to move cephalad **(Fig. 5.136)**.

8. If an anterior innominate dysfunction is present, the symptomatic and restricted side will have a preference to move caudad **(Fig. 5.137)**.

9. The physician will document the findings in the progress note according to the position or freedom of motion elicited.

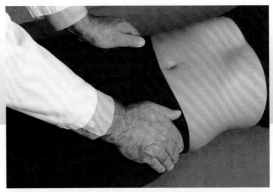

Figure 5.134. Step 3.

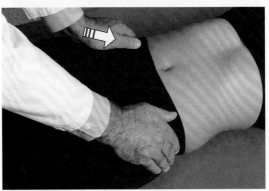

Figure 5.135. A. Step 4, supine short lever with thenar impulse.

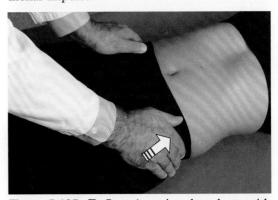

Figure 5.135. B. Step 4, supine short lever with thenar impulse on left.

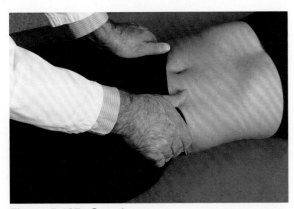

Figure 5.137. Step 8.

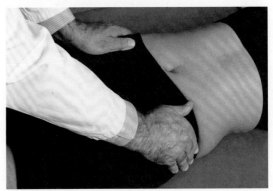

Figure 5.136. Step 7.

References

1. Chila AG, exec. ed. Foundations of Osteopathic Medicine. 3rd ed. Baltimore, MD: Lippincott Williams & Wilkins, 2011.
2. Glossary of Osteopathic Terminology, Educational Council on Osteopathic Principles of the American Association of Colleges of Osteopathic Medicine, www.aacom.org
3. Greenman P. Principles of Manual Medicine. 3rd ed. Philadelphia, PA: Lippincott Williams & Wilkins, 2003.
4. Magee DJ. Orthopedic Physical Assessment. 5th ed. St. Louis, MO: Saunders, 2008.
5. Mitchell F Jr. The Muscle Energy Manual. Vol. 2, Evaluation and Treatment of the Thoracic Spine, Lumbar Spine, & Rib Cage. East Lansing, MI: MET Press, 1998.

PART 2

Osteopathic Manipulative Techniques

Only three or four distinct technique styles were included in the American osteopathic manipulative curriculum prior to late 1950 and mid-1960. Some techniques (i.e., indirect, long-levered articulatory) may have been used earlier, but were not considered in the development of osteopathic principles and practice curriculum of early osteopathic medical schools. Although other osteopathic physicians were developing principles and techniques in other styles (Sutherland, Chapman, Hoover, etc.), the forms that most osteopathic schools taught were relegated to soft tissue, articulatory, HVLA, and various lymphatic/visceral oriented techniques. As the newer techniques became more popular and a critical number of those practitioners joined the faculties of osteopathic medical schools, the techniques taught became more numerous. Patients who previously may not have tolerated OMT could now be treated, or be treated more safely and effectively.

6

Principles of Osteopathic Manipulative Techniques

Osteopathic manipulative techniques (OMTs) are numerous. Some techniques have been known by more than one name, many new techniques have been developed, and some have seen resurgence after years of neglect. They have gone through a metamorphosis in description and, finally, with the advent of the Educational Council on Osteopathic Principles (ECOP) and its *Glossary of Osteopathic Terminology* (www.aacom. org/ome/councils/ecop), have been standardized into the styles described in this text.

Direct and Indirect Technique

It is sometimes easier to understand the principles of OMT according to which barrier and anatomic area the technique primarily affects. The first principle relates to the nature and direction of the restrictive barrier. Using this principle, most techniques can be categorized as direct or indirect. Thus, a technique engaging the most restrictive barrier (bind, tight) is classified as direct, and a technique engaging (or moving toward) the least restrictive barrier (ease, loose) is classified as indirect.

The second principle is associated with which anatomic manifestation of the dysfunction is primary (e.g., muscle vs. joint). To determine that a muscle dysfunction is primary, the second principle directs the physician to use techniques such as soft tissue or muscle energy rather than high-velocity, low-amplitude (HVLA) technique or osteopathic cranial manipulative medicine, formerly referred to as osteopathy in the cranial field.

Generally, direct techniques engage the most restrictive barrier, and indirect techniques engage the least restrictive barrier, which most commonly is described as the edge of the physiologic barrier **(Fig. 6.1)**. However, in some instances (i.e., myofascial release and combined techniques), the physician may interact alternately with the direct and indirect barriers. Frequently, however, a dysfunctional state causes restrictive barriers to each side of the normal resting neutral point. These bilateral restrictive barriers are

most commonly asymmetric in reference to their distance from neutral but may be equally and symmetrically distant **(Figs. 6.2 and 6.3)**. It is important to note that these illustrate two-dimensional representations, and the practitioner must extrapolate this to the three-dimensional (cardinal axes) movements found in a patient.

Examination of the barriers delineated in Figures 6.2 and 6.3 shows that it is possible to treat a restrictive barrier at either the ease or bind quality elicited on the palpatory examination.

In our clinical experience, we have noted other barriers related to symmetrical and asymmetrical motions. These barriers are found between the anatomic limit and the normally described physiologic barriers present in the patient exhibiting mean or averaged physiologic barriers. These barriers are associated with increased ranges of motion in patients typically described as *"hypermobile."* These hypermobile barriers can present

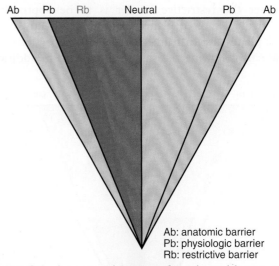

Ab: anatomic barrier
Pb: physiologic barrier
Rb: restrictive barrier

Figure 6.1. Asymmetric range of motion with a normal physiologic barrier (Pb) opposite the side on which a restrictive barrier (Rb) is present. *NOTE: In asymmetric motion patterns, the neutral point will shift toward the range of the most available motion.*

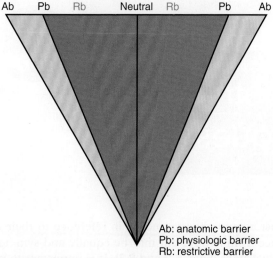

Ab: anatomic barrier
Pb: physiologic barrier
Rb: restrictive barrier

Figure 6.2. Two restrictive barriers (Rb) asymmetrically restricted.

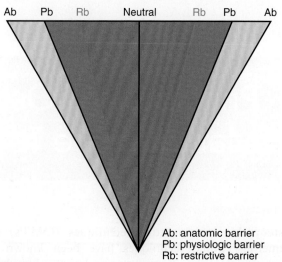

Ab: anatomic barrier
Pb: physiologic barrier
Rb: restrictive barrier

Figure 6.3. Two restrictive barriers (Rb) symmetrically restricted.

symmetrically **(Fig. 6.4)** or asymmetrically **(Fig. 6.5)**. They may also present unilaterally, as hypermobility in one range with a normal physiologic range to its opposing paired range **(Fig. 6.6)**, or they may exhibit restriction within a normal physiologic range with hypermobility to the opposing side **(Fig. 6.7)**. These hypermobile-associated barriers may be found in patients with normal connective tissues; patients with connective tissue abnormalities, such as those seen in *Ehlers-Danlos* syndrome; or patients who have experienced trauma and/or have instability secondary to degenerative joint and/or disk disease.

In implementing an osteopathic technique, it is important to understand the principles that determine safety and success (e.g., see Chapter 11—HVLA) and whether the restrictive barrier is to be approached directly in all three planes of motion, directly in all three planes at the "feather's edge" of the barrier(s), or indirectly following the same procedures. In addition,

the technique may call for balancing between the direct and indirect barriers. In this case, the tissues and/or articulations are positioned so that when reaching a point of balance, movement away from the *balance point* will meet with equal resistance (and motion limitations) in all directions. In a nondysfunctional state, the balance point is located at the neutral point equally between the physiologic barriers. In a dysfunctional state, the original neutral moves away from the restrictive barrier toward the ease or indirect barrier **(Fig. 6.8)**. Techniques that approach the *balance point* in a dysfunctional state would be, by definition, indirect. However, depending on the anatomic location of the dysfunction (e.g., myofascial vs. articular), engaging the balance point may require moving directly through the barrier of one layer of tissue in order to gain control of the dysfunction being treated. Once the dysfunction is controlled, the physician would then carry the dysfunctional tissue or articulation toward the freedom (ease) and determine

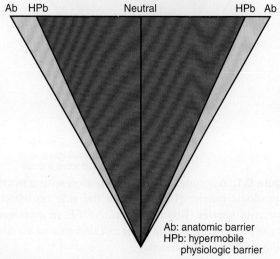

Ab: anatomic barrier
HPb: hypermobile physiologic barrier

Figure 6.4. Symmetrical hypermobility.

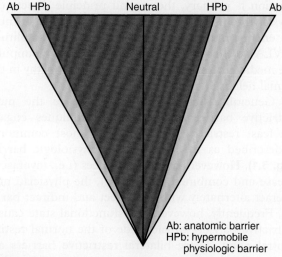

Ab: anatomic barrier
HPb: hypermobile physiologic barrier

Figure 6.5. Asymmetrical hypermobility.

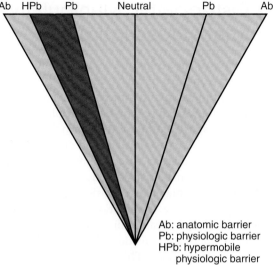

Ab: anatomic barrier
Pb: physiologic barrier
HPb: hypermobile
physiologic barrier

Figure 6.6. Unilateral hypermobility (HPb), making it appear as if there is an asymmetry with a restrictive barrier to the opposite paired range, which is actually the physiologic barrier (PB).

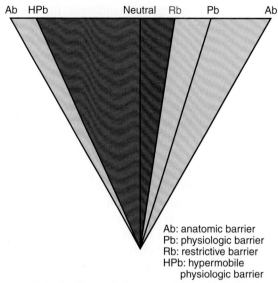

Ab: anatomic barrier
Pb: physiologic barrier
Rb: restrictive barrier
HPb: hypermobile
physiologic barrier

Figure 6.7. Unilateral hypermobility (HPb) in one motion, while its paired motion has a restrictive barrier (Rb) between neutral and the physiologic barrier (Pb).

the location of the balance point. Therefore, by definition, the direction of the technique toward the ease or bind barriers of the dysfunction determines whether it is indirect or direct, respectively, not what occurs before gaining control of the dysfunction.

Many authorities have described physiologic motion of the spine. Most frequently, the principles stated and promoted by Harrison Fryette, D.O., are those taught in osteopathic medical schools (first and second principles [laws] of physiologic motion of the spine). These rules are specific to the thoracic and lumbar spine regions, but they have tangential relation to how the mechanics of the cervical spine are perceived. Our non-American manual medicine associates have added other caveats to Fryette, yet they agree with the basis of these findings, which have been duplicated by others (e.g., White and Panjabi, coupled motions) (1).

Paraphrasing C.R. Nelson (whose principle of motion is considered the third of the three physiologic principles of motion), we see that the initiation of spinal vertebral motion in one plane will affect motion in all other planes (2). Osteopathic texts have described this principle but always within the context of a single restrictive barrier causing asymmetrically restricted findings of motion potential in an articulation. Expanding this statement to what we have observed clinically would therefore correlate with Figures 6.2 and 6.3. This would also make it feasible to orient classically described direct techniques, such as HVLA, in an indirect manner (which we have seen taught and performed internationally). The most important criteria to understand, whether performing direct or indirect techniques, are the normal physiologic motions of the specific area being examined and/or treated and the compliance of the tissues involved (e.g., acute vs. chronic dysfunction).

Somatic Dysfunction

As stated earlier, somatic dysfunction is the diagnostic criterion that calls for OMT. The various qualities elicited on the physical examination of a patient may lead the physician to understand that the nature of a

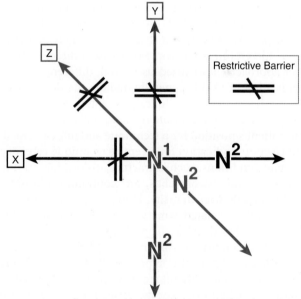

Figure 6.8. Three-dimensional schematic illustrating how, in a simplified cardinal axis (x, y, z) representation, the neutral (midrange) point in a nondysfunctional articulation (N^1) moves away from the restrictive barrier and toward the direction of the free (ease) physiologic barrier (N^2) in a dysfunctional state. In attempting an indirect technique, the physician will attempt to control the segment at the various, new N^2 neutral (balance) points.

dysfunction in one region is different from that of another dysfunction in a different region. Thus, the physician may choose to use one technique for one dysfunction and another technique for the other. If a patient exhibits regional motion disturbance but intersegmental motion is normal, a technique oriented to the articular aspects of the anatomy may not be indicated. Or a patient might present for neck ache that on examination exhibits paravertebral muscle hypertonicity and general tenderness but no specific tender points. This patient may benefit from a myofascial technique but not counterstrain, as no counterstrain tender points are present.

Some patients exhibit somatic components of visceral disease, and the treatment of this component may have only a limited effect, whereas a patient with a primary somatic dysfunction and a secondary visceral component may react well (somatically and viscerally) to a specific OMT. Other factors in the presentation of somatic dysfunction may change the thought process in developing the treatment plan. Other visceral and autonomic effects, lymphatic congestion, and gross edema will all cause the physician to re-evaluate the possibilities for OMT and the potential for a number of techniques that may be indicated in that case.

Contraindications

Contraindications to OMT have changed dramatically during our years of clinical practice because of the development of new and/or modified techniques and better understanding of disease processes. The ability to perform OMT in a range of extremely gentle to more forceful manner, combined with a direct or indirect approach, has caused us to look differently at the application of OMT, generally making the decision on a case-by-case basis of clinical presentation. This case-by-case orientation may often change only the choice of the patient's position for a technique and not be considered a contraindication for an entire technique category. Certain conditions, such as fracture, dislocation, tumor, infection, and osteomyelitis, are contraindications for OMT directly over that site. However, it does not preclude OMT to related somatic dysfunction in areas that are proximal or distal to the problem.

Other conditions that may alter the physician's opinion concerning the appropriateness of OMT are Down syndrome, rheumatoid arthritis, Klippel-Feil syndrome, achondroplastic dwarfism, pregnancy, strains and sprains, acute herniated intervertebral disk, acute inflammatory situations, anatomic instability, hypermobility, joint prosthesis, and severe manifestations of visceral disorders. These conditions may contraindicate OMT in total or may contraindicate only a specific technique in a specific region. The physician's clinical judgment and a complete understanding of the technique are paramount in the final decision as to whether OMT is appropriate.

The Osteopathic Manipulative Treatment Prescription

The selection of the technique to be used is primarily founded in the nature of the somatic dysfunction and its most prominent manifestations. This atlas presents 12 OMT sections. Each section has an explanatory preface for the specific technique and the principles of its use and application. The previously stated areas of dysfunction (articular, myofascial, visceral, vascular, lymphatic, and so on) that can be considered during selection of the treatment plan may affect the decision to use a specific technique at one dysfunctional level or another, depending on the physical findings (i.e., HVLA vs. muscle energy vs. facilitated positional release vs. myofascial release or a combination). This will be discussed further and more specifically in each of the technique sections.

The OMT prescription is similar to that of the pharmacologic prescription: The type of technique is comparable to the category of the pharmacologic agent chosen; the method and position chosen for the OMT technique are comparable to the route of administration of the pharmacologic agent; the forces involved in the OMT and whether they are directly or indirectly applied are comparable to the strength or dose of the medication; and the repetitions, timing, and duration of the OMT are comparable to the amount of medication dispensed and the frequency of its administration.

For example, a 70-year-old patient who complains of chronic low back pain secondary to lumbar discogenic spondylosis, lumbar spinal stenosis, and lumbar somatic dysfunction may be treated with articulatory and myofascial soft tissue techniques weekly over weeks to months. However, a 16-year-old patient who complains of acute low back pain secondary to a sprain during football practice may be treated with a combination of indirect myofascial release, muscle energy, and counterstrain techniques every 2 to 3 days for 2 to 4 weeks.

Simple rules to guide the implementation of OMT are best seen in the dose guidelines outlined in the *Foundations for Osteopathic Medicine* (2). In general, one must understand the nature of the dysfunction and the other clinical manifestations being presented, the severity and energy-depleting effects of the condition, the age of the patient, and whether the condition is acute or chronic. Common medical sense combined with a well-grounded risk-benefit rationale should be the guiding principles.

References

1. White A, Panjabi M. Clinical Biomechanics of the Spine. 2nd ed. Philadelphia, PA: Lippincott Williams & Wilkins, 1990.
2. Ward R, exec.ed. Foundations for Osteopathic Medicine. 2nd ed. Philadelphia, PA: Lippincott Williams & Wilkins, 2003.

Soft Tissue Techniques

7

Technique Principles

Soft tissue technique is defined by the Educational Council on Osteopathic Principles (ECOP) as "a direct technique, which usually involves lateral stretching, linear stretching, deep pressure, traction, and/or separation of muscle origin and insertion while monitoring tissue response and motion changes by palpation; also called myofascial treatment" (1). Some aspects of soft tissue techniques are similar to those of myofascial release in respect to the thermodynamic effects in altering physical states with resultant tissue reactivity (*fascial creep*). However, the specific manual methods by which the physician causes these reactions are slightly different. The most distinguishing aspects of soft tissue technique as compared to myofascial release technique are that with soft tissue technique, the forces are more deeply directed into the patient and that these forces are implemented in a rhythmic, alternating (pressure on, pressure off) fashion. As this is being performed, a constant feedback is occurring, allowing the physician to determine the patient's response and the extent and depth of the dysfunctional component being treated. With this rhythmic style engagement of the tissues, the physician's force and rhythmic cadence may be varied, thereby engaging the joints/articulations of the region being treated. Depending on these forces and rhythms, the soft tissue technique may be expanded into the realm of lymphatic techniques (Chapter 16) and articulatory and combined techniques (Chapter17). (see Chapters 16 and 17).

The forces should be directed deeply enough to engage the tissue being treated, but at the same time, the treatment should be mildly to moderately introduced and comfortably accepted by the patient. The only exception to this rule is the *inhibitory pressure* style, in which the physician may choose to use a constant, deeply introduced force over some time (i.e., more than 30 seconds or until the tissue releases [as noted by an increase in its length or decrease in its tension]) (2).

Technique Classification

Direct Technique

In direct technique, the myofascial tissues are moved toward the restrictive barrier (tension, bind). To use direct technique, the physician must understand the anatomic relationship of the tissues being treated in terms of musculotendinous origin and insertion, depth of the muscle or fascia, and muscle type. The direction, depth, and force of pressure will vary with the specific area being treated because of normal anatomic changes from region to region.

Technique Styles

Parallel Traction

In parallel traction, the myofascial structure being treated is contacted at its origin and insertion, and the treatment force is directed parallel to the musculotendinous axis, causing an overall increase in length of the structure. This may be done by directing a force with the hand that is proximal to the origin, the hand that is proximal to the insertion, or both hands moving opposite each other at the same time. Each of these will cause a relative increase in length of the myofascial tissue being treated.

Perpendicular Traction ("Kneading")

In perpendicular traction, the myofascial structure in question is contacted at its midpoint between the origin and the insertion, and a perpendicular force is directed away from the longitudinal axis.

Direct Inhibitory Pressure

In direct inhibitory pressure, the myofascial structure being treated is contacted over the musculotendinous portion of the hypertonic muscle, and a force is directed into it. However, deep, specific pressure on the muscle belly can cause painful side effects and bruising. Therefore, the pressure should be directed at the tendon or musculotendinous junction. This form of soft tissue technique is particularly useful for painful, hypertonic muscle states in the piriformis, gluteus medius, and levator scapulae muscles and other tissues such as the iliotibial band. In this variation of soft tissue technique, there is not the rhythmic, alternating (pressure on, pressure off) force implementation, but rather a constantly applied force that is begun gently and with patient tolerance, slowly increasing in force penetration until a positive tissue response (release) is palpated.

Indications

1. Use as part of the musculoskeletal screening examination to quickly identify regions of restricted motion, tissue texture changes, and sensitivity.
2. Reduce muscle hypertonicity, muscle tension, fascial tension, and muscle *spasm*.
3. Stretch and increase elasticity of shortened, inelastic, and/or fibrotic myofascial structures to improve regional and/or intersegmental ranges of motion.
4. Improve circulation to the specific region being treated by local physical and thermodynamic effects or by reflex phenomena to improve circulation in a distal area (e.g., through somatic-somatic or somatovisceral reflexes).
5. Increase venous and lymphatic drainage to decrease local and/or distal swelling and edema and potentially improve the overall immune response. This will improve local tissue nutrition, oxygenation, and removal of metabolic wastes.
6. Stimulate the stretch reflex in hypotonic muscles.
7. Promote patient relaxation.
8. Reduce patient *guarding* during implementation of other osteopathic manipulative techniques or additional medical treatment.
9. Potentiate the effect of other osteopathic techniques.
10. Improve the physician-patient relationship, as this technique typically imparts a pleasant sensation to the patient.

Contraindications

Relative Contraindications

Use with caution, as common medical sense is the rule. For example, in an elderly osteoporotic patient, the soft tissue *prone pressure* technique may be contraindicated over the thoracocostal and pelvic regions, but the *lateral recumbent* methods can be more safely applied. Also, contact and stretching over an acutely strained or sprained myofascial, ligamentous, or capsular structure may exacerbate the condition. Therefore, in these situations, caution should prevail, and the soft tissue technique may be withheld until tissue disruption and inflammation have stabilized.

Other precautions in the use of soft tissue technique:

1. Acute sprain or strain
2. Fracture or dislocation
3. Neurologic or vascular compromise
4. Osteoporosis and osteopenia
5. Malignancy. Most restrictions are for treatment in the affected area of malignancy; however, care should be taken in other distal areas depending on the type of malignancy and/or lymphatic involvement.
6. Infection (e.g., osteomyelitis), contagious skin diseases, painful rashes or abscesses, acute fasciitis, and any other conditions that would preclude skin contact
7. Organomegaly secondary to infection, obstruction, or neoplasm
8. Undiagnosed visceral pathology/pain

Absolute Contraindications

None, as the physician may work proximal to the problem above or below the affected area and may alter the patient's position or technique to achieve some beneficial effect.

General Considerations and Rules

1. The patient should be comfortable and relaxed.
2. The physician should be in a position of comfort so as to minimize energy expenditure and whenever possible should use body weight instead of upper extremity strength and energy.
3. Initially, forces must be of low intensity and applied slowly and rhythmically. As heat develops and the tissues begin to react, the pressure may be increased if clinically indicated and well tolerated; however, the cadence should remain slowly rhythmical.
4. The applied forces should always be comfortable and not cause pain. A comfortable and pleasant experience is the intended effect.
5. Never direct forces directly into bone, and limit pressure into the muscle belly.
6. As this is not a massage or friction technique, never rub or irritate the patient's skin by the friction of your hands. The physician's hand should carry the skin with it and not slide across it when applying the directed force.
7. Determine how you would like to employ the force:
   a. By pushing or pulling perpendicular to cause traction to the long axis of the musculotendinous structure
   b. By applying traction in a parallel direction to the long axis, increasing the distance between the origin and the insertion of the muscle fibers

Cervical Region

Supine Traction

 See Video 7.1

1. The patient lies supine on the treatment table.

2. The physician sits or stands at the head of the table.

3. The physician's one hand gently cradles the occiput between the thumb and index finger. The physician's other hand lies across the patient's forehead or grasps under the chin **(Figs. 7.1 and 7.2)**. (Use caution in patients with temporomandibular joint [TMJ] dysfunctions.)

4. The physician exerts cephalad traction with both hands with the head and neck in a neutral to slightly flexed position to avoid extension. The cradling hand must not squeeze the occiput, or the occipitomastoid suture will be compressed **(Fig. 7.3)**.

5. This tractional force is applied and released slowly. It may be increased in amplitude as per patient tolerance.

6. This technique may also be performed using sustained traction.

7. This technique may be performed for 2 to 5 minutes to achieve the desired effects. It may be especially helpful in patients with degenerative disk disease.

8. In patients with TMJ dysfunction, it may be modified by placing one hand on the forehead instead of the mandible **(Fig. 7.4)**.

9. Tissue tension is reevaluated to assess the effectiveness of the technique.

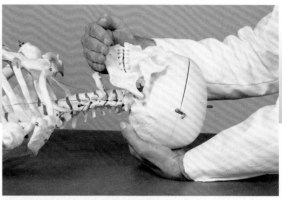

Figure 7.1. Step 3, skeleton.

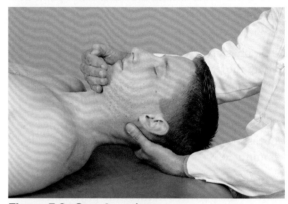

Figure 7.2. Step 3, patient.

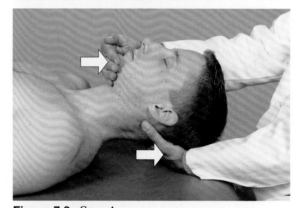

Figure 7.3. Step 4.

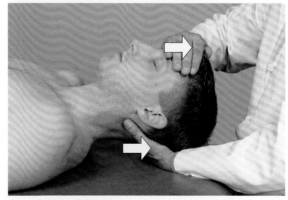

Figure 7.4. Step 8.

Cervical Region

Single Forearm Fulcrum
Forward Bending/Side Bending/Rotation

 See Video 7.2

1. The patient lies supine on the treatment table.

2. The physician is seated at the head of the table.

3. The physician gently flexes the patient's neck with one hand while sliding the other hand palm down under the patient's neck and opposite shoulder **(Fig. 7.5)**.

4. The physician gently rotates the patient's head along the physician's forearm toward the elbow, producing a unilateral stretch of the cervical paravertebral musculature **(Fig. 7.6)**.

5. This stretch can be repeated as many times as necessary to achieve the desired effect, usually 2 to 3 minutes.

6. This procedure is reversed to treat the opposite side of the patient's neck, *or* the physician's hand that was on the table can be lifted onto the patient's shoulder **(Fig. 7.7)**, and steps 4 and 5 can be repeated in the opposite direction **(Fig. 7.8)**.

7. Tissue tension is reevaluated to assess the effectiveness of the technique.

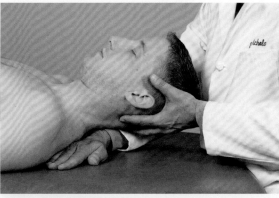
Figure 7.5. Step 3.

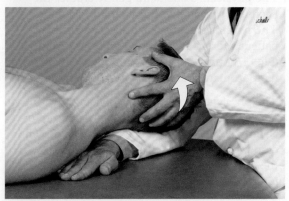
Figure 7.6. Step 4, rotation right.

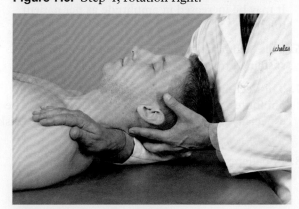
Figure 7.7. Step 6, neutral.

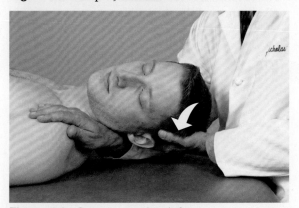
Figure 7.8. Step 6, rotation left.

Cervical Region

Bilateral Forearm Fulcrum
Forward Bending Method

 See Video 7.2

1. The patient lies supine on the treatment table.

2. The physician is seated at the head of the table.

3. The physician's arms are crossed under the patient's head, and the physician's hands are placed palm down on the patient's anterior shoulder region **(Fig. 7.9)**.

4. The physician's forearms gently flex the patient's neck, producing a longitudinal stretch of the cervical paravertebral musculature **(Fig. 7.10)**.

5. This technique may be performed in a gentle, rhythmic fashion or in a sustained manner.

6. Tissue tension is reevaluated to assess the effectiveness of the technique.

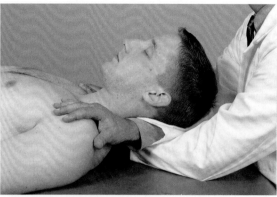
Figure 7.9. Step 3.

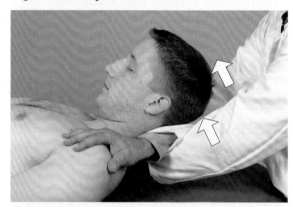
Figure 7.10. Step 4.

Cervical Region

Contralateral Traction
Supine, Unilateral Method

 See Video 7.3

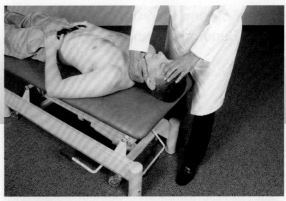

Figure 7.11. Step 3.

1. The patient lies supine on the treatment table.

2. The physician stands at the side of the table opposite the side to be treated.

3. The physician's caudad hand reaches over and around the neck to touch with the pads of the fingers the patient's cervical paravertebral musculature on the side opposite the physician **(Fig. 7.11)**.

4. The physician's cephalad hand lies on the patient's forehead to stabilize the head **(Fig. 7.12)**.

5. Keeping the caudad arm straight, the physician gently draws the paravertebral muscles ventrally (*white arrow*, **Fig. 7.13**), producing minimal extension of the cervical spine.

6. This technique may be performed in a gentle, rhythmic, and kneading fashion or in a sustained manner.

7. Tissue tension is reevaluated to assess the effectiveness of the technique.

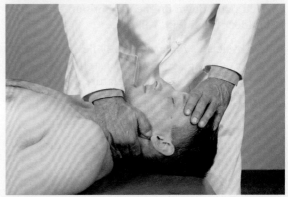

Figure 7.12. Step 4.

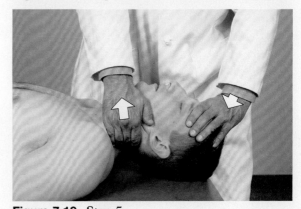

Figure 7.13. Step 5.

Cervical Region

Cradling with Traction
Supine, Bilateral Method

 See Video 7.4

1. The patient lies supine on the treatment table.

2. The physician sits at the head of the table.

3. The physician's fingers are placed under the patient's neck bilaterally, with the fingertips lateral to the cervical spinous processes and the finger pads touching the paravertebral musculature overlying the articular pillars **(Fig. 7.14)**.

4. The physician exerts a gentle to moderate force, ventrally to engage the soft tissues and cephalad to produce a longitudinal tractional effect (stretch) **(Figs. 7.15 and 7.16)**.

5. This traction on the cervical musculature is slowly released.

6. The physician's hands are repositioned to contact different levels of the cervical spine, and steps 4 and 5 are performed to stretch various portions of the cervical paravertebral musculature.

7. This technique may be performed in a gentle rhythmic and kneading fashion or in a sustained manner.

8. Tissue tension is reevaluated to assess the effectiveness of the technique.

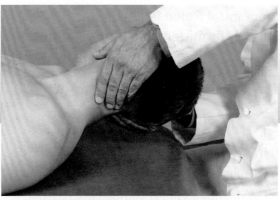

Figure 7.14. Step 3.

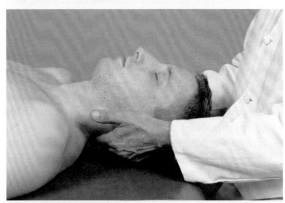

Figure 7.15. Step 4.

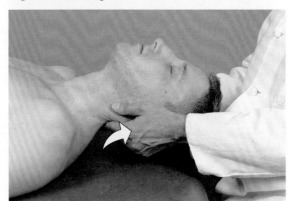

Figure 7.16. Step 4.

Cervical Region

Suboccipital Release
Supine, Intermittent/Inhibitory Method

 See Video 7.5

1. The patient lies supine on the treatment table.

2. The physician sits at the head of the table.

3. The physician's finger pads are placed palm up beneath the patient's suboccipital region, in contact with the trapezius and its immediate underlying musculature **(Fig. 7.17)**.

4. The physician slowly and gently applies pressure upward into the tissues for a few seconds and then releases the pressure **(Figs. 7.18 and 7.19)**.

5. This pressure may be reapplied and released slowly and rhythmically until tissue texture changes occur *or* for 2 minutes. The pressure may also be continued in a more constant inhibitory style for 30 seconds to 1 minute.

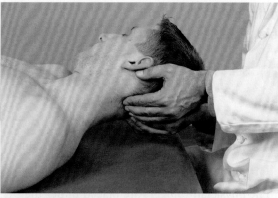
Figure 7.17. Step 3.

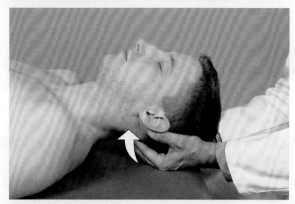
Figure 7.18. Step 4.

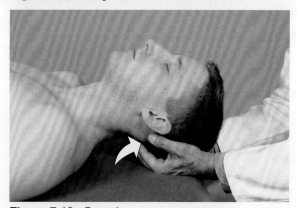
Figure 7.19. Step 4.

Cervical Region

Axial Rotation

 See Video 7.6

1. The patient lies supine on the treatment table.

2. The physician sits at the head of the table.

3. The physician's cupped hands (palmar aspect) are placed to each side of the patient's temporomandibular region, making sure to not compress over the external acoustic meatus **(Fig. 7.20)**.

4. The physician gently and slowly axially rotates the patient's head to the left to the restrictive barrier at its passive tolerable elastic limit and holds this position for 3 to 5 seconds **(Fig. 7.21)**.

5. The physician then slowly rotates the head to the right restrictive barrier at its passive tolerable elastic limit and holds this position for 3 to 5 seconds **(Fig. 7.22)**.

6. This is repeated to each side until release of tissue tension and/or improvement of range of motion.

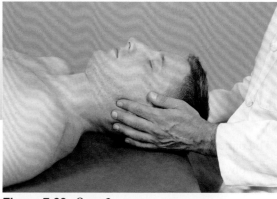

Figure 7.20. Step 3.

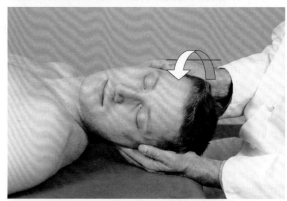

Figure 7.21. Step 4.

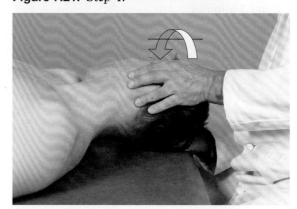

Figure 7.22. Step 5.

Cervical Region

Forefingers Cradling

 See Video 7.7

1. The patient lies supine on the treatment table.

2. The physician sits or stands at the head of the table.

3. The physician's hands cradle the temporal regions (avoiding pressure over the ears) with the fingers over the cervical paraspinal tissues, proximal to the articular processes **(Fig. 7.23)**.

4. The patient's head is bent slightly backward (extended) and taken through a progression of side bending and rotation to one side and then the other with continuing pressure from the finger pads on the posterior cervical tissues **(Figs. 7.24 and 7.25)**.

5. This is repeated in a slow, rhythmic manner until release of tissue tension and/or improvement of range of motion. Normally, this takes between 2 and 3 minutes.

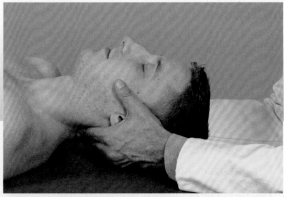
Figure 7.23. Step 3.

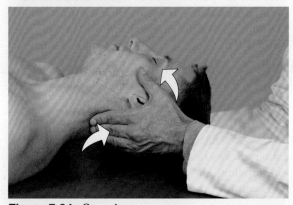
Figure 7.24. Step 4.

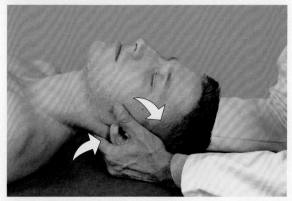
Figure 7.25. Step 4.

Cervical Region

Cervical Thumb Rest

 See Video 7.8

1. The patient lies supine on the treatment table with or without a pillow under the head.

2. The physician sits or stands at the head of the table.

3. The thumb and forefinger of one of the physician's hands cup the posterior cervical area palm up **(Fig. 7.26)**.

4. The physician's other hand is placed over the temporal and frontal regions of the patient's head and gently brings the head into slight backward bending (extension) and rotation against the thumb **(Figs. 7.27 and 7.28)**.

5. The motion is very slight.

6. Tension (pressure) is relaxed slowly and reapplied slowly.

7. The pressure may be reversed to the other side.

8. Tissue tension is reevaluated to assess the effectiveness of the technique.

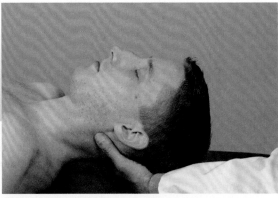

Figure 7.26. Step 3.

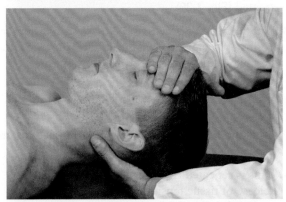

Figure 7.27. Step 4.

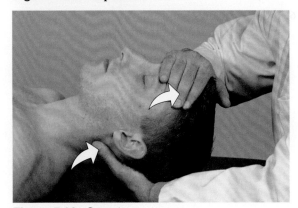

Figure 7.28. Step 4.

Cervical Region

Lateral Traction with Shoulder Block Supine, Side Bending/Rotation Method

 See Video 7.9

1. The patient lies supine on the treatment table and the physician stands or sits at the head of the table.

2. The physician places one hand on top of the patient's acromioclavicular joint on the side to be treated **(Fig. 7.29)**.

3. The physician's other hand crosses the midline to control the patient's head from that same side and gently pushes the head toward the opposite side **(Fig. 7.30)**.

4. The physician moves the head until meeting the restrictive barrier at its passive tolerable elastic limit and holds this position for 3 to 5 seconds and then slowly returns the head to neutral.

5. This is repeated rhythmically and gently until release of tissue tension and/or improvement in range of motion.

6. The physician's hands may be reversed and the process repeated on the opposite side.

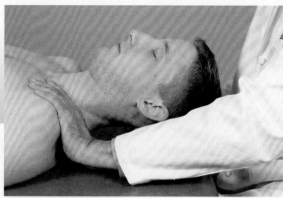

Figure 7.29. Step 2.

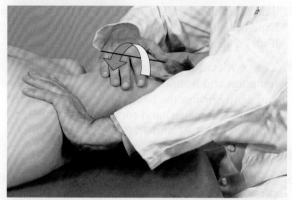

Figure 7.30. A. Steps 3 and 4, anterior head control.

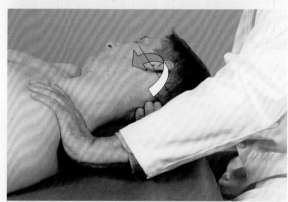

Figure 7.30. B. Steps 3 and 4, alternate, posterior head control.

Cervical Region

Lateral Traction with Shoulder Block
Seated, Side Bending/Rotation Method

 See Video 7.10

1. The patient is seated on the treatment table.

2. The physician stands behind and to the right side of the patient with the patient resting comfortably against the physician's chest.

3. The physician's right cupped hand and forearm are passed under the patient's chin so as to gently touch the patient's left periauricular region **(Fig. 7.31)**.

4. The physician's left hand is placed on top of the patient's left shoulder at the superior trapezius and supraclavicular region **(Fig. 7.32)**.

5. The physician's right hand gently rotates the patient's head to the right and exerts a gentle cephalad traction while the left hand maintains a gentle caudad counterforce on the left shoulder **(Fig. 7.33)**.

6. This technique may be performed in a gentle, rhythmic fashion or in a sustained manner.

7. If indicated, the technique may be reversed to treat the opposite side.

8. Tissue tension is reevaluated to assess the effectiveness of the technique.

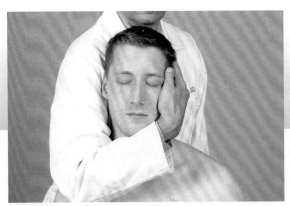

Figure 7.31. Step 3.

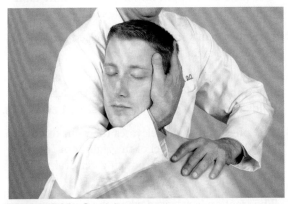

Figure 7.32. Step 4.

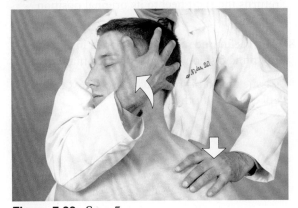

Figure 7.33. Step 5.

Cervical Region

Cervical Traction
Seated, Lower Extremity Assist Method

 See Video 7.11

1. The patient is seated on the treatment table.

2. The physician stands behind and to the left of the patient.

3. The physician's right foot is placed on the table with the right knee and hip flexed.

4. The physician's right elbow is placed on the physician's right thigh.

5. The physician's right hand cradles the occiput with the thumb and index finger while the left hand holds the patient's forehead (**Figs. 7.34 and 7.35**).

6. The physician slowly elevates the right thigh and knee by lifting the heel of the right foot (plantarflexing foot), thereby producing cervical traction (**Fig. 7.36**).

7. The traction is released when the physician slowly returns the right heel to its original position (**Fig. 7.37**).

8. This technique may be performed in a gentle, rhythmic fashion or in a sustained manner.

9. Tissue tension is reevaluated to assess the effectiveness of the technique.

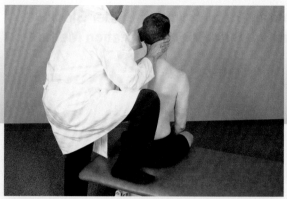

Figure 7.34. Step 5.

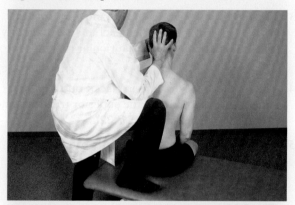

Figure 7.35. Step 5, alternative hand position.

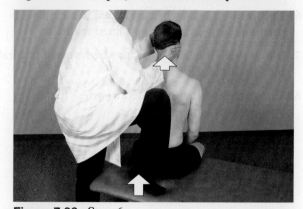

Figure 7.36. Step 6.

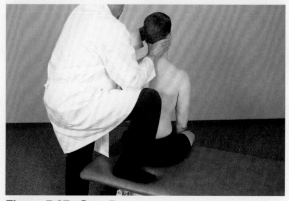

Figure 7.37. Step 7.

Cervical Region

Cradling with Traction
Seated, Head on Chest Method

 See Video 7.12

1. The patient is seated on the treatment table.

2. The physician stands facing the patient with one leg in front of the other for balance.

3. The patient's frontal bone (forehead) is placed against the physician's infraclavicular fossa or sternum **(Fig. 7.38)**.

4. The pads of the physician's fingers contact the medial aspect of the cervical paravertebral musculature overlying the articular pillars **(Fig. 7.39)**.

5. The physician leans backward, drawing the patient toward the physician. This causes the physician's hands to engage the soft tissues, exerting a gentle ventral force with concomitant cephalad traction. This produces a longitudinal tractional effect (stretch) **(Fig. 7.40)**.

6. This technique may be performed in a gentle, rhythmic, and kneading fashion or in a sustained manner.

7. Tissue tension is reevaluated to assess the effectiveness of the technique.

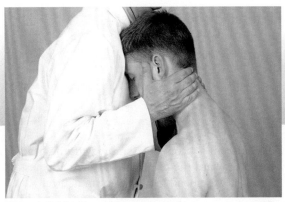
Figure 7.38. Step 3.

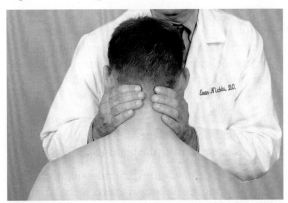
Figure 7.39. Step 4.

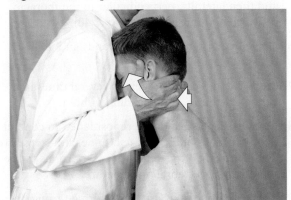
Figure 7.40. Step 5.

Thoracic Region

Unilateral Prone Pressure

 See Video 7.13

1. The patient is prone, preferably with the head turned toward the physician. (If the table has a face hole, the head may be kept in neutral.)

2. The physician stands at the side of the table opposite the side to be treated.

3. The physician places the thumb and thenar eminence of one hand on the medial aspect of the patient's thoracic paravertebral musculature overlying the transverse processes on the side opposite the physician **(Fig. 7.41)**.

4. The physician places the thenar eminence of the other hand on top of the abducted thumb of the bottom hand or over the hand itself **(Fig. 7.42)**.

5. Keeping the elbows straight and using the body weight, the physician exerts a gentle force ventrally (downward) to engage the soft tissues and then laterally, perpendicular to the thoracic paravertebral musculature **(Fig. 7.43)**.

6. This force is held for a few seconds and is slowly released.

7. Steps 5 and 6 can be repeated several times in a gentle, rhythmic, and kneading fashion.

8. The physician's hands are repositioned to contact different levels of the thoracic spine, and steps 5 to 7 are performed to stretch various portions of the thoracic paravertebral musculature.

9. This technique may also be performed using deep, sustained pressure.

10. Tissue tension is reevaluated to assess the effectiveness of the technique.

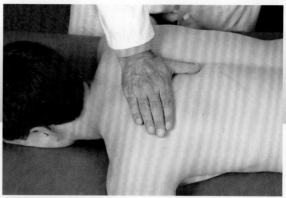

Figure 7.41. Step 3.

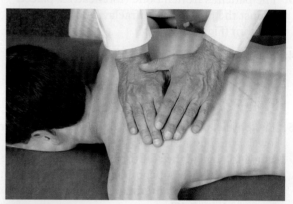

Figure 7.42. Step 4.

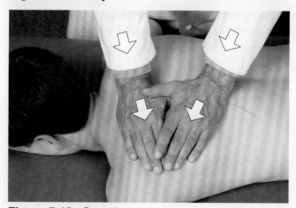

Figure 7.43. Step 5.

Thoracic Region

Unilateral Prone Pressure
Alternating "Catwalk" Variation

1. The patient is prone on the treatment table, preferably with the head turned toward the physician. (If the table has a face hole, the head may be kept in neutral.)

2. The physician stands at the side of the table, opposite the side to be treated.

3. The physician's hands are placed palm down side by side on the medial aspect of the patient's thoracic paravertebral musculature overlying the transverse processes on the side opposite the physician **(Fig. 7.44)**.

4. The physician adds enough downward pressure to engage the underlying fascia and musculature with the caudad hand **(Fig. 7.45)**.

5. The physician adds lateral pressure, taking the myofascial structures to their comfortable elastic limit **(Fig. 7.46)**.

6. This force is held for several seconds and then slowly released.

7. As the pressure is being released with the caudad hand, the physician's cephalad hand begins to add a downward lateral force **(Fig. 7.47)**.

8. The combination of downward and lateral forces and the release of this pressure is alternately applied between the two hands.

9. The downward and lateral pressure directed by each hand should be rhythmically applied for several seconds.

10. Tissue tension is reevaluated to assess the effectiveness of the technique.

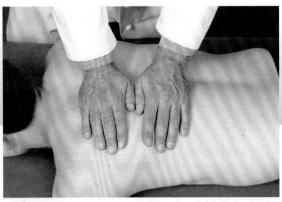

Figure 7.44. Step 3.

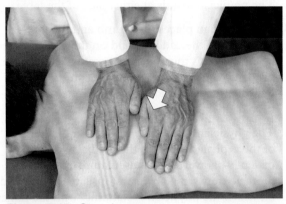

Figure 7.45. Step 4.

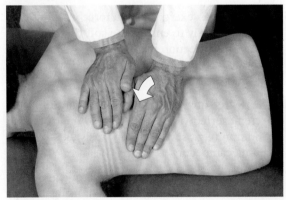

Figure 7.46. Step 5.

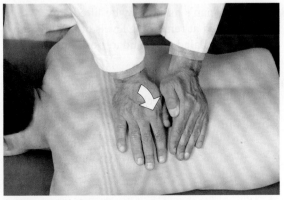

Figure 7.47. Step 7.

Thoracic Region

Bilateral Prone Pressure/Counterpressure

 See Video 7.14

1. The patient lies prone on the treatment table, preferably with the head turned toward the physician. (If the table has a face hole, the head may be kept in neutral.)

2. The physician stands at either side of the table.

3. The physician places the thumb and thenar eminence of the caudad hand on the medial aspect of the patient's thoracic paravertebral musculature overlying the transverse processes on the side opposite the physician with the fingers pointing cephalad.

4. The physician places the hypothenar eminence of the cephalad hand on the medial aspect of the patient's paravertebral musculature overlying the thoracic transverse processes, ipsilateral to the side on which the physician is standing, with the fingers pointing caudad (**Figs. 7.48 and 7.49**).

5. The physician exerts a gentle force with both hands, ventrally to engage the soft tissues and then in the direction the fingers of each hand are pointing, creating a separation and distraction effect (**Fig. 7.50**).

6. The degree of ventral force and longitudinal stretch exerted varies according to the patient's condition (e.g., severe osteoporosis), as rib cage trauma can occur.

7. This technique may be performed in a gentle, rhythmic, and kneading fashion or using a deep, sustained pressure.

8. The physician's hands may be lifted and repositioned at remaining levels of dysfunction and the cephalad and caudad positions may be reversed.

9. Tissue tension is reevaluated to assess the effectiveness of the technique.

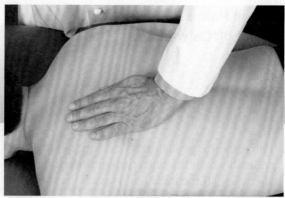
Figure 7.48. Step 4.

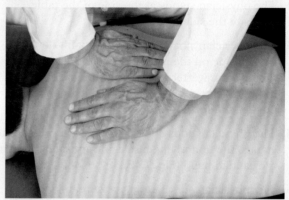
Figure 7.49. Step 4.

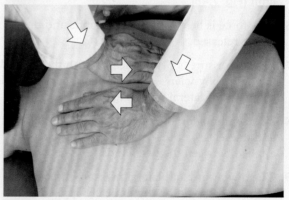
Figure 7.50. Step 5.

Thoracic Region

Unilateral Side Leverage
Short/Long-Lever Method

 See Video 7.15

1. The patient lies in the lateral recumbent (side lying) position, treatment side down.

2. The physician is seated on the side of the table, facing the patient.

3. The physician reaches over the patient's shoulder with the caudad hand and places the thumb and thenar eminence on the medial aspect of the paravertebral muscles overlying the upper thoracic transverse processes at the side on which the patient is lying **(Fig. 7.51)**.

4. The physician reaches under the patient's face with the cephalad hand and contacts the periauricular region, cradling the head **(Fig. 7.52)**.

5. The physician's caudad hand exerts a gentle force ventrally and laterally to engage the soft tissues while the cephalad hand gently lifts the head to produce cervical and upper thoracic side bending. The physician may add slight flexion until meeting the comfortable elastic limit of the tissues **(Fig. 7.53)**.

6. Step 5 can be repeated several times in a gentle, rhythmic, and kneading fashion or using deep, sustained pressure.

7. The physician's caudad hand is repositioned to contact different levels of the upper thoracic spine, and steps 5 and 6 are performed to stretch various portions of the upper thoracic paravertebral musculature **(Fig. 7.54)**.

8. Tissue tension is reevaluated to assess the effectiveness of the technique.

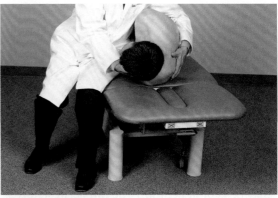
Figure 7.51. Step 3.

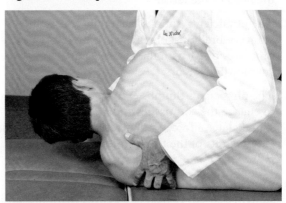
Figure 7.52. Step 4.

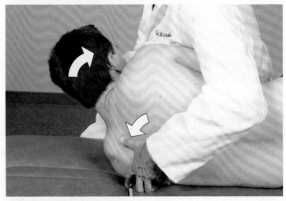
Figure 7.53. Step 5.

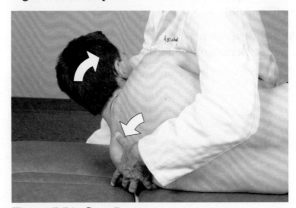
Figure 7.54. Step 7.

Thoracic Region

Bilateral Thumb Pressure

 See Video 7.16

1. The patient lies prone on the treatment table, preferably with the head turned toward the physician. (If the table has a face hole, the head may be kept in neutral.) The physician stands at the head of the table.

2. The physician's thumbs bilaterally contact the paravertebral musculature overlying the transverse processes of T1 with the fingers fanned out laterally **(Fig. 7.55)**.

3. The physician's thumbs exert a gentle ventral force to engage the soft tissues and add a caudal and slightly lateral force until meeting the comfortable elastic limits of the tissues **(Fig. 7.56)**. *Do not rub the skin, as it may be irritated.*

4. This stretch is held for several seconds and then slowly released. Repeat in a gentle, rhythmic, and kneading fashion.

5. The thumbs are repositioned over the transverse processes of each thoracic segment (T2, T3, and so on to T12) continuing this rhythmic kneading procedure to the apex of the thoracic kyphosis (usually T7–T8).

6. The physician then moves to the level of the patient's pelvis and faces the patient's head. The physician's thumbs are placed paraspinally over the transverse processes of T12 pointing cephalad with the fingers fanned out laterally **(Fig. 7.57)**.

7. The physician repeats the kneading procedure from T12 to T1 or uses deep, sustained pressure **(Fig. 7.58)**.

8. Tissue tension is reevaluated to assess the effectiveness of the technique.

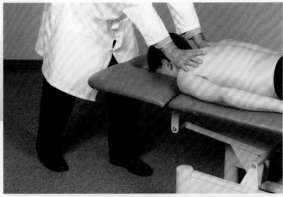

Figure 7.55. Step 2.

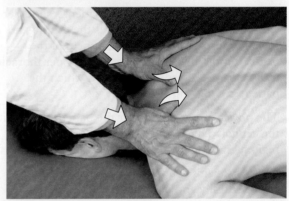

Figure 7.56. Step 3.

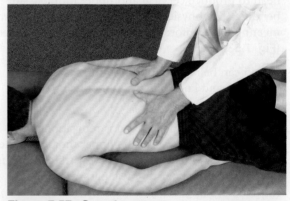

Figure 7.57. Step 6.

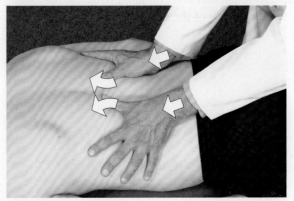

Figure 7.58. Step 7.

Thoracic Region

Bilateral Trapezius Pressure
Direct Inhibitory Method

 See Video 7.17

1. The patient lies supine on the treatment table.

2. The physician sits at the head of the table.

3. The physician's hands are placed on each trapezius so that the thumbs (pads up) lie approximately two thumb breadths inferior to the posterior border of the trapezius and the index and third digits (pads down) rest on the anterior border of the trapezius two finger breadths inferiorly **(Fig. 7.59)**. The thumbs and finger pads may be reversed in position if this is more comfortable for the physician **(Fig. 7.60)**.

4. The physician slowly adds a squeezing force on the trapezius between the thumbs and fingers **(Fig. 7.61)**.

5. This pressure is held until tissue texture changes are palpated or for 1 to 2 minutes.

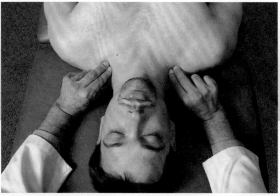

Figure 7.59. Step 3.

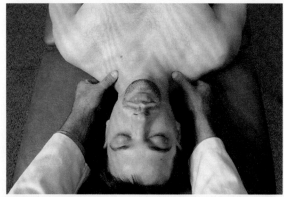

Figure 7.60. Step 3, alternative position.

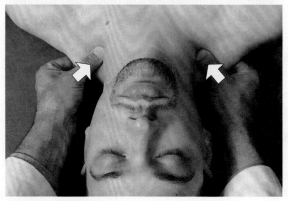

Figure 7.61. Step 4.

Thoracic Region

Upper Thoracic with Shoulder Block Lateral Recumbent Method

 See Video 7.18

1. The patient lies in the lateral recumbent position with the side to be treated up.

2. The physician stands at the side of the table, facing the patient.

3. The physician's caudad hand is passed under the patient's arm, with the pads of the fingers on the medial aspect of the patient's paravertebral muscles overlying the thoracic transverse processes **(Fig. 7.62)**.

4. The physician's cephalad hand contacts the anterior portion of the shoulder to provide an effective counterforce **(Fig. 7.63)**. Note: The patient's arm may be flexed approximately 120 degrees and draped over the physician's shoulder-contacting arm as needed **(Fig. 7.64)**.

5. The physician's caudad hand exerts a gentle force, ventrally to engage the soft tissues and laterally to create a perpendicular stretch of the thoracic paravertebral musculature **(Fig. 7.65)**.

6. This stretch is held for a few seconds and is then slowly released.

7. Steps 5 and 6 are repeated in a gentle, rhythmic, and kneading fashion.

8. The physician's caudad hand is repositioned to another affected level of the thoracic spine, and steps 5 to 7 are performed at each affected level.

9. This technique may also be performed using deep, sustained pressure.

10. Tissue tension is reevaluated to assess the effectiveness of the technique.

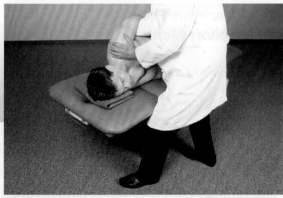

Figure 7.62. Step 3.

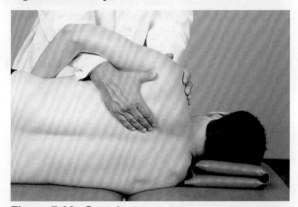

Figure 7.63. Step 4.

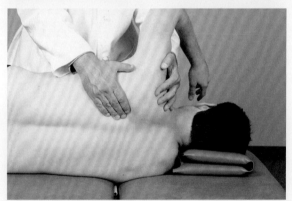

Figure 7.64. Step 4, alternative position.

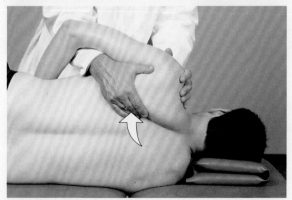

Figure 7.65. Step 5.

Thoracic Region

Mid- and Lower Thoracic Region Lateral Recumbent Method

 See Video 7.19

1. The patient is in a lateral recumbent position with the side to be treated up.

2. The physician stands at the side of the table, facing the front of the patient.

3. The physician reaches both hands under the patient's arm, with the pads of the fingers contacting the medial aspect of the patient's paravertebral muscles, overlying the thoracic transverse processes **(Figs. 7.66 and 7.67)**.

4. The physician's hands exert a gentle force ventrally to engage the soft tissues and laterally to create a perpendicular stretch of the thoracic paravertebral musculature **(Fig. 7.68)**.

5. This stretch is held for a few seconds and is slowly released.

6. Steps 4 and 5 are repeated in a gentle, rhythmic, and kneading fashion.

7. The physician's hands are repositioned to another affected level of the thoracic spine, and steps 4 to 6 are performed to stretch various portions of the thoracic paravertebral musculature.

8. This technique may also be performed using deep, sustained pressure.

9. Tissue tension is reevaluated to assess the effectiveness of the technique.

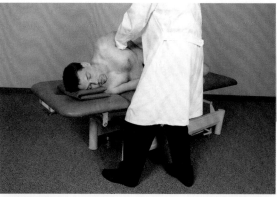
Figure 7.66. Step 3.

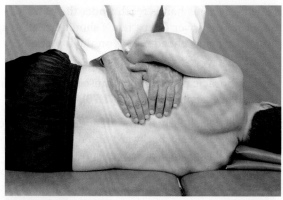
Figure 7.67. Step 3.

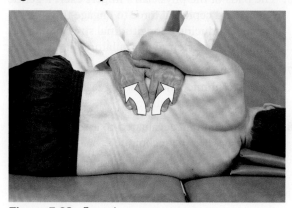
Figure 7.68. Step 4.

Thoracic Region

Upper Thoracic Extension "Under and Over" Technique

 See Video 7.20

1. The patient is seated with the arms crossed and the thumbs hooked into the antecubital fossae **(Fig. 7.69)**.

2. The physician stands facing the patient.

3. The physician's hands reach under the patient's forearms and over the patient's shoulders, allowing the patient's forehead to rest on the forearms.

4. The pads of the physician's fingers contact the upper thoracic paravertebral musculature overlying the transverse processes **(Fig. 7.70)**.

5. With one leg slightly behind the other for balance, the physician leans backward and draws the patient forward. The physician simultaneously raises the patient's forearms, using them as a lever, producing minimal thoracic extension **(Fig. 7.71)**.

6. The pads of the physician's fingers exert a gentle ventral and cephalad force to engage the soft tissues, producing a longitudinal stretch of the thoracic paravertebral musculature **(Fig. 7.72)**.

7. Steps 5 and 6 may be repeated several times in a gentle, rhythmic, and kneading fashion or using deep, sustained pressure.

8. Tissue tension is reevaluated to assess the effectiveness of the technique.

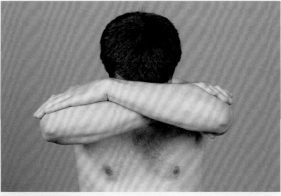

Figure 7.69. Step 1.

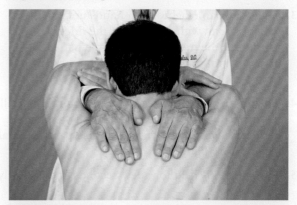

Figure 7.70. Step 4.

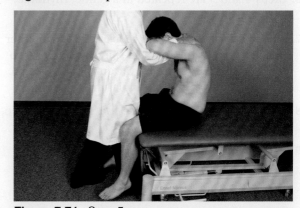

Figure 7.71. Step 5.

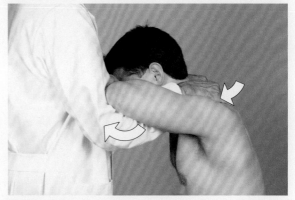

Figure 7.72. Step 6.

Thoracic Region

Midthoracic Extension

 See Video 7.21

1. The patient is seated on the end of the table with the hands clasped behind the neck.

2. The physician stands at the side of the patient.

3. The physician reaches under the patient's upper arms and grasps the patient's far elbow. The patient's other elbow rests on the physician's forearm near the antecubital fossa.

4. With the fingers pointing cephalad, the physician's other hand is cupped over the thoracic spinous processes, contacting the paravertebral musculature of one side with the thenar eminence and the other side with the hypothenar eminence **(Figs. 7.73 and 7.74)**.

5. The physician exerts a gentle force ventrally and cephalad, engaging the soft tissues to produce a longitudinal stretch while the other hand elevates the patient's elbows to produce minimal thoracic extension **(Fig. 7.75)**. *CAUTION: DO NOT push directly down on the spinous processes or hyperextend the thoracic spine.*

6. This technique may be performed in a gentle, rhythmic fashion *or* with deep, sustained pressure.

7. The physician's dorsal hand is repositioned at different levels of the thoracic spine, and steps 5 and 6 are performed to stretch various portions of the thoracic paravertebral musculature.

8. Tissue tension is reevaluated to assess the effectiveness of the technique.

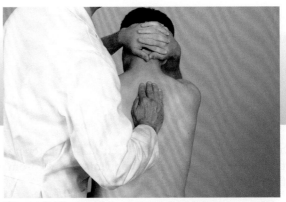

Figure 7.73. Step 4.

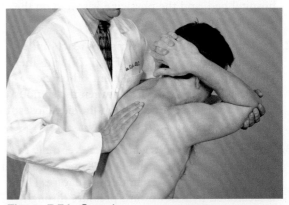

Figure 7.74. Step 4.

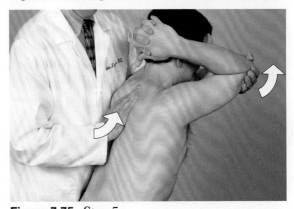

Figure 7.75. Step 5.

Thoracic Region

"Rib Raising"
Supine, Extension Method

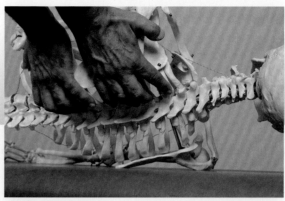

Figure 7.76. Step 2.

This procedure is commonly used in the postoperative setting to treat the somatic components of viscerosomatic reflexes (postsurgical paralytic ileus).

1. The patient is supine on the treatment table or hospital bed, and the physician is seated on the side to be treated.

2. The physician's hands (palms up) reach under the patient's thoracic spine **(Fig. 7.76)** with the pads of the fingers on the patient's thoracic paravertebral musculature between the spinous and the transverse processes on the side closest to the physician **(Fig. 7.77)**.

3. The physician exerts a gentle force ventrally to engage the soft tissues and laterally perpendicular to the thoracic paravertebral musculature. This is facilitated by a downward pressure through the elbows on the table, creating a fulcrum to produce a ventral lever action at the wrists and hands, engaging the soft tissues. The fingers are simultaneously drawn toward the physician, producing a lateral stretch perpendicular to the thoracic paravertebral musculature **(Fig. 7.78)**.

4. This stretch is held for several seconds and is slowly released.

5. Steps 3 and 4 are repeated several times in a gentle, rhythmic, and kneading fashion.

6. The physician's hands are repositioned to contact the different levels of the thoracic spine, and steps 3 to 6 are performed to stretch various portions of the thoracic paravertebral musculature.

7. This technique may also be performed using deep, sustained pressure.

8. Tissue tension is reevaluated to assess the effectiveness of the technique.

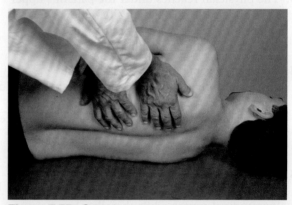

Figure 7.77. Step 2.

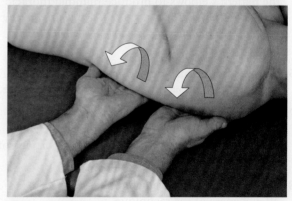

Figure 7.78. Step 3.

Lumbar Region

Unilateral Prone Pressure

 See Video 7.22

1. The patient is prone, with the head turned toward the physician. (If the table has a face hole, keep the head in neutral.)

2. The physician stands at the side of the table opposite the side to be treated **(Fig. 7.79)**.

3. The physician places the thumb and thenar eminence of one hand on the medial aspect of the patient's lumbar paravertebral musculature overlying the transverse processes on the side opposite the physician **(Fig. 7.80)**.

4. The physician places the thenar eminence of the other hand on the abducted thumb of the bottom hand **(Fig. 7.81)**.

5. Keeping the elbows straight and using the body weight, the physician exerts a gentle force ventrally to engage the soft tissues and laterally perpendicular to the lumbar paravertebral musculature **(Fig. 7.82)**.

6. This force is held for several seconds and is slowly released.

7. Steps 5 and 6 can be repeated several times in a gentle, rhythmic, and kneading fashion.

8. The physician's hands are repositioned to contact different levels of the lumbar spine, and steps 5 to 7 are performed to stretch various portions of the lumbar paravertebral musculature.

9. This technique may also be performed using deep, sustained pressure.

10. Tissue tension is reevaluated to assess the effectiveness of the technique.

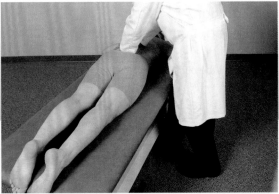
Figure 7.79. Step 2.

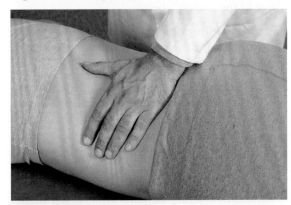
Figure 7.80. Step 3.

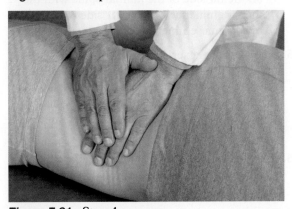
Figure 7.81. Step 4.

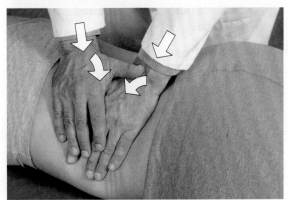
Figure 7.82. Step 5.

Lumbar Region

Prone Traction
Two-Handed, Lumbosacral Method

 See Video 7.23

1. The patient is prone with the head turned toward the physician. (If the table has a face hole, keep the head in neutral.)

2. The physician stands at the side of the table at the level of the patient's pelvis.

3. The heel of the physician's cephalad hand is placed over the base of the patient's sacrum with the fingers pointing toward the coccyx **(Fig. 7.83)**.

4. The physician does one or both of the following:
   a. The physician's caudad hand is placed over the lumbar spinous processes with the fingers pointing cephalad, contacting the paravertebral soft tissues with the thenar and hypothenar eminences **(Fig. 7.84)**.
   b. The hand may be placed to one side of the spine, contacting the paravertebral soft tissues on the far side of the lumbar spine with the thenar eminence or the near side with the hypothenar eminence.

5. The physician exerts a gentle force with both hands ventrally to engage the soft tissues and to create a separation and distraction effect in the direction the fingers of each hand are pointing **(Fig. 7.85)**. Do not push directly down on the spinous processes.

6. This technique may be applied in a gentle, rhythmic, and kneading fashion *or* using deep, sustained pressure.

7. The physician's caudad hand is repositioned at other levels of the lumbar spine, and steps 4 to 6 are repeated.

8. Tissue tension is reevaluated to assess the effectiveness of the technique.

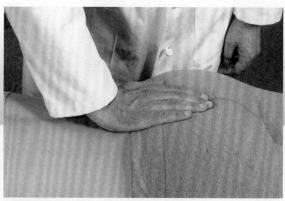

Figure 7.83. Step 3.

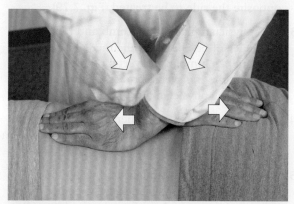

Figure 7.84. Step 4a.

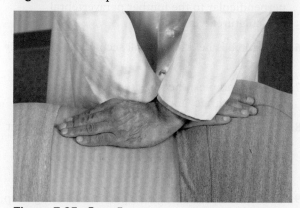

Figure 7.85. Step 5.

Lumbar Region

Bilateral Thumb Pressure

 See Video 7.24

1. The patient is prone, with the head turned toward the physician. (If the table has a face hole, keep the head in neutral.)

2. The physician stands at the side of the table at the level of the patient's thighs or knees.

3. The physician's thumbs are placed on both sides of the spine, contacting the paravertebral muscles overlying the transverse processes of L5 with the fingers fanned out laterally **(Fig. 7.86)**.

4. The physician's thumbs exert a gentle force ventrally to engage the soft tissues cephalad and laterally until the barrier or limit of tissue motion is reached **(Fig. 7.87)**. *Note*: Do not rub the skin with your thumbs, as this will irritate or chafe it.

5. This stretch is held for several seconds, is slowly released, and is then repeated in a gentle, rhythmic, and kneading fashion.

6. The physician's thumbs are repositioned over the transverse processes of each lumbar segment (L4, L3, L2, and then L1), and steps 4 and 5 are repeated to stretch the various portions of the lumbar paravertebral musculature.

7. This technique may also be performed using deep, sustained pressure.

8. Tissue tension is reevaluated to assess the effectiveness of the technique.

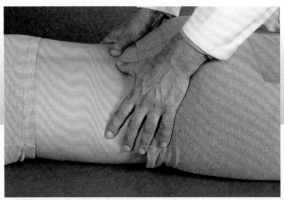

Figure 7.86. Step 3.

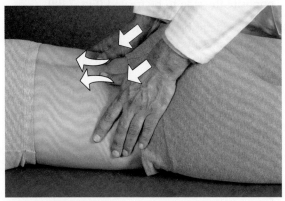

Figure 7.87. Step 4.

Lumbar Region

Unilateral, Prone Scissors Technique

 VIDEO *See Video 7.25*

1. The patient is prone, with the head turned toward the physician. (If the table has a face hole, keep the head in neutral.)

2. The physician stands at the side of the table opposite the side to be treated **(Fig. 7.88)**.

3. On the side to be treated, the physician's caudad hand reaches over to grasp the patient's leg proximal to the knee or at the tibial tuberosity **(Fig. 7.89)**.

4. The physician lifts the patient's leg, extending the hip and adducting it toward the other leg to produce a scissors effect **(Fig. 7.90)**.

5. The physician's caudad hand may be placed under the far leg and then over the proximal leg so that the patient's leg can support the physician's forearm.

6. The physician places the thumb and thenar eminence of the cephalad hand on the patient's paravertebral musculature overlying the lumbar transverse processes to direct a gentle force ventrally and laterally to engage the soft tissues while simultaneously increasing the amount of hip extension and adduction **(Fig. 7.91)**.

7. This force is held for several seconds and is slowly released.

8. Steps 6 and 7 are repeated several times in a slow, rhythmic, and kneading fashion.

9. The physician's cephalad hand is then repositioned to contact other levels of the lumbar spine, and steps 6 to 8 are performed to stretch the various portions of the lumbar paravertebral musculature.

10. This technique may also be performed using deep, sustained pressure.

11. Tissue tension is reevaluated to assess the effectiveness of the technique.

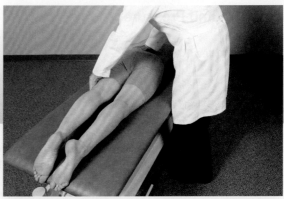
Figure 7.88. Step 2.

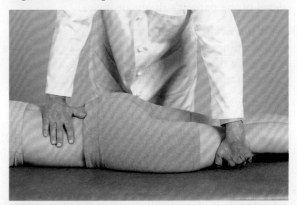
Figure 7.89. Step 3.

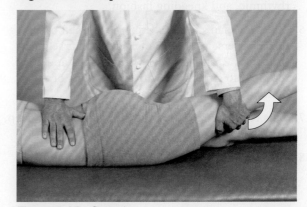
Figure 7.90. Step 4.

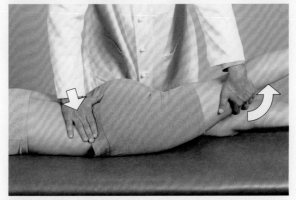
Figure 7.91. Step 6.

Lumbar Region

Prone Pressure with Counterleverage

 See Video 7.26

1. The patient is prone with the head turned toward the physician. (If the table has a face hole, keep the head in neutral.)

2. The physician stands at the side of the table opposite the side to be treated **(Fig. 7.92)**.

3. The physician places the thumb and thenar eminences of the cephalad hand on the medial aspect of the paravertebral muscles overlying the lumbar transverse processes on the side opposite the physician.

4. The physician's caudad hand contacts the patient's anterior superior iliac spine on the side to be treated and gently lifts it toward the ceiling **(Fig. 7.93)**.

5. To engage the soft tissues, the physician's cephalad hand exerts a gentle force ventrally and laterally, perpendicular to the lumbar paravertebral musculature **(Fig. 7.94)**.

6. This force is held for several seconds and is slowly released.

7. Steps 4 to 6 are repeated several times in a slow, rhythmic, and kneading fashion.

8. The physician's cephalad hand is then repositioned to contact different levels of the lumbar spine, and steps 4 to 6 are performed to stretch various portions of the lumbar paravertebral musculature.

9. This technique may also be performed using deep, sustained pressure.

10. Tissue tension is reevaluated to assess the effectiveness of the technique.

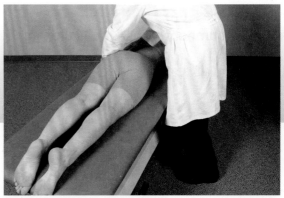
Figure 7.92. Step 2.

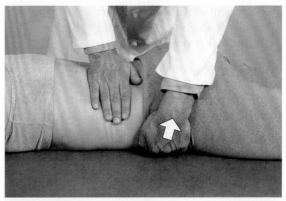
Figure 7.93. Step 4.

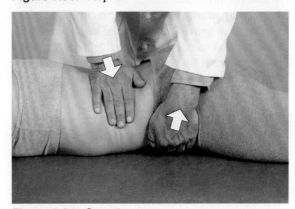
Figure 7.94. Step 5.

Lumbar Region

Unilateral Pressure
Lateral Recumbent (Hips/Knees Flexed)

 See Video 7.27

1. The patient lies in the lateral recumbent position with the treatment side up.

2. The physician stands at the side of the table, facing the front of the patient.

3. The patient's knees and hips are flexed, and the physician's thigh is placed against the patient's infrapatellar region **(Fig. 7.95)**.

4. The physician reaches over the patient's back and places the pads of the fingers on the medial aspect of the patient's paravertebral muscles overlying the lumbar transverse processes **(Fig. 7.96)**.

5. To engage the soft tissues, the physician exerts a gentle force ventrally and laterally to create a perpendicular stretch of the lumbar paravertebral musculature **(Fig. 7.97)**.

6. While the physician's thigh against the patient's knees may simply be used for bracing, it may also be flexed to provide a combined bowstring and longitudinal traction force on the paravertebral musculature. This technique may be applied in a gentle rhythmic and kneading fashion or with deep, sustained pressure.

7. This technique may be modified by bracing the anterior superior iliac spine with the caudad hand while drawing the paravertebral muscles ventrally with the cephalad hand **(Fig. 7.98)**.

8. The physician's hands are repositioned to contact different levels of the lumbar spine, and steps 4 to 6 are performed to stretch various portions of the lumbar paravertebral musculature.

9. Tissue tension is reevaluated to assess the effectiveness of the technique.

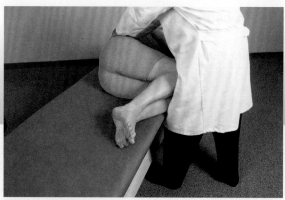
Figure 7.95. Step 3.

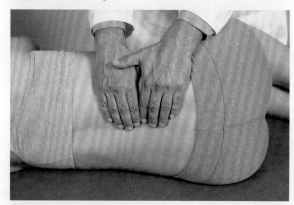
Figure 7.96. Step 4.

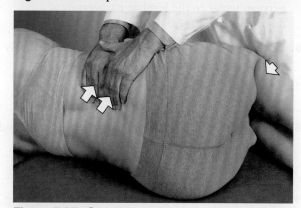
Figure 7.97. Step 5.

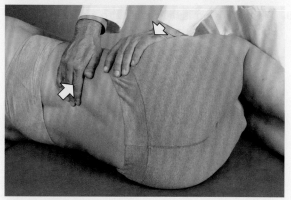
Figure 7.98. Step 7.

Lumbar Region

Supine Extension

 See Video 7.28

1. The patient is supine. (The patient's hips and knees may be flexed for comfort.)

2. The physician is seated at the side to be treated.

3. The physician's hands (palms up) reach under the patient's lumbar spine, with the pads of the physician's fingers on the patient's lumbar paravertebral musculature between the spinous and the transverse processes on the side closest to the physician **(Figs. 7.99 and 7.100)**.

4. To engage the soft tissues, the physician exerts a gentle ventral and lateral force perpendicular to the thoracic paravertebral musculature. This is facilitated by downward pressure through the elbows on the table, creating a fulcrum to produce a ventral lever action at the wrists and hands **(Fig. 7.101)**.

5. The fingers are simultaneously drawn toward the physician, producing a lateral stretch perpendicular to the thoracic paravertebral musculature.

6. This stretch is held for several seconds and is slowly released.

7. Steps 4 to 6 are repeated several times in a gentle, rhythmic, and kneading fashion.

8. The physician's hands are repositioned to contact the different levels of the lumbar spine, and steps 4 to 6 are performed to stretch various portions of the lumbar paravertebral musculature.

9. This technique may also be performed using deep, sustained pressure.

10. Tissue tension is reevaluated to assess the effectiveness of the technique.

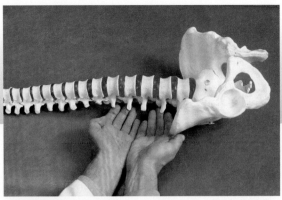
Figure 7.99. Step 3.

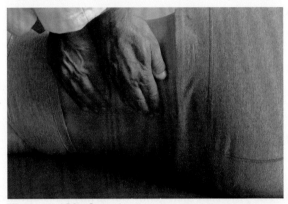
Figure 7.100. Step 3.

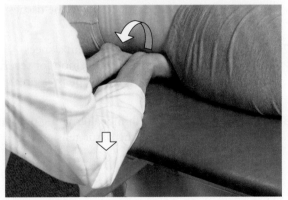
Figure 7.101. Step 4.

Lumbar Region

Long-Lever, Counterleverage

 See Video 7.29

1. The patient lies supine on the treatment table.

2. The physician's caudad hand flexes the patient's hips and knees to approximately 90 degrees each **(Fig. 7.102)**.

3. The physician's cephalad hand reaches over the patient and under the patient's lumbar region in the area of the dysfunction.

4. The physician controls the patient's lower extremities bilaterally at the tibial tuberosities and slowly moves the knees laterally away from the physician **(Fig. 7.103)**.

5. As the patient's knees are moved away from the physician, the physician monitors the tension directed into the paravertebral lumbar tissues.

6. The physician then gently but firmly pulls upward (anteriorly) into the patient's paraspinal tissues until the comfortable elastic limits of the tissues are met **(Fig. 7.104)**.

7. The physician next moves the patient's knees slightly farther away, holds this position for several seconds, and then slowly releases the pressure **(Fig. 7.105)**.

8. This is repeated in a rhythmic, alternating pressure and release fashion until the tissue tension is released or up to 2 minutes.

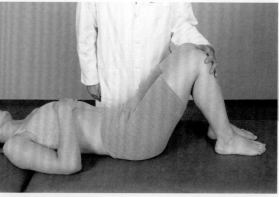

Figure 7.102. Step 2.

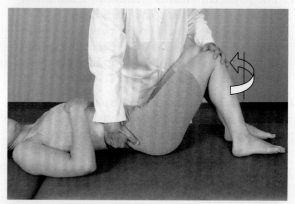

Figure 7.103. Step 4.

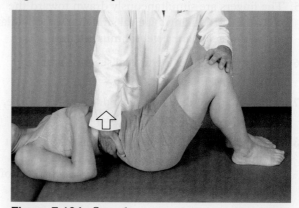

Figure 7.104. Step 6.

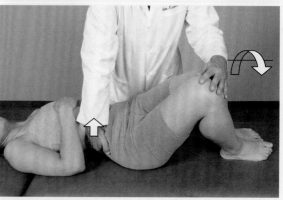

Figure 7.105. Step 7.

Lumbar Region

Unilateral Myofascial Hypertonicity Seated, Rotation Method

 See Video 7.30

1. The patient is seated on the end of the table with the physician standing behind the patient and to the right side, opposite the dysfunction.

2. The patient is instructed to place the left hand behind the neck and grasp the left elbow with the right hand. The physician's right hand reaches under the patient's right axilla and grasps the patient's left upper arm **(Fig. 7.106)**.

3. The physician's left thumb and thenar eminence are placed on the medial aspect of the patient's left paravertebral musculature overlying the lumbar transverse processes **(Fig. 7.107)**.

4. The patient is instructed to lean forward and relax, allowing the body weight to rest onto the physician's right arm.

5. To engage the soft tissues, the physician's left hand directs a gentle ventral and lateral force to create a perpendicular stretch while rotating the patient to the right with the physician's right arm and hand **(Fig. 7.108)**.

6. This stretch is held for several seconds and is slowly released.

7. Steps 5 and 6 are repeated several times in a gentle, rhythmic, and kneading fashion.

8. The physician's left hand is repositioned to contact the remaining dysfunctional levels of the lumbar spine, and steps 5 to 7 are repeated.

9. This technique may also be performed using deep, sustained pressure.

10. Tissue tension is reevaluated to assess the effectiveness of the technique.

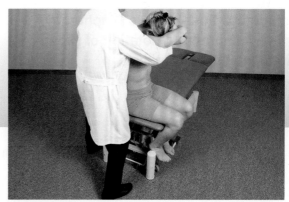

Figure 7.106. Step 2.

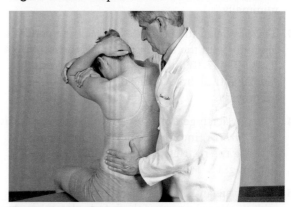

Figure 7.107. Step 3.

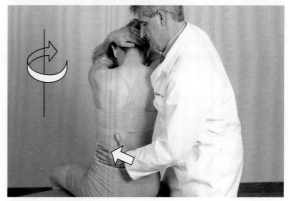

Figure 7.108. Step 5.

Pelvic Region

Ischiorectal Fossa/Pelvic Diaphragm
Prone, with Internal Rotation of Hips
Direct Inhibition Emphasis

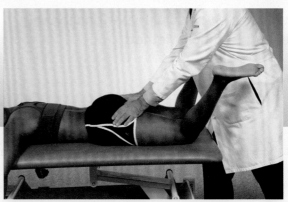

Figure 7.109. Step 1 to 3.

1. The patient lies prone and the physician stands at the foot of the table.

2. The patient's knees are flexed approximately 90 degrees, and the hips are internally rotated minimally.

3. The physician then reaches between the patient's legs and, with the thumbs, palpates the ischiorectal fossae **(Fig. 7.109)** that are located immediately medial and slightly cephalad to the ischial tuberosities.

4. The physician gently but firmly adds a compressive force (*arrows*) into the ischiorectal fossa until meeting the restrictive barrier of the "pelvic diaphragm."

5. The physician directs a laterally directed force with the thumbs toward the inferior lateral angles (ILAs) of the sacrum **(Fig. 7.110)**.

6. This pressure is held until a release is determined, or the patient can be instructed to cough while the physician continues to maintain pressure with the thumbs.

7. The above procedure may be repeated three to five times.

8. Tissue tension is reevaluated to assess the effectiveness of the technique.

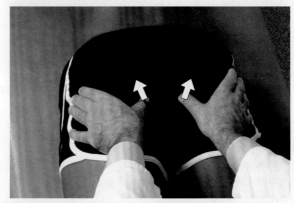

Figure 7.110. Step 5, thumb pressure toward ILAs.

Upper Extremity Region

Levator Scapula Hypertonicity
Direct Inhibition Emphasis

1. The patient is seated and the physician stands behind the patient on the side of the dysfunction.

2. The physician locates the inferior portion of the levator scapula muscle's musculotendinous border near the superior, medial border of the scapula **(Fig. 7.111)**.

3. The physician's thumb or olecranon process of the elbow is placed at the musculotendinous portion of the levator scapula muscle immediately cephalad to its insertion on the scapula **(Figs. 7.112 and 7.113)**.

4. Starting with a gentle pressure over the musculotendinous portion or, pushing perpendicular along the edge of the musculotendinous junction, the physician meets the resistance of the tissue.

5. The physician may alter the vector of the pressure inferiorly, medially, or laterally in order to meet the barrier more effectively.

6. The physician maintains a steady pressure in this manner until a release of the spasm is noted. This may take from 20 seconds to 1 minute.

7. The physician reassesses the tissue texture and other related components of the dysfunction (TART).

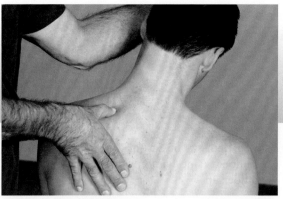

Figure 7.111. Step 2.

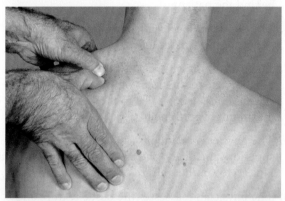

Figure 7.112. Step 3, direct vector toward barrier(s).

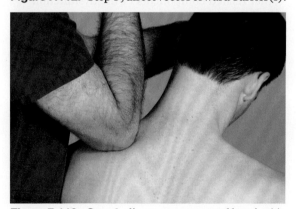

Figure 7.113. Step 3, direct vector toward barrier(s).

Upper Extremity Region

Teres Minor Hypertonicity
Direct Inhibition Emphasis

1. The patient sits or lies (or lies) in the lateral recumbent (side-lying) position with the injured shoulder up.

2. The physician stands at the side of the table behind the patient.

3. The physician locates the teres minor muscle at the posterior axillary fold.

4. The pads of the physician's thumbs are placed at a right angle to the fibers of the muscle (thumb pressure directed parallel to muscle) at the point of maximum hypertonicity **(Fig. 7.114)**.

5. The physician maintains a steady pressure superiorly, medially, and slightly anteriorly (*arrows*, **Fig. 7.115**) until a release of the spasm is noted.

6. The physician reassesses the tissue texture and other related components of the dysfunction (TART).

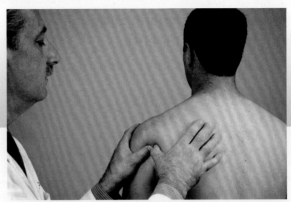

Figure 7.114. Step 4, thumbs at point of greatest tension.

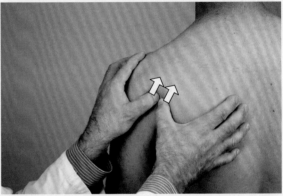

Figure 7.115. Step 5.

Upper Extremity Region

Midhumeral Counterlateral Traction

1. The patient lies supine on the treatment table.

2. The patient's right arm is abducted 60 to 90 degrees so that the physician can stand or sit between the abducted arm and the patient's trunk.

3. The physician's right hand is placed palm down over the lateral humerus at the insertion level of the deltoid muscle and the physician's left hand grasps the patient's right forearm/wrist **(Fig. 7.116)**.

4. The patient's elbow is flexed 45 to 90 degrees and then the physician slowly externally rotates the patient's shoulder/arm while compressing the tendinous insertion of the deltoid muscle and causing a slight medially directed fascial drag of the overlying tissues toward the patient's body **(Fig. 7.117)**.

5. When reaching the restrictive fascial barrier, the physician slowly releases the tension by internally rotating the patient's shoulder and relaxing the compression on the humerus. The shoulder only needs to be internally rotated enough to release the pressure and returning the arm to neutral is not necessary.

6. The maneuver is repeated by externally rotating the patient's arm with concomitant compression and medially directed drag on the humeral fascia.

7. This procedure may be repeated in a slow, rhythmic fashion for 2 to 5 minutes. If the physician thinks a more lengthened time of stretch is advisable, the fascial barrier can be met and the pressure held for 10 to 20 seconds.

8. Tissue tension is reevaluated to assess the effectiveness of the technique.

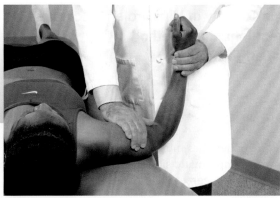

Figure 7.116. Step 3.

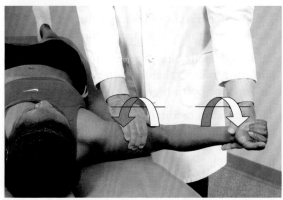

Figure 7.117. Step 4.

Lower Extremity Region

Hypertonicity of Hip Girdle Muscles
Direct Inhibition Method
Ex: Left Piriformis

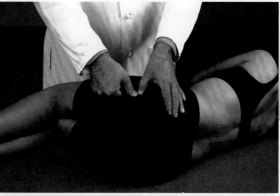

Figure 7.118. Steps 1.5

1. The patient lies in the lateral recumbent position with symptomatic side up and both hips flexed to 90 to 120 degrees.

2. The patient's knees are flexed to approximately 100 degrees.

3. The physician stands in front of the patient at the level of the patient's hip, facing the table.

4. The physician locates the hypertonic or painful piriformis muscle slightly posterior and inferior to the superior portion of the greater trochanter.

5. The physician maintains a firm pressure with the pad of the thumb medially (down toward the table) over the muscle until a release is palpated **(Fig. 7.118)**.

6. Alternative: The physician may use the olecranon process of the elbow instead of the thumbs **(Fig. 7.119)**. The olecranon is sensitive to the pressure (*arrow*) and is able to determine the tendon's resistance and the differential anatomy of the area. It is also easier on the physician, as this style of technique can fatigue the thumbs.

7. The physician reassesses the tissue texture and other related components of the dysfunction (TART).

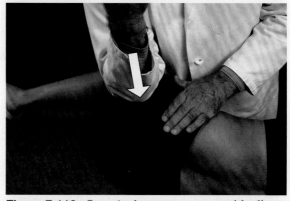

Figure 7.119. Step 6, alternate contact with elbow.

Lower Extremity Region

Iliotibial Band Tension
Prone, Counterleverage

1. The patient lies prone and the physician stands on the left side of the patient.

2. The patient's right knee is flexed to 90 degrees.

3. The physician's right hand grasps the patient's right foot or lower leg while reaching over the patient to place the left hand, palm down, over the patient's right lateral thigh **(Fig. 7.120)**.

4. The physician begins to push the patient's foot and lower leg laterally while simultaneously compressing the right hand into the patient's lateral thigh to engage the iliotibial band (ITB) pulling posteromedially to its restrictive barrier **(Fig. 7.121)**.

5. On meeting the ITB's restrictive barrier, the physician can maintain the tension for 10 to 20 seconds and slowly release the tension and repeat until a maximum release of the tissue is noted or perform this technique in a slow, rhythmic manner, which is repeated over a few minutes or until the tissue texture is maximally improved.

6. To disengage the tension on the ITB, the physician pulls the patient's foot/lower leg back toward the midline while decreasing the pressure on the lateral thigh **(Fig. 7.122)**.

7. Tissue tension is reevaluated to assess the effectiveness of the technique.

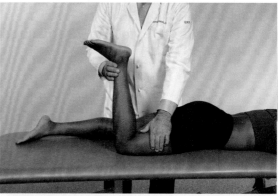

Figure 7.120. Steps 1 to 3.

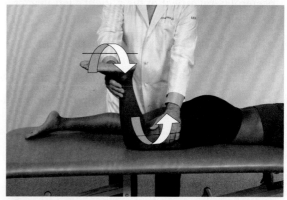

Figure 7.121. Step 4, stretching to ITB.

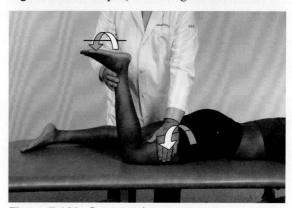

Figure 7.122. Step 6, release pressure.

Lower Extremity Region

Iliotibial Band Tension
Lateral Recumbent, Effleurage/Petrissage

1. The patient lies in the right lateral recumbent position and the physician stands facing the front of the patient.

2. The physician's left hand rests on the posterolateral aspect of the patient's left iliac crest to stabilize the pelvis.

3. The physician makes a "fist" with the right hand and places the flat portion of the proximal phalanges over the distal, lateral thigh (**Fig. 7.123**).

4. The physician adds slight pressure into the distal ITB and begins to slide the hand toward the trochanteric (**Fig. 7.124**).

5. This is repeated for 1 to 2 minutes and then the tissue tension is reevaluated to assess the effectiveness of the technique.

6. If preferred, the physician can alternate from the distal to proximal stroking and perform a proximal to distal stroking, ending at the distal ITB (**Fig 7.125**).

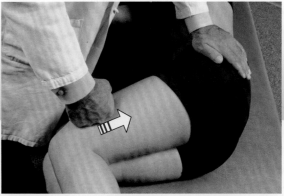

Figure 7.123. Steps 1 to 3, hand position.

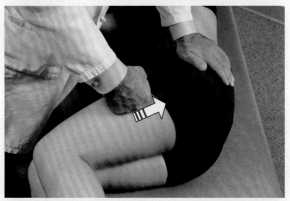

Figure 7.124. Step 4, distal to proximal stroke.

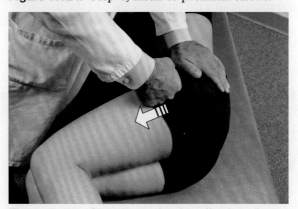

Figure 7.125. Step 6, proximal to distal stroke.

Lower Extremity Region

Plantar Fascia Hypertonicity
Longitudinal Stretch

 See Video 7.31

Indications

Plantar Fasciitis

Rigid Acquired Pes Planus

General Relaxation and Lymphatic Drainage

Technique

1. The patient lies supine and the physician sits at the foot of the table.

2. The physician places one hand over the dorsum of the patient's foot for control/stabilization.

3. The physician makes a closed fist and places the flat portion of the proximal fifth phalanx against the sole of the patient's foot just proximal to the metatarsal **(Fig. 7.126)**.

4. The flat portions of the physician's proximal phalanges are rolled along the plantar aponeurosis toward the calcaneus **(Fig. 7.127)**.

5. The physician slowly, with moderate pressure, begins to drag the hand distal to proximal on the plantar aspect of the foot toward the calcaneus, while incrementally adding contact with the dorsum of each additional phalangeal bone (i.e., 5th → 4th → 3rd → 2nd) **(Figs. 7.128 and 7.129)**.

6. This maneuver is repeated in slow, rhythmic fashion for 1 to 2 minutes or to patient tolerance.

7. Tissue tension and midfoot and forefoot mobility are reevaluated to assess the effectiveness of the technique.

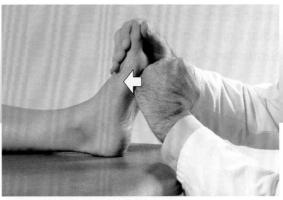

Figure 7.126. Steps 2 to 3.

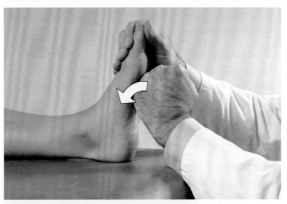

Figure 7.127. Step 4, begin to add pressure.

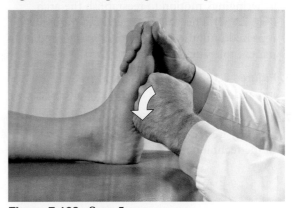

Figure 7.128. Step 5.

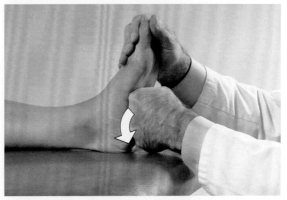

Figure 7.129. Step 5.

Lower Extremity Region

Plantar Fascia Hypertonicity
Medial Longitudinal Arch
Counterforce Springing Emphasis

 See Video 7.32

Indications

Pes Planus

Rigid Midfoot

1. The patient lies supine and the physician stands or sits at the foot of the table.

2. The physician places both thumbs under the longitudinal arc of the patient's foot with the fingers of each hand fanning out on the dorsal surface of the foot **(Fig. 7.130)**.

3. The cephalad hand/thumb lifts the arch with a force that wraps laterally across the top of the foot.

4. The caudad hand wraps medially around the foot creating an arch-raising counterforce.

5. The two hands twist in opposite directions with a "wringing" motion to reestablish the arch **(Fig. 7.131)**. This rolling, stretching motion is repeated until the desired effect is achieved or to patient tolerance.

6. **Figures 7.132 and 7.133** demonstrate a variation in hand placement and acceptable alternative.

7. Tissue tension and motion of the midfoot and forefoot are reevaluated to assess the effectiveness of the technique.

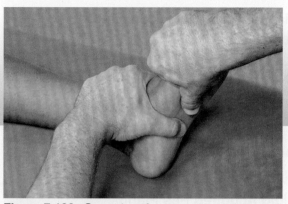

Figure 7.130. Steps 1 to 2.

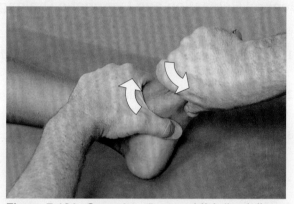

Figure 7.131. Steps 3 to 5, reestablish "arch."

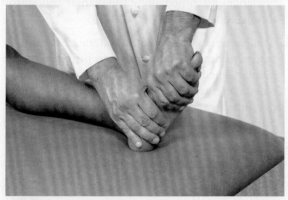

Figure 7.132. Step 6.

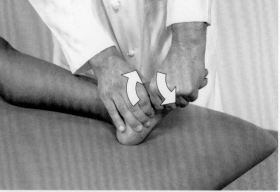

Figure 7.133. Step 6.

References

1. Glossary of Osteopathic Terminology. Educational Council on Osteopathic Principles of the American Association of Colleges of Osteopathic Medicine, http://www.aacom.org

2. Chila AG, exec. ed. Foundations of Osteopathic Medicine. 3rd ed. Baltimore, MD: Lippincott Williams & Wilkins, 2011.

3. Greenman P. Principles of Manual Medicine. 3rd ed. Philadelphia, PA: Lippincott Williams & Wilkins, 2003.

8

Myofascial Release Techniques

Fascia as an Organ System

Until recently, fascia was not recognized as a distinctly important tissue requiring many hours of course study in medical school. Both the Gray and Hollinshead anatomy texts refer to fascia quite generally as a tissue dissected in anatomy labs and during surgery, that is, "Fascia is a term so vague in usage that it signifies little more than collections of connective tissue large enough to be visible to the unaided eye" and "the term fascia is rather loosely applied in anatomy and in surgery," respectively. Hollinshead also remarks that "in one sense, a fascia has no beginning and no end, and any description of fascia is necessarily somewhat arbitrary" (1,2).

More recently, interest in fascia as an *organ system* important in both health maintenance and disease prevention led to the First International Fascia Research Congress (FRC) at Harvard Medical School in 2007. From that meeting came a more universal definition of fascia more closely related to that which the osteopathic profession had held, which can be paraphrased as "The soft tissue component of the connective tissue system that permeates the human body, forming a continuous, whole-body, three-dimensional matrix of structural support. It interpenetrates and surrounds all organs, muscles, bones, and nerve fibers, creating a unique environment for body systems' functioning. As such, it extends to all fibrous connective tissues, including aponeuroses, ligaments, tendons, retinacula, joint capsules, organ and vessel tunics, the epineurium, the meninges, the periosteum, and all the endomysial and intermuscular fibers of the myofasciae."

Technique Principles

Ward describes myofascial release technique as "designed to stretch and reflexively release patterned soft tissue and joint-related restrictions" (3). This style of osteopathic manipulation has historical ties to early osteopathic manipulative treatment and soft tissue technique, but Ward combined principles of many other techniques to develop a distinct technique, even though its roots may go back to early osteopathic physicians (4). The Educational Council on Osteopathic Principles has defined myofascial release technique as a "system of diagnosis and treatment first described by Andrew Taylor Still and his early students, which engages continual palpatory feedback to achieve release of myofascial tissues" (5). In comparing this technique to other osteopathic techniques (especially for soft tissue), it is obvious that hand placement and force vector directions are similar and that the principles used to affect the various anatomic tissue types, muscle origins and insertions, and so on are also important in this style. Whereas soft tissue technique has been historically direct in classification, myofascial release can be performed in either a direct or an indirect manner. Therefore, some would classify it as a combined technique (2). Other differences in comparing myofascial release to soft tissue are the facts that (a) the penetrating pressures in myofascial release are deep enough to only engage the fascial compartments surrounding the musculature, not the more deeply performed muscle engagement of soft tissue and (b) the pressure that is placed at the barrier is constant in myofascial release, whereas classical soft tissue (not its inhibition style) is an alternating, pressure-on, pressure-off, repetitive technique.

Myofascial release technique may be performed with one hand or two. Clinically, a two-handed method may be more effective in diagnosis and treatment. The osteopathic physician will use epicritic palpation to determine the soft tissue compliance (looseness, ease, freedom) and stiffness (tightness, binding, restriction). However, in dysfunctional states, there may be a general or universal barrier (restriction), so that these tissues have an asymmetric quality or quantity of compliance. Thus, a sense of freedom in one or more directions and restriction in the others can exist. These asymmetries are clinically described as having a tight-loose or ease-bind relationship. Ward also points out that the tight-loose asymmetry may be more clinically relevant at the loose sites, where pain and instability may be present (3). Therefore, the physician must be aware that there may be a cause-and-effect situation whereby (a) the tight or direct barrier is causing a secondary loose reaction or (b) the loose site is inherently unstable, and easing the barrier in either direction may not be clinically advisable.

Barriers may be identified with the patient passive or active. The treatment may also consist of these alternatives. The patient's respiratory assistance, specifically directed isometric muscle contractions (e.g., clenching fists or jaw), tongue movements or ocular movements, and so on are often used to potentiate the technique. These are generally referred to as release-enhancing maneuvers (REMS), not to be confused with rapid eye movements. They have also been described as activating forces such as inherent (intrinsic) force of the body's natural tendency to seek homeostasis; respiratory force (cooperation/assist) including coughing; patient cooperation by contracting specific muscles; physician-guided forces; and vibratory force (including oscillations) (4).

As the fascia is so deeply incorporated into the muscles and the rest of the body, any force directed on it may affect the ligamentous and capsular (articular) tissues and structures very distal to the specific area being palpated and treated. Therefore, this technique may effect widespread reactions (i.e., "tensegrity" relationships). For example, releasing the area surrounding T7 and T8 may cause the patient to have less suboccipital symptoms through the positive effect of the technique on the trapezius muscle.

A number of physical and anatomic aspects are important in myofascial release as illustrated by Ward (3). These include Wolff law, Hooke law, and Newton third law. They relate the various reactions to force, such as deformation and the fact that physical contact between the physician and patient has equal and opposite force magnitudes. Therefore, by introducing laws of thermodynamics and energy conservation theories, we can project the changes that occur in the patient's tissues when pressure is initiated into these structures. Joule found that the amount of energy done as work was converted to heat. The resulting changes may occur not only in the fascial structures but also in their cellular components as a result of various physical and bioelectric phenomena, including piezoelectricity, mechanotransduction, and/or hysteresis (6). As these changes in tissue quality occur, the physician, through palpation, can sense this as a softening, elongation, and/or relaxation of the tissues. Or, as the name of the technique implies, a *release* of the tension associated with a simultaneous increased lengthening of the tissues (4,6). This phenomenon may continue over time with subsequent release in changing vectors, which the physician should follow with the appropriate direct or indirect style of myofascial release technique. With continued treatment affecting these tissues, the opportunity may exist to alter the elastic properties permanently (plastic change).

O'Connell includes *piezoelectricity* as another possible basis for the effects of myofascial treatment. This theory also incorporates the process of *mechanotransduction*, whereby mechanical stress or loads can develop bioelectrical reactions causing reactions at the cellular level (fibroblasts, chondrocytes, and osteoblasts). Studies have shown that this may be occurring in bone through the action of collagen, and, as fascia is a collagen-rich tissue, theories extrapolating this process to fascia have been recently promoted (6).

Technique Classification

Direct, Indirect, or Combined with Two-Handed Technique

Myofascial release may be performed directly, so that the restrictive barrier (tension, bind) is engaged, or indirectly, so as to engage the physiologic or restrictive barrier at the ease (loose, free) direction of tension or motion asymmetry (see Chapter 6, "Principles of Osteopathic Manipulative Techniques"). It may also be performed in a simultaneous direct and indirect approach in which the physician uses one hand to approach the tight barrier and the other to approach the loose barrier. Additionally, the physician may alternate between direct and indirect types or, balancing at a "neutral" point between the two barrier extremes (similar to functional technique).

Technique Styles

Light, Moderate, or Heavy in Force Application

Myofascial release technique is interesting and very useful in that the forces may be directed in differentiated levels; also, the physician can direct the force toward (direct) or away from (indirect) the barriers being monitored. Therefore, this technique is useful in acute and chronic clinical presentations with their associated variations in pain level.

Indications

1. Use as part of the musculoskeletal screening examination to quickly identify regions of potential motion restriction and tissue texture changes.
2. Reduce muscle tension and fascial tension.
3. Stretch and increase elasticity of shortened, inelastic, and/or fibrotic myofascial structures to improve regional and/or intersegmental ranges of motion.
4. Reduce the tight-loose asymmetry to improve the tissue consistency in the loose tissues by increasing elasticity in the tight tissues.

5. Improve circulation to the specific region being treated by local physical and thermodynamic effects or by reflex phenomena to improve circulation in a distal area (e.g., through somatosomatic, somatovisceral reflexes).

6. Increase venous and lymphatic drainage to decrease local and/or distal swelling and edema and potentially improve the overall immune response.

7. Potentiate the effect of other osteopathic techniques.

Contraindications

Relative Contraindications

As myofascial technique may be performed with extremely light pressure in a direct or indirect manner, there is little likelihood of adverse effects other than aches posttreatment that are secondary to compensation and decompensation reactions and similar to aches postexercise. As in other techniques, increased water intake and ice pack application as needed posttreatment will generally reduce any such reaction.

1. Acute sprain or strain
2. Fracture or dislocation
3. Neurologic or vascular compromise
4. Osteoporosis and osteopenia
5. *Malignancy*: Most restrictions are for treatment in the affected area of malignancy; however, care should be taken in other distal areas depending on type of malignancy and/or lymphatic involvement.
6. Infection (e.g., osteomyelitis)

Absolute Contraindications

None, as the technique may be performed with very light pressure. The physician may work proximal or distal to the affected area and alter the patient's position or style of technique to achieve some beneficial effect.

General Considerations and Rules

1. The physician palpates the patient using layer-by-layer palpatory principles and with just enough pressure to capture the skin and subcutaneous fascial structures. This is one level of pressure less than that of soft tissue technique. Any movement of the hand on the skin should cause the skin to move along with the hand without sliding the hand over the skin.
2. The physician gently moves the palpating hand or hands in a linear direction of choice (hands of the clock) moving through the x- and y-axes. The

z-axis has already been engaged by the layer-by-layer palpatory pressure into the body, gaining access to the superficial fascia.

3. Symmetry versus asymmetry of tissue compliance is noted in the linear directions tested.

4. The physician may add a variety of directions of motion, including other linear movements in a 360-degree reference and clockwise and counterclockwise rotational movement. Again, symmetry versus asymmetry of tissue compliance is noted.

5. The pressure the physician uses to determine compliance may be minimal or moderate, depending on the clinical presentation of the patient (acute painful vs. chronic minimally painful) and what the physician believes is appropriate for the situation.

6. After determining the ease and bind barriers of the tissue in these directions, the physician determines whether gentle or moderate pressure in a direct (toward bind) or indirect (toward ease) technique is appropriate. Again, this is determined by the clinical presentation and examination findings. In general, the gentlest method is the safest.

7. The physician slowly moves the hand-controlled myofascial tissues toward the appropriate barrier, and on meeting the barrier, he or she holds the tissue at that point without relieving the pressure. The physician should notice that after approximately 20 to 30 seconds, a change of tissue compliance occurs; this is demonstrated by movement of the tissue through the originally determined barrier (creep or fascial creep).

8. The physician follows this change and continues to engage the barrier until no further evidence of creep occurs. There may be a number of compliance changes (creep) before this phenomenon stops.

9. The physician reevaluates the tissue to determine whether the tissue's compliance and quality have improved. The technique may be repeated at the same area or another, and follow-up visits may be prescribed for a 3-day interval or longer, depending on patient reactivity.

Because of the various tissue levels encountered and the proximal-to-distal relationships (tensegrity) associated with the somatic dysfunction, there may be countless ways in which to touch and position the patient when implementing myofascial release technique. We have described a number of commonly used techniques but have also illustrated many others without the descriptive text because the physician may follow the guidelines and develop a particular strategy or treatment protocol that best suits the patient.

Cervical Region

Supine Cradling
Direct or Indirect

1. The patient lies supine, and the physician sits at the head of the table.

2. The physician's hands are placed palms up under the patient's articular process (pillar) at the level of the dysfunction **(Fig. 8.1)**.

3. The physician lifts upward into the patient's posterior cervical tissues with only enough force to control the skin and underlying fascia, so as to not slide the hands across the patient's skin.

4. The physician monitors inferior and superior, left and right circumferential rotation, and torsional (twisting) motion availability for ease-bind symmetric or asymmetric relations **(Fig. 8.2)**.

5. After determining the presence of an ease-bind asymmetry, the physician will either indirectly or directly meet the ease-bind barrier **(Fig. 8.3)**.

6. The force is applied in a very gentle to moderate manner.

7. This force is held for 20 to 60 seconds or until a release is palpated. The physician may continue this and follow any additional release (creep) until it does not recur. Deep inhalation or other release-enhancing mechanisms can be helpful.

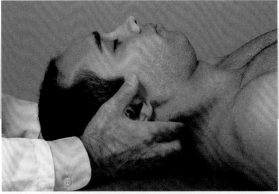

Figure 8.1. Step 2, articular processes.

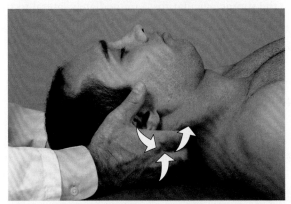

Figure 8.2. Step 4, meeting the barriers.

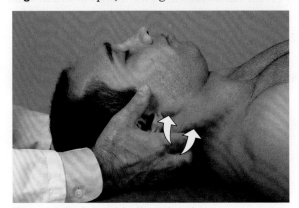

Figure 8.3. Step 5, indirect barrier.

Cervical Region

Anterior Cervical/Supraclavicular Direct

1. The patient lies supine, and the physician sits or stands at the head of the table.

2. The physician abducts the thumbs and places the thumbs and thenar eminences over the clavicles in the supraclavicular fossa immediately lateral to the sternocleidomastoid muscles **(Fig. 8.4)**.

3. The physician applies a downward, slightly posterior force (*arrows*, **Fig. 8.5**) that is vectored toward the feet.

4. The physician moves the hands back and forth from left to right (*arrows*, **Fig. 8.6**) to engage the restrictive barrier.

5. If there appears to be symmetric restriction, both hands can be directed (*arrows*, **Fig. 8.7**) toward the bilateral restriction.

6. As the tension releases, the thumb or thumbs can be pushed farther laterally.

7. This pressure is maintained until no further improvement is noted.

8. The physician reassesses the components of the dysfunction (TART).

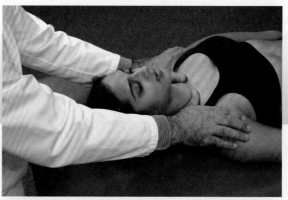

Figure 8.4. Steps 1 and 2.

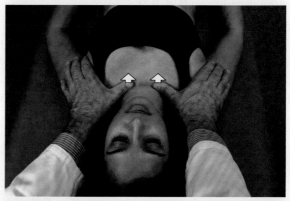

Figure 8.5. Step 3.

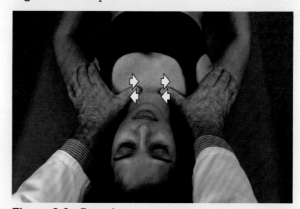

Figure 8.6. Step 4.

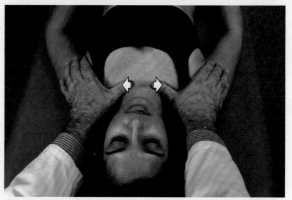

Figure 8.7. Step 5, bilateral tension, if needed.

Thoracic Region

Thoracic Inlet/Outlet
Seated, "Steering Wheel"
Direct or Indirect

 See Video 8.1

1. The patient is seated. The physician stands behind the patient.

2. The physician places the hands palms down over the shoulders, at the angle of the neck and shoulder girdle (cervicothoracic junction) **(Fig. 8.8)**.

3. The physician places the thumbs over the posterior first rib region and places the index and third digits immediately superior and inferior to the clavicle at the sternoclavicular joints bilaterally **(Fig. 8.9)**.

4. The physician lifts upward into the patient's posterior cervical tissues with only enough force to control the skin and underlying fascia so as to not slide across the patient's skin.

5. The physician monitors inferior and superior, left and right circumferential rotation, and torsional (twisting) motion availability for ease-bind symmetric or asymmetric relations.

6. After determining the presence of an ease-bind asymmetry, the physician will either indirectly or directly meet the ease-bind barrier.

7. The force is applied in a very gentle to moderate manner.

8. This force is held for 20 to 60 seconds or until a release is palpated. The physician may continue this and follow any additional release (creep) until it does not recur. Deep inhalation or other release-enhancing mechanisms can be helpful.

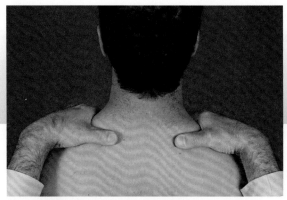

Figure 8.8. Step 2.

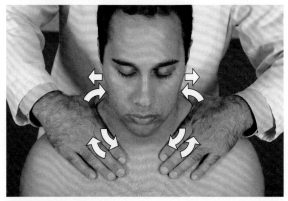

Figure 8.9. Step 3.

Thoracic Region

Prone Regional Thoracic
Direct or Indirect

1. The patient lies prone on the treatment table.

2. The physician stands beside the patient, slightly cephalad to the iliac crests.

3. The physician places both hands palms down with the fingers slightly spread apart immediately paraspinal on each side **(Fig. 8.10)**.

4. The physician imparts a downward force into the patient's thoracic tissues with only enough force to control the skin and underlying fascia so as to not slide across the patient's skin.

5. The physician monitors inferior and superior, left and right circumferential rotation, and torsional (twisting) motion availability for ease-bind clockwise and counterclockwise relations **(Figs. 8.11 and 8.12)**.

6. After determining the presence of an ease-bind asymmetry, the physician will either indirectly or directly meet the ease-bind barrier.

7. The force is applied in a very gentle to moderate manner.

8. This force is held for 20 to 60 seconds or until a release is palpated. The physician may continue this and follow any additional release (creep) until it does not recur. Deep inhalation or other release-enhancing mechanisms can be helpful.

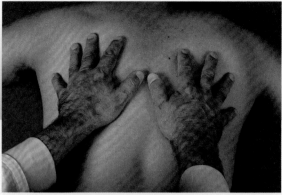

Figure 8.10. Step 3.

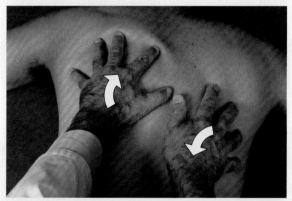

Figure 8.11. Step 5, inferior and superior barriers.

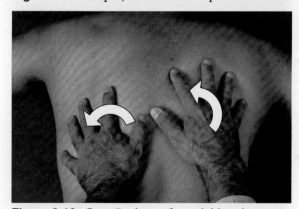

Figure 8.12. Step 5, circumferential barriers.

Thoracic Region

Pectoral, Thoracic/Rib Cage
Supine, Long-Lever Traction
Direct

1. The patient lies supine, and the physician sits or stands at the head of the table.

2. The patient's arms are extended at the elbows and slowly flexed at the shoulder by lifting them upward off the table until meeting a restrictive barrier (normal flexion is approximately 180 degrees) **(Figs. 8.13 and 8.14)**.

3. The physician carefully checks the flexion barrier and then, by adding a traction force in a cephalad direction and rotating the shoulders externally and internally, by extending forearm supination and pronation, attempts to determine where a compound, resultant restrictive barrier exists **(Figs. 8.15 and 8.16)**.

4. The physician is attempting to determine restrictive barriers not only proximally in the shoulder girdle but also in the distal upper extremities as well as the chest cage and abdomen/pelvis. When sensing the restrictive fascial barriers, the physician exerts a force "directly" in a gentle to moderate manner and holds this tension for 20 to 60 seconds or until a release is palpated.

5. To facilitate the reaction, a "*release-enhancing maneuver*" (REM) may be produced by having the patient inhale fully, hold the breath for 5 to 10 seconds, and then exhale.

6. When a release is palpated, the physician should follow it by adding traction and rotational maneuvers to the new restrictive barrier. If preferred, the physician may perform this technique indirectly toward the ease barriers, but in our clinical experience, the direct version is most successful.

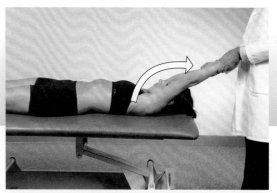

Figure 8.13. Steps 1 and 2, lateral view.

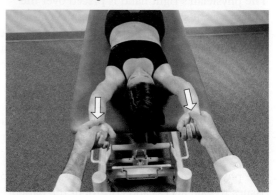

Figure 8.14. Steps 1 and 2, cephalad view.

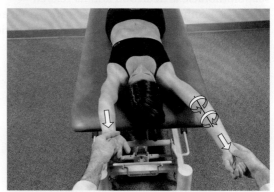

Figure 8.15. Step 3, traction: left abduction; right internal versus external rotation.

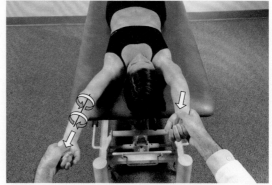

Figure 8.16. Step 3, traction; right abduction; left internal versus external rotation.

Thoracic Region

Scapulothoracic Articulation
Direct

1. The patient lies in the left, lateral recumbent position, and the physician stands facing the patient at the side of the table.

2. The physician's right hand is placed over the patient's right shoulder, anchoring the clavicle with the webbing of the thumb/index finger. The physician's finger pads contact the superior medial angle of the scapula at the insertion of the levator scapula and rhomboid muscles.

3. The physician's left hand is placed under the patient's right arm, and the physician's finger pads are placed at the inferior medial scapular border at the inferior aspect of the scapula **(Fig. 8.17)**.

4. The physician adds a gentle compression into the tissues to gain access and control of the patient's scapulothoracic articulation and its related myofascial components. The physician next takes the scapula inferior/caudal **(Fig. 8.18)** and superior/cephalad **(Fig. 8.19)** and evaluates the ease-bind barrier relationship.

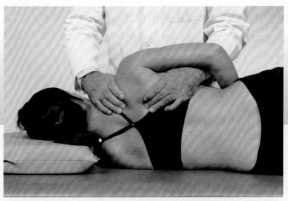

Figure 8.17. Steps 1 to 3, hand placement.

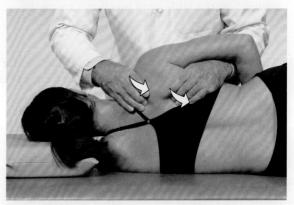

Figure 8.18. Step 4, assess caudal barrier.

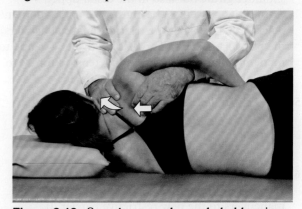

Figure 8.19. Step 4, assess the cephalad barrier.

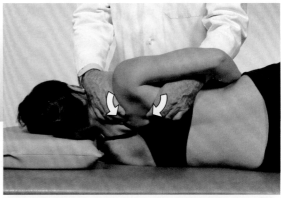

Figure 8.20. Step 5, assess the medial barrier.

5. Next, the physician carries the scapulothoracic articulation toward the spinal midline **(Fig. 8.20)** and then draws the scapula laterally **(Fig. 8.21)** and assesses these ease-bind barriers.

6. After sensing the combined ease-bind relationship, the physician determines the combination of movements that developed the greatest ease-bind asymmetry and then holds the scapulothoracic articulation at the greatest restrictive barrier. When sensing the restrictive fascial barrier(s), the physician exerts a force "directly" in a gentle to moderate manner and holds this tension for 20 to 60 seconds or until a release is palpated.

7. To facilitate the reaction, a "release-enhancing maneuver" (REM) may be produced by having the patient inhale fully, hold the breath for 5 to 10 seconds, and then exhale.

8. When a release is palpated, the physician should follow it by adding tension to the new restrictive barrier. If preferred, the physician may perform this technique indirectly toward the ease barriers, but in our clinical experience, the direct version is most successful.

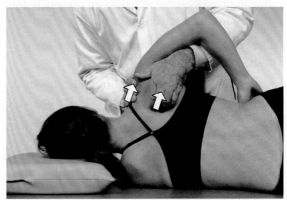

Figure 8.21. Step 5, assess the lateral barrier.

Lumbosacral Region

Lumbosacral/Pelvic Fascia
Supine, Direct or Indirect

1. The patient lies supine, and the physician sits at the side of the patient at the level of the midfemur to knee.

2. The physician asks the patient to bend the knee so the physician's cephalad hand can internally rotate the hip until the pelvis comes off the table.

3. The physician's other hand is placed palm up under the sacrum **(Fig. 8.22)**.

4. After returning the hip to neutral, the physician places the other forearm and hand over the anterior superior iliac spines (ASISs) of the patient's pelvis **(Fig. 8.23)**.

5. The physician leans down on the elbow of the arm that is contacting the sacrum, keeping the sacral hand relaxed and with the forearm monitors for ease-bind asymmetry in left and right rotation **(Fig. 8.24)** and left and right torsion.

6. After determining the presence of an ease-bind asymmetry, the physician will either indirectly or directly meet the ease-bind barrier.

7. The force is applied in a very gentle to moderate manner.

8. This force is held for 20 to 60 seconds or until a release is palpated. The physician may continue this and follow any additional release (creep) until it does not recur. Deep inhalation or other release-enhancing mechanisms can be helpful.

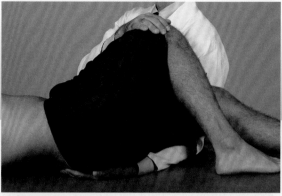

Figure 8.22. Step 3.

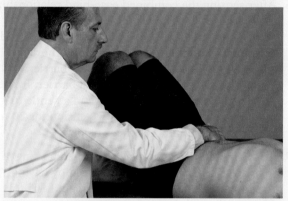

Figure 8.23. Step 4.

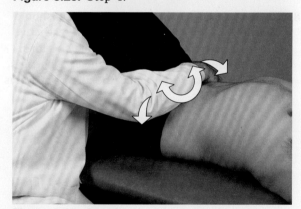

Figure 8.24. Step 5.

Lumbosacral Region

Lumbar/Lumbosacral Fascia
Prone, Direct or Indirect

1. The patient lies prone. The physician stands beside the patient.

2. The physician places one hand over the inferior lumbar segment (e.g., L4–L5) and the other over the superior lumbar segment (e.g., L1–L2) **(Fig. 8.25)**.

3. The physician monitors inferior and superior glide, left and right rotation, and clockwise and counterclockwise motion availability for ease-bind asymmetry **(Fig. 8.26)**.

4. After determining the presence of an ease-bind asymmetry, the physician will either indirectly or directly meet the ease-bind barrier.

5. The force is applied in a very gentle to moderate manner.

6. This force is held for 20 to 60 seconds or until a release is palpated. The physician may continue this and follow any additional release (creep) until it does not recur. Deep inhalation or other release-enhancing mechanisms can be helpful.

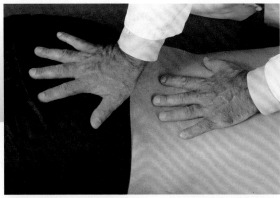

Figure 8.25. Step 2.

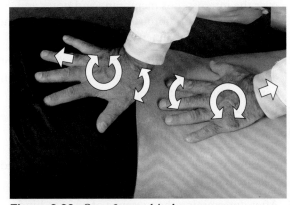

Figure 8.26. Step 3 ease-bind asymmetry.

Upper Extremities

Interosseous Membrane (Radioulnar)
Direct or Indirect

1. The patient is seated or supine. The physician stands or sits in front and to the side of the patient on the affected side.

2. The physician palpates the affected forearm over the interosseous membrane and notes any evidence of a taut, fibrous band, pain, or ease-bind tissue elasticity asymmetry.

3. The physician places the thumbs over the anterior dysfunctional aspect of the interosseous membrane with the palm and fingers encircling the forearm **(Fig. 8.27)**.

4. The physician monitors cephalad and caudad, left and right rotation, and clockwise and counterclockwise motion availability for ease-bind asymmetry **(Fig. 8.28)**.

5. After determining the presence of an ease-bind asymmetry, the physician will either indirectly or directly meet the ease-bind barrier.

6. The force is applied in a very gentle to moderate manner.

7. This force is held for 20 to 60 seconds or until a release is palpated. The physician may continue this and follow any additional release (creep) until it does not recur. Deep inhalation or other release-enhancing mechanisms can be helpful.

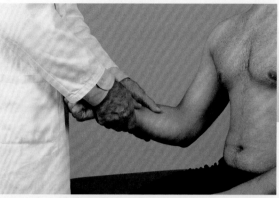

Figure 8.27. Step 3.

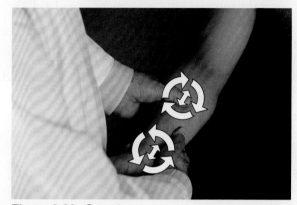

Figure 8.28. Step 4.

Upper Extremities

Wrist, Carpal Tunnel
Direct

 See Video 8.2

1. The patient may sit or lie supine, and the physician stands in front of the patient or at the side, respectively.

2. The patient's hand is placed palm up in the "anatomical position."

3. The physician's thumbs are placed on the medial and lateral attachments of the transverse carpal ligament. On the thenar side, these are the tubercles of the scaphoid and trapezium. On the hypothenar side, they are the pisiform and the hook (hamulus) of the hamate **(Figs. 8.29 and 8.30)**.

4. As the physician's fingers wrap around the dorsal surface of the wrist, the physician exerts tension on the carpal region (especially the flexor retinaculum) by pressing the thumbs into the volar surface of the base of the hand and pushing the thumbs apart (*arrows*), while not sliding the thumbs over the skin, but dragging the skin and superficial fascia with the thumbs **(Fig. 8.31)**.

5. This pressure is maintained for 20 to 60 seconds or until a release of tissue tension is palpated.

6. If the patient has carpal tunnel symptoms of pain or paresthesias during this procedure, the tension should be relaxed, and if symptoms are relieved, repeat the tension holding 20 to 60 seconds or until exacerbation of symptoms, relaxing tension again.

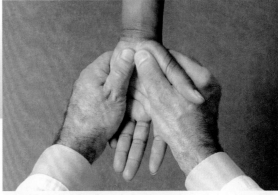
Figure 8.29. Steps 2 and 3.

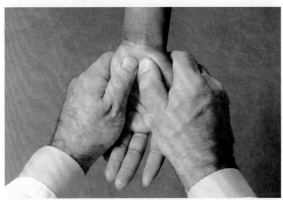
Figure 8.30. Steps 2 and 3, hand placement variation.

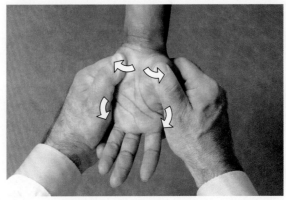
Figure 8.31. Step 4, direct stretching of flexor retinaculum.

Lower Extremities

Gastrocnemius Hypertonicity Direct or Indirect with Traction

1. The patient lies supine, and the physician sits at the side of the table just distal to the patient's calf, facing the head of the table **(Fig. 8.32)**.

2. The physician places both hands side by side under the gastrocnemius muscle. The physician's fingers should be slightly bent (*arrow*, Fig. 14.75) (*arrow*, **Fig. 8.33**), and the weight of the leg should rest on the physician's fingertips.

3. The physician's fingers apply an upward force (*arrow at left*, **Fig. 8.34**) into the muscle and then pull inferiorly (*arrow at right*), using the weight of the leg to compress the area.

4. This pressure is maintained until a release occurs.

5. The physician reassesses the components of the dysfunction (TART).

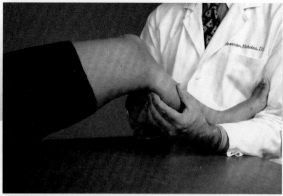

Figure 8.32. Step 1.

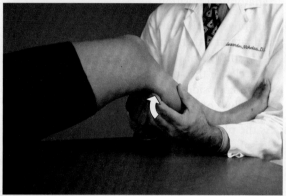

Figure 8.33. Step 2.

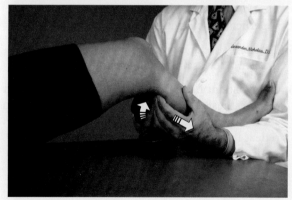

Figure 8.34. Step 3.

Lower Extremities

Supine Leg Traction

1. The patient lies supine on the treatment table, and the physician stands at the patient's feet.

2. The physician's hands (palms up) reach under and control the patient's Achilles and calcaneal region.

3. The physician lifts both lower legs to 20 to 30 degrees off the table **(Fig. 8.35)**.

4. The physician gently leans backward, adding slight traction through the leg, to affect tension in the lower leg, hip, and sacroiliac joints **(Fig. 8.36)**.

5. The physician may add internal and/or external rotation and abduction and/or adduction through the leg and attempt to discern any ease-bind asymmetry in these movements and at what level of the pelvis, hip, knee, or other structures it may be most evident **(Fig. 8.37)**.

6. After determining the presence of an ease-bind asymmetry, the physician will either indirectly or directly meet the ease-bind barrier **(Fig. 8.38)**.

7. The force is applied in a very gentle to moderate manner.

8. This force is held for 20 to 60 seconds or until a release is palpated. The physician may continue this and follow any additional release (creep) until it does not recur. Deep inhalation or other release-enhancing mechanisms can be helpful.

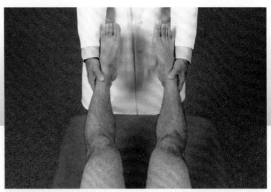
Figure 8.35. Step 3.

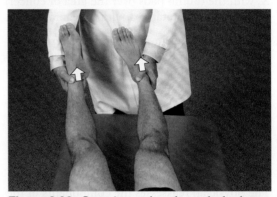
Figure 8.36. Step 4, traction through the leg.

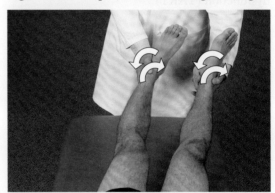
Figure 8.37. Step 5 internal/external rotation and abduction/adduction.

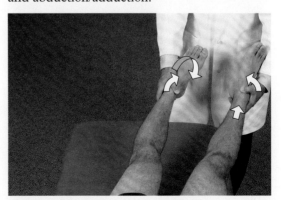
Figure 8.38. Step 6 indirect and direct barriers.

Lower Extremities

Plantar Fasciitis
Direct

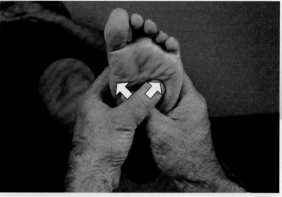

Figure 8.39. Steps 1 to 3.

1. The patient lies supine, and the physician sits at the foot of the table.

2. The physician's thumbs are crossed, making an **X**, with the thumb pads over the area of concern (tarsal to distal metatarsal) at the plantar fascia.

3. The thumbs impart an inward force (*arrows*, **Fig. 8.39**) that is vectored distal and lateral. This pressure is continued until the restrictive (bind) barrier is met.

4. The pressure is held until a release is palpated.

5. This is repeated with the foot alternately attempting plantar flexion **(Fig. 8.40)** and dorsiflexion **(Fig. 8.41)**.

6. The physician reassesses the components of the dysfunction (TART).

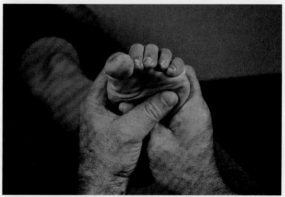

Figure 8.40. Step 5, plantar flexion.

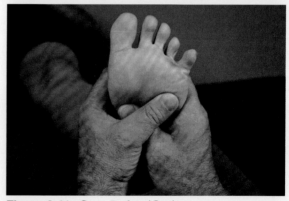

Figure 8.41. Step 5, dorsiflexion.

Cranial Region

Cranial Fascia
Direct or Indirect

1. The patient lies supine, and the physician sits at the head of the table.

2. The physician places the hands palm down on the patient's head in the "vault hold" **(Fig. 8.42)**.

3. The physician gently directs a compression force into the cranial soft tissues to engage the superficial fascia.

4. The physician then adds a right and then left rotation force through the tissues to determine if there are restrictive and/or asymmetric fascial barriers **(Fig. 8.43)**.

5. Next, by guiding the hands superior and inferior, the physician determines if there are side bending **(Fig. 8.44)** components and then, with medial and lateral wrist glide motions, checks for flexion/ extension barriers **(Fig. 8.45)**.

6. These motions can be treated individually or by determining their compound restrictive barriers.

7. After determining the presence of an ease-bind asymmetry, the physician will either indirectly or directly meet the ease-bind barrier.

8. The force is applied in a very gently to moderate manner, and the physician will continue this until a release is palpated (fascial creep) and continue to follow this creep until it does not recur. This is held for 20 to 60 seconds or until a release is palpated.

9. The physician should then reevaluate the patient's fascial barriers to see if a positive change has occurred.

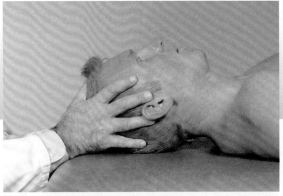

Figure 8.42. Steps 1 and 2, lateral view, "vault hold."

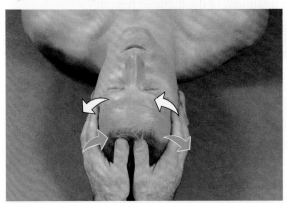

Figure 8.43. Step 4, assess rotational barriers.

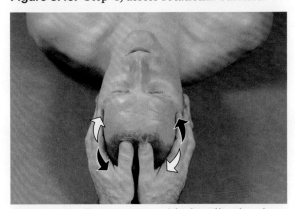

Figure 8.44. Step 5, assess side-bending barriers.

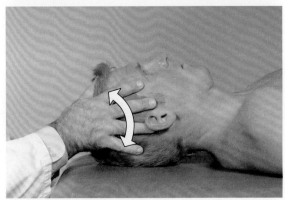

Figure 8.45. Step 5, assess flexion/extension barriers.

Additional Regional Applications

Additional Myofascial Release Techniques

Figures 8.46 to 8.56 show the continued principles of myofascial release (direct, indirect) but are without written descriptions. Just use the *arrows* as a guide to the many vectored force applications that can be effective for treatment of the pictured region.

See Video 8.3
(Thoracolumbar Region)

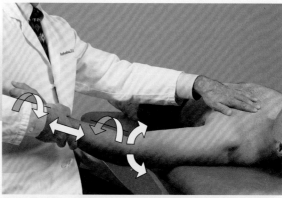

Figure 8.46. Sternoclavicular joint and arm traction.

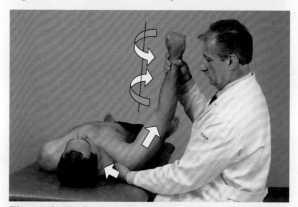

Figure 8.47. Long axis release.

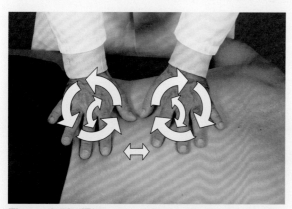

Figure 8.50. Thoracolumbar release.

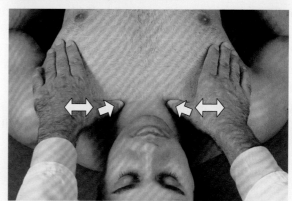

Figure 8.48. Scalene release.

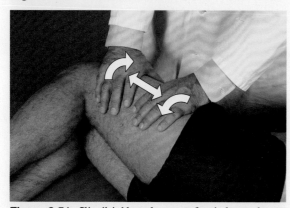

Figure 8.51. Iliotibial band-tensor fascia lata release.

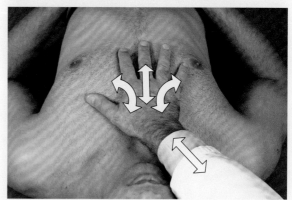

Figure 8.49. Sternal release.

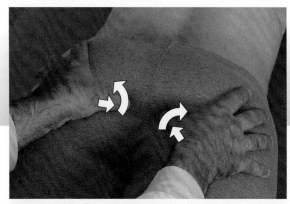

Figure 8.52. Sacral-coccygeal release.

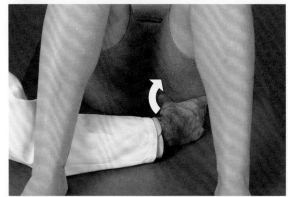

Figure 8.53. Ischiorectal fossa (pelvic diaphragm) release.

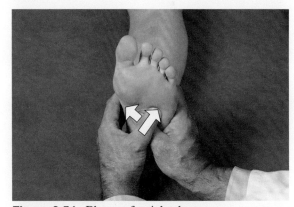

Figure 8.54. Plantar fascial release.

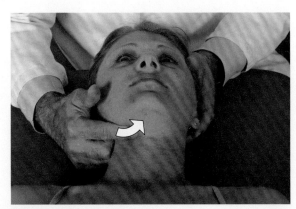

Figure 8.56. Hyoid release.

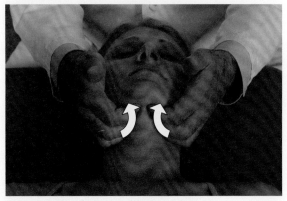

Figure 8.55. Submandibular release.

References

1. Williams PL, ed. Gray's Anatomy. 38th ed. London, UK: Churchill Livingstone, 1995.
2. Rosse C, Gaddum-Rosse P. Hollingshead's Textbook of Anatomy. 5th ed. Philadelphia, PA: Lippincott-Raven, 1997.
3. Ward R, exec. ed. Foundations for Osteopathic Medicine. 2nd ed. Philadelphia, PA: Lippincott Williams & Wilkins, 2003.
4. DeStefano L. Greenman's Principles of Manual Medicine. Baltimore, MD: Lippincott Williams & Wilkins, 2011.
5. Glossary of Osteopathic Terminology. Educational Council on Osteopathic Principles of the American Association of Colleges of Osteopathic Medicine, www.aacom.org
6. Chila AG, exec. ed. Foundations of Osteopathic Medicine. 3rd ed. Baltimore, MD: Lippincott Williams & Wilkins, 2011.

Counterstrain Techniques

Technique Principles

Counterstrain technique was proposed by Lawrence H. Jones, DO, FAAO (1912 to 1996). Jones initially believed that a patient could be placed in a position of comfort so as to alleviate the symptoms. After noticing a dramatic clinical response, he studied the nature of musculoskeletal dysfunctions and determined that tender points could be elicited by prodding with the fingertip (1). These tender points were eventually collated into local areas of tenderness, which are related to segmental and musculotendinous areas of somatic dysfunction. Tender points are usually found within tendinous attachments, the belly of a muscle, and often ligaments. They are described as discrete points, about the size of a fingertip, that are exquisitely tender, tense, and edematous (2). The patient may not have conscious pain at the tender point location, and the area immediately surrounding the tender point, when palpated, is relatively normal and painless in comparison. Tender points may be related to the trigger points proposed by Travell and Simons (3) but are generally discussed as separate entities in the osteopathic community.

This technique was originally termed by Dr. Jones as "Spontaneous Release by Positioning," later termed strain/counterstrain, and also has been referred to as Jones technique. The Educational Council on Osteopathic Principles (ECOP) has defined this technique as "a system of diagnosis and treatment that considers the dysfunction to be a continuing, inappropriate strain reflex, which is inhibited by applying a position of mild strain in the direction exactly opposite to that of the reflex; this is accompanied by specific directed positioning about the point of tenderness to achieve the desired therapeutic response." There are many postulates as to how the technique works, but most involve the alpha Ia afferent and gamma efferent relationships and nociception (1,2). There may be other aspects at play, including the Golgi tendon organ, bioelectric phenomena, and fluid aspects, such as the lymphatics and interstitial fluid exchange.

Jones postulated a mechanism of injury concerning these tender points and theorized how the technique elicits the appropriate response based on the previously mentioned physiologic principles. These ideas were described as follows (2,4):

1. An event produces specific or generalized, rapid shortening in the myofascial component(s), while, simultaneously, the tissues directly opposite may be lengthened.
2. Afferent feedback indicates possible myofascial damage from a "strain" (stress).
3. The body tries to prevent the myofascial damage by rapidly contracting the myofascial tissues affected resulting in relative hypershortening of the stressed myofascial component (agonist).
4. In response, a (rapid) lengthening in the opposing muscle (antagonist) is produced.
5. Thereby, an inappropriate reflex is created that is manifested as a tender point in the antagonist muscle.
6. The end result is hypertonic myofascial tissue and restricted motion.

Glover and Rennie have proposed the following neurophysiologic basis for the development of the tender point (2):

1. Trauma produces change in myofascial tissue at the microscopic and biochemical levels.
2. Force of trauma causes damage to myofibrils and their microcirculation.
3. A neurochemical response is triggered to preserve further tissue injury and repair damaged tissues. Tissue oxygen/pH low—bradykinin formed and substance P released, which results in vasodilation and tissue edema. Prostaglandins are released to further the inflammatory response.
4. Resultant edema from tissue damage reduces normal circulation by compressing arterioles, capillaries, venules, and lymphatic vessels.
5. Tissue injury and the presence of these chemicals lower the sensitization to mechanical stimulation.

151

6. The tissue disruption and the subsequent metabolic and chemical changes produce nociceptive activity, which can result in increased sensitivity to touch or a *tender point*.
7. The damage to the microcirculation changes the intramuscular pressure and can produce muscle fatigue due to decreased cellular metabolism.
8. These metabolic changes affect the chemical matrix around the myofibrils and can produce nociceptive activity resulting in tenderness.

The Educational Council on Osteopathic Principles at its biannual meeting in April 2014, after review of the current research and literature, approved a consensus document that summarizes the various theories for the development of a tender point and the proposed mechanisms for the clinical efficacy of counterstrain.

The proprioceptive theory proposes that tender points develop when local muscle fibers are maintained in a hypertonic state due to an inappropriate proprioceptive reflex during the initiation of somatic dysfunction or an injury.

There are two phases in the development of a tender point:

1. Sudden lengthening of a shortened muscle, or overstretching or overloading of a muscle
2. Defensively initiated contraction of that muscle in an effort to prevent injury

As Muscle A (e.g., the biceps) is suddenly lengthened, its muscle spindles' intrafusal fibers are also stretched. To avoid injury, Muscle A then reflexively contracts through a defensively initiated protective reflex (nocifensive) activation of alpha motor neurons.

The reflexive contraction of Muscle A, such as biceps (and its synergists), results in a sudden lengthening of the opposing muscle, Muscle B (triceps). The sudden lengthening of Muscle B may also cause it to reflexively contract.

This altered motor neuron activity maintains the two opposing muscle contractions and may lead to tender points in Muscle A and/or B. This altered activity can persist after the original injury heals.

Counterstrain treatment uses precise body positioning to shorten the strained muscle and reduce the muscle spindle activity and abnormal muscle contractions of both Muscles A and B.

The sustained abnormal metabolism theory suggests that tissue injury alters local body position, affecting local microcirculation and tissue metabolism. Due to the creation of a degree of localized ischemia, local nutrient supply and metabolic waste removal is reduced. Proinflammatory cytokine production is increased. These changes lower the firing threshold of sensory neurons causing localized neuronal sensitization. During palpation, these changes manifest as localized edema and tenderness. The precise body positioning used in

counterstrain improves local vascular circulation and reduces localized production of inflammatory mediators.

The impaired ligamentomuscular reflex theory is similar to the proprioceptive theory. This theory, however, proposes that dysfunction may result from a protective reflex that occurs when ligaments and related myofascial structures are placed under strain. A localized strain in a ligament can reflexively inhibit muscular contractions that increase the ligamentous strain and can stimulate muscular contractions that reduce the strain.

In summary, counterstrain tender point sensitivity represents an alteration in myofascial tissue function that reflects multiple underlying factors, both local and distant. After injury, nocifensive response is coupled with circulatory alterations, increased muscle tone, and/or ligamentous injury. This creates a degree of ischemia with reduced muscle work capacity, increased tissue sensitivity, and altered muscle spindle and proprioceptive activity in the injured myofascial tissues, resulting in the generation of tender points.

As counterstrain may be described as a technique that identifies and treats tender points associated with a somatic dysfunction, we note that other than the myofascial component, most of the other components of the dysfunction may be inadvertently ignored by some using this technique. Because of this, asymmetry of the structural components, the relationship of tissue texture changes (chronic and acute phenomena), and, most importantly, regional and intersegmental motion restriction/asymmetry tend not to be considered in the "comfort-based" positioning in this style of osteopathic treatment. Therefore, counterstrain tends to be viewed mostly by its myofascial components (the myofascial structure where the tender point is located, etc.), which have been the determining factors for the various classical treatment positions.

Jones believed that putting the joint into its position of greatest comfort would reduce the continuing inappropriate proprioceptor activity. As Glover and Rennie report, Jones made another discovery: the anterior aspects of the body must be evaluated even if the symptoms are posterior (2,5). Jones eventually mapped many local areas of tenderness to which he related segmental and/or myofascial dysfunction. His tender point locations and their relation to dysfunction do not typically use the x-, y-, and z-axis parameters of flexion/extension, rotation, and side bending that are common to articular, positional, and motion-based definitions of somatic dysfunction (describing motion restriction and asymmetry). As counterstrain is also used for muscular (myofascial) dysfunctions and there are overlaps between the two types of dysfunctions, tender points can be confused with one another. This has caused some confusion, and terms like *maverick tender points* have been used to resolve the fact that the classic position does not always eliminate the tender point. For example, a hypertonic deep cervical muscle may be tender in an area similar to that of a superficial or intermediate muscle or the reflex tender point from a cervical dysfunction of a primary articular component. But the positions to alleviate the pain may be opposite each other, or in a totally different position. Therefore, recognizing this fact should dramatically reduce the perception of maverick tender points, and the physician's understanding of tender points should include and recognize the specific superficial to deep muscle–tender point relations as well as the articular relations. Jones refers in some areas to specific muscles, yet in the vertebral regions, he seems to stay more focused on articular spinal segmental levels of dysfunction.

In clinical examination, a tender point often presents on the open-faceted (stretched) side of the dysfunctional segment. For example, a C5, FSRRR dysfunction will most frequently exhibit a tender point on the left side of the patient's cervical spine. Therefore, with an FSRRR dysfunction, the facet on the right side is closed, and the facet on the left side is opened. In this case, the tender point is on the side of the restricted coupled motion.

Therefore, another criterion that we find clinically important in this technique is proper association of the dysfunctional pattern to the treatment position in the various articular types of dysfunctions. As these articular aspects are important components in the complete diagnosis of somatic dysfunction and students must spend much time understanding their neutral and nonneutral coupled relationships, we believe that by including these in the diagnostic and treatment armamentarium, the osteopathic physician may increase the total therapeutic effect. Neutral and nonneutral dysfunctions (Types I and II, respectively) may have specific tender points and positions that alleviate the tender point. Yet, in most published texts (1,2,4–6), there is little mention of the change in position for opposite-sided coupling (Type I) and same-sided coupling (Type II) of rotation and side bending. The most widespread idea is that flexion dysfunctions produce anterior tender points and extension dysfunctions produce posterior tender points. However, in which directions do the neutral dysfunctions exhibit tender points? Over many years of teaching osteopathic manipulative medicine in the laboratory at Philadelphia College of Osteopathic Medicine as well as in our European osteopathic seminars, we have done a number of small, nonblinded surveys of the class attendants when teaching this subject. From our limited findings, we believe that neutral dysfunctions can produce anterior and posterior tender points. This may be an area of further study and potential research.

Review of the many positions for counterstrain treatment shows that some positions are examples of treatment of Type I dysfunctions (e.g., side bend toward, rotate away [STRA]), and others are examples of treatment of Type II dysfunctions (e.g., side bend, rotate away [SARA]). The most important aspect of any technique is the diagnosis. Without a proper diagnosis, the

determination of the key dysfunction, and the determination of whether the primary component is articular, myofascial, or both, the treatment will be less than optimal.

Technique Classification

Indirect

As previously discussed, the patient positioning in counterstrain technique to eliminate the tender point may be directed to a dysfunctional myofascial component that resulted from some stress where an abnormal painful reflex (e.g., alpha-gamma) has been initiated. In treating with counterstrain, the approach would be to shorten and reduce the tension in the lengthened myofascial structure (muscle) or to do the same to the articular dysfunction's components with its -x, y-, and z-axes of motion freedom; thus, the patient positioning is away from the bind or restriction and toward the ease or freedom. By ECOP definitions, this would put counterstrain in the indirect category of treatment. The physician should know, prior to positioning the patient, whether the dysfunction is a primary or secondary myofascial component (e.g., psoas hypertonicity causing lumbar symptoms) and/or whether there is primary articular Type I or II dysfunction, as the corrective positions may vary accordingly.

Technique Styles

Time Defined or Release Defined

The physician may use a time-defined method, in which the treatment position is held for 90 seconds and then repositioned to the neutral starting position for reassessment. Alternatively, the physician may use a palpatory marker of tissue release, which may occur prior to the 90-second time-defined marker. After feeling a sense of release, relaxation, pulsation, or similar phenomenon, the physician may forgo the time definition and reposition the patient for reassessment.

Indications

1. Acute, subacute, and chronic somatic dysfunctions of articular and/or myofascial origin
2. Adjunctive treatment of systemic complaints with associated somatic dysfunction (e.g., viscerosomatic reflex causing rib dysfunction)

Contraindications

Absolute Contraindications

1. Traumatized (sprained or strained) tissues, which would be negatively affected by the positioning of the patient
2. Severe illness in which strict positional restrictions preclude treatment

3. Instability of the area being positioned that has the potential to produce unwanted neurologic or vascular side effects
4. Vascular or neurologic syndromes, such as basilar insufficiency or neuroforaminal compromise whereby the position of treatment has the potential to exacerbate the condition
5. Severe degenerative spondylosis with local fusion and no motion at the level where treatment positioning would normally take place

Relative Contraindications/Precautions

1. Patients who cannot voluntarily relax, so that proper positioning is difficult
2. Stoic patients who cannot discern the level of pain or its change secondary to positioning
3. Patients who cannot understand the instructions and questions of the physician (e.g., patient 6 months of age)
4. Patients with connective tissue disease, arthritis, Parkinson disease, and so on, in whom positioning for tender point pain reduction exacerbates the distal connective tissue or arthritic problem or no motion is available for positioning

General Considerations and Rules

The physician must ascertain the somatic dysfunction, its severity, its tissue location and type, and whether any of these precautions or contraindications are present. If warranted, the following sequence is necessary:

1. Find the most significant tender point with the patient in a neutral, comfortable position.
    a. Locate one or more tender points associated with the previously diagnosed somatic dysfunction by testing with a few ounces of firm but discreet finger pad or thumb pressure. No circular motion should be part of this pressure; it is straight into the tender point.
    b. If multiple tender points exist, treat the most painful first. When several tender points lie in a row, first treat the one in the middle. In addition, treat proximal before distal (2).
    c. Quantify the tender point's pain level for the patient as 100%, 10, or a monetary unit such as $1. We have found that the monetary unit works best in the teaching of counterstrain, as physicians and physicians in training tend to confuse the analog pain scale, in which the patient is asked to gauge his or her pain on a scale of 0 to 10, with the assigned pain of 10. With use of the analog scale, the tendency is to ask, "What is your pain?" instead of saying, "This pain is a 10." With the monetary scale, this does not occur.

2. Slowly and carefully, place the patient in the position of ease or optimal comfort.
    a. First obtain a gross reduction of tenderness in the classic treatment position recommended for the level of dysfunction and tender point location and then fine-tune through small arcs of motion until the tenderness (pain) is *completely alleviated.*
    b. If the tender point cannot be eliminated, a 70% reduction of pain may be acceptable for treatment effect. However, for every ascending numeric level of pain that remains, an associated 10% of treatment effectiveness is lost. For example, if the tender point is reduced only by 70%, there is only a 70% potential for a good treatment effect. Anything <70% reduction causes an even greater potential for treatment failure. Therefore, the goal is 100% pain reduction by positioning whenever possible.
    c. In general, anterior points require some level of flexion, depending on the segmental level involved, and posterior points require some level of extension, depending on the segment involved.
    d. As tender points move away from the midline, the greater is the possibility for necessity of more side bending. However, the nature of the dysfunction (Type I or II) and its motion parameters dictate the proper positioning.

3. Maintain the position for 90 seconds. It had been reported that 120 seconds is necessary for costal dysfunctions. Personal communication with various members of ECOP and with those who worked closely with Jones shows that costal dysfunctions also take 90 seconds. Jones believed that the positions for treatment of costal dysfunctions caused the patient to be unable to easily relax, and therefore, he gave them an additional 30 seconds to relax. Therefore, the 120-second period has been promoted as the classically described time-defined method for rib dysfunctions, whereas clinically, 90 seconds will suffice. The 90-second time frame is now the standard for all dysfunctions treated with counterstrain technique (7). In our hands and experience, the time-defined method works better than feeling for a tissue release. We believe that Jones's attempts at various time increments and his conclusion that holding the position for 90 seconds was the most effective method must have a reason. We believe that most problems diagnosed and successfully treated with this technique involve the resetting of neurologic feedback mechanisms earlier identified and that use of these mechanisms requires an optimum amount of time to achieve the desired clinical outcome. Other techniques that may appear similar to counterstrain

(e.g., facilitated positional release) use different release-enhancing mechanisms, and so they cannot be compared exactly with counterstrain.

4. While maintaining the effective position, the finger pad should remain at the site of the tender point for the entire treatment period whenever possible, so the physician may intermittently throughout the treatment period (perhaps every 30 seconds) recheck the level of pain at the tender point.
   a. The finger pad is not putting any therapeutic pressure into the tissues.
   b. If the finger pad is removed, the physician loses control of the tender point, rendering the evaluation useless, as the tender point location may not be exactly relocated. Also, the patient often does not believe the physician is on the original tender point and may question the exact location of the monitoring finger. Staying vigilant at the site, you can confidently assure the patient that you are indeed on the original site.
   c. Also, if using the tissue release marker instead of time, the physician must have the finger pad on the tender point site to constantly sense the tissue reaction.
5. After 90 seconds (time-defined treatment) or when tissue appears to release (release-defined treatment), slowly return the passive patient through a path of least resistance to the original neutral position in which the tender point was elicited. The patient must not help, so if you feel that the patient is helping you, stop and ask him or her to relax.
6. Recheck the tender point. If the tender point was reduced to 0 initially, there is a good chance that it will remain at 0. It is possible, however, that the pain will elevate somewhat posttreatment. If the posttreatment pain is rated at 3 compared to the originally assigned level of 10 prior to treatment, 70% effectiveness was achieved in only 90 seconds. The effect may continue to improve the patient's symptoms over time, or the patient may need follow-up in a few days for reevaluation and treatment.
7. Recheck the somatic dysfunction parameters originally present (e.g., the segmental or myofascial dysfunction).

The shorthand rules are as follows:

1. Find the tender point associated with the dysfunction.
2. Tell the patient the tender point is a 10 or 100 or a dollar's worth of pain.
3. Place the patient in the position that reduces the pain of the tender point 100%, or as close to 100% as possible, but at least 70%.

4. Hold this position for 90 seconds.
5. Slowly, through a path of least resistance, return the relaxed patient to neutral.
6. Recheck the tender point and the other diagnostic components of the dysfunction (ART).

Posttreatment reaction may include general soreness through the following 24 to 48 hours. This is unusual in our clinical experience but has been reported by others (1). Treating more than six tender points at one visit appears to be correlated to this reaction. If this occurs, instruct the patient to increase fluids and use ice packs over the sore areas for 15 to 20 minutes every 3 hours as needed. Treatments should be prescribed according to the physician's clinical judgment, but 3-day intervals are appropriate. The patient's response will determine how often the patient needs treatment.

Abbreviations for Counterstrain Technique

Yates and Glover introduced a shorthand description that many students use to help remember the positioning for specifically located tender points. This shorthand uses the initials for types of motions (directions of movement) and upper and lower case for greater and lesser movement in the direction identified, respectively. The common abbreviations of this shorthand method are A, anterior; P, posterior; F or f, flexion; E or e, extension; SR or Sr, side bending right; SL or Sl, side bending left; RR or Rr, rotation right; RL or Rl, rotation left; IR or ir, internal rotation; ER or er, external rotation; ABD or Abd, abduction; ADD or Add, adduction; SUP or sup, supination; and PRO or pro, pronation. Specific abbreviations refer to motion toward (t-T) or away (a-A) from the side of the tender point. Uppercase letters mean more of that particular motion and lower case means less (6). Other abbreviations refer to obvious bony landmarks, such as spinous process (SP), transverse process (TP), iliac crest (CR), and occiput (OCC).

The following techniques are described and illustrated in a stepwise sequence. We have abridged the text describing each individual technique, as the counterstrain sequence is the same for each dysfunction. The unique factors of each dysfunction are the location of the tender point and the classic treatment position. This first technique will illustrate the complete counterstrain sequence with the unique aspect of the technique highlighted. All of the following techniques will be described with only the information unique to that specific somatic dysfunction and its tender point. The tender point locations are a compilation of descriptions from Jones et al. (1), Rennie and Glover (5), Yates and Glover (6), Myers (4), Snider and Glover (10) and our clinical findings.

Anterior Cervical Region

Anterior Cervical Tender Points

Anterior cervical (AC) counterstrain tender points are outlined in Table 9.1 and illustrated in **Figure 9.1**.

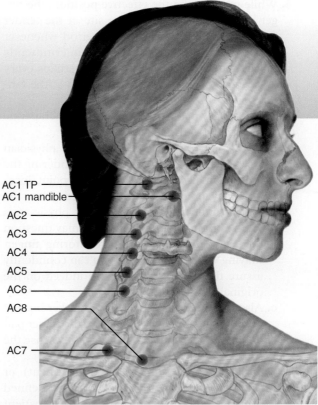

Figure 9.1. Anterior cervical counterstrain tender points. (Modified with permission from Ref. (8).)

Table 9.1 Common Anterior Cervical Tender Points

Tender Point	Location	Classic Treatment Position	Acronym
Anterior cervical 1 AC1 mandible AC1 transverse process	On the posterior aspect of the ascending ramus of the mandible at the level of the earlobe On the lateral aspect of the C1 transverse process midway between the ramus of the mandible and the mastoid process	Marked rotation away; fine-tune with minimal flexion and side bending away	RA
Anterior cervical 2–6 AC2–AC6	On the anterior lateral aspect of the anterior/posterior tubercles of the transverse process of the corresponding cervical vertebrae	Flex to level of the dysfunctional segment; side bend away, rotate away	F Sa Ra
Anterior cervical 7 AC7	On the posterosuperior surface of the clavicle at the clavicular attachment of the sternocleidomastoid muscle	Flex to the level of C7; side bend toward, rotate way	F St Ra
Anterior cervical 8 AC8	On the superior medial end of the clavicle at the sternal attachment of the sternocleidomastoid muscle	Flex, but less than AC7; side bend away, rotate away	f-F Sa Ra

Anterior Cervical Region

AC1 Mandible, AC1 Transverse Process

 See Video 9.1

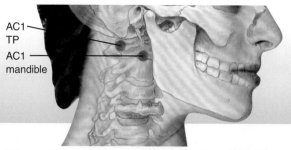

Figure 9.2. AC1 tender point location. (Modified with permission from Ref. (8).)

Indication for Treatment

Somatic dysfunction of the cervical spine (C1). The patient may present with frontal or migraine headaches and blurring of vision and may mimic temporomandibular joint dysfunction (4,5).

Tender Point Location

AC1 Mandible: On the posterior surface of the ascending ramus of the mandible at or just below the level of the earlobe associated with the rectus capitis anterior muscle (4) **(Fig. 9.2)**. Press posterior to anterior.
AC1 Transverse Process: On the lateral aspect of the C1 transverse process midway between the ramus of the mandible and the mastoid process associated with the rectus capitis lateralis muscle (4,5). Press lateral to medial.

Counterstrain Sequence

1. The patient is supine, and the physician sits at the head of the treatment table.
2. The physician presses the appropriate tender point with the pad of one finger with a few ounces of pressure to quantify the initial level of tenderness at 100% or 10 on a scale of 0 to 10.
3. The physician releases the pressure but maintains light contact on the tender point, monitoring it throughout the treatment.
4. The patient's head is rotated 90 degrees away from the tender point.
5. The physician fine-tunes through small arcs of motion (more or less rotation with slight flexion and/or side bending away) until the tenderness has been *completely alleviated* or reduced as close to 100% as possible, but at least 70% **(Figs. 9.3 to 9.5)**.
6. The physician maintains this position for at least 90 seconds while the patient remains totally relaxed.
7. After 90 seconds, the physician slowly returns the patient passively to the neutral position, through the path of least resistance. The physician reminds the patient to remain totally relaxed and not assist in any way.
8. The physician reevaluates the tender point and the other diagnostic components of the dysfunction (ART) to determine the effectiveness of the technique. Typically, at least 70% reduction of the original tenderness is required for successful treatment of the dysfunction.

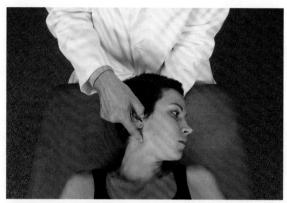

Figure 9.3. AC1: RA.

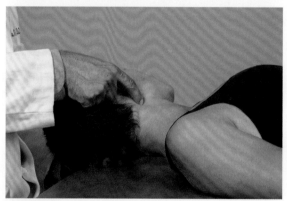

Figure 9.4. AC1: RA.

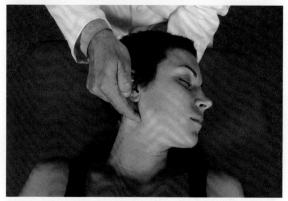

Figure 9.5. AC1: f RA.

Anterior Cervical Region

AC2–AC6

 See Video 9.2

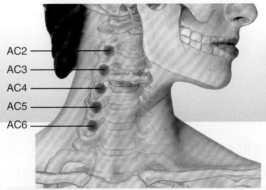

Figure 9.6. AC2–AC6 tender points. (Modified with permission from Ref. (8).)

Indication for Treatment

Somatic dysfunction of the cervical spine (C2 to C6). The patient may present with posterolateral neck pain.

Tender Point Location

On the anterior lateral aspect of the anterior/posterior tubercles of the transverse process of the corresponding dysfunctional cervical vertebrae. **AC2** is associated with the middle scalene and longus colli muscles; **AC3 and AC4** are associated with the anterior, middle scalenes; longus capitis and longus colli muscles; **AC5 and AC6** are associated with anterior, middle, posterior scalenes; longus capitis and longus colli muscles. Press posterior and medial **(Fig. 9.6)**.

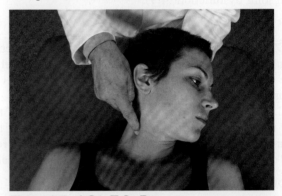

Figure 9.7. AC4: F Sa Ra.

Treatment Position: F Sa Ra

1. The patient's head and neck are flexed to the level of the dysfunctional segment, side bent, and rotated away from the tender point **(Figs. 9.7 to 9.10)**.

2. The physician fine-tunes through small arcs of motion (more or less flexion, side bending and rotation away) until the tenderness has been *completely alleviated* or reduced as close to 100% as possible, but at least 70%.

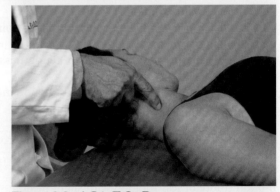

Figure 9.8. AC4: F Sa Ra.

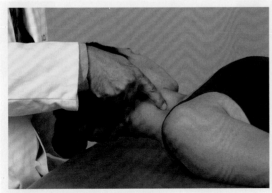

Figure 9.10. AC6: F Sa Ra.

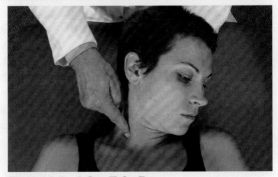

Figure 9.9. AC6: F Sa Ra.

Anterior Cervical Region

AC7

See Video 9.3

Indication for Treatment

Somatic dysfunction of the cervical spine. The patient may present with pain in the lower cervical region.

Tender Point Location

On the posterosuperior surface of the clavicle at the clavicular attachment of the sternocleidomastoid muscle. Press superior to inferior **(Fig. 9.11)**.

Treatment Position: F St Ra

1. The patient's head and neck are markedly flexed to the level of C7, rotated away, and side bent toward the side of the tender point **(Figs. 9.12 to 9.14)**.

2. The physician fine-tunes through small arcs of motion (more or less flexion, side bending toward and rotation away) until the tenderness has been *completely alleviated* or reduced as close to 100% as possible, but at least 70%.

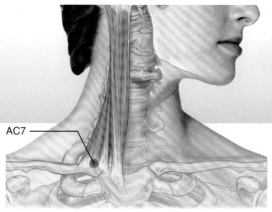
Figure 9.11. AC7 tender point. (Modified with permission from Ref. (8).)

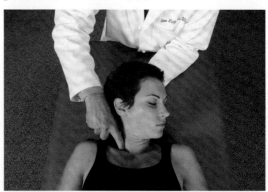
Figure 9.12. AC7: F St Ra.

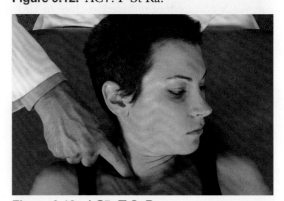
Figure 9.13. AC7: F St Ra.

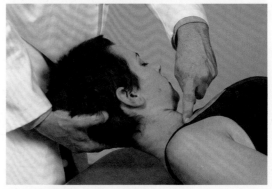
Figure 9.14. AC7: F St Ra (alternative hand placement).

Anterior Cervical Region

AC8

 See Video 9.3

Indication for Treatment

Somatic dysfunction of the cervical spine. Clinical presentation is similar to that of AC7.

Tender Point Location

On the superior medial end of the clavicle at the sternal attachment of the sternocleidomastoid muscle. Press posterior, inferior, and lateral **(Fig. 9.15)**.

Treatment Position: f-F Sa Ra

1. The patient's head and neck are flexed (<C7), rotated away, and side bent away from the side of tender point **(Figs. 9.16 to 9.18)**.

2. The physician fine-tunes through small arcs of motion (more or less flexion, side bending, and rotation away) until the tenderness has been *completely alleviated* or reduced as close to 100% as possible, but at least 70%.

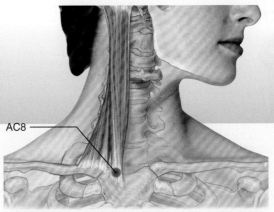

Figure 9.15. AC8 tender point. (Modified with permission from Ref. (8).)

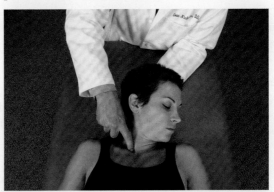

Figure 9.16. AC8: f-F Sa Ra.

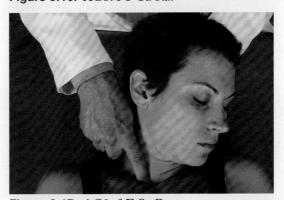

Figure 9.17. AC8: f-F Sa Ra.

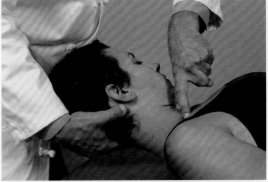

Figure 9.18. AC8: f-F Sa Ra (alternative hand placement).

Posterior Cervical Region

Posterior Cervical Tender Points

Posterior cervical tender points are outlined in Table 9.2 and illustrated in **Figure 9.19**.

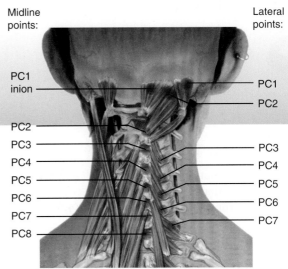

Figure 9.19. Posterior cervical counterstrain tender points. (Modified with permission from Ref. (8).)

Table 9.2 Common Posterior Cervical Tender Points

Tender Point	Location	Classic Treatment Position	Acronym
PC1 inion	On the inferior nuchal line, lateral to the inion	Flexion of the occipitoatlantal articulation; fine-tune with side bending toward, rotation away	F St Ra
PC1 (occiput)	On the inferior nuchal line midway between inion and mastoid, associated with the splenius capitis and/or rectus capitis posterior major/minor and obliquus capitis superior muscles (4,5)	Extension of occipitoatlantal articulation with mild compression on the head to reduce myofascial tension of the suboccipital tissues (slight side bending and rotation away, as needed)	e-E Sa Ra
PC2 (occiput)	On the inferior nuchal line within the semispinalis capitis muscle associated with the greater occipital nerve (5)	Extension of occipitoatlantal articulation with mild compression on the head to reduce myofascial tension of the suboccipital tissues (slight side bending and rotation away, as needed)	e-E Sa Ra
PC2 midline spinous process	On the superior or superior lateral aspect/tip of the spinous process of C2	Same as above	e-E Sa Ra
PC3 midline spinous process	On the inferior or inferolateral aspect/tip of the spinous process of C2	Flex, side bend away, and rotate away	f-F Sa Ra
PC4–PC8 midline spinous process	On the inferior or inferolateral aspect of the spinous process. PC4 is inferior to the C3 spinous process. Remainder of tender points follow this pattern	Extend to the level of the dysfunctional segment with minimal to moderate side bending directed at the segment and minimal to moderate rotation away	e-E Sa Ra
PC3–PC7 lateral	On the posterolateral aspect of the articular process associated with the dysfunctional segment	Extend to the level of the dysfunctional segment with minimal to moderate side bending directed at the segment and minimal to moderate rotation away	e-E Sa Ra

Posterior Cervical Region

PC1 Inion

 See Video 9.4

Indication for Treatment

Somatic dysfunction of the occiput and/or cervical spine. Patient may present with pain in the suboccipital region and frontal/periorbital headache (4,5).

Tender Point Location

On the inferior nuchal line just inferior and lateral to the inion associated with the medial border of the semispinalis capitis and rectus capitis posterior minor **(Fig. 9.20)**. Press anterior and laterally into muscle mass.

Treatment Position: F occiput (F St Ra)

1. The physician flexes the patient's head by inducing cephalad traction on the patient's occiput while inducing caudad motion on patient's frontal area **(Figs. 9.21 to 9.23)**.

2. The physician fine-tunes through small arcs of motion (more or less flexion; may require minimal side bending toward and rotation away) until the tenderness has been *completely alleviated* or reduced as close to 100% as possible, but at least 70%.

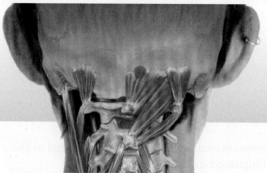

Figure 9.20. PC1 inion tender point. (Modified with permission from Ref. (8).)

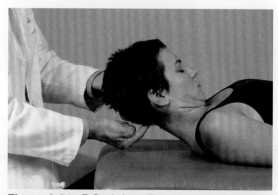

Figure 9.21. PC1 inion: F occiput (F St Ra).

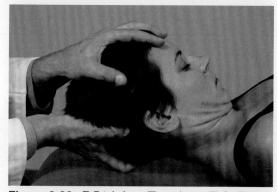

Figure 9.22. PC1 inion: F occiput (F St Ra).

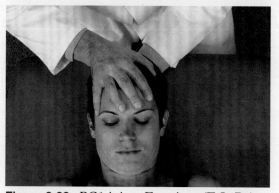

Figure 9.23. PC1 inion: F occiput (F St Ra).

Posterior Cervical Region

PC1 Occiput, PC2 Occiput

 See Video 9.5

Indication for Treatment

Somatic dysfunction of the occiput or cervical spine. The patient may present with posterolateral headache and pain behind the eye. PC2 will give more periorbital and/or temporal headaches (4,5).

Tender Point Locations

PC1 (occiput): On the inferior nuchal line midway between inion and mastoid associated with the splenius capitis and/or the rectus capitis posterior major/minor and obliquus capitis superior muscles (4,5).

PC2 (occiput): On the inferior nuchal line within the semispinalis capitis muscle associated with the greater occipital nerve (5). Press anteriorly! **(Fig. 9.24).**

Treatment Position: e-E Sa Ra

1. The patient's head is extended to the level of the dysfunctional vertebra; slight occipitoatlantal compression may be needed **(Figs. 9.25 and 9.26).**

2. The physician fine-tunes through small arcs of motion (more or less extension, slight side bending, and rotation away) until the tenderness has been *completely alleviated* or reduced as close to 100% as possible, but at least 70%.

3. Alternative: Extension, rotate away, and fine-tune **(Figs. 9.27 and 9.28).**

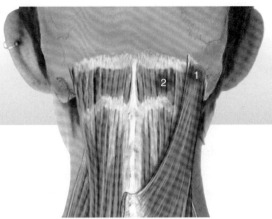

Figure 9.24. PC1 occiput; PC2 occiput tender points. (Modified with permission from Ref. (8).)

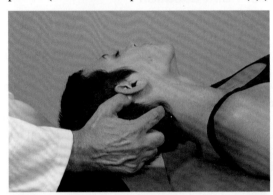

Figure 9.25. PC1 occiput: e-E Sa Ra.

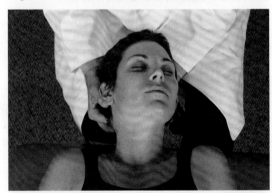

Figure 9.26. PC1 occiput; PC2 occiput: e-E Sa Ra.

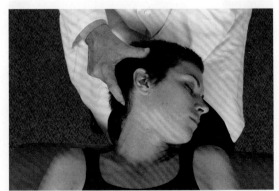

Figure 9.28. PC1 occiput; PC2 occiput: e RA, alternative.

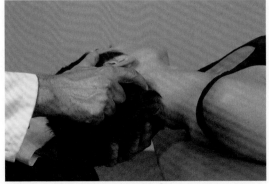

Figure 9.27. PC1 occiput; PC2 occiput: e RA, alternative.

Posterior Cervical Region

PC2, PC4–PC8 Spinous Process (Midline)

 See Video 9.6

Indication for Treatment

Somatic dysfunction of the cervical spine. The patient may present with posterior neck pain and generalized headache.

Tender Point Location

PC2 midline: On the superior or superior lateral aspect/tip of the spinous process of C2. Anatomically may correlate with rectus capitis posterior major/minor (4) and obliquus capitis inferior muscles **(Fig. 9.29)**.
PC4–PC8 midline: On the inferior or inferolateral aspect (tip) of the spinous process. PC4 is inferior to the C3 spinous process. PC5 is inferior to the spinous process of C4. Remainder of tender points follow this pattern. Anatomically may correlate with semispinalis capitis, multifidus, or rotatores (4,5).

Treatment Position: e-E Sa Ra

1. The patient's head is extended to the level of the dysfunctional segment (PC2, **Fig. 9.30**; PC5, **Figs. 9.31 and 9.32**; PC7, **Fig. 9.33**); minimal side bending and rotation away may be needed.

2. The physician fine-tunes through small arcs of motion (more or less extension, with minimal side bending and rotation away) until the tenderness has been *completely alleviated* or reduced as close to 100% as possible, but at least 70%.

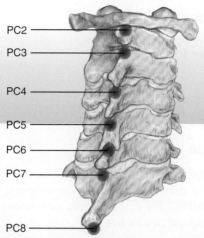

Figure 9.29. PC2–PC8 midline tender points. (Modified with permission from Ref. (8).)

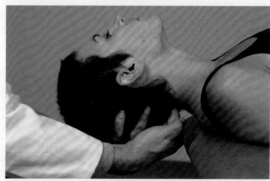

Figure 9.30. PC2: e Sa Ra.

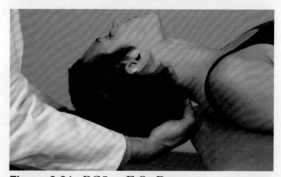

Figure 9.31. PC5: e-E Sa Ra.

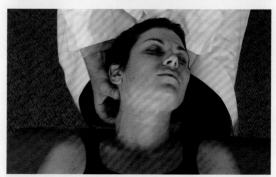

Figure 9.32. PC5: e-E Sa Ra.

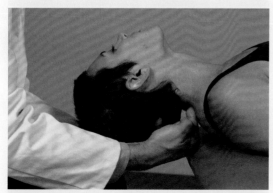

Figure 9.33. PC7: e-E Sa Ra.

Posterior Cervical Region

PC3 Spinous Process (Midline)

 See Video 9.7

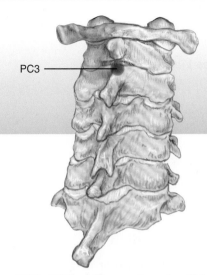

Indication for Treatment

Somatic dysfunction of the cervical spine. The patient may present with suboccipital headache, earache, tinnitus, and/or vertigo (4,5).

Tender Point Location

On the inferior tip or inferolateral aspect of the spinous process of C2. Anatomically may correlate with irritation of the greater and/or third occipital nerve and/or muscles innervated by the C3 nerve root (i.e., middle scalene, longus capitis, longus colli) (5). Press posterior to anterior **(Fig. 9.34)**.

Figure 9.34. PC3 midline tender point. (Modified with permission from Ref. (8).)

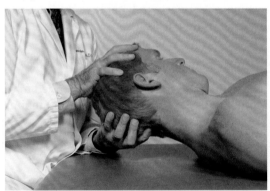

Treatment Position: f-F Sa Ra

1. The patient's head is flexed to the level of the dysfunctional segment, with minimal side bending and rotation away from the tender point **(Fig. 9.35)**.

2. The physician fine-tunes through small arcs of motion (more or less flexion, side bending, and rotation away) until the tenderness has been *completely alleviated* or reduced as close to 100% as possible, but at least 70%.

Figure 9.35. PC3: f-F Sa Ra.

Posterior Cervical Region

PC3–PC7 Articular Process (Lateral)

 See Video 9.6

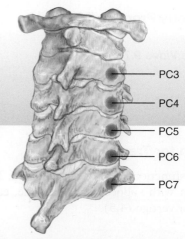

Figure 9.36. PC3–PC7 lateral tender points. (Modified with permission from Ref. (8).)

Indication for Treatment

Somatic dysfunction of the cervical spine. The patient may present with neck pain and headache.

Tender Point Location

On the posterolateral aspect of the articular process associated with the dysfunctional segment. Anatomically may correlate with transversospinalis muscle group (semispinalis cervicis and capitis, multifidus, and rotatores) (4,5) **(Fig. 9.36)**.

Treatment Position: E Sa-A Ra-A

1. The patient's head and neck are extended to the level of the dysfunctional segment with minimal to moderate side bending and rotation away (**Figs. 9.37 to 9.40**, PC3, PC3, PC6, and PC6, respectively).

2. The physician fine-tunes through small arcs of motion (more or less extension, side bending, and rotation away) until the tenderness has been *completely alleviated* or reduced as close to 100% as possible, but at least 70%.

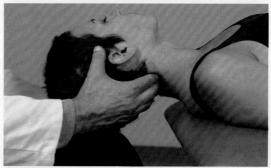

Figure 9.37. PC3: e-E Sa Ra.

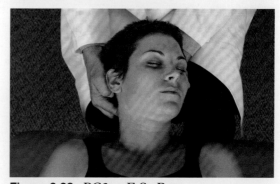

Figure 9.38. PC3: e-E Sa Ra.

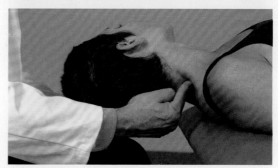

Figure 9.39. PC6: e-E Sa Ra.

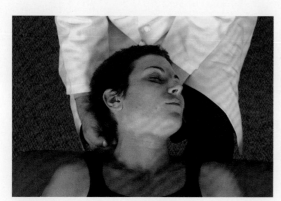

Figure 9.40. PC6: e-E Sa Ra.

Anterior Thoracic Region

Anterior Thoracic Tender Points

Anterior thoracic counterstrain tender points are outlined in Table 9.3 and illustrated in **Figure 9.41**.

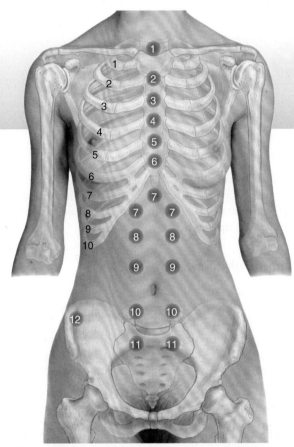

Figure 9.41. Anterior thoracic counterstrain tender points. (Modified with permission from Ref. (8).)

Table 9.3 Common Anterior Thoracic Tender Points

Tender Point	Location	Classic Treatment Position	Acronym
AT1 midline AT2 midline	Midline or just lateral to the episternal notch Midline or just lateral to the junction of manubrium and sternum (angle of Louis)	Flex to dysfunctional level Fine-tune with side bending and/or rotation	f-F
AT3–AT6	On the sternum at the corresponding costal level (midline or lateral to midline)	Flex to dysfunctional level Fine-tune with side bending and/or rotation	f-F
AT7–AT9	Points are lateral to the midline within the rectus abdominis. AT7: inferior tip of xiphoid and/or 1/4 distance from tip of xiphoid and umbilicus AT8: halfway between tip of xiphoid and umbilicus AT9: 3/4 distance from tip of xiphoid and umbilicus	Patient seated Flex to dysfunctional level, side bend toward, and rotate torso away	F St Ra
AT10–AT12	AT10: 1/4 distance from the umbilicus and pubic symphysis AT11: halfway between the umbilicus and pubic symphysis AT12: on the anterior superior surface of the iliac crest at the midaxillary line	Patient supine with hips and knees flexed; flex to spinal level, knees (pelvis) toward which rotates torso away; side bend (ankles/feet) toward	F St Ra

Anterior Thoracic Region

AT1, AT2

 See Video 9.8

Indication for Treatment

Somatic dysfunction of the thoracic spine. The patient may present with anterior chest wall pain and upper back pain associated with anterior head and neck carriage and upper thoracic kyphosis (5).

Tender Point Location

AT1: Midline or just lateral to the episternal notch associated with sternal fascia and pectoralis major muscle (5) **(Fig. 9.42)**.
AT2: Midline or just lateral to the junction of the manubrium and sternum (angle of Louis) associated with sternal fascia and pectoralis major muscle (5).

Treatment Position: f-F

1. The patient is seated on the treatment table with hands interlaced behind the head/neck.

2. The physician stands behind the patient and wraps arms under the patient's axillae and around the chest and places hands over the manubrium.

3. The patient leans back against the physician's chest and thigh, causing marked flexion of the neck to the level of the dysfunctional thoracic segment **(Figs. 9.43 to 9.45)**.

4. The physician fine-tunes through small arcs of motion (more or less flexion; may require minimal side bending and/or rotation if the tender point is to the left or right of midline) until the tenderness has been *completely alleviated* or reduced as close to 100% as possible, but at least 70%.

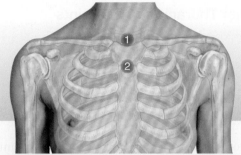

Figure 9.42. AT1–AT2 tender points. (Modified with permission from Ref. (8).)

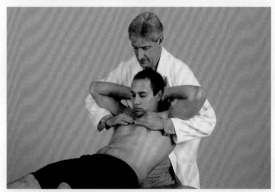

Figure 9.43. AT1–AT2: f-F.

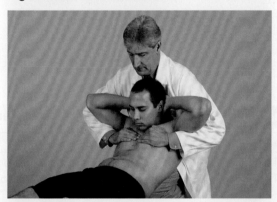

Figure 9.44. AT1–AT2: f-F.

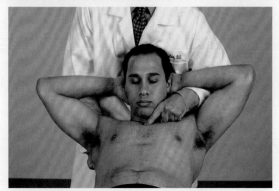

Figure 9.45. AT1–AT2: f-F, alternative hand placement.

Anterior Thoracic Region

AT3–AT6

 See Video 9.9

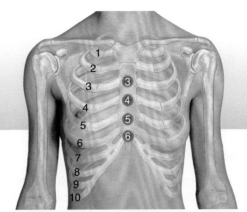

Figure 9.46. AT3–AT6 tender points. (Modified with permission from Ref. (8).)

Indication for Treatment

Somatic dysfunction of the thoracic spine. Clinical presentation is similar to that of AT1–AT2 and may include gastroesophageal reflux (5).

Tender Point Location

AT3–AT6: On the sternum at the level of corresponding costal cartilage/rib (midline or lateral to the midline) and may be associated with sternal fascia and pectoralis major muscle (4,5) **(Fig. 9.46)**.

Treatment Position: f-F

1. The patient lies supine with the arms off the side of the table, and the physician's thigh is behind the patient's upper thoracic region.

2. While the physician's index finger pad palpates the tender point, the patient is elevated from the table with the physician's thigh toward the level of the dysfunctional segment.

3. The physician places the other hand behind the patient's head and neck and carefully forward bends the patient's chest (physician may use chest or abdomen instead of hand). The physician should sense a concavity developing at the fingertip location as the proper vector of flexion is developed **(Figs. 9.47 and 9.48)**.

4. Alternative technique: The patient lies supine with the arms off the side of the table, and the physician's chest is behind the patient's upper thoracic region. The physician leans forward with the chest and abdomen while pulling backward on the patient's arms to flex the thoracic spine to the desired level **(Fig. 9.49)**. Using this variation, the physician is unable to monitor the tender point throughout the treatment sequence.

5. The physician fine-tunes through small arcs of motion (more or less flexion, minimal or no side bending, or rotation) until the tenderness has been *completely alleviated* or reduced as close to 100% as possible, but at least 70%.

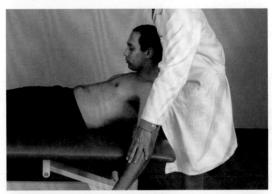

Figure 9.47. AT3–AT6: F IR (arms).

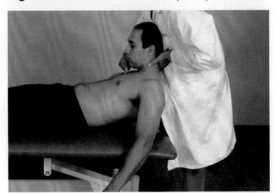

Figure 9.48. AT3–AT6: FIR alternative hand placement.

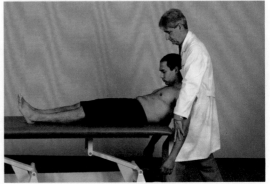

Figure 9.49. AT3–AT4: F IR (arms).

Anterior Thoracic Region

AT7–AT9

 See Video 9.10

Indication for Treatment

Somatic dysfunction of the thoracic spine. Patient may complain of midthoracic pain, epigastric or flank pain, and gastroesophageal reflux.

Tender Point Location

Anatomically, may correlate with the rectus abdominis (4,5), external/internal oblique and transversus abdominis muscles (5). **(Fig. 9.50).**
AT7: inferior tip of xiphoid and/or ¼ distance from the tip of the xiphoid and the umbilicus, lateral to the midline **(Fig. 9.50).**
AT8: halfway between the tip of the xiphoid and the umbilicus, lateral to the midline.
AT9: ¾ distance from the tip of the xiphoid and the umbilicus, lateral to the midline.

Treatment Position: F St Ra

1. The patient is seated on the treatment table with the physician standing behind the patient.

2. The physician's foot on the side opposite the tender point is placed on the table with the patient's arm resting on a pillow on the physician's thigh.

3. The patient leans back against the physician's abdomen, and the arm on the side of the tender point is adducted across the patient's chest to induce flexion and rotation to the desired level **(Fig. 9.51).**

4. The physician side bends the patient's thoracic spine to the side of the tender point and desired level by elevating the thigh and translating the patient's shoulders to the side of the tender point **(Fig. 9.52).**

5. The physician fine-tunes through small arcs of motion (more or less flexion, side bending, and rotation) until the tenderness has been *completely alleviated* or reduced as close to 100% as possible, but at least 70%.

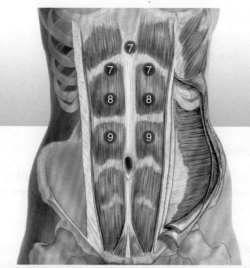

Figure 9.50. AT7–AT9 tender points. (Modified with permission from Ref. (8).)

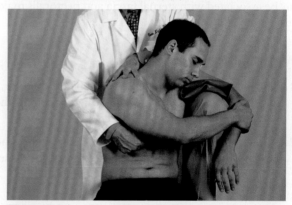

Figure 9.51. AT7–AT9: F St Ra.

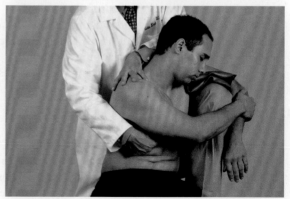

Figure 9.52. AT7–AT9: F St Ra (fine-tune).

Anterior Thoracic Region

AT9–AT12

 See Videos 9.11 and 9.12

Indication for Treatment

Somatic dysfunction of the thoracic and/or lumbar region. The patient may present with lower thoracic or upper lumbar pain, lower abdominal pain, or flank pain (5).

Tender Point Location

Anatomically, may correlate with the rectus abdominis (4,5), external/internal oblique and transversus abdominis muscles (5). **(Fig. 9.53)**.

AT9: ¾ distance from the tip of the xiphoid and the umbilicus, lateral to the midline.

AT10: ¼ distance from the umbilicus and the pubic symphysis, lateral to the midline.

AT11: halfway between the umbilicus and the pubic symphysis, lateral to the midline.

AT12: superior and anterior surface of the iliac crest at the midaxillary line.

Treatment Position: F ST (Ankles) RT (knees/pelvis) RA (Torso)

1. The patient lies supine, and the physician stands on the side of the tender point and places the foot on the table.
2. The patient's hips and knees are flexed, placed on the physician's thigh, and then flexed further to the desired level. The end of the table may be elevated or a pillow placed under the patient's pelvis to provide additional flexion.
3. The patient's knees are pulled toward the side of the tender point, causing the pelvis and the lower segment to rotate toward the tender point and the torso and upper segment to rotate away.
4. The patient's ankles are brought toward the side of the tender point, which side bends the dysfunctional segment toward the tender point (AT9–AT11, **Fig. 9.54**; AT12, **Figs. 9.55 and 9.56**). The side-bending component may vary depending on which myofascial structures are involved, the direction of their fibers, or whether there is an articular component to the dysfunction.
5. The physician fine-tunes through small arcs of motion (more or less hip flexion, rotation, and side bending) until the tenderness has been *completely alleviated* or reduced as close to 100% as possible, but at least 70%.

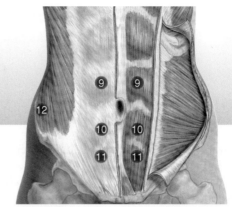

Figure 9.53. AT9–AT12 tender points. (Modified with permission from Ref. (8).)

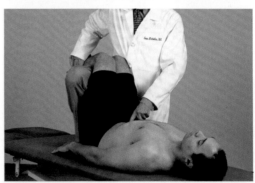

Figure 9.54. AT9–AT11: F St (ankles) RT (knees/pelvis) Ra (torso).

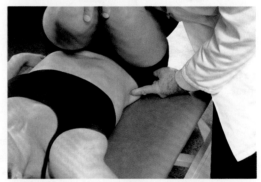

Figure 9.55. AT12: F St (ankles) RT (knees/pelvis) Ra(torso).

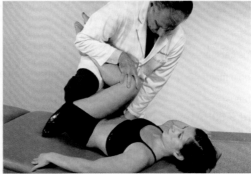

Figure 9.56. AT12: F St (ankles) RT (knees/pelvis) Ra(torso).

Posterior Thoracic Region

Anatomy of the Thoracic and Lumbar Regions

Muscle layers of the thoracic and lumbar region are illustrated in **Figures 9.57 to 9.59.**

Muscle attachments of the upper four thoracic vertebrae are illustrated in **Figure 9.60.**

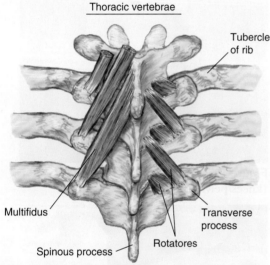

Figure 9.59. Multifidus and rotatores of the thoracic vertebrae.

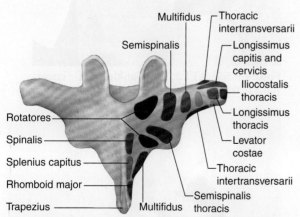

Figure 9.60. Muscle attachments of the upper four thoracic vertebrae.

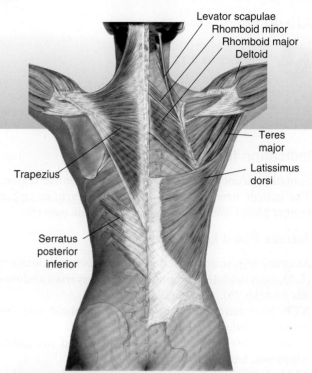

Figure 9.57. Superficial muscles of the back.

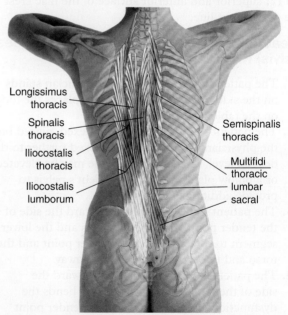

Figure 9.58. Intermediate muscles of the back.

Posterior Thoracic Region

Posterior Thoracic Tender Points

Posterior thoracic counterstrain tender points are outlined in Table 9.4 and illustrated in **Figure 9.61**.

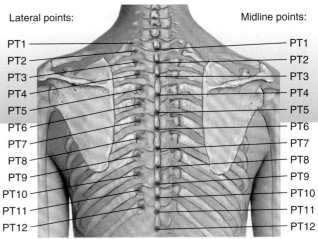

Figure 9.61. Posterior thoracic counterstrain tender points. (Modified with permission from Ref. (8).)

Table 9.4 Common Posterior Thoracic Tender Points

Tender Point	Location	Classic Treatment Position	Acronym
PT1–PT12 midline	Midline, on the inferior aspect/tip of the spinous process of the dysfunctional segment	Extend to dysfunctional level Rotation and side bending are minimal. Avoid extension of the occipitoatlantal and cervical region	e-E
PT1–PT12 posterior	On the inferolateral aspect/tip of the deviated spinous process of the dysfunctional segment *Vertebral rotation is opposite the side of spinous process deviation	Extend to dysfunctional level, side bend, and rotate away	e-E SA RA
PT1–PT12 transverse process	On the posterolateral aspect of the transverse process of the dysfunctional segment	Extend, side bend away, rotate toward	e-E SA RT

Posterior Thoracic Region

PT1–PT12 Spinous Process (Midline)

 See Videos 9.13 and 9.14

Indication for Treatment

Somatic dysfunction of the thoracic spine. The patient may present with tenderness in the center of the back and flattening of the thoracic kyphosis (5).

Tender Point Location

In the midline, on the inferior tip of the spinous process of the dysfunctional segment and may be associated with the supraspinous ligament, or the interspinales, spinalis, or semispinalis thoracic muscles (5) **(Fig. 9.62)**.

Treatment Position: e-E

1. The patient lies prone, and the physician stands at the head of the treatment table and may place his/her knee/thigh on the table next to the patient for added control and comfort during the treatment.

2. The patient's arms hang over the sides of the table, and the physician, supporting the patient's head and neck by cupping the chin, gently lifts and extends the neck and thoracic spine to the level of the dysfunctional thoracic segment (PT3, **Fig. 9.63**; PT6, **Fig. 9.64**).

3. Minimal or no side bending or rotation is needed.

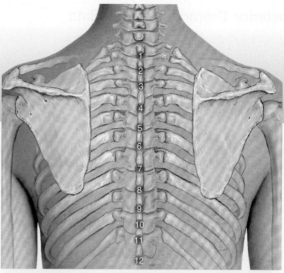

Figure 9.62. PT1–PT12 midline tender points. (Modified with permission from Ref. (8).)

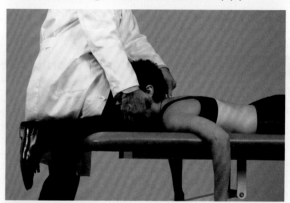

Figure 9.63. PT3: e-E.

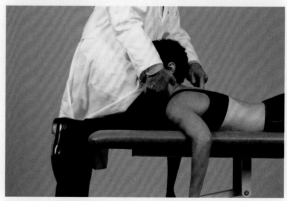

Figure 9.64. PT6: e-E.

4. When treating midline points in the lower thoracic region, the patient's arms and shoulders are flexed forward parallel to the table, and the physician's thigh is positioned to provide the extension required (PT9, **Fig. 9.65**).

5. A supine alternative to avoid hyperextension of the occipitoatlantal (O–A) and upper cervical region may be preferable for physician control and patient comfort (PT1–PT4, **Fig. 9.66**).

6. The physician fine-tunes through small arcs of motion (more or less extension) until the tenderness has been *completely alleviated* or reduced as close to 100% as possible, but at least 70%.

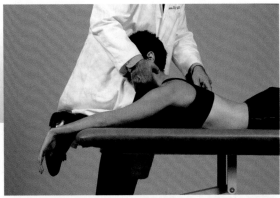

Figure 9.65. PT9: E.

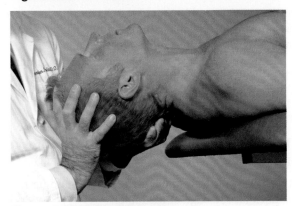

Figure 9.66. PT1–PT4: e-E.

Posterior Thoracic Region

PT1–PT9 Spinous Process (Inferolateral)

 See Video 9.15

Indication for Treatment

Somatic dysfunction of the thoracic region.

Tender Point Location

On the inferolateral aspect of the deviated spinous process of the dysfunctional segment. Press from inferior to superior at a 45 degree angle **(Fig. 9.67)**.

Hypertonicity of the right semispinalis and multifidi will side bend the vertebral segment to the right, rotate it to the left, and deviate the spinous process to the right (5).

Treatment Position: E Sa Ra

PT1–PT4 (e.g., T2 tender point right inferolateral aspect T2 spinous process, deviated to the right).

1. The patient lies supine with the neck and upper back off the edge of the table.

2. The physician sits at the head of the table supporting the patient's head to prevent hyperextension of the occipitoatlantal and cervical region.

3. The physician extends to the level of the dysfunction and fine-tunes with side bending and rotation away until the tenderness has been *completely alleviated* or reduced as close to 100% as possible, but at least 70% **(Fig. 9.68)**.

PT5–PT9 (e.g., T6 tender point right inferolateral aspect T6 spinous process, deviated to the right)

1. The patient lies prone, and the physician stands or sits at the side of the tender point.

2. The patient rotates the head/neck to the left (side opposite tender point).

3. The patient's right arm/shoulder (side of tender point) is flexed, resting comfortably on the side of the head and the left arm along the side of the body.

4. The patient's left shoulder is pulled posterior and caudad, which produces extension, rotation away, and side bending away from the side of the tender point and deviated spinous process **(Fig. 9.69)**.

5. The physician fine-tunes through small arcs of motion (more or less extension, rotation, and side bending) until the tenderness has been *completely alleviated* or reduced as close to 100% as possible, but at least 70%.

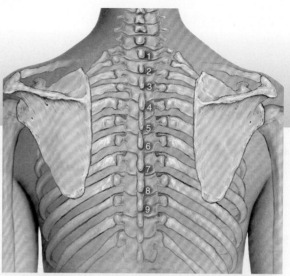
Figure 9.67. PT1–PT9 posterior tender points.

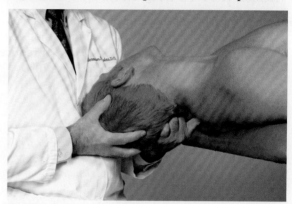
Figure 9.68. PT2 right spinous process tender point.

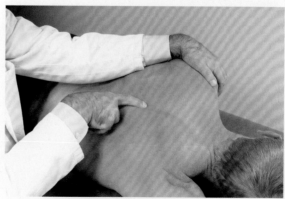
Figure 9.69. PT6 right spinous process tender point.

Posterior Thoracic Region

PT4–PT9 Transverse Process

 See Video 9.16

Indication for Treatment

Somatic dysfunction of the thoracic spine.

Tender Point Location

On the posterolateral aspect of the transverse process associated with the longissimus thoracis, levatores costarum, semispinalis, multifidus, or rotatores (5) **(Fig. 9.70)**.

Treatment Position: E Sa RT

1. The patient lies prone, the head rotated to the side of the tender point, and the physician sits at the head of the table. The physician's forearm is placed under the patient's axilla on the side of the tender point with the hand on the posterolateral chest wall. The physician's forearm lifts patient's shoulder to produce extension and rotation to the side of the tender point and side bends the torso by adding more shoulder abduction **(Fig. 9.71)**.

2. The patient lies prone, the head rotated to the side of the tender point, and physician stands at the side opposite the tender point. The patient's torso may be side bent away and the arm on the side of the tender point abducted to produce even more side bending away. The patient's left shoulder is pulled posterior and cephalad, which produces extension and rotation toward and side bending away from the side of the tender point **(Fig. 9.72)**.

3. The side bending component may vary depending on which specific myofascial structures are involved, the direction of their fibers, or whether there is an articular component to the dysfunction.

4. The physician fine-tunes through small arcs of motion (more or less extension, rotation, and side bending) until the tenderness has been *completely alleviated* or reduced as close to 100% as possible, but at least 70%.

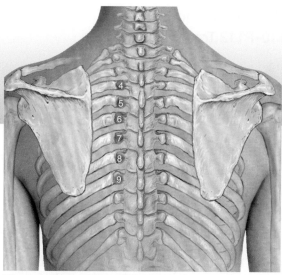

Figure 9.70. PT4–PT9 lateral tender points. (Modified with permission from Ref. (8).)

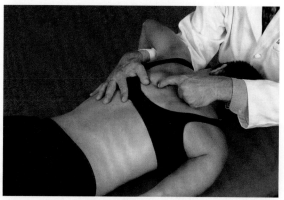

Figure 9.71. PT6: e-E Sa-A Rt-T.

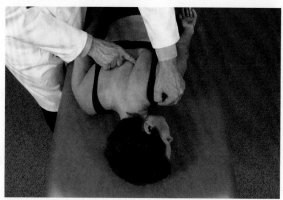

Figure 9.72. PT6: e-E Sa-A Rt-T.

Posterior Thoracic Region

PT10–PT12 Spinous Process (Inferolateral)
PT10–PT12 Transverse Process

 See Video 9.17

Indication for Treatment

Somatic dysfunction of the thoracic region.

Tender Point Location

PT10–PT12 Spinous Process (Inferolateral): On the inferolateral aspect of the deviated spinous process of the dysfunctional segment **(Fig. 9.73)**.

PT10–PT12 Transverse Process: Posterolateral aspect of the transverse process of the dysfunctional segment **(Fig. 9.73)**.

Treatment Position: e-E Sa Rt (pelvis) Ra (torso)

T10–T12 (e.g., T11 tender point left; T11 spinous process, deviated to the left, rotated right).

1. The patient lies prone, and the physician may stand on either side of the tender point. The patient's legs are positioned to the side which produces the greatest reduction of tenderness. The side bending component may vary depending on which myofascial structures are involved, the direction of their fibers, or whether there is an articular component to the dysfunction. The physician grasps the anterior superior iliac spine (ASIS) on the side of the tender point; leans back, gently lifting upward to induce extension and rotation of the pelvis (lower segment) toward the side of the tender point; and rotates the torso (upper segment) away **(Fig. 9.74)**.

T10–T12 (e.g., T11 tender point right; T11 transverse process, rotated to the right).

1. The patient lies prone, and the physician may stand on either side of the tender point. The patient's legs are positioned to the side which produces the greatest reduction of tenderness. The side bending component may vary depending on which myofascial structures are involved, the direction of their fibers, or whether there is an articular component to the dysfunction. The physician grasps the ASIS on the side opposite the tender point; leans back, gently lifting upward to induce extension and rotation of the pelvis (lower segment) away from the side of the tender point; and rotates the torso (upper segment) toward the side of the tender point **(Fig. 9.75)**.

2. The physician fine-tunes through small arcs of motion (extension, rotation, and side bending) until the tenderness has been *completely alleviated* or reduced as close to 100% as possible, but at least 70%.

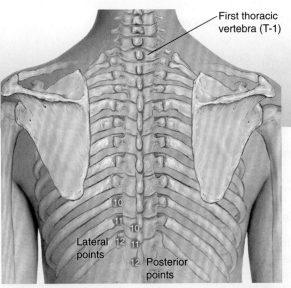

Figure 9.73. PT9–PT12 posterior and lateral tender points. (Modified with permission from Ref. (8).)

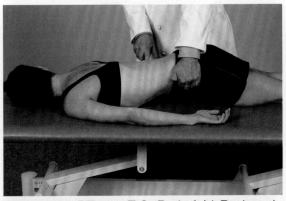

Figure 9.74. PT11: e-E Sa Rt (pelvis) Ra (torso).

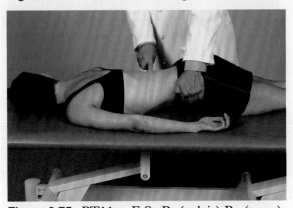

Figure 9.75. PT11: e-E Sa Rt (pelvis) Ra (torso).

Anterior Costal Region

Anterior Coastal Tender Points

Anterior costal counterstrain tender points are outlined in Table 9.5 and illustrated in **Figure 9.76**.

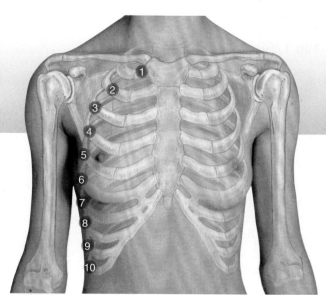

Figure 9.76. Anterior costal counterstrain tender points. (Modified with permission from Ref. (8).)

Table 9.5 Common Anterior Costal Tender Points (Jones Term "Depressed Ribs")

Tender Point	Location	Classic Treatment Position	Acronym
AR1	Below the clavicle on the first chondro-sternal articulation	Patient supine—using the cervical-thoracic spine, flex, side bend, and rotate toward the tender point.	f-F St RT
AR2	On the superior aspect of the second rib at the midclavicular line	Same as above	Same as above
AR3–AR10	On the dysfunctional rib at the anterior axillary line	Patient seated flex, side bend, and rotate toward	f-F ST RT

Anterior Costal Region

AR1, AR2
Rib 1, Rib 2 Depressed (Exhaled)

 See Videos 9.18 and 9.19

Indication for Treatment

Somatic dysfunction of ribs 1 and 2 (exhalation, depressed). The patient may complain of pain in the anterior chest wall due to excessive coughing, sneezing, or anterior head carriage (5).

Tender Point Location

AR1: Below the clavicle on the first chondrosternal articulation associated with the pectoralis major and internal intercostal muscles (5) **(Fig. 9.77)**.
AR2: On the superior aspect of the second rib at the midclavicular line.

Treatment Position: f-F St RT

1. The patient lies supine, and the physician stands or sits at the head of the table.

2. The patient's head and neck are flexed to engage the level of the dysfunctional rib.

3. The patient's head and neck are side bent and rotated toward the tender point **(Figs. 9.78 to 9.80)**.

4. The physician fine-tunes through small arcs of motion (more or less flexion, side bending, or rotation) until the tenderness has been *completely alleviated* or reduced as close to 100% as possible, but at least 70%.

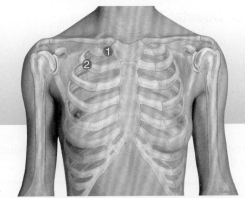

Figure 9.77. AR12 tender points. (Modified with permission from Ref. (8).)

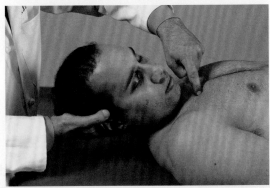

Figure 9.78. AR12: f-F St RT.

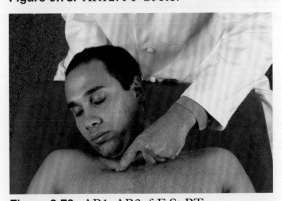

Figure 9.79. AR1–AR2: f-F St RT.

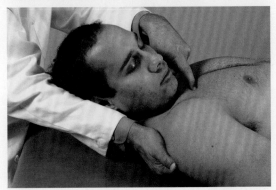

Figure 9.80. AR1–AR2: f-F St RT (alternative hand placement).

Anterior Costal Region

AR3–AR10
Rib 3–Rib 10 Depressed (Exhaled)

 See Video 9.20

Indication for Treatment

Somatic dysfunction, ribs 3 to 10 (exhalation, depressed). The patient may complain of pain in the lateral chest wall from strain due to excessive coughing, sneezing, or overuse of the upper extremity (4,5).

Tender Point Location

AR3–AR10: On the dysfunctional rib at the anterior axillary line. AR3-AR8 are associated with the internal intercostals (5) and serratus anterior muscles (4,5). AR9-AR10 are associated with the internal intercostal muscles (5). **(Fig. 9.81)**.

Treatment Position: f-F St-T Rt-T

1. The patient is seated with the hips and knees flexed on the table on the side of the tender point. For comfort, the patient may let the leg on the side of the tender point hang off the front of the table, the other leg crossed under it.

2. The physician stands behind the patient with the foot opposite the tender point on the table and the thigh under the patient's axilla (induces side bending toward tender point).

3. The patient's thorax is slightly flexed to the level of the dysfunctional rib.

4. The patient's arm on the side of the tender point is extended and allowed to hang off the edge of the table behind the patient, inducing rotation and further side bending toward the tender point **(Figs. 9.82 and 9.83)**.

5. The physician fine-tunes through small arcs of motion (more or less flexion, side bending, and rotation) until the tenderness has been *completely alleviated* or reduced as close to 100% as possible, but at least 70%.

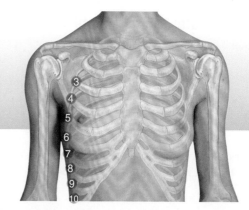

Figure 9.81. AR3–AR6 tender points. (Modified with permission from Ref. (8).)

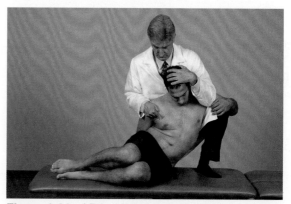

Figure 9.82. AR3–AR6: f-F St-T Rt-T.

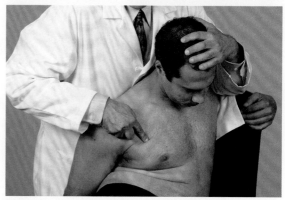

Figure 9.83. AR3–AR6: f-F St-T Rt-T.

Posterior Costal Region

Posterior Costal Tender Points

Posterior costal counterstrain tender points are outlined in Table 9.6 and illustrated in **Figure 9.84**.

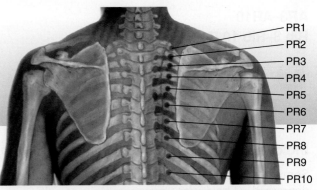

Figure 9.84. Posterior costal counterstrain tender points. (Modified with permission from Ref. (8).)

Table 9.6 | Common Posterior Costal Tender Points (Jones Term "Elevated Ribs")

Tender Point	Location	Classic Treatment Position	Acronym
PR1	On posterosuperior aspect of rib 1 just lateral to the costo-transverse articulation	Patient seated: using the cervical-thoracic spine, side bend away, rotate toward, and slightly extend	e SA Rt
PR2–PR10	On the posterosuperior angle of the corresponding rib	Patient seated: flex, side bend, and rotate away	f SA RA

Posterior Costal Region

PR1
Rib 1 Elevated (Inhaled)

 See Video 9.21

Indication for Treatment

Somatic dysfunction at rib 1 (inhalation, elevated). The patient may complain of pain at the cervicothoracic junction caused by trauma, overhead sleeping position, or sudden movement of the neck and upper thoracic region (5).

Tender Point Location

PR1: On the posterior superior angle of the first rib just lateral to the costotransverse articulation **(Fig. 9.85)**.

Treatment Position: e-E SA Rt

1. The patient is seated. The physician stands behind the patient.

2. The physician's foot opposite the tender point is placed on the table under the patient's axilla.

3. The physician monitors the first rib tender point with the pad of the index finger **(Fig. 9.86)**.

4. With the other hand, the physician gently extends the patient's head and neck to engage the first rib and then side bends the head and neck away from the tender point, carefully monitoring the movement, so it is vectored to engage the first rib.

5. The physician rotates the head toward the tender point **(Figs. 9.87 and 9.88)**.

6. The physician fine-tunes through small arcs of motion (more or less extension, rotation, and side bending) until the tenderness has been *completely alleviated* or reduced as close to 100% as possible, but at least 70%.

7. Alternate position: The patient is supine with the physician seated at the head of the treatment table. Follow steps 3 to 6 as described above.

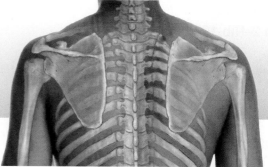

Figure 9.85. PR1 tender point. (Modified with permission from Ref. (8).)

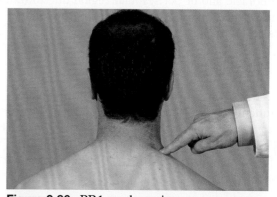

Figure 9.86. PR1 tender point.

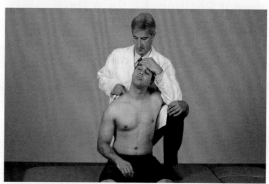

Figure 9.87. PR1: e SA Rt.

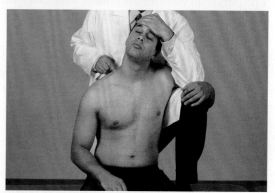

Figure 9.88. PR1: e SA Rt.

Posterior Costal Region

PR2–PR10
Rib 2–Rib 10 Elevated (Inhaled)

 See Video 9.22

Indication for Treatment

Somatic dysfunction of ribs 2 to 10 (inhalation, elevated). The patient may complain of pain in the upper midthoracic and/or periscapular region due to trauma, overhead sleeping position, or sudden movement of the neck and thoracic region (5).

Tender Point Location

PR2–PR6: On the superior aspect of the angle of the dysfunctional rib associated with the levatores costarum and/or serratus posterior superior muscles (5) **(Fig. 9.89)**.
PR7–PR10: On the superior aspect of the angle of the dysfunctional rib associated with the levatores costarum muscles (5) **(Fig. 9.89)**.

Treatment Position: f-F Sa-A Ra-A

1. The patient is seated with legs on the side of table (for comfort, the patient may hang the leg opposite the tender point off the table).

2. The physician stands behind patient with the foot ipsilateral to the tender point on the table with the thigh under the patient's axilla.

3. The physician gently flexes patient's head, neck, and thorax to engage the level of the dysfunctional rib.

4. The physician elevates the patient's shoulder with the axilla resting on the thigh, which side bends the trunk away from the tender point.

5. The patient is asked to slowly extend the shoulder and arm opposite the tender point and allow the arm to hang down. This induces side bending and rotation away from the tender point **(Figs. 9.90 and 9.91)**.

6. The physician fine-tunes through small arcs of motion (more or less flexion, rotation, and side bending) until the tenderness has been *completely alleviated* or reduced as close to 100% as possible, but at least 70%.

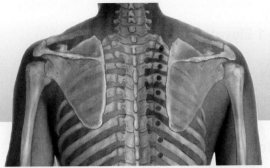

Figure 9.89. PR2–PR10 tender points. (Modified with permission from Ref. (8).)

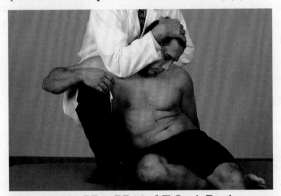

Figure 9.90. PR2–PR10: f-F Sa-A Ra-A.

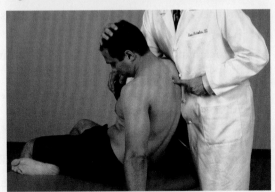

Figure 9.91. PR2–PR10: f-F Sa-A Ra-A.

Anterior Lumbar Region

Anterior Lumbar Tender Points

Anterior lumbar counterstrain tender points are outlined in Table 9.7 and illustrated in **Figure 9.92**.

Note: The acronyms for the classic positions represent the point of reference related to the movement of the upper of the two segments involved in the dysfunction. Therefore, the physician may stand on either side of the patient and depending on the dysfunction may alter the side bending and rotational elements. In these supine techniques with motion initiated from below the dysfunction, when the knees and pelvis are directed toward the physician, the segment that has not been engaged yet (i.e., upper of the two) is relatively rotated away. In other words, when the physician initiates rotational motion from below the dysfunctional segment without incorporating it into this motion, the dysfunctional segment is relatively rotated in the opposite direction. For example, if the physician stands on the right of the patient and pulls the knees toward the right (physician), the pelvis and sacrum rotate toward the physician, while L5 remains relatively static and therefore is rotated left. As the physician pulls the knees farther to the right, the next superior segment (L5) rotates to the right, and thus, the segment above (L4) is rotated to the left.

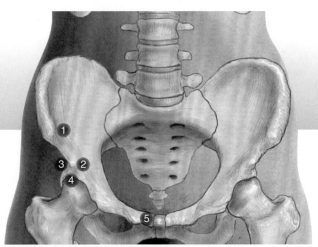

Figure 9.92. Anterior lumbar counterstrain tender points. (Modified with permission from Ref. (8).)

Due to the various layers of myofascial structures in the spinal regions, the direction of their fibers, and the physiologic motion pattern of articular dysfunctions, the "classic treatment position" may not always completely alleviate the tender point. Based on the indirect nature of counterstrain technique, if a tender point is related to a Type I or Type II dysfunction, the segment should be placed in its position of "ease" in all three planes to alleviate the tenderness.

Table 9.7 Common Anterior Lumbar Tender Points

Tender Point	Location	Classic Treatment Position	Acronym
		Physician stands on same side of tender point for AL1, AL5; opposite side for AL2–AL4. Patient supine with hips and knees flexed to shorten tissues around the tender point	
AL1	Medial to the anterior superior iliac spine (ASIS)	Flex to L1, side bend (ankles) toward, knees (pelvis) toward which rotates torso and L1 away	F St RA
AL2	Medial to the anterior inferior iliac spine (AIIS)	Flex to spinal level, side bend (ankles) away, knees (pelvis) away which rotates torso and lumbar segment toward	F Sa RT
AL3	Lateral to the anterior inferior iliac spine (AIIS)	Same as above (AL2)	F SA RT
AL4	Inferior to the anterior inferior iliac spine (AIIS)	Same as above (AL2)	F SA RT
AL5	Anterior, superior aspect of the pubic ramus just lateral to the symphysis	Flex, side bend (ankles) away, knees (pelvis) toward which rotates torso and lumbar segment away	F SA Ra

Anterior Lumbar Region

AL1

 See Video 9.23

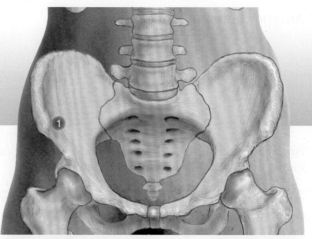

Figure 9.93. AL1 tender point. (Modified with permission from Ref. (8).)

Indication for Treatment

Somatic dysfunction of the lumbar and/or pelvic region. The patient may complain of pain in the thoracolumbar region, lower lateral abdominal wall, and anterior thigh (4,5).

Tender Point Location

Medial to the anterior superior iliac spine (ASIS); Press medial to lateral; anatomically may correlate with the transversus abdominis and internal oblique muscles (ilioinguinal nerve = L1 root) as well as the iliopsoas muscle group (4,5) **(Fig. 9.93)**.

Treatment Position: F St (ankles) RA (torso)

1. The patient lies supine, and the physician stands at the side of the tender point.

2. The patient's hips and knees are flexed, placed on the physician's thigh, and then flexed further to the desired level, to engage the lower of the two segments involved (L2).

3. The patient's knees are pulled toward the physician, rotating the pelvis and lumbar spine up to the level of L2, leaving L1 rotated away from the tender point.

4. The patient's ankles and feet are pulled toward the physician, to the level of L2, which side bends the lumbar spine to the side of the tender point **(Figs. 9.94 and 9.95)**.

5. The physician fine-tunes through small arcs of motion (more or less flexion, rotation, and side bending) until the tenderness has been *completely alleviated* or reduced as close to 100% as possible, but at least 70%.

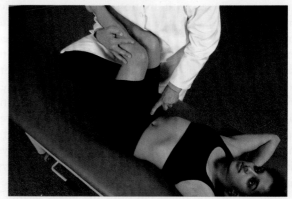

Figure 9.94. AL1: F St (ankles) RT (knees/pelvis) RA (torso).

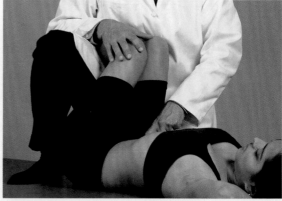

Figure 9.95. AL1: F St (ankles) RT (knees/pelvis) RA (torso).

Anterior Lumbar Region

AL2

 See Video 9.24

Indication for Treatment

Somatic dysfunction of the lumbar region. The patient may complain of lower back and anterior lateral hip pain.

Tender Point Location

Medial to the anterior inferior iliac spine (AIIS); press medial to lateral **(Fig. 9.96)**; anatomically may correlate with the external oblique (4), the genitofemoral nerve (L1–L2 nerve root); and the iliopsoas muscle group (5).

Treatment Position: F SA (ankles) RA (torso)

1. The patient lies supine, and the physician stands at the side of the table opposite the tender point.

2. The patient's hips and knees are flexed to the level of L3. The patient's knees may be placed on the physician's thigh for control and patient comfort.

3. The patient's hips and knees are pulled toward the physician, rotating the pelvis and lumbar spine to the level of L3, leaving L2 rotated toward the tender point.

4. The patient's ankles and feet are brought toward the physician (away from the tender point) to the level of L3, which side bends the lumbar spine away from the tender point **(Figs. 9.97 and 9.98)**.

5. The physician fine-tunes through small arcs of motion (more or less flexion, rotation, and side bending) until the tenderness has been *completely alleviated* or reduced as close to 100% as possible, but at least 70%.

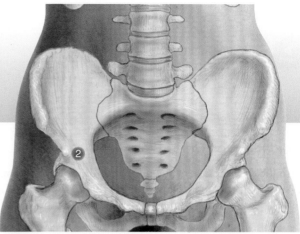
Figure 9.96. AL2 tender point. (Modified with permission from Ref. (8).)

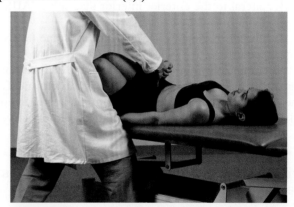
Figure 9.97. AL2: F SA (ankles) RT (knees/pelvis) RA (torso).

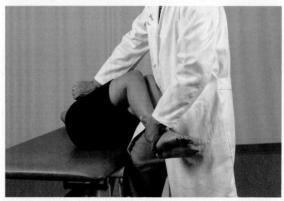
Figure 9.98. AL2: F SA (ankles) RT (knees/pelvis) RA (torso).

Anterior Lumbar Region

AL3, AL4

 See Video 9.25

Indication for Treatment

Somatic dysfunction of the lumbar and/or pelvic region. The patient may complain of lower back, groin, and/or anterior lateral hip pain (4,5).

Tender Point Location

AL3: Lateral to the anterior inferior iliac spine (AIIS); press medially.
AL4: Inferior to the anterior inferior iliac spine (AIIS); press cephalad.

Anatomically may correlate with the lateral border of the iliacus muscle (4); the psoas muscle and L3 and L4 spinal root contributions from the lateral femoral cutaneous (L2–L3), femoral, and obturator nerves (L2–L4) (5) **(Fig. 9.99)**.

Treatment Position: F SA (ankles) RA (knees/pelvis) RT (torso)

1. The patient lies supine, and the physician stands at the side of the tender point.

2. The physician may place the caudad leg on the table and lay the patient's legs on the physician's thigh.

3. The patient's hips and knees are flexed enough to engage the lower of the two segments involved.

4. The patient's hips and knees are pulled toward the physician, rotating the pelvis and lumbar spine to the level of the lower segment, leaving the upper segment rotated toward the tender point.

5. The patient's ankles and feet are brought toward the physician (away from the tender point), which side bends the lumbar spine away from the tender point **(Figs. 9.100 and 9.101)**.

6. The physician fine-tunes through small arcs of motion (more or less flexion, rotation, and side bending) until the tenderness has been *completely alleviated* or reduced as close to 100% as possible, but at least 70%.

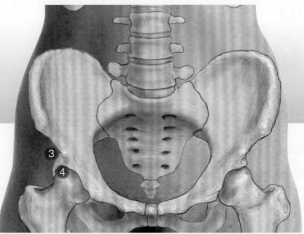

Figure 9.99. AL3–AL4 tender points. (Modified with permission from Ref. (8).)

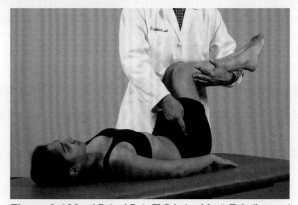

Figure 9.100. AL3–AL4: F SA (ankles) RA (knees/pelvis) RT (torso).

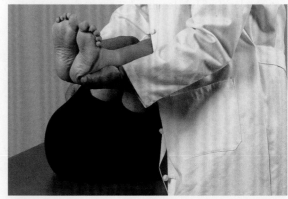

Figure 9.101. AL3–AL4: F SA (ankles) RA (knees/pelvis) RT (torso).

Anterior Lumbar Region

AL5

 See Video 9.26

Indication for Treatment

Somatic dysfunction of the lumbar, sacral, or pelvic region. The patient may complain of tenderness in the pubic region due to a pubic shear dysfunction or obturator nerve entrapment (5) or complain of low back, sacral, or pelvic pain (4).

Tender Point Location

On the anterior superior aspect of the pubic ramus just lateral to the symphysis. Press posterior **(Fig. 9.102)**. Anatomically may correlate with the rectus abdominis (4), adductor longus, pubic shear dysfunction or the referral site of obturator nerve entrapment (5).

Treatment Position: F SA (ankles) RA (torso)

1. The patient lies supine, and the physician stands at the side of the tender point.

2. The physician places the caudad foot leg on the table and lays the patient's legs on the physician's thigh.

3. The patient's hips and knees are flexed enough to engage the sacrum (S1).

4. The patient's hips and knees are pulled slightly toward the physician, rotating the pelvis/sacrum toward the tender point but leaving L5 rotated away from the side of the tender point.

5. The patient's ankles and feet are pushed slightly away from the physician, which produces side bending away from the tender point **(Fig. 9.103)**.

6. The physician fine-tunes through small arcs of motion (more or less flexion, rotation, and side bending) until the tenderness has been *completely alleviated* or reduced as close to 100% as possible, but at least 70%.

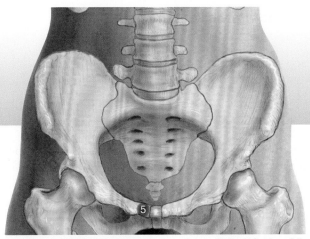
Figure 9.102. AL5 tender point. (Modified with permission from Ref. (8).)

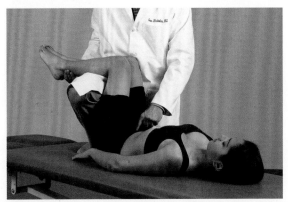
Figure 9.103. AL5: F SA (ankles) RT (knees/pelvis) RA (torso).

Anterior Pelvic Region

Anterior Pelvic Tender Points

Anterior pelvic counterstrain tender points are outlined in Table 9.8 and illustrated in **Figure 9.104**.

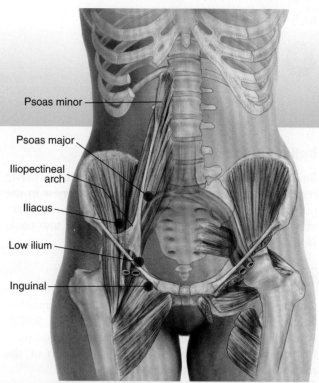

Psoas minor

Psoas major

Iliopectineal arch

Iliacus

Low ilium

Inguinal

Figure 9.104. Anterior pelvic counterstrain tender points. (Modified with permission from Ref. (8).)

Table 9.8	Common Anterior Pelvic Tender Points		
Tender Point	**Location**	**Classic Treatment Position**	**Acronym**
Psoas	⅔ of the distance from the ASIS to the midline; press deep in a posterior direction toward the belly of the psoas	Marked bilateral hip flexion; side bend lumbar spine toward; may require some external rotation of the hip	F ST
Iliacus	⅓ of the distance from the ASIS to the midline; press deep in a posterior lateral direction toward the iliacus	Marked bilateral flexion and external rotation of the hips with the knees flexed	F ER
Low ilium	Superior surface of the iliopectineal (iliopubic) eminence associated with the attachment of psoas minor	Marked ipsilateral hip flexion	F
Inguinal	On the lateral aspect of the pubic tubercle associated with the attachment of the pectineus muscle and/or the inguinal ligament	Flexion of thighs with contra-lateral thigh crossed over the ipsilateral thigh. Ipsilateral lower leg pulled laterally to create slight internal rotation of the hip on the affected side	F ADD IR

Anterior Pelvic Region

Psoas Major

 See Video 9.27

Indication for Treatment

Somatic dysfunction of the lumbar and/or pelvic region. The patient may complain of pain in the thoracolumbar region and/or the anterior hip, thigh, or groin (5).

Tender Point Location

The tender point is found ⅔ of the distance from the ASIS to the midline; press deep in a posterior direction toward the belly of the psoas **(Fig. 9.105)**.

Treatment Position: F ST er

1. The patient lies supine, and the physician stands at the side of the tender point.

2. The physician markedly flexes the patient's hips/knees and adds slight external rotation of the hips. Pulling the knees toward the tender point to side bend the lumbar spine may also be required **(Fig. 9.106)**.

3. The physician fine-tunes through small arcs of motion (more or less hip flexion, side bending, and rotation) until the tenderness is *completely alleviated* or reduced as close to 100% as possible, but at least 70%.

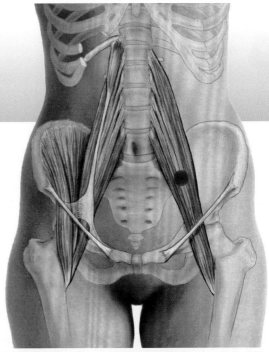

Figure 9.105. Psoas major tender point. (Modified with permission from Ref. (8).)

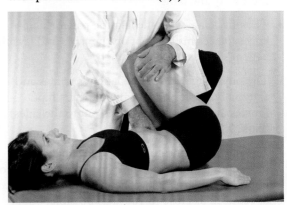

Figure 9.106. Psoas: F ST.

Anterior Pelvic Region

Iliacus

 See Video 9.28

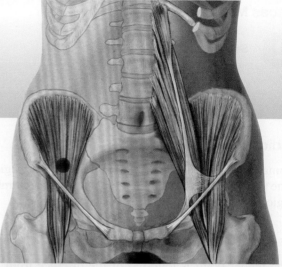

Figure 9.107. Iliacus tender point. (Modified with permission from Ref. (8).)

Indication for Treatment

Somatic dysfunction of the lumbar and/or pelvic region. The patient may complain of pain in the thoracolumbar region and/or anterior hip/thigh (5).

Tender Point Location

The tender point is found ⅓ of the distance from the ASIS to the midline; press deep in a posterolateral direction toward the iliacus **(Fig. 9.107)**.

Treatment Position: F ER (hips) Abd (knees)

1. The patient lies supine, and the physician stands at the side of the table.

2. The physician, while flexing the patient's hips/knees, places his/her foot on the table and lays the patient's knees on his/her thigh.

3. The physician crosses the patient's ankles and externally rotates both of the patient's hips (ankles are crossed with knees out to the sides) **(Figs. 9.108 and 9.109)**.

4. The physician fine-tunes through small arcs of motion (more or less hip flexion, external rotation) until the tenderness has been *completely alleviated* or reduced as close to 100% as possible, but at least 70%.

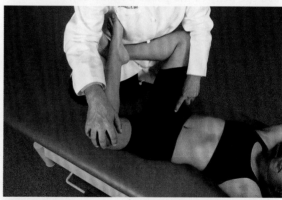

Figure 9.108. Iliacus: F ER (hips) Abd (knees).

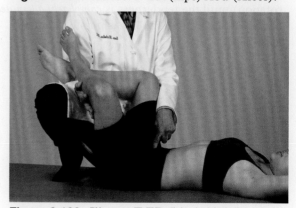

Figure 9.109. Iliacus: F ER (hips) Abd (knees).

Anterior Pelvic Region

Low Ilium (*Psoas Minor*)

 See Video 9.29

Indication for Treatment

Somatic dysfunction of the lumbar and/or pelvic region. The patient may complain of pain in the anterior hip and/or groin (4).

Tender Point Location

On the superior surface of the iliopectineal (iliopubic) eminence associated with the attachment of psoas minor muscle **(Fig. 9.110)**.

Treatment Position: F

1. The patient lies supine, and the physician stands at the side of the tender point.

2. The patient's hip on the side of the tender point is markedly flexed **(Fig. 9.111)**.

3. The physician fine-tunes through small arcs of motion (more or less hip flexion) until the tenderness is *completely alleviated* or reduced as close to 100% as possible, but at least 70%.

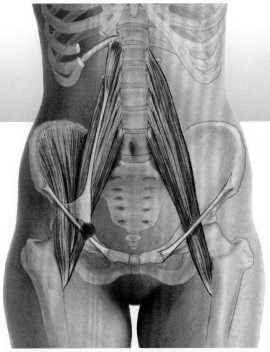

Figure 9.110. Low ilium tender point. (Modified with permission from Ref. (8).)

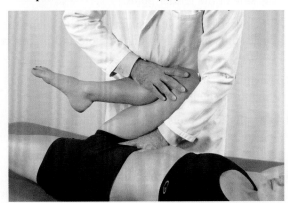

Figure 9.111. Low ilium: F.

Anterior Pelvic Region

Inguinal (*Pectineus*)

 See Video 9.30

Indication for Treatment

Somatic dysfunction of the pelvic region. The patient may complain of pain in the anterior hip, thigh, or groin.

Tender Point Location

The tender point is found on the lateral aspect of the pubic tubercle associated with the attachment of the pectineus muscle and/or the inguinal ligament. Press posterior and medially **(Fig. 9.112)**.

Treatment Position: F ADD IR

1. The patient lies supine, and the physician stands at the side of the tender point.

2. The physician, while flexing the patient's hips/knees, puts his/her foot on the table and places the patient's knees on his/her thigh.

3. The physician places the patient's contralateral thigh over the ipsilateral thigh.

4. The physician pulls the patient's ipsilateral lower leg laterally (toward TPt./Dr.) to induce adduction and internal rotation of the hip **(Fig. 9.113)**.

5. The physician fine-tunes (more or less hip flexion, internal rotation, and adduction) until the tenderness is *completely alleviated* or reduced as close to 100% as possible, but at least 70%.

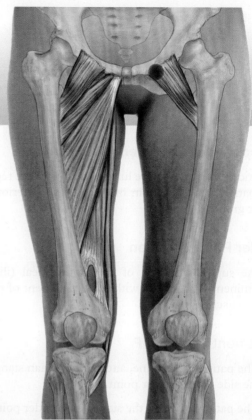

Figure 9.112. Inguinal tender point. (Modified with permission from Ref. (8).)

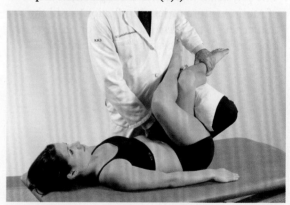

Figure 9.113. Inguinal: F ADD IR.

Posterior Lumbar Region

Posterior Lumbar Tender Points

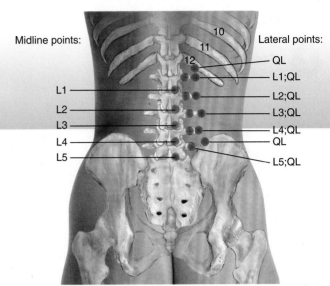

Posterior lumbar tender points are outlined in Table 9.9 and illustrated in **Figure 9.114**.

Figure 9.114. Posterior lumbar counterstrain tender points. (Modified with permission from Ref. (8).)

Table 9.9 Common Posterior Lumbar Tender Points

Tender Point	Location	Classic Treatment Position	Acronym
PL1–PL5 spinous process	On the inferolateral aspect/tip of the deviated spinous process of the dysfunctional segment *Vertebral rotation is opposite the side of spinous process deviation.	Patient prone: Extend to spinal level by lifting extremity or ASIS on side of tender point, which also rotates pelvis/lower segment toward and upper segment away; side bend away (adduct lower extremity)	e-E Sa Ra
PL1–PL5 transverse process	On the posterolateral aspect of the transverse process of the dysfunctional segment	As above	e-E SA RA
Quadratus lumborum	On the inferior aspect of the 12th rib On the lateral tips of the lumbar transverse processes On the superior aspect of the iliac crest	Hip/thigh extension, abduction, and external rotation. May require side bending of lumbar spine toward	E ABD ER

Posterior Lumbar Region

PL1–PL5

 See Video 9.31

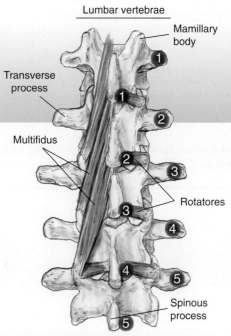

Figure 9.115. PL1–PL5 posterior and lateral tender points. (Modified with permission from Ref. (8).)

Indication for Treatment

Somatic dysfunction of the lumbar region. The patient may present with lower back pain in the area of the tender point.

Tender Point Location

PL1–PL5 Spinous Process: On the inferolateral aspect of the deviated spinous process of dysfunctional segment.
PL1–PL5 Transverse Process: On the posterolateral aspect of the transverse process of the dysfunctional segment **(Fig. 9.115).**

Treatment Position: e-E Add RT (pelvis) RA (torso)

1. The patient lies prone, and the physician stands at the side of the table that offers optimal control and ease of positioning.

2. The patient's thigh/hip is extended, adducted, and externally rotated. This rotates the pelvis and lower segment toward the side of the tender point, leaving the upper segment rotated away from the side of the tender point **(Figs. 9.116 and 9.117).**

3. The physician fine-tunes through small arcs of motion (more or less hip extension, adduction, and external rotation) until the tenderness has been *completely alleviated* or reduced as close to 100% as possible, but at least 70%.

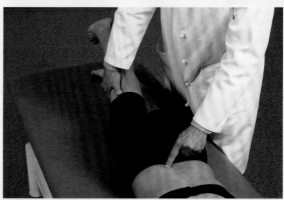

Figure 9.116. PL4: e-E Add RT (pelvis) RA (torso).

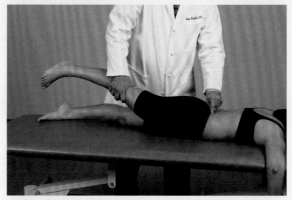

Figure 9.117. PL4: e-E Add RT (pelvis) RA (torso).

Posterior Lumbar Region

PL1–PL5 (Alternate)

 See Video 9.32

Indication for Treatment

Somatic dysfunction of the lumbar region. The patient may present with lower back pain in the area of the tender point.

Tender Point Location

PL1–PL5 Spinous Process: On the inferolateral aspect of the deviated spinous process of dysfunctional segment.
PL1–PL5 Transverse Process: On the posterolateral aspect of the transverse process of the dysfunctional segment **(Fig. 9.118)**.

Treatment Position: E Sa RT (pelvis) RA (torso)

1. The patient lies prone, and the physician stands on the side opposite the tender point.

2. The patient's legs are positioned to the side that produces the greatest reduction in tenderness. The side bending component may vary depending on which myofascial structures are involved, the direction of their fibers, or whether there is an articular component to the dysfunction.

3. The physician grasps the ASIS on the side of the tender point and leans back, gently lifting upward to induce extension and rotation of the pelvis and lower segment toward the side of the tender point, leaving the upper segment rotated away from the side of the tender point **(Figs. 9.119 and 9.120)**.

4. The physician fine-tunes through small arcs of motion (more or less extension) until the tenderness has been *completely alleviated* or reduced as close to 100% as possible, but at least 70%.

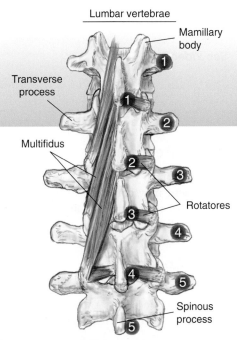

Figure 9.118. PL1–PL5 posterior and lateral tender points. (Modified with permission from Ref. (8).)

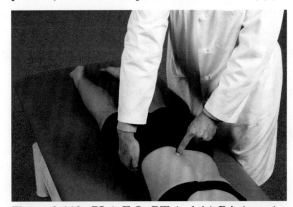

Figure 9.119. PL4: E Sa RT (pelvis) RA (torso).

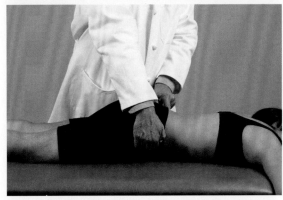

Figure 9.120. PL4: E Sa RT (pelvis) RA (torso).

Posterior Lumbar Region

Quadratus Lumborum

 See Video 9.33

Indication for Treatment

Somatic dysfunction of the 12th rib, lumbar, or pelvic region. The patient may complain of pain in the lower back, at the top of the iliac crest, and in the posterior hip/buttock/sacroiliac region (4,5).

Tender Point Location

On the inferior aspect of the 12th rib (4).
On the lateral tips of the lumbar transverse processes (4).
On the superior aspect of the iliac crest (4) **(Fig. 9.121)**.

Treatment Position: E ABD ER

1. The patient lies prone, and the physician stands on the side of the tender point.

2. The physician side bends the trunk toward the side of the tender point.

3. The physician extends, abducts, and externally rotates the patient's hip **(Fig. 9.122)**.

4. The physician fine-tunes through small arcs of motion (more or less hip extension, abduction, and external rotation) until the tenderness is *completely alleviated* or reduced as close to 100% as possible, but at least 70%.

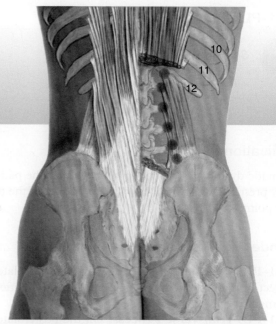

Figure 9.121. Quadratus lumborum tender point. (Modified with permission from Ref. (8).)

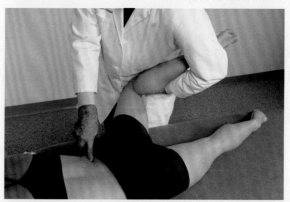

Figure 9.122. Quadratus lumborum: E ABD ER.

Posterior Pelvic Region

Posterior Pelvic Tender Points

Posterior pelvic counterstrain tender points are outlined in Table 9.10 and illustrated in **Figure 9.123**.

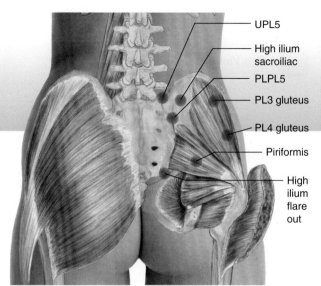

Figure 9.123. Posterior pelvic counterstrain tender points. (Modified with permission from Ref. (8).)

Table 9.10 Common Posterior Pelvic Tender Points

Tender Point	Location	Classic Treatment Position	Acronym
Upper pole L5 UPL5	Superior medial surface of the posterior superior iliac spine (PSIS)	Hip extension, fine-tune with adduction, internal/external rotation	E Add er/ir
High ilium sacroiliac	2–3 cm lateral to the PSIS pressing medially toward the PSIS	Hip extension, fine-tune with abduction, external rotation	E Abd ER
Lower pole L5 LPL5	On the ilium just inferior to PSIS pressing superiorly	Hip flexed 90, slight internal rotation, and adduction	F IR Add
High ilium flare out	Lateral aspect of the ILA and/or lateral aspect of the coccyx *Note:* Jones 1 describes three separate locations for this point: lateral margin of the coccyx, ILA, and inferior aspect of the buttock. Jones 2 calls the ILA point HIFO, then drops the point at the coccyx, and renames the buttocks point as the gemelli point.	Hip extension, adduction	E Add E ADD
PL3 lateral PL4 lateral (gluteus medius)	Upper outer portion of the gluteus medius at the level of the PSIS PL3— ⅔ lateral from PSIS to tensor fasciae latae PL4—posterior margin of tensor fasciae latae	Hip extension with fine-tuning in abduction and external rotation	E Abd er
Piriformis	Midpoint between the lower half of the lateral aspect of the sacrum and ILA and the greater trochanter	Marked flexion of the hip and abduction. Fine-tune with external or internal rotation	F ABD er/ir

Posterior Pelvic Region

Lower Pole L5 (LPL5)

 See Videos 9.34 and 9.35

Indication for Treatment

Somatic dysfunction of the lumbar spine and/or pelvis. The patient may complain of low back pain and/or pelvic pain.

Tender Point Location

On the ilium just inferior to the PSIS associated with the posterior sacroiliac ligaments, the erector spinae or biceps femoris muscles (5), or a referral site from the iliopsoas muscle group (4) **(Fig. 9.124)**.

Treatment Position: F IR Add

1. The patient lies prone close to the edge of the table, and the physician stands or sits at the side of the tender point.

2. The patient's lower extremity is suspended off the edge of the table, with the knee and hip flexed 90 degrees **(Fig. 9.125)**.

3. The patient's hip is internally rotated and the knee is adducted slightly under the table **(Fig. 9.126)**.

4. **Alternate technique:** The patient lies in the lateral recumbent position on the side opposite the tender point. The patient's hip and knee are flexed 90 degrees, and the hip is internally rotated and the knee/thigh is adducted **(Fig. 9.127)**.

5. The physician fine-tunes (more or less hip flexion, internal rotation, adduction) until the tenderness is *completely alleviated* or reduced as close to 100% as possible, but at least 70%.

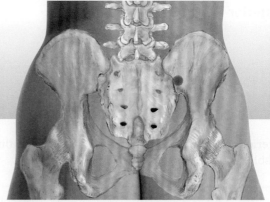

Figure 9.124. Lower pole L5 tender point. (Modified with permission from Ref. (8).)

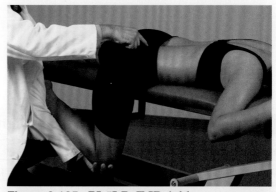

Figure 9.125. PL5LP: F IR Add.

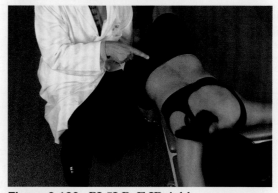

Figure 9.126. PL5LP: F IR Add.

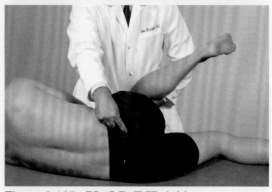

Figure 9.127. PL5LP: F IR Add.

Posterior Pelvic Region

Upper Pole L5 (UPL5)

 See Video 9.36

Indication for Treatment

Somatic dysfunction of the lumbar spine and/or pelvis. The patient may complain of low back and pelvic pain.

Tender Point Location

On the superior medial aspect of the posterior superior iliac spine (PSIS) between the L5 spinous process and the PSIS **(Fig. 9.128)**. Anatomically may correlate the multifidus and rotatores muscles and/or the iliolumbar ligament (4,5).

Treatment Position: E Add ir/er

1. The patient lies prone, and the physician stands at the side of the tender point.

2. The physician extends and adducts the patient's hip and fine-tunes through small arcs of motion (more or less hip extension, adduction, external or internal rotation) until the tenderness is *completely alleviated* or reduced as close to 100% as possible, but at least 70% **(Fig. 9.129)**.

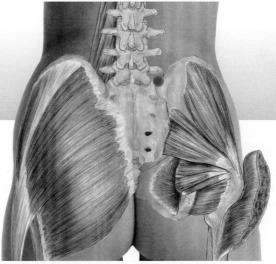

Figure 9.128. Upper pole L5 tender point. (Modified with permission from Ref. (8).)

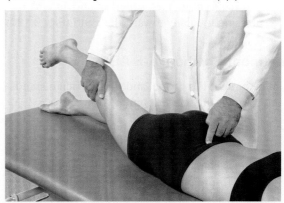

Figure 9.129. UPL5: E Add ir/er.

Posterior Pelvic Region

High Ilium Sacroiliac

 See Video 9.37

Indication for Treatment

Somatic dysfunction of the lumbar and/or pelvic region. The patient may complain of pain in the buttock associated with strain of the quadratus lumborum (5) or the gluteus maximus muscle (4) or sprain of the iliolumbar ligament (5).

Tender Point Location

Two to three centimeters superior and lateral to the PSIS, pressing medially toward the PSIS **(Fig. 9.130)**.

Treatment Position: e-E ABD ER

1. The patient lies prone, and the physician stands on the side of the tender point.

2. The patient's hip/lower extremity is extended, abducted, and externally rotated **(Fig. 9.131)**.

3. The physician fine-tunes through small arcs of motion (more or less hip extension, external rotation, abduction) until the tenderness is *completely alleviated* or reduced as close to 100% as possible, but at least 70%.

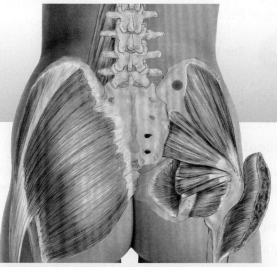

Figure 9.130. High ilium sacroiliac tender point. (Modified with permission from Ref. (8).)

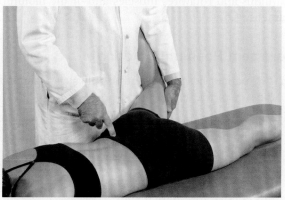

Figure 9.131. HI SI gluteus e-E ABD ER.

Posterior Pelvic Region

High Ilium Flare Out (*Coccygeus*)

 See Video 9.38

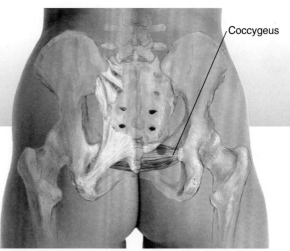

Coccygeus

Figure 9.132. High ilium flare out tender point. (Modified with permission from Ref. (8).)

Indication for Treatment

Somatic dysfunction of the pelvic region or sacrum. The patient may complain of pain in the lower medial portion of the gluteus maximus (4) or deep within the coccygeus muscle and pelvic floor (5).

Tender Point Location

On the lateral aspect of the inferior angle of the sacrum (ILA) associated with the attachment of the coccygeus muscle (5) **(Fig. 9.132)**.

Treatment Position: E ADD

1. The patient lies prone, and the physician stands at the side of the table opposite the tender point.

2. The patient's hip/lower extremity is extended and adducted enough to cross over the contralateral leg **(Fig. 9.133)**.

3. The physician fine-tunes through small arcs of motion (more or less hip extension, adduction) until the tenderness is *completely alleviated* or reduced as close to 100% as possible, but at least 70%.

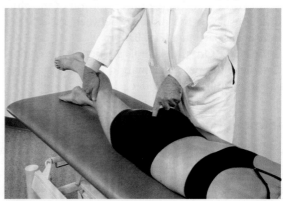

Figure 9.133. HI IL FO: E ADD.

Posterior Pelvic Region

PL3 Lateral, PL4 Lateral (*Gluteus Medius*)

 See Video 9.39

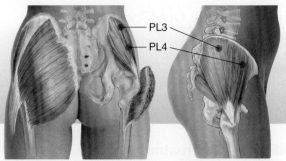

Figure 9.134. PL3, PL4 lateral (gluteus medius) tender points. (Modified with permission from Ref. (8).)

Indication for Treatment

Somatic dysfunction of the lumbar and/or pelvic region. The patient may complain of pain below the iliac crest in the posterior gluteal region while walking or getting up from seated position (5).

Tender Point Location

PL3 lateral: On the upper outer portion of the gluteus medius muscle, ⅔ the distance between the PSIS and the tensor fasciae latae **(Fig. 9.134)**.
PL4 lateral: On the lateral portion of the gluteus medius near the posterior margin of the tensor fasciae latae **(Fig. 9.134)**.

Treatment Position: E Abd er

1. The patient lies prone, and the physician stands at the side of the tender point.

2. The patient's hip/thigh is extended and abducted. May require external rotation or internal rotation of the hip **(Figs. 9.135 and 9.136)**.

3. The physician fine-tunes through small arcs of motion (more or less hip extension, abduction, internal/external rotation) until the tenderness is *completely alleviated* or reduced as close to 100% as possible, but at least 70%.

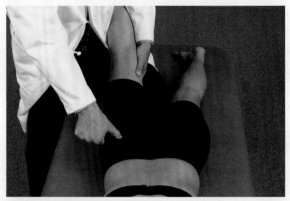

Figure 9.135. PL3, PL4 lateral: E Abd er.

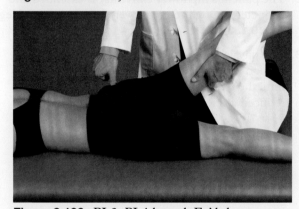

Figure 9.136. PL3, PL4 lateral: E Abd er.

Posterior Pelvic Region

Piriformis

See Videos 9.40 and 9.41

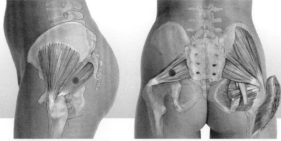

Figure 9.137. Piriformis tender point. (Modified with permission from Ref. (8).)

Indication for Treatment

Somatic dysfunction of the pelvic region. The patient may complain of pain in the buttock and the posterior thigh (sciatic neuritis).

Tender Point Location

Classically found at the midpoint between the lower half of the lateral aspect of the sacrum (ILA) and the greater trochanter **(Fig. 9.137)**. This is near the sciatic notch, and therefore, to avoid sciatic irritation, we have commonly used the tender points either proximal to the sacrum or the trochanter. If both of these can be simultaneously reduced effectively, the treatment can be extremely successful.

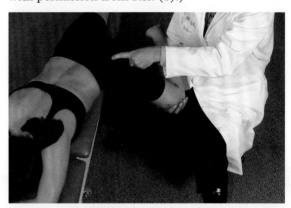

Figure 9.138. Piriformis: F abd-ABD er.

Treatment Position: F ABD ER

1. The patient lies prone, and the physician stands or sits on the side of the tender point.

2. The patient's leg (on the side of the tender point) is off the edge of the table; the hip is markedly flexed and abducted. The patient's leg rests on the physician's thigh/knee **(Fig. 9.138)**.

3. The physician fine-tunes through small arcs of motion (more or less hip flexion, abduction, external or internal rotation) until the tenderness is *completely alleviated* or reduced as close to 100% as possible, but at least 70%.

4. Alternate position No. 1: patient supine, marked flexion of the hip, abduction, and external or internal rotation **(Fig. 9.139)**.

5. Alternate position No. 2: patient lateral recumbent, marked flexion of the hip, abduction, and external or internal rotation **(Fig. 9.140)**.

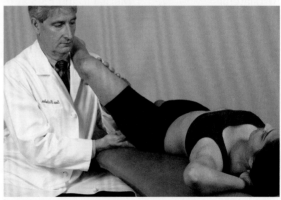

Figure 9.139. Piriformis: F abd-ABD er.

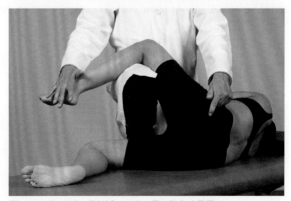

Figure 9.140. Piriformis: F abd-ABD er.

Sacral Region

Sacral Tender Points

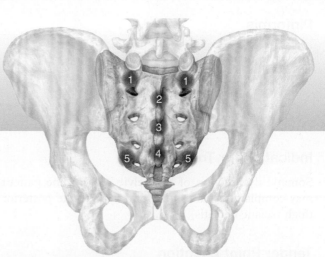

Sacral counterstrain tender points are outlined in Table 9.11 and illustrated in **Figure 9.141**.

Figure 9.141. Sacral counterstrain tender points. (Modified with permission from Ref. (9).)

Table 9.11 Common Sacral Tender Points

Tender Point	Location	Classic Treatment Position
PS1 bilateral	Medial to the PSIS at the level S1 (sacral sulcus/base)	Apply a posterior-to-anterior pressure on the opposite ILA, which rotates the sacrum around the oblique axis
PS2; PS3; PS4 midline	Midline on the sacrum at the corresponding sacral level	2: Apply a posterior-to-anterior pressure midline to the apex of the sacrum (extend sacrum) 3: May require flexion or extension 4: Apply posterior-to-anterior pressure midline on the base of the sacrum (flex sacrum) Note: This produces rotation of the sacrum around the transverse axis.
PS5 bilateral	Just medial and superior to the ILA of the sacrum	Apply a posterior-to-anterior pressure on the opposite sacral base, which rotates sacrum around the oblique axis

Source: Myers HL. Clinical Application of Counterstrain. Tucson, AZ: Osteopathic Press, A Division of Tucson Osteopathic Medical Foundation, 2006.

Sacral Region

PS1 Bilateral

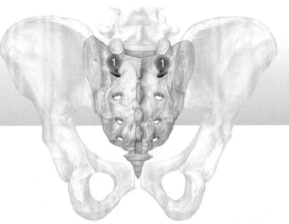

Figure 9.142. PS1 bilateral tender points. (Modified with permission from Ref. (9).)

Indication for Treatment

Somatic dysfunction of the lumbar spine, pelvis, or sacrum. The patient may complain of pain in the sacral or pelvic region associated with the attachment of the erector spinae and transversospinalis muscle group (4).

Tender Point Location

Medial to the PSIS at the level of S1 (sacral base) **(Fig. 9.142)**.

Treatment Position

1. The patient lies prone, and the physician stands at the side of the table.

2. The physician applies a posterior to anterior pressure on the inferolateral angle (ILA) of the sacrum diagonally opposite the tender point. This produces rotation of the sacrum around the oblique axis (4) **(Figs. 9.143 and 9.144)**.

3. The physician fine-tunes with more or less pressure of the opposite ILA until the tenderness is *completely alleviated* or reduced as close to 100% as possible, but at least 70%.

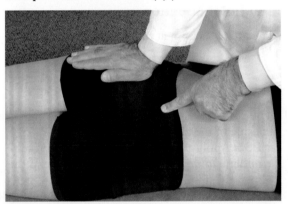

Figure 9.143. PS1.

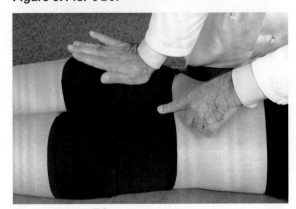

Figure 9.144. PS1.

Sacral Region

PS2–PS4 Midline

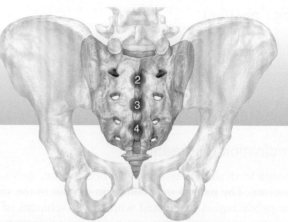

Figure 9.145. PS2; PS3; PS4 tender points. (Modified with permission from Ref. (9).)

Indication for Treatment

Somatic dysfunction of the lumbar region, pelvis, or sacrum. The patient may complain of pain in sacral or pelvic region associated with the attachment of the erector spinae and transversospinalis muscle group (4).

Tender Point Location

Midline on the sacrum at the corresponding sacral level **(Fig. 9.145)**.

Treatment Position

1. The patient lies prone, and the physician stands at the side of the table.
   - **PS2:** Apply a posterior to anterior pressure midline to the apex of the sacrum (extend the sacrum) **(Fig. 9.146)**.
   - **PS3:** May require flexion/extension **(Figs. 9.146 and 9.147)**.
   - **PS4:** Apply a posterior to anterior pressure midline on the base of the sacrum (flex the sacrum) **(Fig. 9.147)**.

   Note: This produces rotation of the sacrum around the transverse axis (4).

2. The physician fine-tunes with more or less pressure on the sacrum until the tenderness is *completely alleviated* or reduced as close to 100% as possible, but at least 70%.

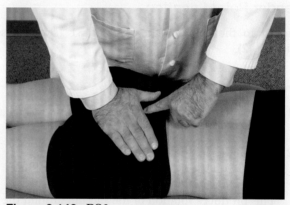

Figure 9.146. PS2.

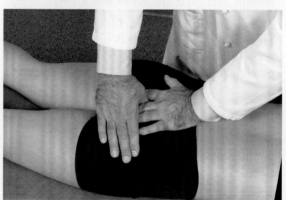

Figure 9.147. PS4.

Sacral Region

PS5 Bilateral

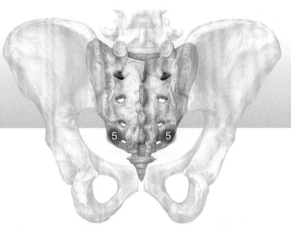

Figure 9.148. PS5 bilateral tender points. (Modified with permission from Ref. (9).)

Indication for Treatment

Somatic dysfunction of the lumbar region, pelvis, or sacrum. The patient may complain of pain in the sacral or pelvic region associated with the attachment of the erector spinae and transversospinalis muscle group (4).

Tender Point Location

Just medial and superior to the ILA of the sacrum **(Fig. 9.148)**.

Treatment Position

1. The patient lies prone, and the physician stands at the side of the table.

2. The physician applies a posterior to anterior pressure on the sacral base/sulcus diagonally opposite the tender point. This produces rotation of the sacrum around the oblique axis (4) **(Fig. 9.149)**.

3. The physician fine-tunes with more or less pressure on the sacral base until the tenderness is *completely alleviated* or reduced as close to 100% as possible, but at least 70%.

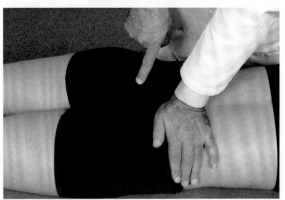

Figure 9.149. PS5.

Lower Extremity Region

Lower Extremity Tender Points

Lower extremity counterstrain tender points are outlined in Table 9.12.

Table 9.12 Common Lower Extremity Tender Points

Tender Point	Location	Classic Treatment Position	Acronym
Tensor fascia latae	Inferior to the crest of the ilium in the body of the tensor fascia latae muscle	Abduction of the hip/thigh, slight flexion	f ABD
Lateral trochanter Iliotibial band	Along the iliotibial band distal to the greater trochanter	Moderate abduction of the hip/thigh, slight flexion	f ABD
Lateral hamstring Biceps femoris	In the posterior thigh lateral to the midline approximately halfway down the shaft of the femur	Flexion of the knee with external rotation and slight abduction of the tibia and plantar flexion of the ankle by compression on the calcaneus	F ER Abd
Lateral meniscus Lateral collateral ligament	Lateral aspect of the meniscus on the joint line	Moderate knee flexion, slight abduction, internal or external rotation of the tibia. May require ankle dorsiflexion and eversion	F Abd ir/er
Medial hamstring Semimembranosus Semitendinosus	In the posterior thigh medial to the midline approximately halfway down the shaft of the femur	Flexion of the knee with internal rotation and slight adduction of the tibia and plantar flexion of the ankle by compression on the calcaneus	F IR Add
Medial meniscus Medial collateral ligament	Anteromedial aspect of the meniscus on the joint line	Moderate knee flexion, internal rotation, and slight adduction of the tibia	F IR Add
Anterior cruciate	Superior aspect of the popliteal fossa on the hamstring tendons, either medially or laterally	Place an object/pillow under the distal femur to create a fulcrum. Apply a shearing force by moving the proximal tibia posteriorly on the femur *Note:* Classic Jones treatment	

Table 9.12 Common Lower Extremity Tender Points (Continued)

Tender Point	Location	Classic Treatment Position	Acronym
Posterior cruciate	In the center or slightly below the center of the popliteal fossa	Place an object/pillow under the distal femur to create a fulcrum. Apply a shearing force by moving the distal femur posteriorly on the proximal tibia *Note:* Classic Jones treatment	
Popliteus	In the belly of the popliteus muscle just inferior to the popliteal space	Slight flexion of the knee with internal rotation of the tibia	F IR
Extension ankle Gastrocnemius	Within the proximal gastrocnemius muscles distal to the popliteal margin	Marked plantar flexion of the ankle with knee flexion	
Medial ankle Tibialis anterior	Inferior to the medial malleolus along the deltoid ligament	Place a fulcrum on the medial aspect of the ankle. Apply an inversion force with slight shear/internal rotation of foot.	INV ir
Lateral ankle fibularis/ peroneus longus, brevis, tertius	Inferior and anterior to the lateral malleolus in the sinus tarsi (talocalcaneal sulcus)	Place a fulcrum on the lateral aspect of the ankle. Apply an eversion force with slight shear /external rotation of foot	EV er
Flexion calcaneus Quadratus plantae	Anterior aspect of the calcaneus on the plantar surface of the foot at the attachment of the plantar fascia	Marked flexion of the forefoot approximating the forefoot to the calcaneus	F

Lower Extremity Region

Lateral Trochanter (*Tensor Fasciae Latae*)

 See Video 9.42

Indication for Treatment

Somatic dysfunction of the pelvic region or lower extremity. The patient may complain of pain in the lateral hip or thigh (4,5).

Tender Point Location

Just inferior to the crest of the ilium in the body of the tensor fasciae latae muscle **(Fig. 9.150)**.

Treatment Position: f ABD

1. The patient lies prone or supine, and the physician stands or sits at the side of the tender point.

2. The patient's hip/thigh is abducted and slightly flexed until the tenderness is *completely alleviated* or reduced as close to 100% as possible, but at least 70%. May require slight internal rotation of the hip (4) **(Fig. 9.151)**.

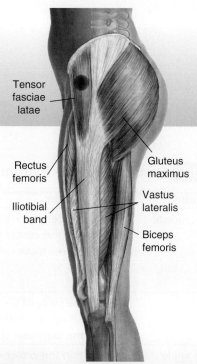

Tensor fasciae latae

Rectus femoris

Iliotibial band

Gluteus maximus

Vastus lateralis

Biceps femoris

Figure 9.150. Tensor fasciae latae tender point. (Modified with permission from Ref. (8).)

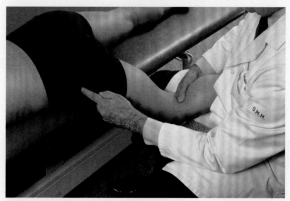

Figure 9.151. Tensor fasciae latae: f ABD.

Lower Extremity Region

Lateral Trochanter (*Iliotibial Band*)

 See Video 9.42

Indication for Treatment

Somatic dysfunction of the pelvis and/or lower extremity. The patient may present with pain in the lateral hip/thigh (4).

Tender Point Location

Along the iliotibial band distal to the lateral trochanter **(Fig. 9.152)**.

Treatment Position: f ABD

1. The patient lies supine or prone, and the physician stands or sits at the side of the tender point.

2. The patient's hip/thigh is abducted and slightly flexed until the tenderness is *completely alleviated* or reduced as close to 100% as possible, but at least 70%. May require slight internal or external rotation of the hip **(Fig. 9.153)**.

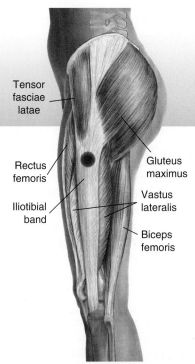

Figure 9.152. Iliotibial band tender point. (Modified with permission from Ref. (8).)

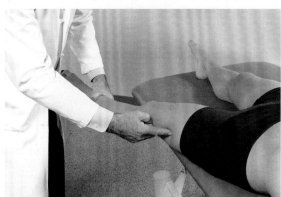

Figure 9.153. Iliotibial band: f ABD.

Lower Extremity Region

Lateral Hamstring (*Biceps Femoris*)

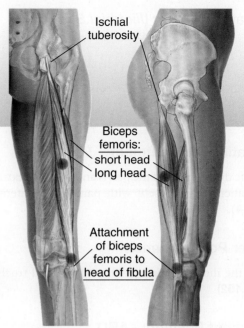

Figure 9.154. Lateral hamstring tender point. (Modified with permission from Ref. (8).)

Indication for Treatment

Somatic dysfunction of the lower extremity. The patient may present with pain in posterolateral aspect of the knee, which may be associated with strain of the biceps femoris tendon or sprain of the anterior cruciate or fibular (lateral) collateral ligaments (1,4,5).

Tender Point Location

On the distal aspect of the biceps femoris muscle near its attachment to the posterolateral surface of the fibular head. May also be found in the posterior thigh, lateral to the midline, approximately halfway down the shaft of the femur **(Fig. 9.154)**.

Treatment Position: F ER abd

1. The patient lies supine or prone, and the physician stands or sits at the side of the tender point.

2. The physician grasps the patient's lateral ankle/foot to control the lower leg.

3. The patient's knee is flexed and the tibia is externally rotated with slight abduction; compression on the calcaneus is added to plantar flex the ankle **(Figs. 9.155 and 9.156)**.

4. The physician fine-tunes (more or less flexion, external rotation, abduction) until the tenderness is *completely alleviated* or reduced as close to 100% as possible, but at least 70%.

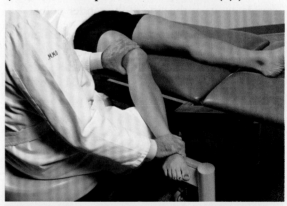

Figure 9.155. Lateral hamstring: F ER Abd.

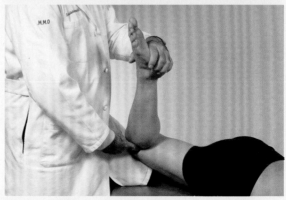

Figure 9.156. Lateral hamstring: F ER Abd.

Lower Extremity Region

Lateral Meniscus
Lateral (Fibular) Collateral Ligament

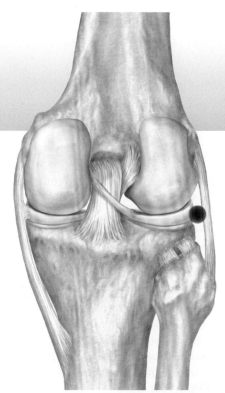

Figure 9.157. Lateral meniscus/collateral ligament tender point. (Modified with permission from Ref. (9).)

Indication for Treatment

Somatic dysfunction of the lower extremity. The patient may present with pain along the lateral aspect of the knee associated with sprain of the fibular (lateral) collateral ligament and/or inflammation of the lateral meniscus (1,4,5).

Tender Point Location

On the lateral aspect of the knee at the lateral joint line associated with fibular (lateral) collateral ligament and lateral meniscus **(Fig. 9.157)**.

Treatment Position: F Abd ir/er

1. The patient lies supine, and the physician stands or sits on the side of the tender point.

2. The patient's hip/thigh is abducted so that the leg hangs off the edge of the table.

3. The physician grasps the patient's lateral ankle/foot to control the lower leg.

4. The patient's knee is flexed approximately 35 to 40 degrees with slight abduction and internal or external rotation of the tibia. May require ankle dorsiflexion and eversion (10) **(Fig. 9.158)**.

5. The physician fine-tunes (more or less flexion, abduction, and internal or external rotation) until the tenderness is *completely alleviated* or reduced as close to 100% as possible, but at least 70%.

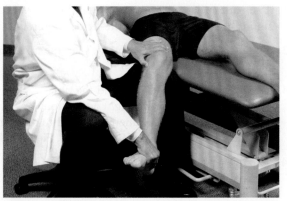

Figure 9.158. Lateral meniscus/collateral ligament: F Abd ir/er.

Lower Extremity Region

Medial Hamstring (*Semimembranosus*)

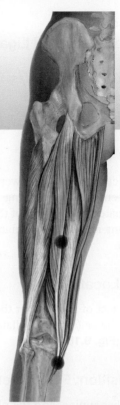

Indication for Treatment

Somatic dysfunction of the lower extremity. The patient may present with pain in the posterior medial aspect of the knee, which may be associated with strain of the semimembranosus and/or semitendinosus tendons and/or sprain of the anterior cruciate ligament (1,4,5).

Tender Point Location

On the distal aspect of the medial hamstring tendons (semimembranosus/semitendinosus) near their attachment to the posterior medial surface of the tibial condyle. May also be found in the posterior thigh medial to the midline, approximately halfway down the shaft of the femur **(Fig. 9.159)**.

Figure 9.159. Medial hamstring tender point. (Modified with permission from Ref. (8).)

Treatment Position: F IR Add

1. The patient lies supine or prone, and the physician stands or sits at the side of the tender point.

2. The physician grasps the patient's lateral ankle/foot to control the lower leg.

3. The patient's knee is flexed and the tibia is internally rotated with slight adduction; compression on the calcaneus is added to plantar flex the ankle (*supine*, **Fig. 9.160**; *prone*, **Fig. 9.161**).

4. The physician fine-tunes (more or less flexion, internal rotation, adduction) until the tenderness is *completely alleviated* or reduced as close to 100% as possible, but at least 70%.

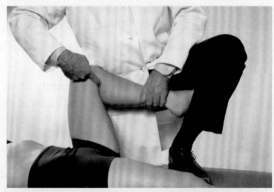

Figure 9.160. Medial hamstring: F IR Add.

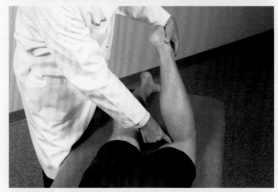

Figure 9.161. Medial hamstring: F IR Add.

Lower Extremity Region

Medial Meniscus
Medial (Tibial) Collateral Ligament

Indication for Treatment

Somatic dysfunction of the lower extremity. The patient may present with pain along the medial aspect of the knee associated with sprain of the tibial (medial) collateral ligament and/or inflammation of the medial meniscus (1,4,5).

Tender Point Location

On the medial aspect of the knee at the medial joint line associated with tibial (medial) collateral ligament and medial meniscus (**Fig. 9.162**).

Treatment Position: F IR Add

1. The patient lies supine, and the physician stands or sits on the side of the tender point.

2. The patient's hip/thigh is abducted so the leg hangs off the edge of the table.

3. The physician grasps the patient's lateral ankle/foot to control the lower leg.

4. The patient's knee is flexed approximately 35 to 40 degrees, and the tibia is adducted and internally rotated. May require plantar flexion and inversion of the ankle (10) (**Fig. 9.163**).

5. The physician fine-tunes (more or less flexion, adduction, and internal rotation) until the tenderness is *completely alleviated* or reduced as close to 100% as possible, but at least 70%.

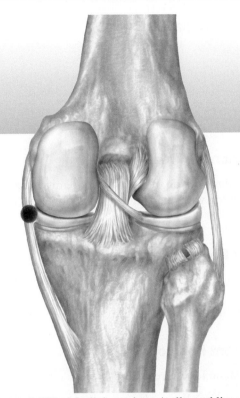

Figure 9.162. Medial meniscus/collateral ligament tender point. (Modified with permission from Ref. (9).)

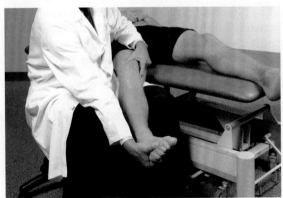

Figure 9.163. Medial meniscus/collateral ligament: F IR Add.

Lower Extremity Region

Anterior Cruciate

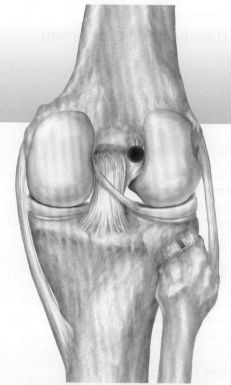

Indication for Treatment

Somatic dysfunction of the lower extremity. The patient may present with pain in the posterior aspect of the knee.

Tender Point Location

On the superior aspect of the popliteal fossa adjacent to the hamstring tendons, either medially or laterally **(Fig. 9.164)**.

Treatment Position

Note: Classic Jones Treatment

1. The patient lies supine, and the physician places a towel roll or pillow under the distal femur to create a fulcrum.

2. The physician places a hand over the anterior proximal tibia (tibial tuberosity) and applies a posterior force that moves the proximal tibia posteriorly on the distal femur **(Fig. 9.165)**.

3. The physician fine-tunes (more or less pressure on the proximal tibia) until the tenderness is *completely alleviated* or reduced as close to 100% as possible, but at least 70%.

Figure 9.164. Anterior cruciate tender point. (Modified with permission from Ref. (9).)

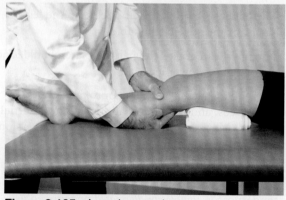

Figure 9.165. Anterior cruciate.

Lower Extremity Region

Posterior Cruciate

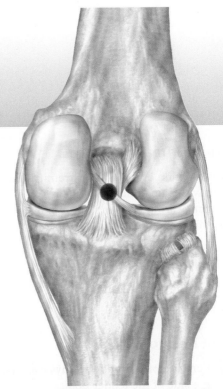

Indication for Treatment

Somatic dysfunction of the lower extremity. The patient may present with pain in the posterior aspect of the knee.

Tender Point Location

In the center or slightly below the center of the popliteal fossa **(Fig. 9.166)**.

Treatment Position

Note: Classic Jones Treatment

1. The patient lies supine, and the physician places a towel roll or pillow under the proximal tibia (calf) to create a fulcrum.

2. The physician places a hand over the anterior thigh (distal femur) and applies a posterior force that moves the distal femur posteriorly on the proximal tibia **(Fig. 9.167)**.

3. The physician fine-tunes (more or less pressure on the distal femur) until the tenderness is *completely alleviated* or reduced as close to 100% as possible, but at least 70%.

Figure 9.166. Posterior cruciate tender point. (Modified with permission from Ref. (9).)

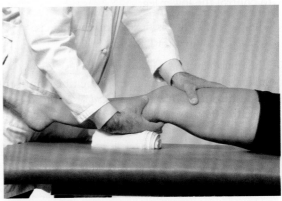

Figure 9.167. Posterior cruciate.

Lower Extremity Region

Popliteus

Indication for Treatment

Somatic dysfunction of the lower extremity. The patient may present with pain in the posterior aspect of the knee during weight bearing (walking or running) associated with strain of the popliteus muscle (4,5).

Tender Point Location

In the belly of the popliteus muscle just inferior to the popliteal space **(Fig. 9.168)**.

Treatment Position: F IR

1. The patient lies prone, and the physician stands or sits on the side of the tender point.

2. The physician grasps the patient's lateral ankle/foot to control the lower leg.

3. The patient's knee is flexed and the tibia is internally rotated **(Fig. 9.169)**.

4. The physician fine-tunes (more or less knee flexion and internal rotation of the tibia) until the tenderness is *completely alleviated* or reduced as close to 100% as possible, but at least 70%.

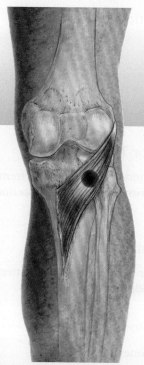

Figure 9.168. Popliteus tender point. (Modified with permission from Ref. (8).)

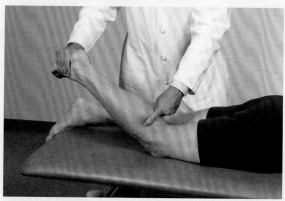

Figure 9.169. Popliteus: F IR.

Lower Extremity Region

Extension Ankle (*Gastrocnemius*)

Indication for Treatment

Somatic dysfunction of the lower extremity. The patient may present with pain in the posterior aspect of the knee and calf region.

Tender Point Location

Within the proximal gastrocnemius muscles distal to the popliteal margin **(Fig. 9.170)**.

Treatment Position

1. The patient lies prone, and the physician stands at the side of the tender point and places his/her foot on the edge of the table.

2. The patient's knee is flexed and the dorsum of the foot is placed on the physician's thigh.

3. The physician applies a compressive force on the patient's calcaneus to produce marked plantar flexion of the ankle **(Fig. 9.171)**.

4. The physician fine-tunes (more or less plantar flexion) until the tenderness is *completely alleviated* or reduced as close to 100% as possible, but at least 70%.

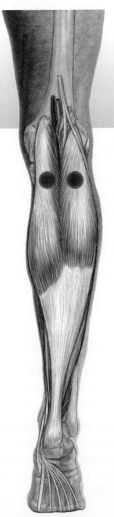

Figure 9.170. Extension ankle tender point. (Modified with permission from Ref. (8).)

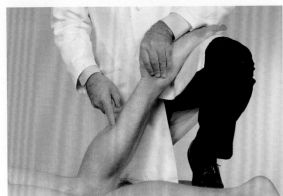

Figure 9.171. Extension ankle: plantar flexion.

Lower Extremity Region

Medial Ankle (*Tibialis Anterior*)

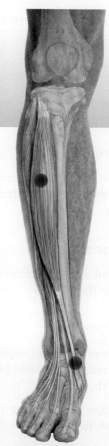

Indication for Treatment

Somatic dysfunction of the lower extremity. The patient may present with pain in the medial aspect of the lower leg or medial ankle.

Tender Point Location

Anterior and inferior to the medial malleolus along the deltoid ligament. May also be found along the anterior surface of tibia in the tibialis anterior muscle **(Fig. 9.172)**.

Treatment Position: INV ir

1. The patient lies in the lateral recumbent position, and the physician places a pillow under the medial aspect of the distal tibia to create a fulcrum.

2. The physician applies an inversion force to the foot and ankle with slight internal rotation of the foot until the tenderness is *completely alleviated* or reduced as close to 100% as possible, but at least 70% **(Fig. 9.173)**.

Figure 9.172. Medial ankle tender point. (Modified with permission from Ref. (8).)

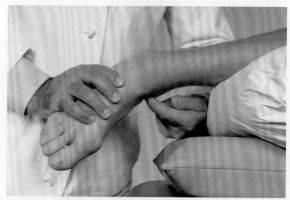

Figure 9.173. Medial ankle: INV ir.

Lower Extremity Region

Lateral Ankle *Fibularis* (*Peroneus*) *Longus, Brevis, Tertius*

Indication for Treatment

Somatic dysfunction of the lower extremity. The patient may present with pain along the lateral aspect of the lower leg or ankle.

Tender Point Location

Anterior and inferior to the lateral malleolus in the sinus tarsi (talocalcaneal sulcus). May also be found on the lateral surface of the leg below the fibular head in the peroneus longus, brevis, or tertius muscles (**Fig. 9.174**).

Treatment Position: EV er

1. The patient lies in lateral recumbent position, and the physician places a pillow under the lateral aspect of the tibia to create a fulcrum.

2. The physician applies an eversion force to the foot and ankle with slight external rotation of the foot until the tenderness is *completely alleviated* or reduced as close to 100% as possible, but at least 70% (**Fig. 9.175**).

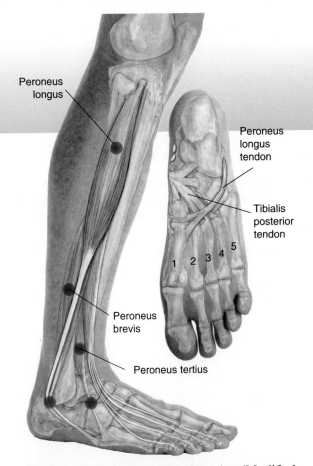

Figure 9.174. Lateral ankle tender point. (Modified with permission from Ref. (8).)

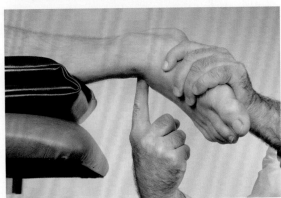

Figure 9.175. Lateral ankle: EV er.

Lower Extremity Region

Flexion Calcaneus (*Quadratus Plantae*)

Indication for Treatment

Somatic dysfunction of the lower extremity. The patient may present with pain on the bottom of the heel and commonly associated with plantar fasciitis (4,5).

Tender Point Location

Anterior aspect of the calcaneus on the plantar surface of the foot at the attachment of the quadratus plantae **(Fig. 9.176)**.

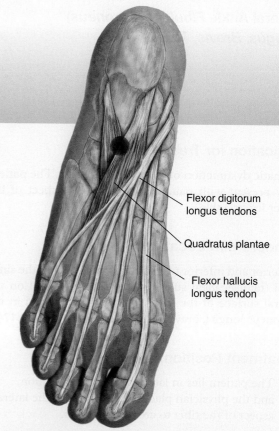

Flexor digitorum longus tendons

Quadratus plantae

Flexor hallucis longus tendon

Figure 9.176. Flexion calcaneus tender point. (Modified with permission from Ref. (8).)

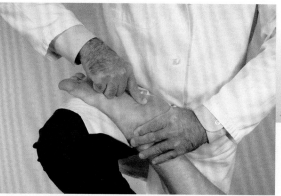

Figure 9.177. Flexion calcaneus: flexion forefoot.

Treatment Position: F

1. The patient lies prone, and the physician stands at the side of the tender point and places his/her foot on the edge of the table.

2. The patient's knee is flexed, and the dorsum of the foot is placed on the physician's thigh.

3. The physician applies a compressive force on the patient's calcaneus to produce marked flexion of the forefoot, approximating the calcaneus and the forefoot **(Fig. 9.177)**.

4. The physician fine-tunes (more or less flexion of the forefoot) until the tenderness is *completely alleviated* or reduced as close to 100% as possible, but at least 70%.

Upper Extremity Region

Upper Extremity Tender Points

Upper extremity counterstrain tender points are outlined in Table 9.13.

Table 9.13 Common Upper Extremity Tender Points

Tender Point	Location	Classic Treatment Position	Acronym
Supraspinatus	In the belly of the supraspinatus muscle	Flexion of shoulder, abduction, with marked external rotation	F Abd ER
Infraspinatus	Upper: Inferior and lateral to the spine of the scapula at the posterior medial aspect of the glenohumeral joint Lower: In the lower portion of the muscle inferior to the spine and lateral to the medial border of the scapula	Flexion of shoulder to 90–120 degrees and abduction; may require external rotation or internal rotation Flexion of shoulder to 135 degrees with slight abduction and external rotation or internal rotation	F Abd er/ir F Abd er/ir
Rhomboid minor/major	Along the medial border of the scapula at the attachment of the rhomboid muscles	Patient seated or prone: Shoulder extension with adduction by pulling arm posterior and medial	E Add
Levator scapulae	On the superior medial border of the scapula at the attachment of the levator scapula	Glide the scapula superiorly and medially to shorten the muscle. May alternatively be treated by marked internal rotation of the shoulder with traction and slight abduction	Scap Sup Med IR Abd traction
Subscapularis	At the anterolateral border of the scapula on the subscapularis muscle pressing from an anterior lateral to posteromedial direction	Shoulder extension and internal rotation	E IR
Long head of biceps	Over the tendon of the biceps muscle in the bicipital groove	Flexion of elbow, shoulder flexion, abduction, internal rotation	F Abd ir
Short head of biceps/coracobrachialis	At the inferolateral aspect of the coracoid process	Flexion of elbow, shoulder flexion, adduction, and internal rotation	F Add ir
Pectoralis minor	Inferior and medial to the coracoid process	Adduction of the arm; protract scapula (medial and caudad)	f-F Add

Table 9.13 Common Upper Extremity Tender Points (Continued)

Tender Point	Location	Classic Treatment Position	Acronym
Radial head lateral	On the anterolateral aspect of the radial head at the attachment of the supinator	Elbow in full extension, forearm in marked supination, and slight valgus force	E SUP Val
Medial epicondyle	On the medial epicondyle of the humerus at the common flexor tendon and the attachment of pronator teres	Flexion, marked pronation, and slight adduction of the forearm with slight flexion of the wrist	F PRO Add
Dorsal wrist	On the dorsal surface of the second metacarpal in the extensor carpi radialis muscle	Wrist extension, with slight abduction	E Abd
	On the dorsal surface of the fifth metacarpal in the extensor carpi ulnaris muscle	Wrist extension, with slight adduction	E Add
Palmar wrist	At the palmar base of the second or third metacarpal in the flexor carpi radialis muscle	Wrist flexion, with slight abduction	F Abd
	At the palmar base of the fifth metacarpal in the flexor carpi ulnaris muscle	Wrist flexion, with slight adduction	F Add
Palmar wrist First carpometacarpal	At the palmar base (radial aspect) of the first metacarpal in the abductor pollicis brevis muscle	Wrist flexion with abduction of the thumb	F Abd

Upper Extremity Region

Supraspinatus

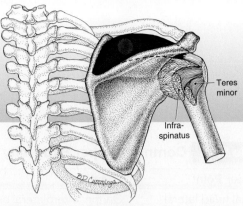

Figure 9.178. Supraspinatus counterstrain tender point. (Modified with permission from Ref. (3).)

Indication for Treatment

Somatic dysfunction of the upper extremity.

Tender Point Location

The tender point lies at the midsupraspinatus muscle just superior to the spine of the scapula **(Fig. 9.178)**.

Treatment Position: F Abd ER

1. The patient lies supine on the treatment table.

2. The physician sits beside the patient at the level of the shoulder girdle.

3. The physician may palpate the tender point with either hand's fingertip pad or control the patient's ipsilateral arm with the other **(Fig. 9.179)**.

4. The patient's arm is flexed to approximately 45 degrees, abducted approximately 45 degrees, and externally rotated **(Figs. 9.180 and 9.181)**.

5. The physician fine-tunes through small arcs of motion (more or less flexion, abduction, and external rotation) until the tenderness has been *completely alleviated* or reduced as close to 100% as possible, but at least 70%.

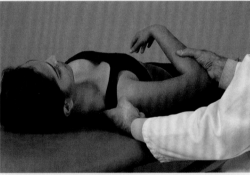

Figure 9.179. Palpation of supraspinatus tender point.

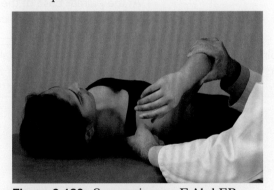

Figure 9.180. Supraspinatus: F Abd ER.

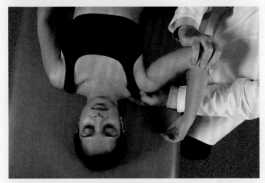

Figure 9.181. Supraspinatus: F Abd ER.

Upper Extremity Region

Infraspinatus

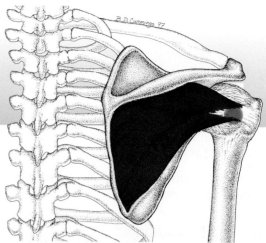

Figure 9.182. Infraspinatus counterstrain tender point. (Modified with permission from Ref. (3).)

Indications for Treatment

Somatic dysfunction of the upper extremity.

Tender Point Location

Upper infraspinatus: Inferior and lateral to the spine of the scapula at the posterior medial aspect of the glenohumeral joint.

Lower infraspinatus: In the lower portion of the muscle inferior to the spine and lateral to the medial border of the scapula **(Fig. 9.182).**

Treatment Position

Upper Infraspinatus Tender Point: F Abd er/ir

1. The patient lies supine on the treatment table, and the physician sits at the side of the table.

2. The patient's shoulder is flexed approximately 90 to 120 degrees and abducted. May require some external or internal rotation depending on the muscle fibers involved (4) **(Figs. 9.183 and 9.184).**

Lower Infraspinatus Tender Point: F Abd er

1. The patient lies in the lateral recumbent position on the side opposite the tender point. The physician may stand or sit either facing the patient or behind the patient.

2. The patient's shoulder is flexed approximately 135 to 150 degrees, abducted, and externally rotated (5) **(Fig. 9.185).**

3. The physician fine-tunes through small arcs of motion (more or less flexion, abduction, internal or external rotation) until the tenderness has been *completely alleviated* or reduced as close to 100% as possible, but at least 70%.

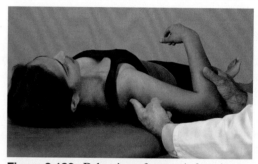

Figure 9.183. Palpation of upper infraspinatus tender point.

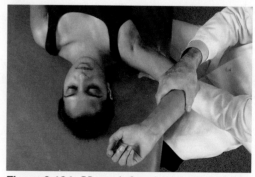

Figure 9.184. Upper infraspinatus: F Abd er/ir.

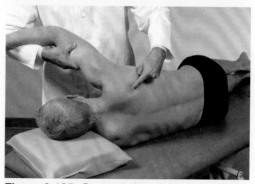

Figure 9.185. Lower infraspinatus: F Abd er.

Upper Extremity Region

Levator Scapulae

Indications for Treatment

This treatment is appropriate for somatic dysfunction of the levator scapulae muscle.

Tender Point Location

The tender point lies at the superior angle of the scapula **(Fig. 9.186)**.

Treatment Position: IR Abd traction

1. The patient lies prone, head rotated away, with the arms at the sides. The physician sits at the side of the affected shoulder.

2. The physician's caudad hand grasps the patient's wrist while the other hand palpates the tender point **(Fig. 9.187)**.

3. The physician internally rotates the patient's shoulder and then adds mild to moderate traction and minimal abduction **(Fig. 9.188)**.

4. The physician fine-tunes through small arcs of motion (more or less internal rotation and abduction) until the tenderness has been *completely alleviated* or reduced as close to 100% as possible, but at least 70%.

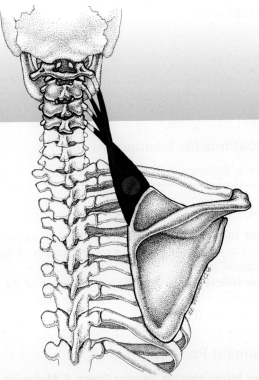

Figure 9.186. Levator scapulae counterstrain tender point. (Modified with permission from Ref. (3).)

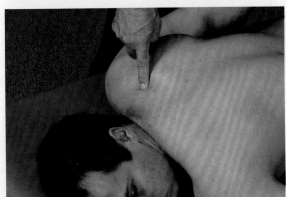

Figure 9.187. Palpation of levator scapulae tender point.

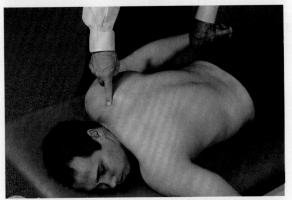

Figure 9.188. Levator scapulae: IR Abd traction.

Upper Extremity Region

Rhomboid Minor/Major

Indications for Treatment

Somatic dysfunction of the upper extremity and/or thoracic spine. The patient typically will complain of pain in the upper thoracic region along the medial border of the scapula.

Tender Point Location

Along the medial border of the scapula at the attachment of the rhomboid muscles. Press medial to lateral **(Fig. 9.189)**.

Treatment Position: E Add

1. The patient may be seated or lie prone, and the physician stands on either side of the patient.

2. The physician locates and monitors the tender point with the pad of the index finger **(Fig. 9.190)**.

3. The patient's shoulder is extended and adducted by pulling the arm/elbow posterior and medial, which retracts the scapula, shortening the fibers of the rhomboid muscle(s) **(Figs. 9.191 and 9.192)**.

4. The physician fine-tunes through small arcs of motion (more or less extension, adduction, and scapular retraction) until the tenderness has been *completely alleviated* or reduced as close to 100% as possible, but at least 70%.

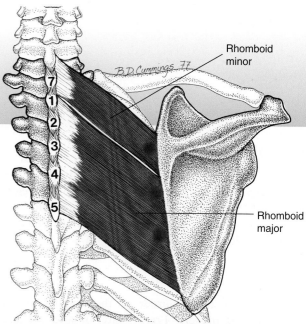

Figure 9.189. Rhomboid minor/major counterstrain tender point. (Modified with permission from Ref. (3).)

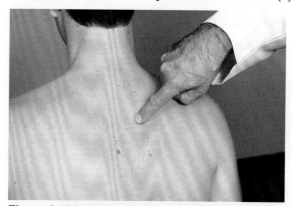

Figure 9.190. Palpation Rhomboid tender point.

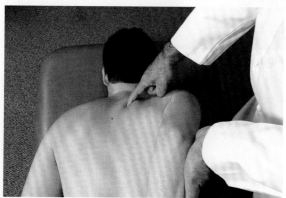

Figure 9.192. Rhomboid minor/major: Prone E Add.

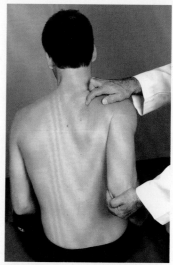

Figure 9.191. Rhomboid minor/major: Seated E Add.

Upper Extremity Region

Subscapularis

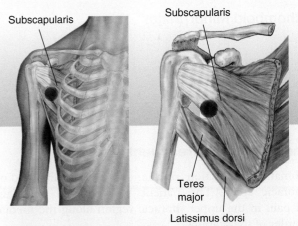

Figure 9.193. Subscapularis counterstrain tender point. (Modified with permission from Ref. (8).)

Indications for Treatment

Somatic dysfunction of the upper extremity. The patient may complain of pain in the posterior shoulder region and restricted range of motion due to rotator cuff tendonitis, adhesive capsulitis, or degenerative changes of the glenohumeral joint.

Tender Point Location

At the anterolateral border of the scapula on the subscapularis muscle. Press posterior and medially **(Fig. 9.193)**.

Treatment Position: E IR

1. The patient lies supine, and the physician sits or stands at the side of the tender point **(Fig. 9.194)**.

2. The patient's shoulder is extended and internally rotated **(Fig. 9.195)**.

3. The physician fine-tunes through small arcs of motion (more or less shoulder extension and internal rotation) until the tenderness is *completely alleviated* or reduced as close to 100% as possible, but at least 70%.

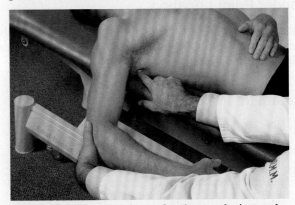

Figure 9.194. Palpation of subscapularis tender point.

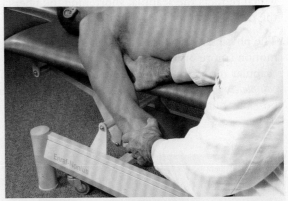

Figure 9.195. Subscapularis: E IR.

Upper Extremity Region

Biceps Brachii (Long Head)

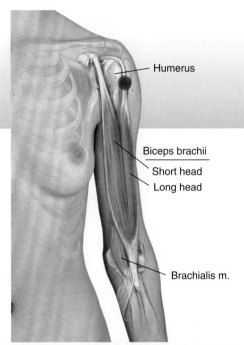

Figure 9.196. Long head of the biceps counterstrain tender point. (Modified with permission from Ref. (8).)

Indications for Treatment

Somatic dysfunction of the upper extremity. The patient may present with pain in the anterior aspect of the shoulder and upper arm associated with strain of the long head tendon of the biceps muscle.

Tender Point Location

Over the long head tendon of the biceps muscle in the bicipital groove **(Fig. 9.196)**.

Treatment Position: F Abd ir

1. The patient lies supine, and the physician stands at the side of the tender point **(Fig. 9.197)**.

2. The patient's elbow and shoulder are flexed, and the shoulder is minimally abducted and internally rotated **(Fig. 9.198)**.

3. The physician fine-tunes through small arcs of motion (more or less shoulder flexion, adduction, and internal rotation) until the tenderness is *completely alleviated* or reduced as close to 100% as possible, but at least 70%.

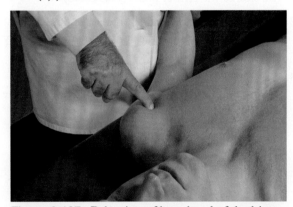

Figure 9.197. Palpation of long head of the biceps tender point.

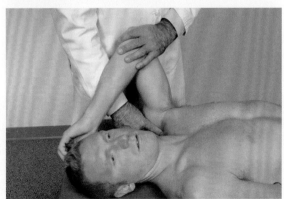

Figure 9.198. Long head of the biceps: F Abd ir.

Upper Extremity Region

Biceps Brachii (Short Head)
Coracobrachialis

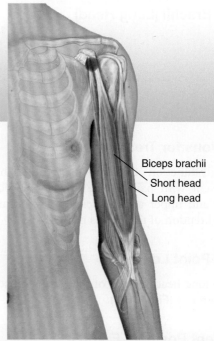

Indications for Treatment

Somatic dysfunction of the upper extremity. The patient may complain of pain in the anterior aspect of the shoulder.

Tender Point Location

At the inferolateral aspect of the coracoid process on the short head tendon of the biceps or the coracobrachialis muscle **(Fig. 9.199)**.

Treatment Position: F Add ir

1. The patient lies supine, and the physician stands at the side of the tender point **(Fig. 9.200)**.

2. The patient's elbow and shoulder are flexed, and the shoulder is minimally adducted and internally rotated **(Fig. 9.201)**.

3. The physician fine-tunes (more or less shoulder flexion, adduction, and internal rotation) until the tenderness is *completely alleviated* or reduced as close to 100% as possible, but at least 70%.

Figure 9.199. Short head of the biceps/coraco-brachialis counterstrain tender point. (Modified with permission from Ref. (8).)

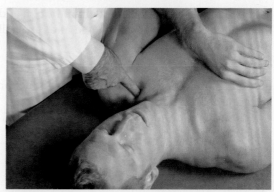

Figure 9.200. Palpation of short head of biceps/coracobrachialis tender point.

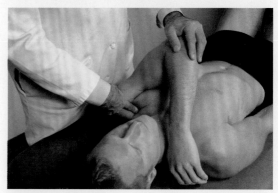

Figure 9.201. Short head of the biceps/coraco-brachialis: F Add ir.

Upper Extremity Region

Pectoralis Minor

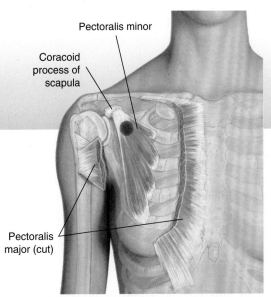

Figure 9.202. Pectoralis minor counterstrain tender point. (Modified with permission from Ref. (8).)

Indications for Treatment

Somatic dysfunction of the upper extremity. The patient may complain of pain in the anterior shoulder region and anterior chest wall/ribs.

Tender Point Location

Inferior and medial to the coracoid process **(Fig. 9.202)**.

Treatment Position: f-F ADD

1. The patient lies supine, and the physician stands at the side of the table opposite the tender point **(Fig. 9.203)**.

2. The patient's arm is adducted across the chest, and the shoulder/scapula is pulled anterior, inferior, and medial to shorten the fibers of the pectoralis minor **(Fig. 9.204)**.

3. The physician fine-tunes through small arcs of motion (more or less adduction and scapular protraction) until the tenderness has been *completely alleviated* or reduced as close to 100% as possible, but at least 70%.

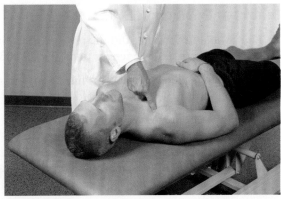

Figure 9.203. Palpation of pectoralis minor tender point.

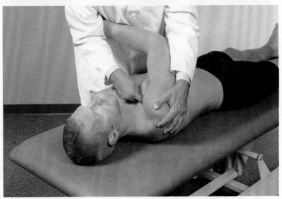

Figure 9.204. Pectoralis minor: f-F Add.

Upper Extremity Region

Radial Head–Lateral (*Supinator*)

Indications for Treatment

Somatic dysfunction of the upper extremity. The patient may complain of pain at the lateral aspect of the elbow commonly associated with excessive supination and pronation.

Tender Point Location

On the anterolateral aspect of the radial head at the attachment of the supinator **(Fig. 9.205)**.

Treatment Position: E SUP Val

1. The patient lies supine, and the physician sits or stands at the side of the tender point **(Fig. 9.206)**.

2. The patient's elbow is placed in full extension, and the forearm is markedly supinated **(Fig. 9.207)**.

3. The physician fine-tunes with more or less supination and applies a slight lateral to medial (valgus) force to the elbow until the tenderness is *completely alleviated* or reduced as close to 100% as possible, but at least 70%.

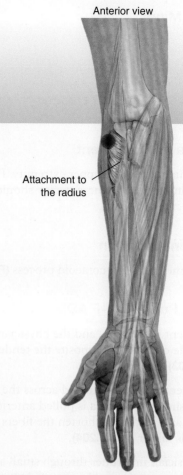

Anterior view

Attachment to the radius

Figure 9.205. Radial head (lateral) counterstrain tender point. (Modified with permission from Ref. (8).)

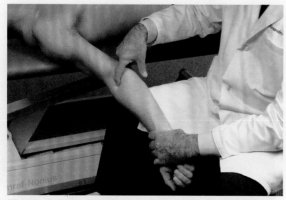

Figure 9.207. Radial head (lateral): E SUP Val.

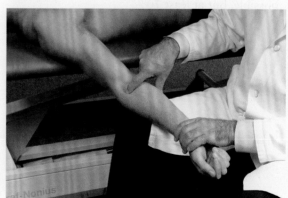

Figure 9.206. Palpation of radial head (lateral) tender point.

Upper Extremity Region

Medial Epicondyle (*Pronator Teres*)

Indications for Treatment

Somatic dysfunction of the upper extremity. The patient may complain of pain in the anterior medial aspect of the elbow near the medial epicondyle.

Tender Point Location

At or near the medial epicondyle of the humerus associated with common flexor tendon and the attachment of the pronator teres muscle **(Fig. 9.208)**.

Treatment Position: F PRO Add

1. The patient lies supine, and the physician sits or stands at the side of the tender point **(Fig. 9.209)**.

2. The patient's elbow is flexed, the wrist is markedly pronated, and the forearm is slightly adducted **(Fig. 9.210)**.

3. The physician fine-tunes (more or less elbow flexion, wrist pronation, and forearm adduction) until the tenderness is *completely alleviated* or reduced as close to 100% as possible, but at least 70%.

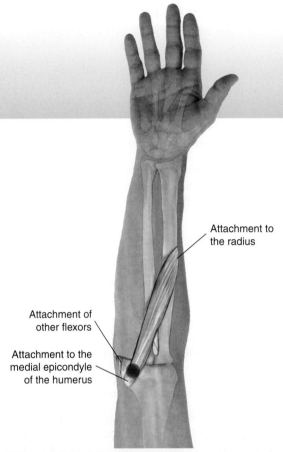

Attachment to
the radius

Attachment of
other flexors

Attachment to the
medial epicondyle
of the humerus

Figure 9.208. Medial epicondyle counterstrain tender point. (Modified with permission from Ref. (8).)

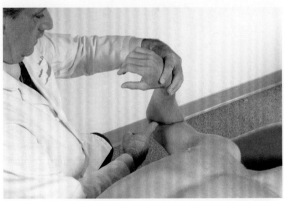

Figure 9.210. Medial epicondyle: F PRO Add.

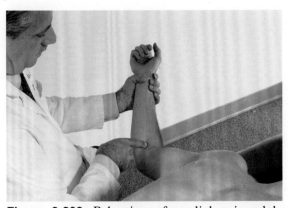

Figure 9.209. Palpation of medial epicondyle tender point.

Upper Extremity Region

Dorsal Wrist (*Extensor Carpi Radialis*)

Indications for Treatment

Somatic dysfunction of the upper extremity. The patient may complain of pain in the forearm and wrist associated with strain of the extensor tendons of the wrist.

Tender Point Location

On the dorsal surface of the second metacarpal associated with the extensor carpi radialis muscle **(Fig. 9.211)**. May also be found in any of the extensor muscles in the forearm.

Treatment Position: E Abd/rd

1. The patient may sit or lie supine on the table, and the physician faces the patient **(Fig. 9.212)**.

2. The patient's wrist is passively extended and abducted (radial deviation) until the tenderness has been *completely alleviated* or reduced as close to 100% as possible, but at least 70% **(Fig. 9.213)**.

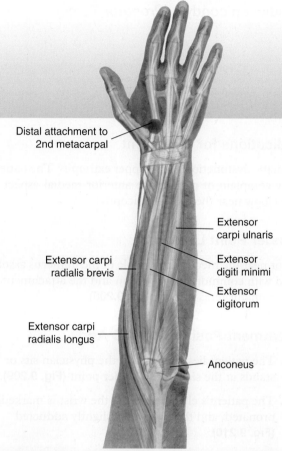

Labels:
Distal attachment to 2nd metacarpal
Extensor carpi ulnaris
Extensor digiti minimi
Extensor digitorum
Extensor carpi radialis brevis
Extensor carpi radialis longus
Anconeus

Figure 9.211. Dorsal wrist (extensor carpi radialis) counterstrain tender point. (Modified with permission from Ref. (8).)

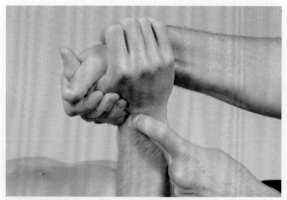

Figure 9.213. Extensor carpi radialis: E Abd/rd.

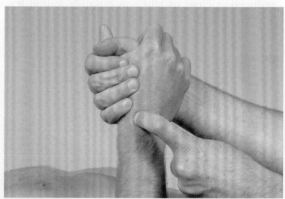

Figure 9.212. Palpation of extensor carpi radialis tender point.

Upper Extremity Region

Dorsal Wrist (*Extensor Carpi Ulnaris*)

Indications for Treatment

Somatic dysfunction of the upper extremity. The patient may complain of pain in the forearm and wrist associated with strain of the extensor tendons of the wrist.

Tender Point Location

On the dorsal surface of the fifth metacarpal associated with the extensor carpi ulnaris muscle **(Fig. 9.214)**. May also be found in any of the extensor muscles in the forearm.

Treatment Position: E Add/ud

1. The patient may sit or lie supine on the table, and the physician faces the patient **(Fig. 9.215)**.

2. The patient's wrist is passively extended and adducted (ulnar deviation) until the tenderness has been *completely alleviated* or reduced as close to 100% as possible, but at least 70% **(Fig. 9.216)**.

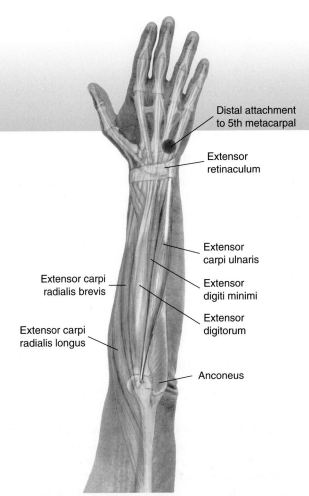

Distal attachment to 5th metacarpal

Extensor retinaculum

Extensor carpi ulnaris

Extensor digiti minimi

Extensor digitorum

Anconeus

Extensor carpi radialis brevis

Extensor carpi radialis longus

Figure 9.214. Dorsal wrist (extensor carpi ulnaris) counterstrain tender point. (Modified with permission from Refs. (8).)

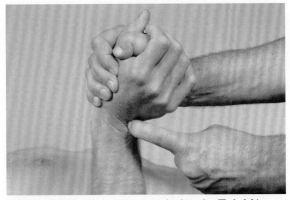

Figure 9.216. Extensor carpi ulnaris: E Add/ur.

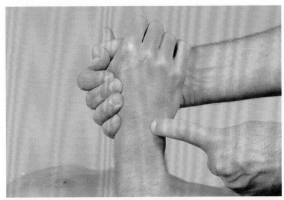

Figure 9.215. Palpation of extensor carpi ulnaris tender point.

Upper Extremity Region

Palmar Wrist (*Flexor Carpi Radialis*)

Indications for Treatment

Somatic dysfunction of the upper extremity. The patient may complain of pain in the forearm and wrist associated with strain of the flexor tendons of the wrist.

Tender Point Location

At the palmar base of the second or third metacarpal in the flexor carpi radialis muscle **(Fig. 9.217)**.
May also be found in any of the flexor muscles in the forearm.

Treatment Position: F Abd/rd

1. The patient may sit or lie supine on the table, and the physician faces the patient.

2. The patient's wrist is passively flexed and abducted (radial deviation) until the tenderness has been *completely alleviated* or reduced as close to 100% as possible, but at least 70% **(Fig. 9.218)**.

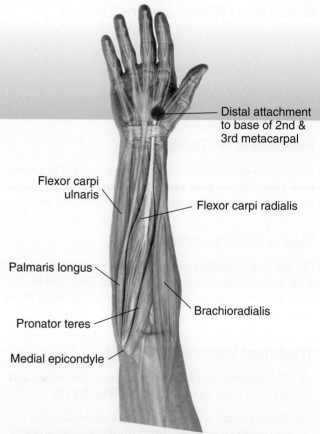

Distal attachment to base of 2nd & 3rd metacarpal

Flexor carpi ulnaris

Flexor carpi radialis

Palmaris longus

Brachioradialis

Pronator teres

Medial epicondyle

Figure 9.217. Palmar wrist (flexor carpi radialis) counterstrain tender point. (Modified with permission from Ref. (8).)

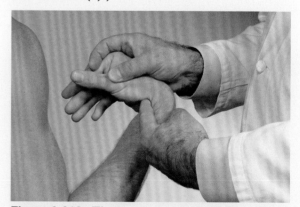

Figure 9.218. Flexor carpi radialis: F Abd/rd.

Upper Extremity Region

Palmar Wrist (*Flexor Carpi Ulnaris*)

Indications for Treatment

Somatic dysfunction of the upper extremity. The patient may complain of pain in the forearm and wrist associated with strain of the flexor tendons of the wrist.

Tender Point Location

At the palmar base of the fifth metacarpal in the flexor carpi ulnaris muscle **(Fig. 9.219)**.
May also be found in any of the flexor muscles in the forearm.

Treatment Position: F Add/ud

1. The patient may sit or lie supine on the table, and the physician faces the patient.

2. The patient's wrist is passively flexed and adducted (ulnar deviation) until the tenderness has been *completely alleviated* or reduced as close to 100% as possible, but at least 70% **(Fig. 9.220)**.

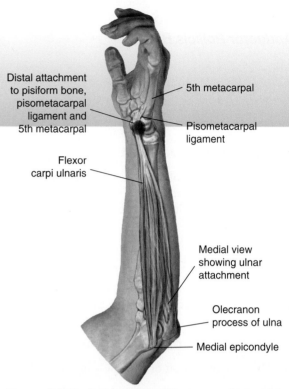

Distal attachment to pisiform bone, pisometacarpal ligament and 5th metacarpal

5th metacarpal

Pisometacarpal ligament

Flexor carpi ulnaris

Medial view showing ulnar attachment

Olecranon process of ulna

Medial epicondyle

Figure 9.219. Palmar wrist (flexor carpi ulnaris) counterstrain tender point. (Modified with permission from Ref. (8).)

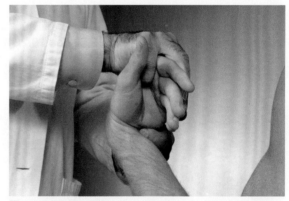

Figure 9.220. Flexor carpi ulnaris: F Add/ud.

Upper Extremity Region

First Carpometacarpal (*Abductor Pollicis Brevis*)

Indications for Treatment

Somatic dysfunction of the upper extremity. The patient may complain of pain in the forearm, wrist, and/or thumb associated with strain of the abductor pollicis brevis muscle.

Tender Point Location

At the palmar base (radial aspect) of the first metacarpal in the abductor pollicis brevis muscle **(Fig. 9.221)**.

Treatment Position: F (wrist) Abd (thumb)

1. The patient may sit or lie supine on the table.

2. The physician locates and monitors the tender point with the pad of the index finger **(Fig. 9.222)**.

3. The patient's wrist is passively flexed, and the thumb is abducted until the tenderness has been *completely alleviated* or reduced as close to 100% as possible, but at least 70% **(Figs. 9.223 and 9.224)**.

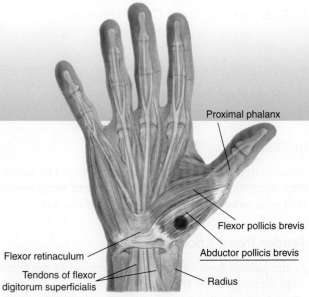

Figure 9.221. Abductor pollicis brevis counterstrain tender point. (Modified with permission from Ref. (8).)

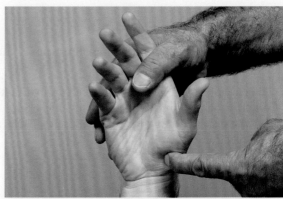

Figure 9.222. Palpation of Abductor pollicis brevis (first carpometacarpal) tender point.

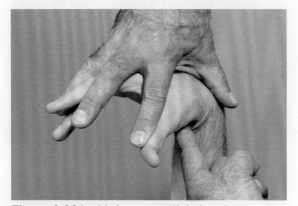

Figure 9.224. Abductor pollicis brevis: F (wrist) Abd (thumb).

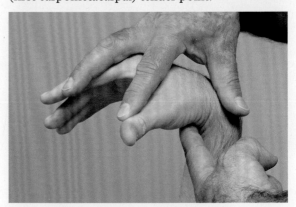

Figure 9.223. Abductor pollicis brevis: F (wrist) Abd (thumb).

Temporomandibular Joint

Masseter

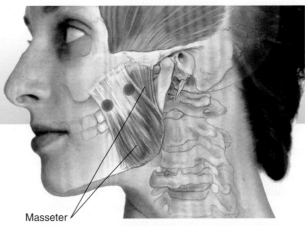

Figure 9.225. Masseter tender point. (Modified with permission from Ref. (8).)

Indication for Treatment

Somatic dysfunction of the head/cranium and/or cervical region. The patient may complain of pain in the neck, face, jaw, ear, or temporomandibular joint and have difficulty opening mouth fully. Mandible may deviate or shift to the side of dysfunction (4).

Tender Point Location

Masseter: Just inferior to the zygoma in the belly of the masseter muscle typically found on the side of mandibular deviation **(Fig. 9.225)**.

Treatment Position

1. The patient lies supine, and the physician sits at the head of the table **(Fig. 9.226)**.

2. The physician gently glides the patient's slightly opened jaw/mandible laterally toward the side of the tender point **(Fig. 9.227)**.

3. Fine-tune until the tenderness is *completely alleviated* or reduced as close to 100% as possible, but at least 70%.

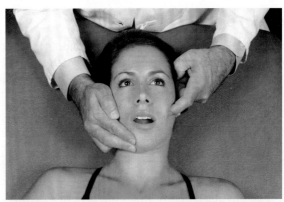

Figure 9.226. Palpation of left masseter tender point.

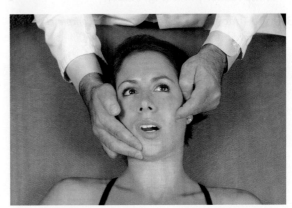

Figure 9.227. Masseter.

Temporomandibular Joint

Jaw Angle Point (*Medial Pterygoid*)

Indication for Treatment

Somatic dysfunction of the head/cranium and/or cervical region. The patient may complain of pain in the neck, face, jaw, ear, or temporomandibular joint and have difficulty opening mouth fully. Mandible may deviate or shift to the side of dysfunction (4).

Tender Point Location

Jaw angle point (1) or medial pterygoid (4): On the posterior surface of the ascending ramus of the mandible about 2 cm. above the angle of the mandible on the side opposite of mandibular deviation **(Fig. 9.228)**.

Treatment Position

1. The patient lies supine, and the physician sits at the head of the table.

2. The physician gently glides the patient's slightly opened jaw/mandible laterally away from the side of the tender point **(Fig. 9.229)**.

3. Fine-tune until the tenderness is *completely alleviated* or reduced as close to 100% as possible, but at least 70%.

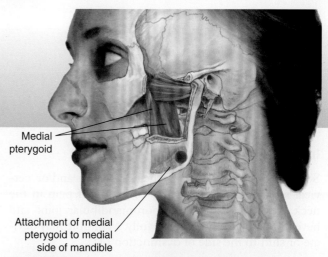

Medial pterygoid

Attachment of medial pterygoid to medial side of mandible

Figure 9.228. Jaw angle/medial pterygoid tender point. (Modified with permission from Ref. (8).)

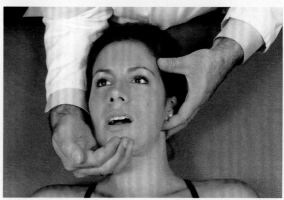

Figure 9.229. Jaw angle/medial pterygoid.

References

1. Jones LH, Kusunose RS, Goering EK. Jones Strain-Counterstrain. Carlsbad, CA: Jones Strain-Counterstrain, 1995.
2. Ward R, exec.ed. Foundations for Osteopathic Medicine. 2nd ed. Philadelphia, PA: Lippincott Williams & Wilkins, 2003.
3. Simons DG, Travell JG, Simons LS. Myofascial Pain and Dysfunction: The Trigger Point Manual. Vol. 1. Baltimore, MD: Lippincott Williams & Wilkins, 1999.
4. Myers HL. Clinical Application of Counterstrain. Tucson, AZ: Osteopathic Press, A Division of Tucson Osteopathic Medical Foundation, 2006.
5. Rennie P, Glover J. Counterstrain and Exercise: An Integrated Approach. 2nd ed. Williamstown, MI: RennieMatrix, 2004.
6. Yates H, Glover J. Counterstrain: A Handbook of Osteopathic Technique. Tulsa, OK: Y Knot, 1995.
7. Chila AG, exec.ed. Foundations of Osteopathic Medicine. 3rd ed. Baltimore, MD: Lippincott Williams & Wilkins, 2011.
8. Clay JH, Pounds DM. Basic Clinical Massage Therapy: Integrating Anatomy and Treatment. Baltimore, MD: Lippincott Williams & Wilkins, 2003.
9. Tank P, Gest T. Lippincott Williams & Wilkins Atlas of Anatomy. Philadelphia, PA: Lippincott Williams & Wilkins, 2009.
10. Snider K, Glover J. Atlas of Common Counterstrain Tender Points. Kirksville, MO: A.T. Still University—Kirksville College of Osteopathic Medicine, 2014.

Muscle Energy Techniques

Technique Principles

Muscle energy technique (MET) is a form of osteopathic manipulative treatment developed by Fred L. Mitchell, Sr., DO (1909–1974). It is defined by the Education Council on Osteopathic Principles (ECOP) as "a form of osteopathic manipulative diagnosis and direct treatment in which the patient's muscles are actively used on request, from a precisely controlled position, in a specific direction, and against a distinctly executed physician counterforce" (1). Some osteopathic physicians (e.g., Hollis Wolf, Nicholas S. Nicholas) have suggested that this technique is a variation of a technique performed by T. J. Ruddy, DO (personal communication). Ruddy developed a technique called rhythmic (rapid) resistive duction (1961) in which repetitive muscle contraction was used to promote lymphatic and venous circulation, resulting in reduction of edema, congestion, and inflammation. His technique used the patient's muscle contraction against a physician's counterforce before the development of MET (2–4). In MET, the physician positions the patient so as to engage the restrictive barrier. Fred Mitchell, Jr., uses the term "feather's edge" to refer to the level of engagement (5,6). This term refers to the initial sense of meeting the restriction with slightly more motion available before meeting the hard end feel of restriction. If the physician engages the barrier to the end point of its restriction, it causes the patient to guard, and it becomes difficult to correct the dysfunction. Additionally, engaging all three axes of motion (x, y, and z) at the feather's edge may also cause a locking up of the dysfunction, resulting in difficulty of treatment and resistant dysfunction. This was one of the first osteopathic techniques to use known and accepted physiologic principles as its major protocol of treatment.

Technique Classification

Direct

In MET, as in other direct techniques, the patient's dysfunction is positioned toward the restrictive barrier. Recent attempts by some manual medicine practitioners, especially outside the United States, have begun to describe indirect technique.

Technique Styles

The following styles are described by the various principles and mechanisms of action by which MET can be used to treat the effects of impaired *myofascial tissues* (hypertonicity, spasm, and fibrosis). Also described is a style (joint mobilization using muscle force) by which MET can mobilize a restricted joint that is impaired due to changes within the articulation itself (inflammation, hyperpositioning, osteoarthritis, etc.), but *not* caused by myofascial etiologies by using the muscle's contraction forces against the boney articulation and by a combination of positioning and contraction force vectors to move the articulation through its restrictive barrier.

Post-Isometric Relaxation

In this form of MET, the physician instructs the patient to *isometrically* contract the dysfunctional muscle(s) (agonist). Therefore, both the origin and insertion attachment points of the contracting muscle must be restrained (anchored) from moving/shortening by placing the physician's hand, fingers, thumbs, etc., over these osseous locations. During this contraction, increased tension is placed on the Golgi tendon organ proprioceptors within the muscle tendon. This can cause a reflex inhibition and subsequent increase in muscle length within a hypertonic muscle. Mitchell believed that after the contraction a refractory period occurred during which the physician could sense relaxation and a temporary increase in muscle length (1,4). This may be an oversimplified explanation, and we believe that additional effects are at play. Most likely, the effects common to soft tissue and myofascial release are also involved in this style of muscle energy.

Heat is generated during isometric muscle contraction; this heat has the same effect on the myofascial structures as proposed in the chapters on myofascial and soft tissue treatment. The heat generation is likely to cause the connective tissues and collagen base, which are under tension, to change to colloidal state (gel to sol). As a result, the fascial envelope may lengthen, also permitting the muscle to lengthen. During this isometric contraction, the tension building up in the muscle is also expressing fluids (e.g., venous blood, lymph) from the belly of the muscle and surrounding interstitial compartment, which potentiates an increase in overall length and/or perceived *relaxation*. As the agonist muscle being contracted is most likely the dysfunctional muscle involved in acute strains, this style of technique is most useful in subacute to chronic conditions, in which muscle shortening and fibrosis may be present, rather than in acute conditions. The force of contraction may vary, but it should be tolerable to both the patient and the physician. The force of the patient's contraction is the least amount necessary to produce a palpable muscle twitch at the segmental level the physician is monitoring (5).

Note: The patient's contraction and the physician's resistance should be performed in a sustained, gentle manner, and not as a competition to see who is stronger.

Reciprocal Inhibition

This form of muscle energy uses the physiologic principle of reciprocal inhibition and relaxation. When an agonist contracts, the antagonist should relax (e.g., brachialis and biceps contract and triceps relaxes). The force of contraction in this style of technique should be very light, only slightly more than the thought to contract, as with a strong muscle contraction the agonist and antagonist may both contract (as occurs during a Valsalva maneuver), thus eliminating the inhibitory reflex and rendering the technique ineffective.

In this form of MET, the physician instructs the patient to very lightly contract the nonaffected muscle. This is done by placing the patient's dysfunctional region *toward* the restrictive barrier's "feather's edge" and then instructing the patient to very gently push toward the barrier. The physician's counterforce is directed away from the patient's restrictive barrier. This technique, as it can use a functional agonist to relax a dysfunctional antagonist, is strongly indicated in acute conditions of musculotendinous strain, so that no further strain is placed on the injured tissues. If performing a post-isometric relaxation technique and the patient has increased pain, it may be because the agonist was strained (injured) and causing it to contract irritating the traumatized myofascial tissues. Therefore, by reversing the patient's direction of contraction and causing the opposing muscle to now become the agonist, the technique becomes more tolerable to the patient. Although this has been one of the basic principles by which osteopathic physicians used MET (especially for acute muscle strains), what may have been lost is the fact that this type of muscle energy style is extremely effective in both subacute and chronic conditions. Its effect in these

conditions could be that of reducing chronic musculotendinous "reflexing," which has caused the muscle to be continuously hypertonic.

Joint Mobilization Using Muscle Force

Muscle force uses patient positioning and muscle contraction to restore limited joint motion. As the muscles are the primary movers of joints, use of a specific muscle contraction with the patient in a specific position allows the forces at play to become very powerful and be vectored specifically to a local area. This is similar to the long-levered style of high-velocity, low-amplitude (HVLA) therapy, except that the patient is actively contracting muscles instead of the physician pulling them to cause movement. In these techniques, the longer the lever, the more powerful the technique becomes. Therefore, this style of muscle energy could be thought of as *low* velocity, low amplitude (LVLA). The resulting contraction may become minimally isotonic.

As stated earlier, motion in joints can be improved by use of forces that are vectored directly or indirectly. MET is classically described as a direct technique and can be used to mobilize a restricted joint; therefore, positioning of the patient is similar to the reciprocal inhibition style of positioning. However, in this case, the muscle contractions can be more powerful (possibly isotonic) up to many pounds of resistance and in contrast to producing a postisometric muscle relaxation/lengthening effect where both ends of the contracting muscle are held in place (anchored), the physician only resists movement at one end but permits motion at the level of the dysfunction, thereby pulling the articulation through the restrictive barrier. By reversing the anchored and nonanchored points, the physician could produce an indirect technique; which, as stated previously, is not classically part of this techniques description.

As in other long-levered style techniques, for example, HVLA, the lower of the two segments involved in spinal dysfunctions must be anchored so that only the dysfunctional segment moves. In other areas (e.g., innominate dysfunctions), the boney segment superior (or cephalad) to the articulation, as well at the distal insertion must be anchored. For the physician's comfort, the patient should be positioned to encourage the development of the most appropriate longest levered force with the least amount of counterforce from the physician necessary for success.

Respiratory Assistance

Respiratory assistance may be used in a number of osteopathic manipulative techniques (e.g., myofascial release, soft tissue, counterstrain, balanced ligamentous tension, ligamentous articular strain). When respiratory assistance is used to help augment a corrective force toward a restrictive barrier, it has been commonly referred to as "a release enhancing maneuver" (effect) or REM, not to be confused with rapid eye movement. In this style of MET, the physician positions the patient to best direct the forces of respiration toward the area of dysfunction and simultaneously use a fulcrum (e.g., the physician's hand) as a counterforce to help direct the dysfunctional region through the restrictive barrier. As diaphragmatic excursion during inhalation may affect muscles very distally because of fascial continuity, motion, and tissue changes may be appreciated locally or peripherally.

Oculocephalogyric (Oculocervical) Reflex

When a patient is asked to make specific eye movements, certain cervical and truncal muscles contract, which reflexively relax the antagonist muscles (1). The patient may be asked to look toward either the restriction (reciprocal inhibitory effect) or the freedom (postisometric effect). Therefore, it is possible to minimally induce Post-isometric relaxation effects or, by reversing the patient's gaze, develop a reciprocal inhibitory effect, if this is indicated. This style is most useful in very severe, acute cervical and upper thoracic conditions when other techniques are impossible due to severity of pain, muscle spasm, or strain.

Indications

Primary Indications

1. Somatic dysfunction of myofascial origin, especially to reduce hypertonic muscles, lengthen shortened muscles, or stretch and improve elasticity in fibrotic muscles
2. Somatic dysfunction of articular origin to mobilize restricted joints and improve the range of motion

Secondary Indications

1. To improve local circulation and respiratory function
2. To balance neuromuscular relationships by altering muscle tone
3. To increase tone in hypotonic or weak muscles

Contraindications

Relative Contraindications

1. Moderate to severe muscle strains
2. Severe osteoporosis in which the physician believes that a risk of tendinous evulsion could occur with the correction
3. Severe illness (i.e., postsurgical or intensive care patient)

Absolute Contraindications

1. Fracture, dislocation, or moderate to severe joint instability at treatment site

2. Lack of cooperation or a patient who cannot understand the instructions of the technique (i.e., an infant or young child or a patient who does not understand the physician's language)

General Considerations and Rules

Depending on the patient's presentation, the style of muscle energy used may vary. Additionally, the nature and length of contraction may be altered from patient to patient and between anatomic regions. Muscles may be morphologically different, one to another. Therefore, the way they respond to isometric contractions may differ. In some areas, holding a muscle contraction for five or more seconds may be necessary; in others, 3 seconds may suffice. Clinical experience will teach this.

The essential steps for most styles of this technique are as follows:

1. The physician positions the bone, joint, or muscle to be treated at the feather's edge of the restrictive barrier (point of initial resistance) in all three planes of motion (x-, y-, z-axes). However, it may be more effective to keep one axis slightly loose (lax), as the dysfunction may become very recalcitrant if simultaneously held at all three axis limits.
2. The physician instructs the patient to contract a specific muscle in a specific direction against the physician's unyielding counterforce for 3 to 5 seconds.
3. The patient ceases all muscle contraction when instructed by the physician to relax or "go to sleep."
4. After sensing that the patient is not guarding and is completely relaxed (may take 1 to 2 seconds), the physician slowly repositions the patient to the feather's edge of the new restrictive barrier.
5. Steps 1 to 4 are repeated until the best possible increase in motion is obtained. This usually requires three to seven repetitions, depending on the affected body region and tolerance of the patient.
6. The physician reevaluates the diagnostic parameters of the original dysfunction to determine the effectiveness of the technique.

Muscle energy may, like most other osteopathic techniques, be used in conjunction with other techniques. It is especially beneficial in potentiating soft tissue, myofascial release, counterstrain, and HVLA techniques. As the treatment positions are so similar to those of HVLA, it is natural to go from MET to HVLA if the MET is not completely successful; MET often makes HVLA more readily successful.

If the physician is unsuccessful with MET, it is most likely because of either a very severe chronic dysfunction or an inaccurate diagnosis. During the corrective procedure, success may be diminished by inaccurate localization of corrective forces (force at a segment too high or low; positioning causing the vectored force at too high or too low a segment). It is important to understand the specificity of the patient's positioning in this technique. The physician must palpate the motion in the exact segmental or muscular tissue that is being treated. Incorrect force of contraction by the patient (too forceful or too gentle) may hinder the successful completion of the technique. If the patient's contraction is too short in duration (i.e., 1 second), it will decrease effectiveness. Other problems may develop if the patient does not completely relax prior to repositioning. Furthermore, if the physician fails to reevaluate the diagnostic findings after treatment, the dysfunction may still be present and prevent a positive response.

Cervical Region

Regional (Long) Restrictor, Subacute/Chronic Post-Isometric Relaxation
Ex: Trapezius Muscle Hypertonicity

 See Video 10.1

1. The patient lies supine, and the physician sits at the head of the table.

2. The physician gently flexes the patient's neck to the edge of the restrictive barrier **(Fig. 10.1)**.

3. The physician instructs the patient to extend or backward bend the head and neck (*black arrow*, **Fig. 10.2**) while the physician applies an equal counterforce (*white arrow*).

4. This isometric contraction is maintained for 3 to 5 seconds, and then the patient is instructed to *stop and relax*.

5. Once the patient has completely relaxed, the physician gently flexes the neck (*white arrow*, **Fig. 10.3**) to the edge of the new restrictive barrier.

6. Steps 3 to 5 are repeated three to five times or until motion is maximally improved.

7. The same sequence is repeated for left and right side bending and rotation.

8. Cervical regional range of motion is retested to determine the effectiveness of the technique.

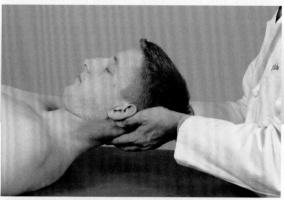

Figure 10.1A. Steps 1 and 2, flexion barrier.

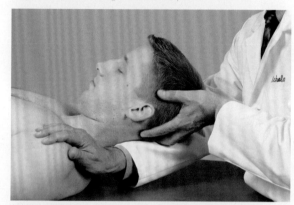

Figure 10.1B. Alternative hand placement.

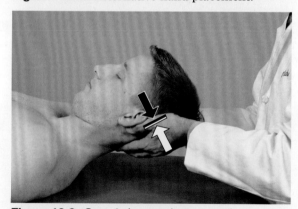

Figure 10.2. Step 3, isometric contraction.

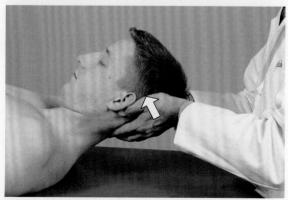

Figure 10.3. Step 5, flexion barrier.

Cervical Region

Sternocleidomastoid (SCM) Dysfunction
Reciprocal Inhibition
Ex: Left SCM Spasm *(Acute Torticollis)*

 See Video 10.2

1. The patient lies supine, and the physician sits at the head of the table supporting the patient's head with the hand and/or resting the patient's head on the knee or thigh.

2. The physician gently rotates the patient's head to the right to position the hypertonic left sternocleidomastoid muscle ventrally **(Fig. 10.4)**.

3. The physician gently extends the patient's head to the edge of the restrictive barrier **(Fig. 10.5)**.

4. The physician instructs the patient to *very gently* extend the head (*black arrow*, **Fig. 10.6**) while the physician applies an equal counterforce (*white arrow*). Alternative method: The physician may also tap the patient's right mastoid process and instruct the patient to "*think* about pushing down against my finger."

5. The physician palpates the left sternocleidomastoid muscle to ensure that adequate relaxation is occurring.

6. This isometric contraction is maintained for 3 to 5 seconds, and then the patient is instructed to *stop and relax*.

7. Once the patient has completely relaxed, the physician gently extends the patient's head (*white arrow*, **Fig. 10.7**) to the edge of the new restrictive barrier.

8. Steps 4 to 7 are repeated three to five times or until motion is maximally improved.

9. To determine the effectiveness of the technique, the physician palpates the left sternocleidomastoid muscle for reduction in tone and observes the patient's head position in the erect posture for improved body carriage.

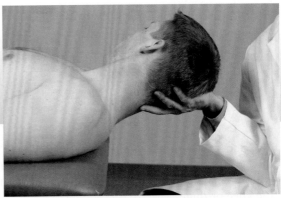

Figure 10.4. Steps 1 and 2.

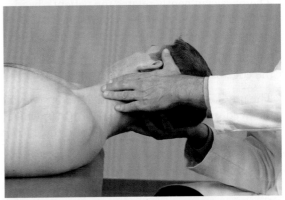

Figure 10.5. Step 3, extension barrier.

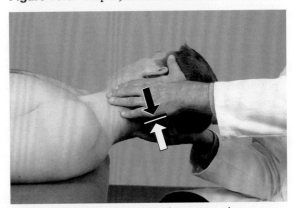

Figure 10.6. Step 4, isometric contraction.

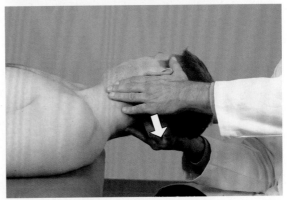

Figure 10.7. Step 7, extension barrier.

Cervical Region

Sternocleidomastoid Dysfunction
Post-Isometric Relaxation
Ex: Hypertonic Left SCM *(Subacute/Chronic)*

 See Video 10.3

1. The patient lies supine, and the physician sits at the head of the table supporting the patient's head with the hand and/or resting the patient's head on the knee or thigh.

2. The physician gently rotates the patient's head to the right to position the hypertonic left sternocleidomastoid muscle ventrally **(Fig. 10.8)**.

3. The physician gently extends the patient's head to the edge of the restrictive barrier **(Fig. 10.9)**.

4. The physician instructs the patient to lift (elevate) the head upward (*black arrow*, **Fig. 10.10**) while the physician applies an equal counterforce (*white arrow*).

5. The physician palpates the left sternocleidomastoid muscle to ensure that adequate contraction is occurring.

6. This isometric contraction is maintained for 3 to 5 seconds, and then the patient is instructed to *stop and relax.*

7. Once the patient has completely relaxed, the physician gently extends the patient's head (*white arrow*, **Fig. 10.11**) to the edge of the new restrictive barrier.

8. Steps 4 to 7 are repeated three to five times or until motion is maximally improved.

9. To determine the effectiveness of the technique, the physician palpates the left sternocleidomastoid muscle for reduction in tone and observes the patient's head position in the erect posture for improved body carriage.

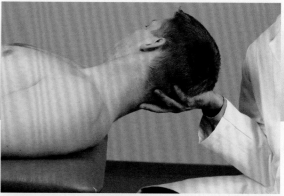

Figure 10.8. Steps 1 and 2.

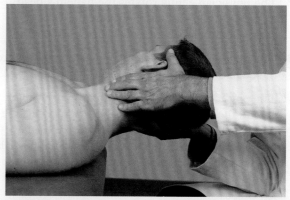

Figure 10.9. Step 3, extension barrier.

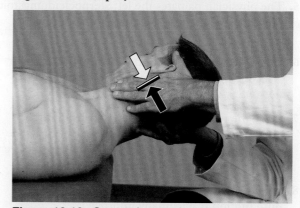

Figure 10.10. Step 4, isometric contraction.

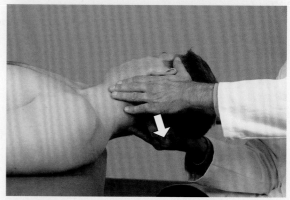

Figure 10.11. Step 7, extension barrier.

Cervical Region

Regional Range of Motion Restriction, Acute Oculocephalogyric *(Oculocervical)* Reflex

 See Video 10.4

The oculocervical reflex can be combined with any of the cervical METs using the following guidelines:

1. To produce extension of the neck: Instruct the patient to look up toward the top of the head for 3 to 5 seconds. After 3 to 5 seconds, tell the patient to *stop and relax* (close the eyes). The physician slowly and gently extends the patient's head and neck to the edge of the new restrictive barrier. This may be repeated three to five times or until motion is maximally improved **(Fig. 10.12)**.

2. To produce flexion of the neck: Instruct the patient to look down at the feet for 3 to 5 seconds. After 3 to 5 seconds, tell the patient to *stop and relax* (close the eyes). The physician slowly and gently flexes the patient's head and neck to the edge of the new restrictive barrier. This may be repeated three to five times or until motion is maximally improved **(Fig. 10.13)**.

3. To produce right side bending: Instruct the patient to look up and to the right for 3 to 5 seconds. After 3 to 5 seconds, tell the patient to *stop and relax* (close the eyes). The physician slowly and gently side bends the patient's head and neck to the edge of the new restrictive barrier. This may be repeated three to five times or until motion is maximally improved **(Fig. 10.14)**.

4. To produce left side bending: Instruct the patient to look up and to the left for 3 to 5 seconds. After 3 to 5 seconds, tell the patient to *stop and relax* (close the eyes). The physician slowly and gently side bends the patient's head and neck to the edge of the new restrictive barrier. This may be repeated three to five times or until motion is maximally improved **(Fig. 10.15)**.

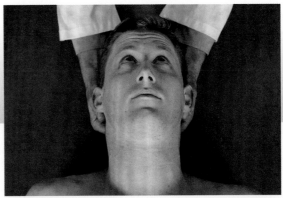

Figure 10.12. Step 1.

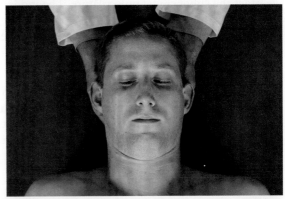

Figure 10.13. Step 2.

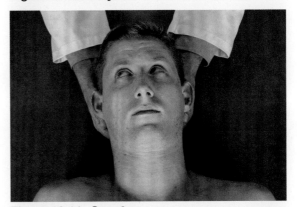

Figure 10.14. Step 3.

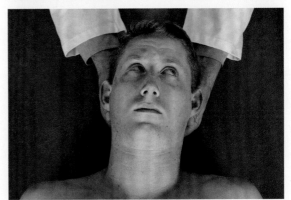

Figure 10.15. Step 4.

Cervical Region

Occipitoatlantal (OA, C0–C1) Dysfunction
Post-Isometric Relaxation
Ex: C0 ESLRR

 See Video 10.5

1. The patient is supine, and the physician sits at the head of the table.

2. One of the physician's hands is placed under the patient's occiput, and the pads of the fingers contact the suboccipital musculature. The index and middle fingers of the physician's opposite hand are placed on the patient's chin beneath the lower lip **(Figs. 10.16 and 10.17)**.

3. The physician gently flexes (*white arrow*, **Fig. 10.18**) and side bends the patient's occiput to the right to the edge of the restrictive barriers. The physician is isolating motion to the occipitoatlantal articulation only. The physician may add rotation left if desired.

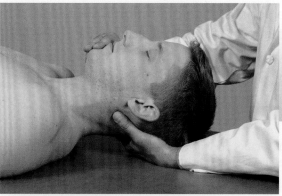

Figure 10.16. Steps 1 and 2, lateral view.

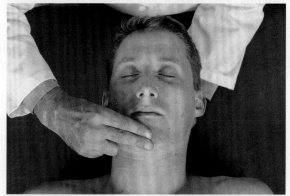

Figure 10.17. Steps 1 and 2, anterior view.

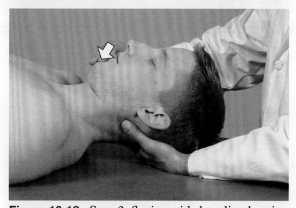

Figure 10.18. Step 3, flexion, side bending barrier.

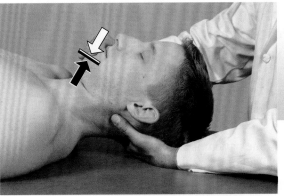

Figure 10.19. Step 4, isometric contraction.

4. The physician instructs the patient to gently lift the chin (*black arrow*, **Fig. 10.19**) up into the physician's fingers, which apply an equal counterforce (*white arrow*). During this action, which attempts to extend the occiput, the physician's hand beneath the occiput should be able to palpate the contraction of the suboccipital muscles.

5. This isometric contraction is maintained for 3 to 5 seconds, and then the patient is instructed to *stop and relax.*

6. Once the patient has completely relaxed, the physician flexes the patient's occiput to the edge of the new restrictive barrier by pulling cephalad on the patient's occiput (*curved white arrow,* **Fig. 10.20**) and pressing gently downward with the fingers on the patient's chin (*straight white arrow*).

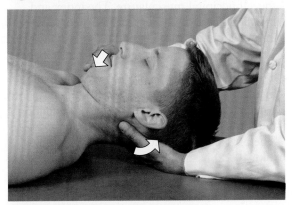

Figure 10.20. Step 6, flexion barrier.

7. Steps 4 to 6 are repeated three to five times or until motion is maximally improved at the dysfunctional segment.

8. The diagnostic parameters of the dysfunction (TART) are reevaluated to determine the effectiveness of the technique.

Cervical Region

Occipitoatlantal (OA, C0–C1) Dysfunction
Post-Isometric Relaxation
Ex: C0 FSLRR

 See Video 10.6

1. The patient is supine, and the physician sits at the head of the table.

2. One of the physician's hands is placed under the occiput, and the pads of the fingers touch the suboccipital musculature. The index and middle fingers of the physician's opposite hand lie immediately beneath the patient's chin **(Fig. 10.21)**. The physician is careful not to choke the patient.

3. The physician extends (*white arrow*) and side bends the occiput to the right until the restrictive barriers are engaged. The physician is isolating motion to occipitoatlantal articulation only. The physician may add rotation left if desired **(Fig. 10.22)**.

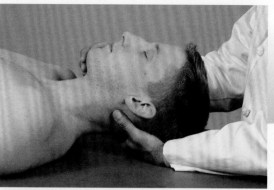

Figure 10.21. Steps 1 and 2.

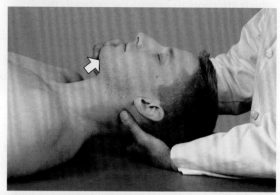

Figure 10.22. Step 3, extension, side bending barrier.

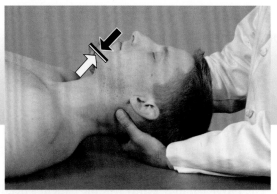

Figure 10.23. Step 4, isometric contraction.

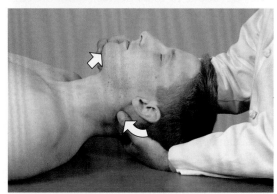

Figure 10.24. Step 6, extension barrier.

4. The physician instructs the patient to gently nod the head forward (*black arrow*, **Fig. 10.23**) so that the chin pulls down into the physician's restraining fingers while the physician applies an equal counterforce (*white arrow*). During this action, which attempts to flex the occiput, the physician's hand beneath the occiput should be able to palpate relaxation of the suboccipital muscles.

5. This isometric contraction is maintained for 3 to 5 seconds, and then the patient is instructed to *stop and relax*.

6. Once the patient has completely relaxed, the physician extends the head (*white arrow*, **Fig. 10.24**) to the edge of the new restrictive barrier by pressing to the ceiling with the hand under the occiput and lifting the cephalad with the fingers beneath the chin.

7. Steps 4 to 6 are repeated three to five times or until motion is maximally improved at the dysfunctional segment.

8. The diagnostic parameters of the dysfunction (TART) are reevaluated to determine the effectiveness of the technique.

Cervical Region

Atlantoaxial (AA, C1–C2) Dysfunction
Post-Isometric Relaxation
Ex: C1 RL

 See Video 10.7

1. The patient is supine, and the physician sits at the head of the table.

2. The physician may gently flex the patient's head (C0–C1, about 15 to 25 degrees) until the edge of the restrictive barrier is reached, or the patient's head may remain in neutral.

3. The physician rotates the patient's head to the right (*white arrow*, **Fig. 10.25**) until the edge of the restrictive barrier is reached.

4. The physician instructs the patient to rotate the head to the left (*black arrow*, **Fig. 10.26**) while the physician applies an equal counterforce (*white arrow*). Note: In acute painful dysfunctions, the patient can very gently rotate or look to the right (reciprocal inhibition, oculocervical).

5. This isometric contraction is maintained for 3 to 5 seconds, and then the patient is instructed to *stop and relax*.

6. Once the patient has completely relaxed, the physician rotates the patient's head (*white arrow*, **Fig. 10.27**) to the right to the edge of the new restrictive barrier.

7. Steps 4 to 6 are repeated three to five times or until motion is maximally improved at the dysfunctional segment.

8. The diagnostic parameters of the dysfunction (TART) are reevaluated to determine the effectiveness of the technique.

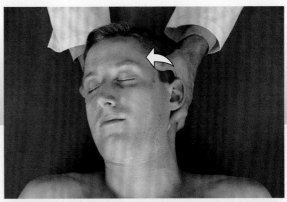
Figure 10.25. Steps 1 to 3, rotation barrier.

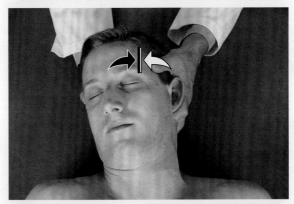
Figure 10.26. Step 4, isometric contraction.

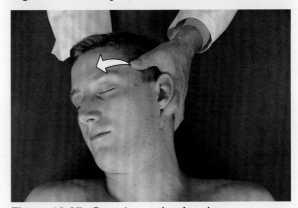
Figure 10.27. Step 6, rotation barrier.

Cervical Region

C2–C7 Dysfunctions
Post-Isometric Relaxation
Ex: C3 FSRRR

 See Video 10.8

1. The patient lies supine, and the physician is seated at the head of the table on the side of the rotational component.

2. The first metacarpal-phalangeal joint of the physician's right hand is placed at the articular pillar of the segment being treated. The heel of the physician's hand closes in against the occiput.

3. The physician cradles the patient's head between the hands (may cup the chin with the left hand). The occiput, C1, C2, and C3 are flexed until the dysfunctional C3 engages C4; the segments are then extended slightly to meet the extension barrier. C3 is then rotated and side bent to the left until the edge of the restrictive barriers are reached in all three planes **(Fig. 10.28)**.

4. The physician instructs the patient to rotate the head (*black arrow*, **Fig. 10.29**) to the right while the physician applies an equal counterforce (*white arrow*). Note: In acute, painful dysfunctions, the physician may instruct the patient to *very gently* rotate or *look* to the left while the physician applies an equal counterforce (*reciprocal inhibition, oculocervical*).

5. This isometric contraction is maintained for 3 to 5 seconds, and then the patient is instructed to *stop and relax.*

6. Once the patient has completely relaxed, the physician repositions the dysfunctional segment to the edge of the new restrictive barriers in all three planes: first, left rotation, then left side bending and, finally, extension (*white arrows*) **(Fig. 10.30)**.

7. Steps 4 to 6 are repeated three to five times or until motion is maximally improved at the dysfunctional segment.

8. The diagnostic parameters of the dysfunction (TART) are reevaluated to determine the effectiveness of the technique.

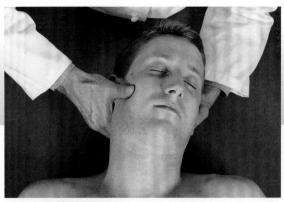

Figure 10.28. Steps 1 to 3.

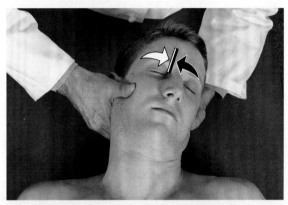

Figure 10.29. Step 4, isometric contraction.

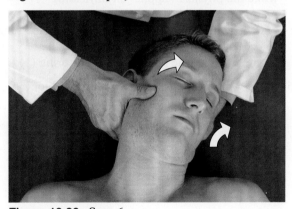

Figure 10.30. Step 6.

Thoracic Region

T1–T4 "Extension" Dysfunctions
Post-Isometric Relaxation
Ex: T4 ESRRR

 See Videos 10.9 and 10.10

1. The patient is seated at the end of the table, and the physician stands at the side of the patient, which offers best control of patient positioning.

2. The physician's left hand palpates the spinous processes of T4 and T5 or the T4–T5 interspace to monitor flexion and extension as the right hand flexes the patient's head and neck (*white arrow,* **Fig. 10.31**) to the edge of the restrictive barrier.

3. The physician's left hand monitors the transverse processes of T4 and T5 to localize side bending and rotation as the right hand side bends (*white arrow,* **Fig. 10.32**) and rotates (*white arrow,* **Fig. 10.33**) the patient's head and neck to the left until the edge of the restrictive barrier is reached.

4. The patient is instructed to extend the head and neck and turn to the right (*black arrow,* **Fig. 10.34**) while the physician applies an unyielding counterforce (*white arrow*). The force of the patient's contraction is the least amount necessary to produce a palpable muscle twitch at the segmental level the physician is monitoring (5).

5. This isometric contraction is maintained for 3 to 5 seconds, and then the patient is instructed to *stop and relax.*

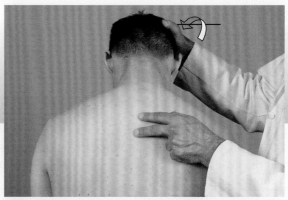

Figure 10.31. Steps 1 and 2, flexion barrier.

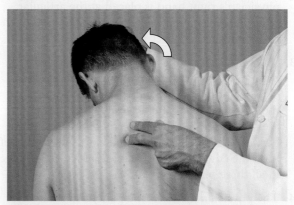

Figure 10.32. Step 3, left side bending barrier.

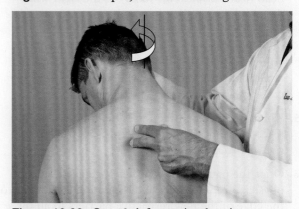

Figure 10.33. Step 3, left rotation barrier.

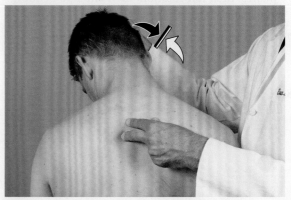

Figure 10.34. Step 4, isometric contraction.

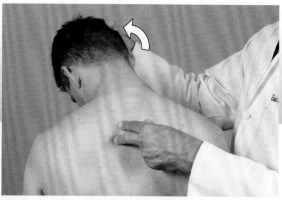

Figure 10.35. Step 6, left side bending barrier.

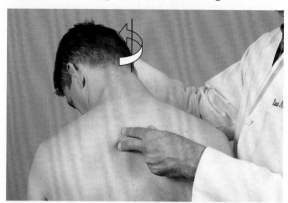

Figure 10.36. Step 6, left rotation barrier.

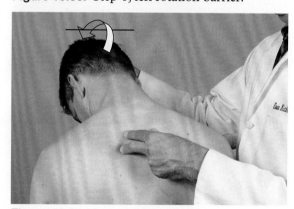

Figure 10.37. Step 6, flexion barrier.

6. Once the patient has completely relaxed, the physician repositions the patient's head and neck to the edge of the new restrictive barriers in all three planes: first, left side bending (*white arrow*, **Fig. 10.35**), then left rotation (*white arrow*, **Fig. 10.36**) and, finally, flexion (*white arrow*, **Fig. 10.37**).

7. Steps 4 to 6 are repeated three to five times or until motion is maximally improved at the dysfunctional segment.

8. The diagnostic parameters of the dysfunction (TART) are reevaluated to determine the effectiveness of the technique.

Thoracic Region

T1–T6 "Flexion" Dysfunctions
Post-Isometric Relaxation
Ex: T4 FSRRR

 See Video 10.11

1. The patient is seated with the right hand on the left shoulder, and the physician stands close to the patient on the side opposite to the rotational component.

2. The physician's left hand reaches under the patient's elbow and grasps the patient's right shoulder. The physician's right hand palpates the spinous processes of T4 and T5 or T4–T5 interspace, and then the physician instructs the patient to relax and rest the full weight of the head and elbow on the physician's arm **(Fig. 10.38)**.

3. Starting with the patient in extreme flexion, the physician slowly raises the left elbow (*white arrow*) as the right hand gently translates the dysfunctional vertebra forward (*white arrow*) to the edge of the extension barrier **(Fig. 10.39)**.

4. The physician's right hand now monitors the transverse processes of T4 and T5 to localize side bending and rotation, as the left arm and hand reposition the patient's left shoulder down (*white arrow*) to engage the edge of the left side bending barrier **(Fig. 10.40)**.

5. The physician then gently rotates the patient's shoulders left (*white arrow*) to engage the edge of the left rotation barrier **(Fig. 10.41)**.

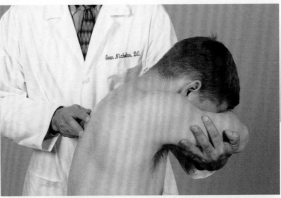

Figure 10.38. Steps 1 and 2.

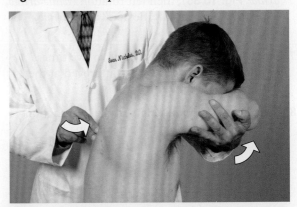

Figure 10.39. Step 3, extension barrier.

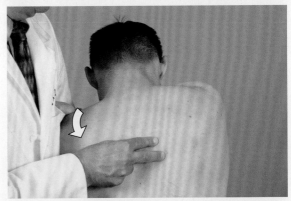

Figure 10.40. Step 4, left side bending barrier.

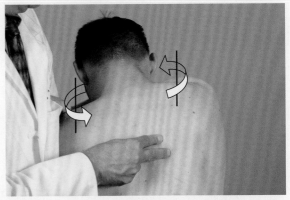

Figure 10.41. Step 5, left rotation barrier.

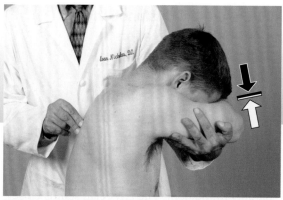

Figure 10.42. Step 6, isometric contraction.

6. The patient is instructed to push the elbows and forehead down against the physician's arm and turn to the right (*black arrow*) as the physician applies an unyielding counterforce (*white arrow*, **Fig. 10.42**). The force of the patient's contraction is the least amount necessary to produce a palpable muscle twitch at the segmental level the physician is monitoring (5).

7. This isometric contraction is maintained for 3 to 5 seconds, and then the patient is instructed to *stop and relax*.

8. Once the patient has completely relaxed, the physician repositions the patient to the edge of the new restrictive barriers in all three planes: first, left side bending **(Fig. 10.43)**, then left rotation **(Fig. 10.44)** and, finally, extension **(Fig. 10.45)**.

9. Steps 6 to 8 are repeated three to five times or until motion is maximally improved at the dysfunctional segment.

10. The diagnostic parameters of the dysfunction (TART) are reevaluated to determine the effectiveness of the technique.

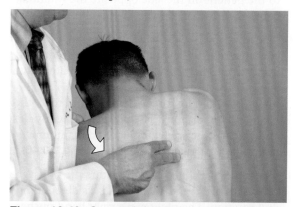

Figure 10.43. Step 8, left side bending barrier.

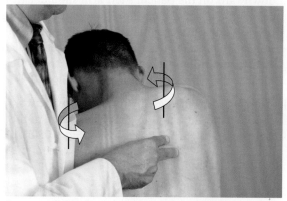

Figure 10.44. Step 8, left rotation barrier.

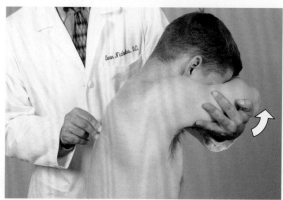

Figure 10.45. Step 8, extension barrier.

Thoracic Region

T5–T12 "Neutral" Dysfunctions
Post-Isometric Relaxation
Ex: T8 NSRRL

 See Video 10.12

1. The patient is seated with the left hand grasping the back of the head/neck and the right hand grasping the left elbow. The right forearm is parallel to the floor. The physician stands close to the patient on the side opposite the rotational component.

2. The physician's right hand passes under the patient's right axilla and grasps the patient's left upper arm. The physician's left hand palpates the spinous processes of T8 and T9, or the T8–T9 interspace, and instructs the patient to relax the head and upper body. The physician slightly flexes and extends the spine, finding and maintaining neutral at that given segment (T8) **(Fig. 10.46)**.

3. The physician's left hand monitors the transverse processes of T8 and T9 to localize side bending and rotation. The physician's right hand pushes downward on the patient's left arm/shoulder (*white arrow*) to engage the edge of the left side bending barrier. The physician may lift the right elbow under the patient's right axilla (*white arrow*) to add translation of the patient's upper body to further localize the left side bending barrier **(Fig. 10.47)**.

4. The physician then gently rotates the patient's shoulders to the right, to engage the edge of the right rotation barrier (*white arrow*, **Fig. 10.48**).

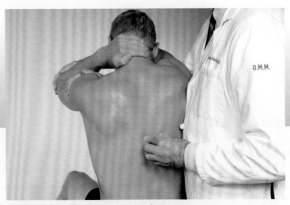

Figure 10.46. Steps 1 and 2.

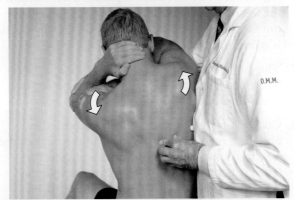

Figure 10.47. Step 3, left side bending barrier.

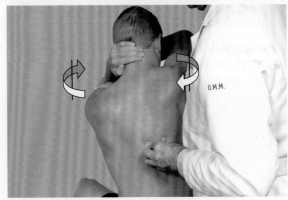

Figure 10.48. Step 4, right rotation barrier.

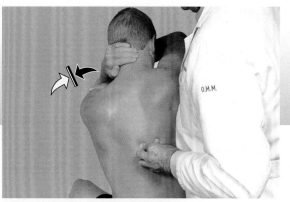

Figure 10.49. Step 5, isometric contraction.

5. The physician instructs the patient to "turn your shoulders to the left" (*black arrow*) as the physician applies an unyielding counterforce (*white arrow*) **(Fig. 10.49)**. The force of the patient's contraction is the least amount necessary to produce a palpable muscle twitch at the segmental level that the physician is monitoring (5).

6. This isometric contraction is maintained for 3 to 5 seconds, and then the patient is instructed to *stop and relax*.

7. Once the patient has completely relaxed, the physician repositions the patient to the edge of the new restrictive barriers: first, left side bending and then right rotation while maintaining neutral in the sagittal plane (*white arrows*, **Fig. 10.50**).

8. Steps 5 to 7 are repeated three to five times or until motion is maximally improved at the dysfunctional segment.

9. Intersegmental motion of the dysfunctional segment and the other diagnostic parameters of the dysfunction (TART) are reevaluated to determine the effectiveness of the technique.

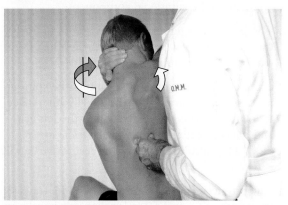

Figure 10.50. Step 7.

Thoracic Region

T5–T12 "Extension" Dysfunctions
Post-Isometric Relaxation
Ex: T8 ESRRR

 See Video 10.13

1. The patient is seated at the end of the table, the left side close to the edge. The patient's arms are folded across the chest, right over left.

2. The physician stands at the side of the patient opposite to the rotational component.

3. The physician's left arm reaches across in front of the patient's elbows and places the left hand on the patient's right shoulder.

4. The physician's right hand monitors the spinous processes of T8 and T9 or the T8–T9 interspace to localize flexion and extension as the left arm and hand flex the patient's torso (*white arrow*, **Fig. 10.51**) until the edge of the restrictive barrier is reached.

5. The physician's right hand monitors the transverse processes of T8 and T9 to localize side bending and rotation as the left arm and hand position the patient's torso to engage the edge of the left side bending (*white arrow*, **Fig. 10.52**) and left rotation barriers (*white arrow*, **Fig. 10.53**).

6. The physician instructs the patient to sit up and turn to the right (*black arrow*) as the physician's left hand applies an unyielding counterforce (*white arrow*, **Fig. 10.54**). The force of the patient's contraction is the least amount necessary to produce a palpable muscle twitch at the segmental level the physician is monitoring (5).

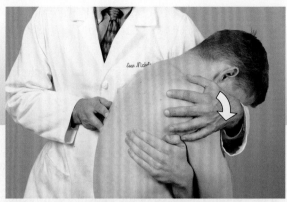
Figure 10.51. Steps 1 to 4, flexion barrier.

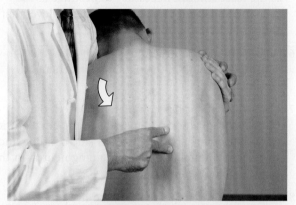
Figure 10.52. Step 5, left side bending barrier.

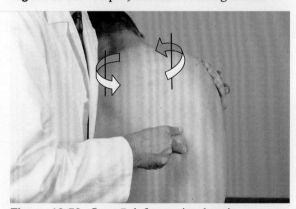
Figure 10.53. Step 5, left rotation barrier.

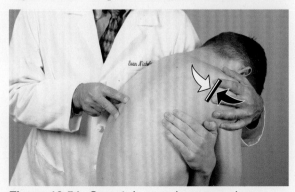
Figure 10.54. Step 6, isometric contraction.

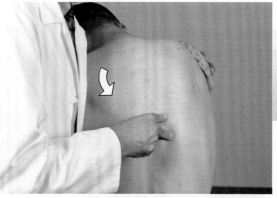

Figure 10.55. Step 8, left side bending barrier.

7. This isometric contraction is maintained for 3 to 5 seconds, and then the patient is instructed to *stop and relax*.

8. Once the patient has completely relaxed, the physician repositions the patient to the edge of the new restrictive barriers in all three planes: first, left side bending **(Fig. 10.55)**, then left rotation **(Fig. 10.56)** and, finally, flexion **(Fig. 10.57)**.

9. Steps 6 to 8 are repeated three to five times or until motion is maximally improved at the dysfunctional segment.

10. The diagnostic parameters of the dysfunction (TART) are reevaluated to determine the effectiveness of the technique.

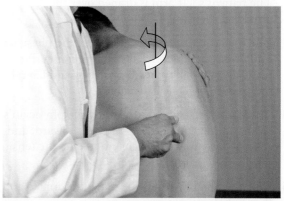

Figure 10.56. Step 8, left rotation barrier.

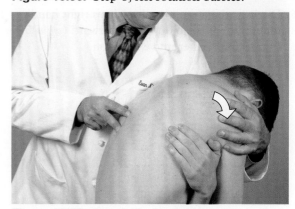

Figure 10.57. Step 8, flexion barrier.

Costal Region

Rib 1 Inhalation Dysfunction
Seated, Respiratory Assist
Ex: Right Rib 1 Inhaled (Elevated)

 See Video 10.14

1. The patient is seated. The physician stands behind the patient, placing the left foot on the table to the left side of the patient and keeping the hip and knee flexed at about 90 degrees.

2. The patient's left arm is draped over the physician's left thigh.

3. The metacarpal-phalangeal joint of the physician's right index finger contacts the superior surface of the dysfunctional right rib posterior and lateral to the costotransverse articulation.

4. The patient's head, controlled by the physician's left hand, is gently flexed, side bent toward, and rotated away from the right rib to take the tension off the scalene musculature **(Fig. 10.58)**.

5. The physician instructs the patient to inhale and then exhale deeply.

6. During exhalation, the physician's right hand follows the first rib down and forward (*white arrow*, **Fig. 10.59**) further into exhalation.

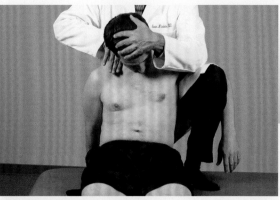

Figure 10.58. Steps 1 to 4.

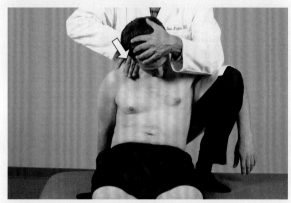

Figure 10.59. Step 6, exhalation.

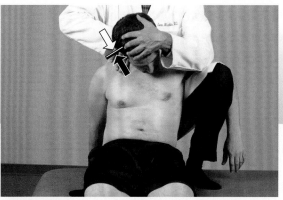

Figure 10.60. Step 7, resist inhalation.

7. The physician instructs the patient to inhale deeply (*black arrow*, **Fig. 10.60**), as the physician's right hand resists (*white arrow*) the inhalation motion of the first rib.

8. The physician then instructs the patient to exhale deeply as the physician's right hand follows the first rib down and forward (*white arrow*, **Fig. 10.61**) toward exhalation.

9. Steps 7 and 8 are repeated five to seven times or until motion is maximally improved at the dysfunctional rib.

10. Motion of the dysfunctional rib is reevaluated to determine the effectiveness of the technique.

11. An alternative technique is to have the patient lift the right shoulder against resistance for 3 to 5 seconds and then carry the rib toward exhalation during the relaxation phase.

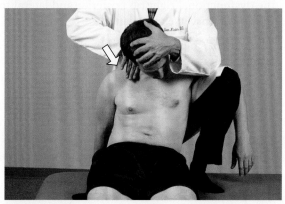

Figure 10.61. Step 8, exaggerate exhalation.

Costal Region

Rib 1 Inhalation Dysfunction
Respiratory Assist, Supine
Ex: Right Rib 1 Inhaled (Elevated)

 See Video 10.15

1. The patient lies supine, and the physician stands or sits behind the patient.

2. The metacarpal-phalangeal joint of the physician's right index finger contacts the superior surface of the dysfunctional right rib posterior and lateral to the costotransverse articulation.

3. The patient's head, controlled by the physician's left hand, is gently flexed, side bent toward, and rotated away from the right rib to take the tension off the scalene musculature (**Fig. 10.62**).

4. The patient inhales and then exhales deeply.

5. During exhalation, the physician's right hand follows the first rib down and forward (*white arrow*, **Fig. 10.63**) further into exhalation.

6. The patient is instructed to inhale deeply (*black arrow*, **Fig. 10.64**) as the physician's right hand resists (*white arrow*) the inhalation motion of the first rib.

7. The patient is then instructed to exhale deeply as the physician's right hand follows the first rib down and forward (*white arrow*, **Fig. 10.65**) toward exhalation.

8. Steps 6 and 7 are repeated five to seven times or until motion is maximally improved at the dysfunctional rib.

9. Motion of the dysfunctional rib is reevaluated to determine the effectiveness of the technique.

10. An alternative technique is to have the patient lift the right shoulder against resistance for 3 to 5 seconds and then carry the rib toward exhalation during the relaxation phase.

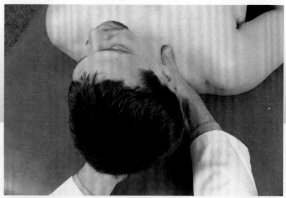

Figure 10.62. Steps 1 to 3.

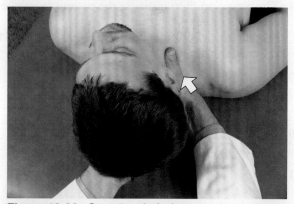

Figure 10.63. Step 5, exhalation.

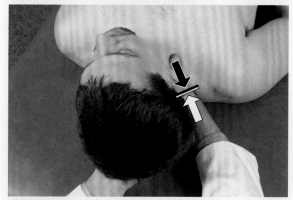

Figure 10.64. Step 6, resist inhalation.

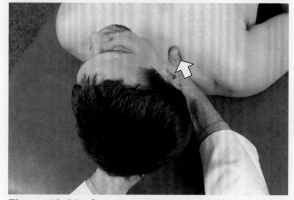

Figure 10.65. Step 7, exaggerate exhalation.

Costal Region

Rib 1, Rib 2 Inhalation Dysfunctions
Post-Isometric Relaxation, Seated
Ex: Right Rib 1 Inhaled (Elevated)

1. The patient is seated, and the physician stands behind the patient, placing the left foot on the table to the left side of the patient and keeping the hip and knee flexed at about 90 degrees.

2. The physician's right thumb is placed over the anteromedial aspect of the dysfunctional right rib.

3. The physician's left hand controls the patient's forehead, rotates it 30 to 45 degrees to the left (*white arrow*), and adds slight extension until meeting the edge of the restrictive barrier **(Fig. 10.66)**.

4. The physician instructs the patient to push the head forward into the physician's left hand (*black arrow*, **Fig. 10.67**), which applies an equal counterforce (*long white arrow*). The right hand (*short white arrow*) simultaneously resists any inhalation movement of the dysfunctional rib.

5. This isometric contraction is held for 3 to 5 seconds, and then the patient is instructed to *relax*.

6. Once the patient has completely relaxed, the physician's left hand minimally extends the patient's head (*white arrow*, **Fig. 10.68**) to the edge of the new restrictive barrier.

7. Steps 4 to 6 are repeated three to five times or until motion is maximally improved at the dysfunctional rib.

8. Motion of the dysfunctional rib is reevaluated to assess the effectiveness of the technique.

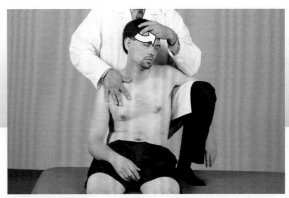

Figure 10.66. Steps 1 to 3.

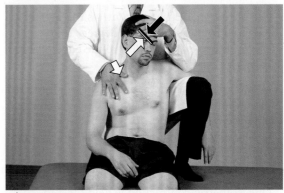

Figure 10.67. Step 4, isometric contraction.

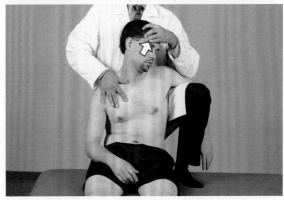

Figure 10.68. Step 6, extension barrier.

Costal Region

Rib 1, Rib 2 Inhalation Dysfunctions
Post-Isometric Relaxation, Supine
Ex: Right Rib 1 Inhaled (Elevated)

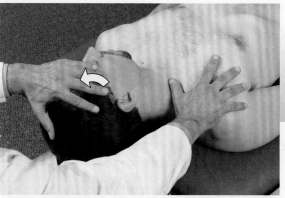

Figure 10.69. Steps 1 to 3, rotation and extension barrier.

1. The patient lies supine, and the physician sits at the head of the table.

2. The physician's right thumb is placed over the anteromedial aspect of the dysfunctional rib.

3. The physician's left hand controls the patient's head and rotates it 30 to 45 degrees to the left (*white arrow*, **Fig. 10.69**) to the edge of the restrictive barrier.

4. The physician instructs the patient to lift the head forward and to the right into the physician's left hand (*black arrow*, **Fig. 10.70**), which applies an equal counterforce (*long white arrow*). The right thumb (*short white arrow*) simultaneously resists any inhalation movement of the dysfunctional ribs.

5. This isometric contraction is held for 3 to 5 seconds, and then the patient is instructed to *relax*.

6. Once the patient has completely relaxed, the physician's left hand minimally extends the patient's head (*white arrow*, **Fig. 10.71**) until a new restrictive barrier is reached.

7. Steps 4 to 6 are repeated three to five times until motion is maximally improved at the dysfunctional rib.

8. Motion of the dysfunctional rib is reevaluated to assess the effectiveness of the technique.

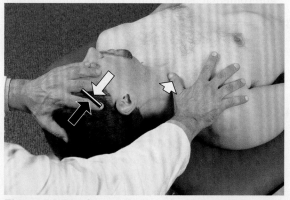

Figure 10.70. Step 4, isometric contraction.

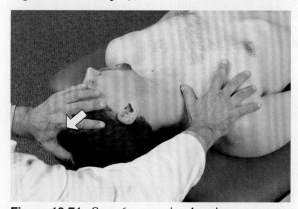

Figure 10.71. Step 6, extension barrier.

Costal Region

Rib 2–Rib 6 Inhalation Dysfunctions
Respiratory Assist
Ex: Right Rib 3 Inhaled (Elevated)

 See Video 10.16

1. The patient lies supine, and the physician's flexed right knee is placed on the table underneath the patient's right upper thoracic region at the level of the dysfunctional rib.

2. The patient's upper body is side bent to the side of the dysfunction (right side) until tension is taken off the dysfunctional rib.

3. The web formed by the physician's right thumb and index finger is placed in the intercostal space above the dysfunctional rib on its superior surface **(Fig. 10.72)**.

4. The patient inhales and exhales deeply.

5. During exhalation, the physician's right hand exaggerates the exhalation motion (*white arrow*, **Fig. 10.73**) of the dysfunctional rib.

6. The patient inhales again (*black arrow*, **Fig. 10.74**) as the physician's right hand resists (*white arrow*) the inhalation motion of the dysfunctional rib.

7. The patient exhales, and the physician exaggerates the exhalation motion (*white arrow*, **Fig. 10.75**) of the dysfunctional rib.

8. Steps 6 and 7 are repeated five to seven times or until motion is maximally improved at the dysfunctional rib.

9. Motion of the dysfunctional rib is reevaluated to assess the effectiveness of the technique.

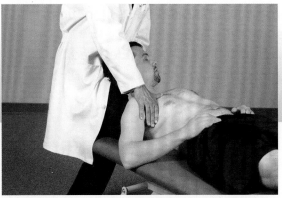
Figure 10.72. Steps 1 to 3.

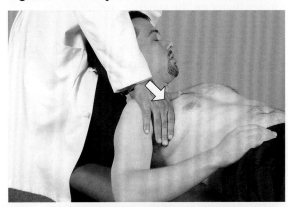
Figure 10.73. Step 5, exaggerate exhalation.

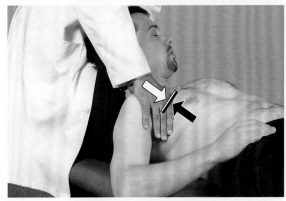
Figure 10.74. Step 6, resist inhalation.

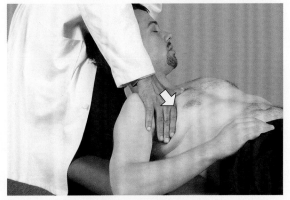
Figure 10.75. Step 7, exaggerate exhalation.

Costal Region

Rib 7–Rib 10 Inhalation Dysfunctions
Respiratory Assist
Ex: Right Rib 9 Inhaled (Elevated)

 See Video 10.17

1. The patient lies supine, and the physician stands at the side of the dysfunctional rib.

2. The physician's left hand abducts the patient's right shoulder and places the right thumb and index finger on the superior surface of the dysfunctional rib.

3. The physician side bends the patient's thoracic spine to the level of the dysfunctional rib **(Fig. 10.76)**.

4. The patient inhales and exhales deeply as the physician's right hand exaggerates (*white arrow*, **Fig. 10.77**) the exhalation motion of the dysfunctional rib.

5. On inhalation (*black arrow*, **Fig. 10.78**), the physician's right hand resists (*white arrow*) the inhalation motion of the dysfunctional rib.

6. The patient exhales, and the physician exaggerates the exhalation motion (*white arrow*, **Fig. 10.79**) of the dysfunctional rib.

7. Steps 5 and 6 are repeated five to seven times or until motion is maximally improved at the dysfunctional rib.

8. Motion of the dysfunctional rib is reevaluated to assess the effectiveness of the technique.

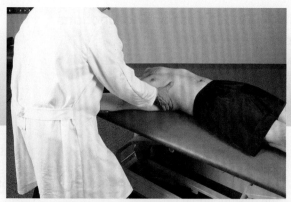
Figure 10.76. Steps 1 to 3.

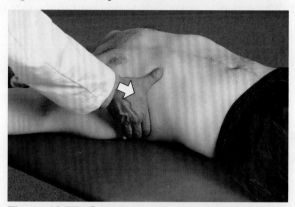
Figure 10.77. Step 4, exaggerate exhalation.

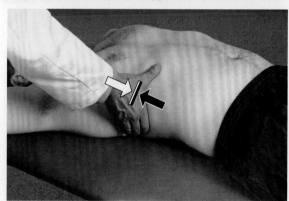
Figure 10.78. Step 5, resist inhalation.

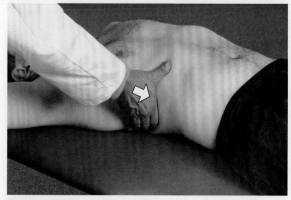
Figure 10.79. Step 6, exaggerate exhalation.

Costal Region

Rib 11, Rib 12 Inhalation Dysfunctions
Respiratory Assist
Ex: Right Rib 12 Inhaled

 See Video 10.18

1. The patient lies prone, and the physician stands at the left side of the table and positions the patient's legs 15 to 20 degrees to the right, taking tension off the quadratus lumborum.

2. The physician places the left hypothenar eminence medial and inferior to the angle of the dysfunctional rib and exerts gentle, sustained lateral and cephalad traction.

3. The physician may grasp the patient's right anterior superior iliac spine with the right hand to stabilize the pelvis **(Fig. 10.80)**.

4. The patient inhales and exhales deeply.

5. During exhalation, the physician's left hand exaggerates (*white arrow*, **Fig. 10.81**) the exhalation motion of the dysfunctional rib by exerting cephalad and lateral traction.

6. On inhalation (*black arrow*, **Fig. 10.82**), the physician's right hand resists (*white arrow*) the inhalation motion of the dysfunctional rib.

7. The patient then exhales, and the physician exaggerates the exhalation motion (*white arrow*, **Fig. 10.83**) of the dysfunctional rib.

8. Steps 6 and 7 are repeated five to seven times or until motion is maximally improved at the dysfunctional rib.

9. Motion of the dysfunctional rib is reevaluated to assess the effectiveness of the technique.

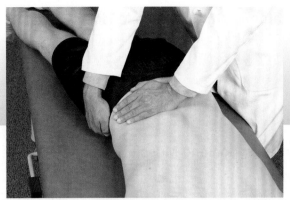

Figure 10.80. Steps 1 to 3.

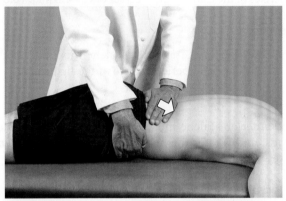

Figure 10.81. Step 5, exaggerate exhalation.

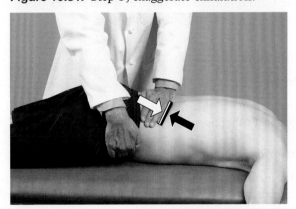

Figure 10.82. Step 6, resist inhalation.

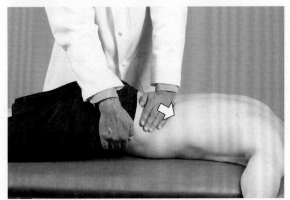

Figure 10.83. Step 7, exaggerate exhalation.

Costal Region

Anatomy of the Scalene Muscles

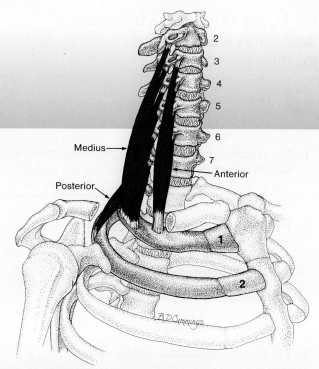

Anterior Scalene Muscle

Origin

The origin of the anterior scalene muscle is at the anterior tubercles of the transverse processes of C3–C6 **(Fig. 10.84)**.

Insertion

The insertion of the anterior scalene muscle is at the scalene tubercle, superior surface of the first rib.

Action

The anterior scalene muscle elevates the first rib, side bends, and rotates the neck (same side/unilateral) and flexes the neck (bilateral).

Innervation

The ventral rami of the cervical spinal nerves (C4–C6) innervate the anterior scalene muscle.

Middle Scalene Muscle

Origin

The origin of the middle scalene muscle is at the posterior tubercles of the transverse processes of C2–C7.

Insertion

The insertion of the middle scalene muscle is on the superior surface of the first rib, posterior to the groove for the subclavian artery.

Action

The middle scalene muscle elevates the first rib during forced inspiration and flexes the neck laterally.

Innervation

The ventral rami of cervical spinal nerves C3–C8 innervate the middle scalene muscle.

Figure 10.84. Anatomy of the scalenes and thoracic outlet (Reprinted with permission from Ref. (7).)

Posterior Scalene Muscle

Origin

The origin of the posterior scalene muscle is at the posterior tubercles of the transverse processes of C5–C7.

Insertion

The insertion of the posterior scalene muscle is at the second rib.

Action

The posterior scalene muscle elevates the second rib during forced inspiration and flexes the neck laterally.

Innervation

The ventral rami of cervical spinal nerves (C6–C8) innervate the posterior scalene muscle.

Costal Region

Rib 1, Rib 2 Exhalation Dysfunctions
Scalene(s) Contraction Mobilizes Rib
Ex: Right Rib 1 Exhaled (Depressed)

 See Videos 10.19 and 10.20

1. The patient lies supine, and the physician stands on the left side of the patient.

2. The patient's head is rotated approximately 30 degrees to the left.

3. The patient's right wrist (dorsal surface) is placed against the forehead **(Fig. 10.85)**.

4. The physician's left hand reaches under the patient, grasps the superior angle of the right dysfunctional rib, and exerts a caudad and lateral traction (*white arrow*, **Fig. 10.86**).

5. The physician instructs the patient to flex the head and neck (*black arrow*, **Fig. 10.87**) without altering the rotation of the head while the physician's right hand applies an unyielding counterforce (*white arrow*). The patient may be asked to slowly inhale during the contraction to enhance the effectiveness of the technique.

6. This isometric contraction is maintained for 3 to 5 seconds, and the patient is instructed to *relax*.

7. Once the patient has completely relaxed, the physician's left hand exerts increased caudad and lateral traction on the angle of the dysfunctional rib (*white arrow*, **Fig. 10.88**).

8. Steps 5 to 7 are repeated five to seven times or until motion is maximally improved at the dysfunctional rib.

9. Motion of the dysfunctional rib is reevaluated to assess the effectiveness of the technique.

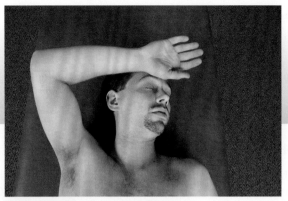
Figure 10.85. Steps 1 to 3.

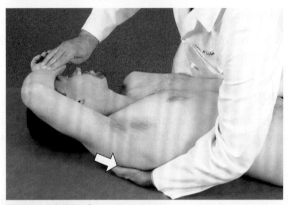
Figure 10.86. Step 4.

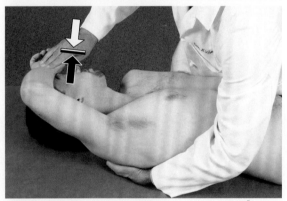
Figure 10.87. Step 5, isometric contraction.

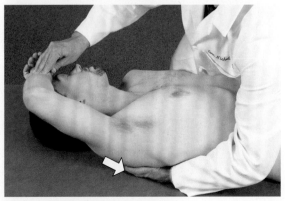
Figure 10.88. Step 7.

Costal Region

Pectoralis Minor Muscle

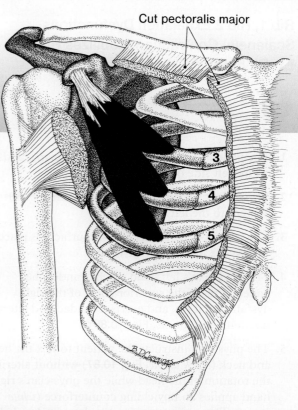

Cut pectoralis major

Origin

The origin of the pectoralis minor muscle is at the anterior superior surface of ribs 3, 4, and 5 **(Fig. 10.89)**.

Insertion

The insertion of the pectoralis minor muscle is at the coracoid process of the scapula.

Action

The pectoralis minor muscle stabilizes the scapula by drawing it inferiorly and anteriorly against thoracic wall.

Innervation

The medial pectoral nerve (C8, T1) innervates the pectoralis minor muscle.

Figure 10.89. Pectoralis minor muscle. (Reprinted with permission from Ref. (7).)

Costal Region

Rib 3–Rib 5 Exhalation Dysfunctions
Pectoralis Minor Contraction Mobilizes Rib
Ex: Right Rib 3 Exhaled (Depressed)

 See Video 10.21

1. The patient lies supine, and the physician stands on the left side of the table.

2. The patient raises the right arm and places the hand over the head **(Fig. 10.90)**.

3. The physician's left hand reaches under the right side of the patient, grasps the superior angle of the dysfunctional rib, and exerts caudad and lateral traction.

4. The physician's right hand is placed over the anterior aspect of the patient's right elbow **(Fig. 10.91)**.

5. The physician instructs the patient to push the elbow against the physician's right hand (*black arrow*, **Fig. 10.92**), which applies an unyielding counterforce (*white arrow*). The patient may be asked to slowly inhale during the contraction to enhance the effectiveness of the technique.

6. This isometric contraction is held for 3 to 5 seconds, and then the patient is instructed to *stop and relax.*

7. Once the patient has completely relaxed, the physician's left hand exerts increased caudad and lateral traction on the angle of the dysfunctional rib (*white arrow*, **Fig. 10.93**).

8. Steps 5 to 7 are repeated five to seven times or until motion is maximally improved at the dysfunctional rib.

9. Motion of the dysfunctional rib is reevaluated to assess the effectiveness of the technique.

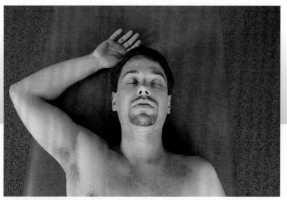

Figure 10.90. Steps 1 and 2.

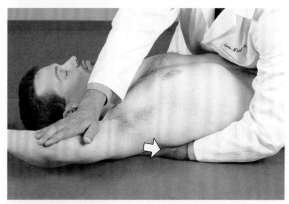

Figure 10.91. Steps 3 and 4.

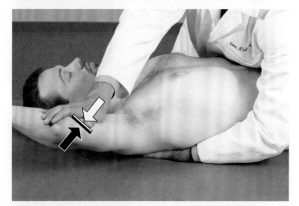

Figure 10.92. Step 5, isometric contraction.

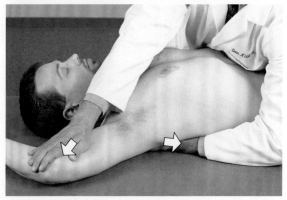

Figure 10.93. Step 7.

Costal Region

Serratus Anterior Muscle

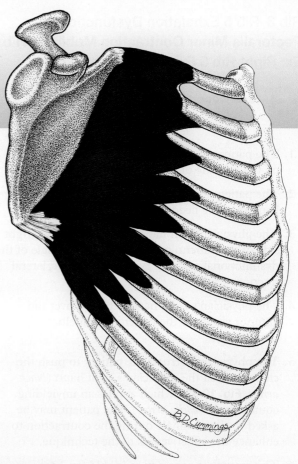

Origin

The origin of the serratus anterior muscle is at the anterior surface of the medial border of the scapula **(Fig. 10.94)**.

Insertion

The insertion of the serratus anterior muscle is at the superior lateral surface of ribs 2 to 8.

Action

The serratus anterior muscle protracts the scapula and holds it against the thoracic wall.

Innervation

The long thoracic nerve (C5 to C7) innervates the serratus anterior muscle.

Figure 10.94. Serratus anterior muscle. (Reprinted with permission from Ref. (7).)

Costal Region

Rib 6–Rib 8 Exhalation Dysfunctions
Serratus Anterior Contraction Mobilizes Rib
Ex: Right Rib 6 Exhaled (Depressed)

 See Video 10.22

1. The patient lies supine, and the physician stands or sits at the side of the dysfunctional rib.

2. The patient's right shoulder is flexed 90 degrees; the elbow may be flexed for better control by the physician.

3. The physician's left hand reaches under the patient and grasps the superior angle of the dysfunctional rib, exerting caudad and lateral traction (*white arrow*, **Fig. 10.95**).

4. The physician instructs the patient to push the elbow toward the ceiling (scapular protraction) (*black arrow*, **Fig. 10.96**) while the physician applies an unyielding counterforce (*white arrow*). The patient may be asked to slowly inhale during the contraction to enhance the effectiveness of the technique.

5. This isometric contraction is held for 3 to 5 seconds, and then the patient is instructed to *stop and relax*.

6. Once the patient has completely relaxed, the physician's left hand exerts increased caudad and lateral traction (*white arrow*, **Fig. 10.97**) on the angle of the dysfunctional rib.

7. Steps 4 to 6 are repeated five to seven times or until motion is maximally improved at the dysfunctional rib.

8. Motion of the dysfunctional rib is reevaluated to assess the effectiveness of the technique.

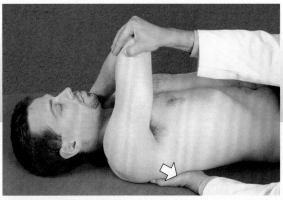
Figure 10.95. Steps 1 to 3.

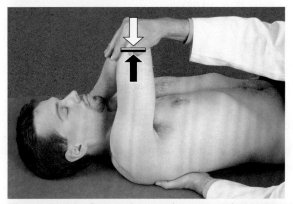
Figure 10.96. Step 4, isometric contraction.

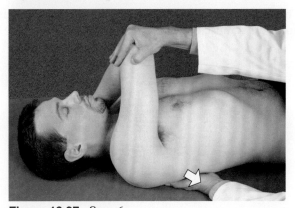
Figure 10.97. Step 6.

Costal Region

Latissimus Dorsi Muscle

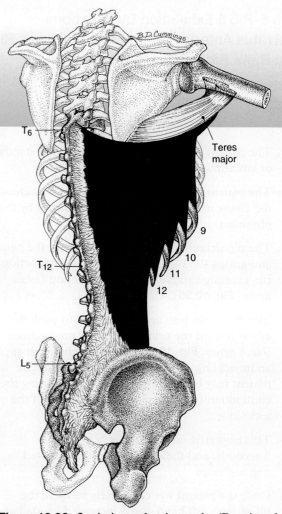

Origin

The origin of the latissimus dorsi muscle is at spinous processes of T7 to S3, the thoracolumbar fascia, the inferior angle of the scapula, the lower four ribs, and the iliac crest **(Fig. 10.98)**.

Insertion

The insertion of the latissimus dorsi muscle is at the intertubercular (bicipital) groove of the humerus.

Action

The latissimus dorsi muscle extends, adducts, and medially rotates the humerus.

Innervation

The thoracodorsal nerve (C6–C8) innervates the latissimus dorsi muscle.

Figure 10.98. Latissimus dorsi muscle. (Reprinted with permission from Ref. (7).)

Costal Region

Rib 9, Rib 10 Exhalation Dysfunctions
Latissimus Dorsi Contraction Mobilizes Rib
Ex: Right Rib 10 Exhaled/Depressed

 See Video 10.23

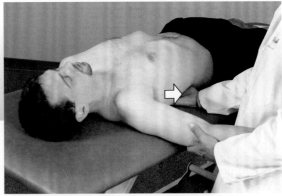

Figure 10.99. Step 3.

1. The patient lies supine, and the physician stands or sits at the side of the dysfunctional rib.

2. The physician's left hand abducts the patient's right shoulder 90 degrees, and the right hand reaches under the patient and grasps the superior angle of the dysfunctional rib, exerting caudad and lateral traction.

3. The physician's left lateral thigh or knee is placed against the patient's right elbow **(Fig. 10.99)**.

4. The physician instructs the patient to push the right arm into the physician's thigh (*black arrow*, **Fig. 10.100**) while the physician's left thigh or arm applies an unyielding counterforce (*white arrow*). The patient may be asked to slowly inhale during the contraction to enhance the effectiveness of the technique.

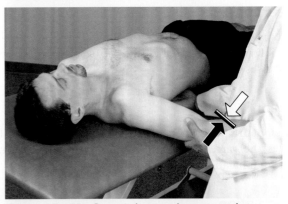

Figure 10.100. Step 4, isometric contraction.

5. This isometric contraction is held for 3 to 5 seconds, and then the patient is instructed to *stop and relax.*

6. Once the patient has completely relaxed, the physician's right hand exerts increased caudad and lateral traction (*white arrow*, **Fig. 10.101**) on the angle of the dysfunctional rib.

7. Steps 4 to 6 are repeated five to seven times or until motion is maximally improved at the dysfunctional rib.

8. Motion of the dysfunctional rib is reevaluated to assess the effectiveness of the technique.

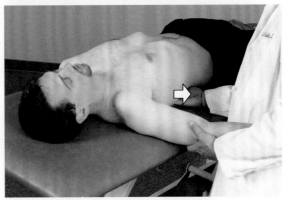

Figure 10.101. Step 6.

Costal Region

Quadratus Lumborum Muscle

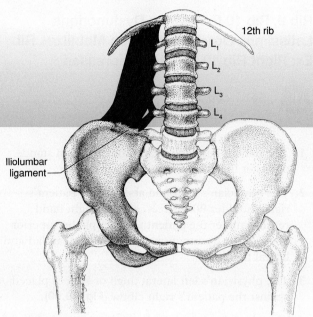

Figure 10.102. Quadratus lumborum. (Reprinted with permission from (7).)

Origin

The origin of the quadratus lumborum muscle is at the iliac crest and the iliolumbar ligament **(Fig. 10.102)**.

Insertion

The insertion of the quadratus lumborum muscle is at the inferior aspect of the 12th rib and the transverse processes of L1–L4.

Action

The quadratus lumborum muscle extends and laterally flexes the vertebral column; it also fixes the 12th rib during inhalation.

Innervation

The ventral branches of T12–L4 innervate the quadratus lumborum muscle.

Costal Region

Rib 11, Rib 12 Exhalation Dysfunctions
Quadratus Lumborum Contraction Mobilizes Rib
Ex: Right Rib 12 Exhaled

 See Video 10.24

1. The patient lies prone, and the physician stands at the left side of the table and positions the patient's legs 15 to 20 degrees to the left, putting tension on the quadratus lumborum.

2. The physician's left hypothenar eminence is placed inferior to the 11th rib and exerts a gentle pressure cephalad to stabilize the 11th rib (*white arrow*, **Fig. 10.103**).

3. The physician's right hand grasps the patient's right iliac crest and gently pulls caudad, which puts additional tension on the quadratus lumborum (*white arrow*, **Fig. 10.103**).

4. The patient inhales, exhales, and then inhales deeply.

5. During inhalation, the physician instructs the patient to pull the right iliac crest toward the patient's right shoulder (*black arrow*, **Fig. 10.104**) as the physician's right hand applies an unyielding counterforce (*opposing white arrow*). At the same time, the physician's left hand maintains cephalad pressure on the inferior aspect of the 11th rib (*left-pointing white arrow*).

6. This isometric contraction is maintained for 3 to 5 seconds, and then the patient is instructed to *stop and relax.*

7. Once the patient has completely relaxed, the physician's right hand gently pulls caudad, which puts additional tension on the quadratus lumborum, while the physician's left hand maintains cephalad pressure on the inferior aspect of the 11th rib (*white arrow*, **Fig. 10.105**).

8. Steps 5 to 7 are repeated five to seven times or until motion is maximally improved at the dysfunctonal rib.

9. Motion of the dysfunctional rib is reevaluated to assess the effectiveness of the technique.

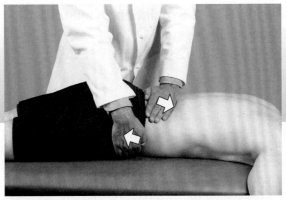

Figure 10.103. Steps 1 to 3.

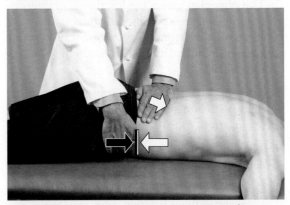

Figure 10.104. Step 5, isometric contraction.

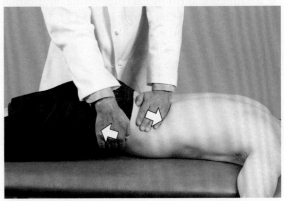

Figure 10.105. Step 7.

Costal Region

Rib 11, Rib 12 Exhalation Dysfunction
Respiratory Assist
Ex: Right Rib 12 Exhaled

1. The patient lies prone, and the physician stands at the left side of the table. The patient's legs are positioned 15 to 20 degrees to the left, putting tension on the quadratus lumborum.

2. The physician places the left thenar eminence or index finger superior and lateral to the angle of the dysfunctional rib and exerts gentle sustained caudad and lateral traction (*white arrow*, **Fig. 10.106**).

3. The physician's right hand grasps the patient's right ASIS and gently lifts toward the ceiling (*white arrow*, **Fig. 10.106**).

4. The patient inhales, exhales, and then inhales deeply.

5. During inhalation, the physician's left hand exaggerates the inhalation motion of the dysfunctional rib by exerting medial and caudad traction (*left-pointing white arrow*, **Fig. 10.107**) as the right hand gently lifts the patient's right anterior superior iliac spine (*upward-pointing white arrow*) toward the ceiling.

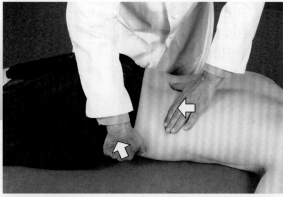

Figure 10.106. Steps 1 to 3.

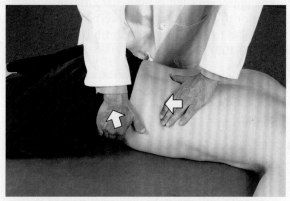

Figure 10.107. Step 5, exaggerate inhalation.

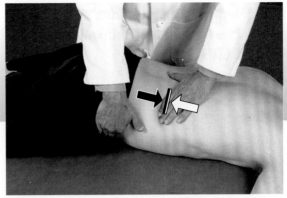

Figure 10.108. Step 6, resist exhalation.

6. On exhalation, the physician's left hand resists (*white arrow*) the exhalation motion of the rib (*black arrow*, **Fig. 10.108**).

7. Steps 5 and 6 are repeated five to seven times or until motion is maximally improved at the dysfunctional rib.

8. Motion of the dysfunctional rib is reevaluated to assess the effectiveness of the technique.

Lumbar Region

L1–L5 "Neutral" Dysfunctions
Seated, Post-Isometric Relaxation
Ex: L2 NSLRR

 See Video 10.25

1. The patient is seated at the end of the table. The physician stands to the side opposite to the rotational component of the dysfunction.

2. The patient places the right hand behind the neck and the left hand on the right elbow.

3. The physician passes the left arm under the patient's left arm and grasps the patient's right upper arm **(Fig. 10.109)**.

4. The physician's right hand monitors the spinous processes of L2 and L3 or the L2–L3 interspace as the left arm and hand flex and extend the patient's torso (*white arrow*, **Fig. 10.110**) until L2 is neutral in relation to L3.

5. The physician's right hand monitors the transverse processes of L2 and L3 to localize side bending and rotation as the left arm and hand position the patient's torso to the edge of the right side bending (*white arrow*, **Fig. 10.111**) and then the left rotation barrier (*white arrow*, **Fig. 10.112**).

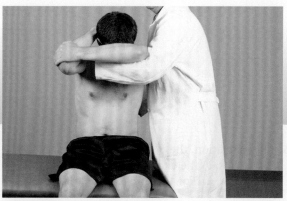

Figure 10.109. Steps 1 to 3.

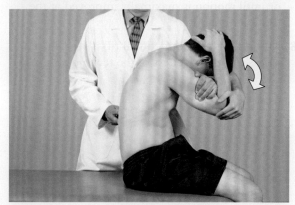

Figure 10.110. Step 4, L2–L3 neutral.

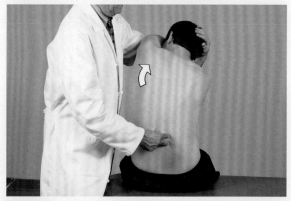

Figure 10.111. Step 5, right side bending barrier.

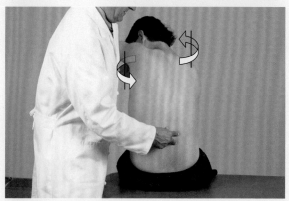

Figure 10.112. Step 5, left rotation barrier.

6. The physician instructs the patient to turn or pull the right shoulder back to the right (*black arrow*, **Fig. 10.113**) while the physician's left hand applies an unyielding counterforce (*white arrow*). The force of the patient's contraction is the least amount necessary to produce a palpable muscle twitch at the segmental level that the physician is monitoring.

7. This isometric contraction is maintained for 3 to 5 seconds, and then the patient is instructed to *stop and relax*.

8. Once the patient has completely relaxed, the physician, keeping L2 neutral, repositions the patient to the edge of the right side bending barrier (*white arrow*, **Fig. 10.114**) and left rotation barrier (*white arrow*, **Fig. 10.115**).

9. Steps 6 to 8 are repeated three to five times or until motion is maximally improved at the dysfunctional segment.

10. Motion of the dysfunctional segment is reevaluated to assess the effectiveness of the technique.

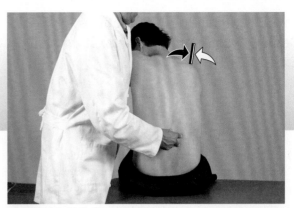

Figure 10.113. Step 6, isometric contraction.

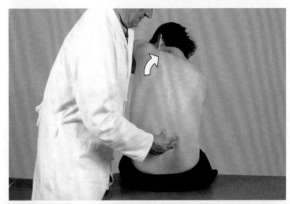

Figure 10.114. Step 8, right side bending barrier.

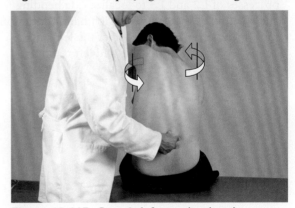

Figure 10.115. Step 8, left rotation barrier.

Lumbar Region

L1–L5 "Extension" Dysfunctions
Seated, Post-Isometric Relaxation
Ex: L2 ESRRR

1. The patient is seated, and the physician stands to the left of the patient (side opposite to the rotational component of the dysfunction).

2. The patient places the right hand behind the neck and the left hand on the right elbow. (Variation: the patient may place the hands behind the neck and approximate the elbows anteriorly.)

3. The physician passes the left arm over or under the patient's left arm and grasps the patient's right upper arm **(Fig. 10.116)**.

4. The physician's right hand monitors the spinous processes of L2 and L3 or the L2–L3 interspace to localize flexion and extension as the physician's left hand positions the patient's trunk to the edge of the restrictive flexion barrier **(Fig. 10.117)**.

5. The physician's right hand monitors the transverse processes of L2 and L3 to localize side bending and rotation as the physician's left hand repositions the patient's trunk to the edge of the left side bending barrier **(Fig. 10.118)** and left rotation barrier **(Fig. 10.119)**.

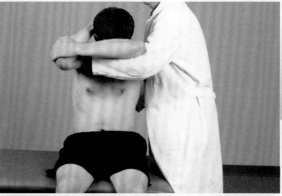

Figure 10.116. Steps 1 to 3.

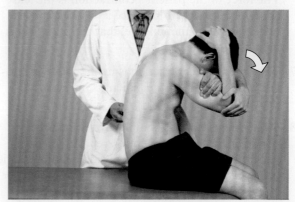

Figure 10.117. Step 4, flexion barrier.

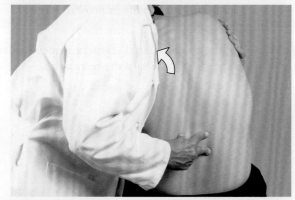

Figure 10.118. Step 5, left side bending barrier.

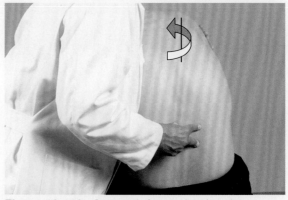

Figure 10.119. Step 5, left rotation barrier.

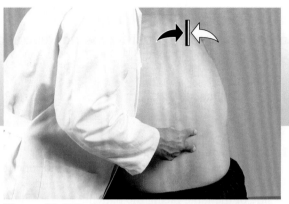

Figure 10.120. Step 6, isometric contraction.

6. The physician instructs the patient to sit up and gently pull the right shoulder backward (*black arrow*, **Fig. 10.120**) while the physician's left hand applies an unyielding counterforce (*white arrow*). The force of the patient's contraction is the least amount necessary to produce a palpable muscle twitch at the segmental level the physician is monitoring.

7. This isometric contraction is maintained for 3 to 5 seconds, and then the patient is instructed to *stop and relax.*

8. Once the patient has completely relaxed, the physician repositions the patient to the edge of the left side bending (*white arrows*, **Fig. 10.121**), left rotation (**Fig. 10.122**), and flexion barrier (**Fig.10.123**).

9. Steps 6 to 8 are repeated three to five times or until motion is maximally improved at the dysfunctional segment.

10. Motion of the dysfunctional segment is reevaluated to assess the effectiveness of the technique.

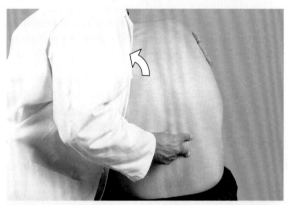

Figure 10.121. Step 8, left side bending barrier.

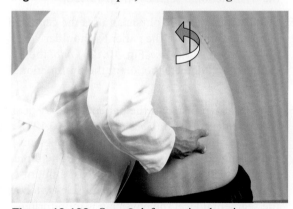

Figure 10.122. Step 8, left rotation barrier.

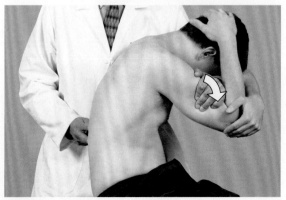

Figure 10.123. Step 8, flexion barrier.

Lumbar Region

L1–L5 "Neutral" Dysfunctions
Lateral Recumbent, Post-Isometric Relaxation
Ex: L4 NSLRR

 See Video 10.26

1. The patient lies in a right lateral recumbent position on the side of the rotational component of the dysfunction, and the physician stands at the side of the table facing the patient.

2. The physician's caudad hand or thigh controls the patient's flexed knees and hips while the cephalad hand palpates the L4 and L5 spinous processes or the L4–L5 interspace.

3. The physician's caudad hand or thigh gently flexes and extends the patient's hips until the physician's cephalad hand determines the dysfunctional segment (L4–L5) to be positioned in neutral **(Fig. 10.124)**.

4. The patient's left leg is lowered off the edge of the table, causing anterior rotation of the pelvis, *until* the physician's cephalad hand detects motion at the dysfunctional segment **(Fig. 10.125)**.

5. Switching hands, the physician uses the cephalad hand to gently move the patient's shoulder posteriorly (*white arrow*, **Fig. 10.126**) *until* the caudad hand detects motion at the dysfunctional segment.

6. The physician instructs the patient to *gently* push the shoulder forward (*black arrow*, **Fig. 10.127**) while the physician's cephalad hand applies an unyielding counterforce (*white arrow*). The force of the patient's contraction is the least amount necessary to produce a palpable muscle twitch at the segmental level the physician is monitoring.

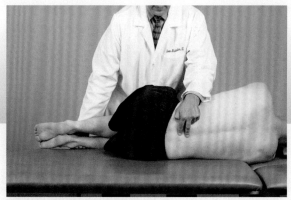
Figure 10.124. Steps 1 to 3.

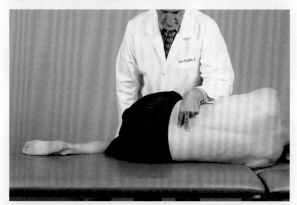
Figure 10.125. Step 4.

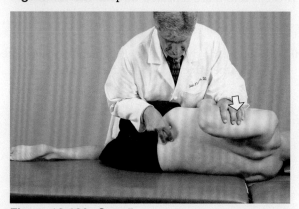
Figure 10.126. Step 5.

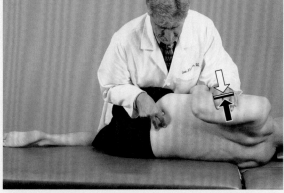
Figure 10.127. Step 6, isometric contraction.

7. This isometric contraction is held for 3 to 5 seconds, and then the patient is told to *stop and relax*.

8. Once the patient has completely relaxed, the physician gently moves the patient's shoulder posteriorly (*white arrow*, **Fig. 10.128**), rotating the thoracic and lumbar spine to the edge of the new restrictive barrier.

9. The patient is instructed to *gently* pull the hip and pelvis cephalad up toward the shoulder (*black arrow*, **Fig. 10.129**) while the physician's caudad hand applies an unyielding counterforce (*white arrow*).

10. This isometric contraction is held for 3 to 5 seconds, and then the patient is told to *stop and relax*.

11. Once the patient has completely relaxed, the physician gently moves the patient's pelvis caudad (*white arrow*, **Fig. 10.130**) to the edge of the new restrictive barrier.

12. Steps 6 to 11 are repeated three to five times or until motion is maximally improved at the dysfunctional segment (L4–L5).

13. Steps 6, 7, 9, and 10 may be performed simultaneously, after which the physician repositions the patient to the edge of the new restrictive barriers.

14. Motion of the dysfunctional segment is reevaluated to assess the effectiveness of the technique.

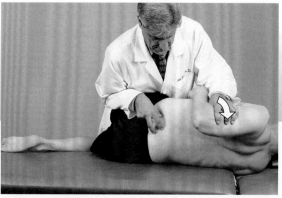

Figure 10.128. Step 8.

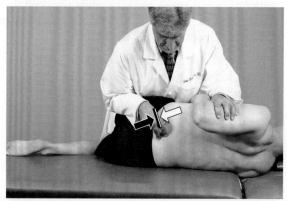

Figure 10.129. Step 9, isometric contraction.

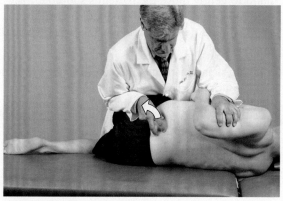

Figure 10.130. Step 11.

Lumbar Region

L1–L5 "Non-Neutral" Dysfunctions
Lateral Recumbent, Post-Isometric Relaxation
Ex: L4 F/E SRRR

 See Video 10.27

1. The patient lies on the side of the rotational component, and the physician stands facing the patient.

2. The physician's caudad hand or thigh controls the patient's flexed knees and hips while the cephalad hand palpates the L4 and L5 spinous processes or the L4–L5 interspace.

3. The physician's caudad hand or thigh gently flexes and extends the patient's hips until the physician's cephalad hand determines the dysfunctional segment (L4–L5) to be positioned in neutral **(Fig. 10.131)**.

4. The physician's caudad hand places the patient's left foot behind the right knee in the popliteal fossa **(Fig. 10.132)**.

5. Switching hands, the physician uses the cephalad hand to gently move the patient's shoulder posteriorly (*white arrow*, **Fig. 10.133**) until the caudad hand detects motion at the dysfunctional segment.

6. The physician instructs the patient to *gently* push the shoulder forward (*black arrow*, **Fig. 10.134**) against the physician's cephalad hand, which applies an unyielding counterforce (*white arrow*). The force of the patient's contraction is the least amount necessary to produce a palpable muscle twitch at the segmental level the physician is monitoring (5).

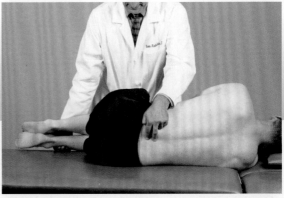

Figure 10.131. Steps 1 to 3.

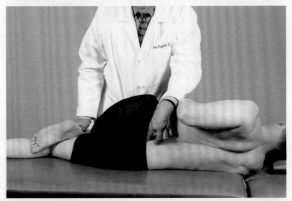

Figure 10.132. Step 4.

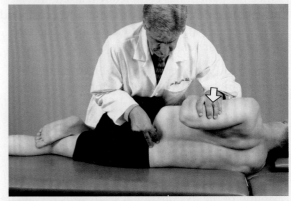

Figure 10.133. Step 5.

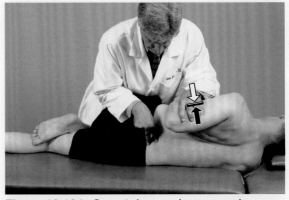

Figure 10.134. Step 6, isometric contraction.

7. This isometric contraction is held for 3 to 5 seconds, and then the patient is told to *stop and relax*.

8. Once the patient has completely relaxed, the physician gently moves the patient's shoulder posteriorly (*white arrow*, **Fig. 10.135**), rotating the thoracic and lumbar spine to the edge of the new restrictive barrier.

9. The patient *gently* pushes the hip and pelvis backward (*black arrow*, **Fig. 10.136**) against the unyielding counterforce of the physician's caudad hand (*white arrow*).

10. This isometric contraction is held for 3 to 5 seconds, and then the patient is told to *stop and relax*.

11. Once the patient has completely relaxed, the physician gently moves the patient's pelvis forward (*white arrow*, **Fig. 10.137**) to the edge of the new restrictive barrier.

12. Steps 6 to 11 are repeated three to five times or until motion is maximally improved at the dysfunctional segment (L4–L5).

13. Steps 6, 7, 9, and 10 may be performed simultaneously, after which the physician repositions the patient to the edge of the new restrictive barriers.

14. Motion of the dysfunctional segment is reevaluated to assess the effectiveness of the technique.

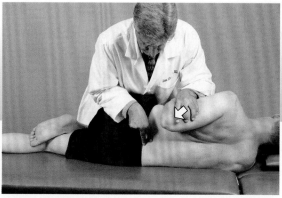

Figure 10.135. Step 8.

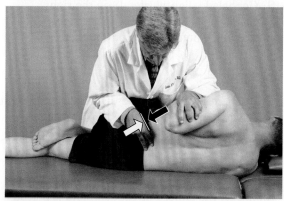

Figure 10.136. Step 9, isometric contraction.

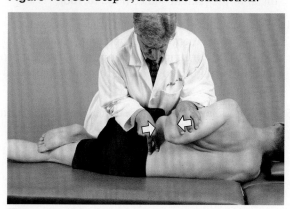

Figure 10.137. Step 11.

Pelvic Region

Iliosacral (Innominate) Dysfunction
Ex: Right Posterior Innominate Rotation
Supine, Combined Mechanisms of Action

 See Videos 10.28 and 10.29

Diagnosis

Standing flexion test: Positive (right posterior superior iliac spine [PSIS] rises)
Loss of passively induced right sacroiliac motion
ASIS: Cephalad (slightly lateral) on the right
PSIS: Caudad (slightly medial) on the right
Sacral sulcus: Anterior, deep on the right

Technique

1. The patient lies supine on a diagonal, so the right sacroiliac joint is off the edge of the table.

2. The physician stands at the right side of the table.

3. The physician's cephalad hand is placed over the patient's left ASIS to prevent the patient from rolling off the table. The caudad hand is placed distal to the patient's knee **(Fig. 10.138)**.

4. The physician's caudad (right) hand passively extends the patient's right hip (*white arrow*, **Fig. 10.139**), bringing the innominate into anterior rotation, until the edge of the restrictive barrier is reached.

5. The physician instructs the patient to lift the right leg (*black arrow*, **Fig. 10.140**) toward the ceiling while the physician applies an equal counterforce (*white arrow*).

6. This isometric contraction is maintained for 3 to 5 seconds, and then the patient is instructed to *stop and relax*.

7. Once the patient has completely relaxed, the physician extends the patient's right hip (*white arrow*, **Fig. 10.141**) to the edge of the new restrictive barrier.

8. Steps 5 to 7 are repeated three to five times.

9. The diagnostic parameters of the dysfunction (TART) are reevaluated to determine the effectiveness of the technique.

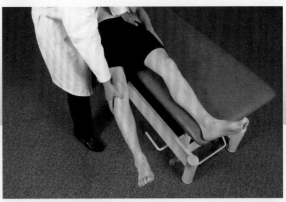

Figure 10.138. Steps 1 to 3.

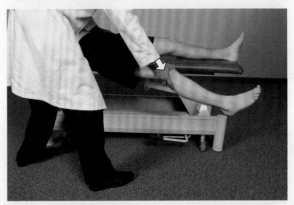

Figure 10.139. Step 4.

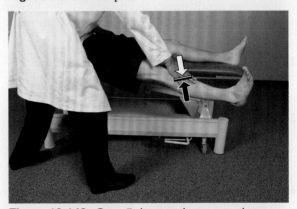

Figure 10.140. Step 5, isometric contraction.

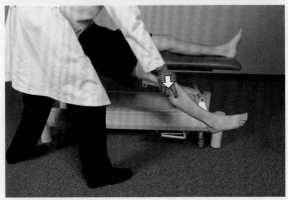

Figure 10.141. Step 7.

Pelvic Region

Iliosacral (Innominate) Dysfunction
Ex: Right Posterior Innominate Rotation
Sims, Combined Mechanisms of Action

 See Videos 10.30 and 10.31

Diagnosis

Standing flexion test: Positive (right PSIS rises)
Loss of passively induced right sacroiliac motion
ASIS: Cephalad (slightly lateral) on the right
PSIS: Caudad (slightly medial) on the right
Sacral sulcus: Anterior, deep on the right

Technique

1. The patient is placed in a left lateral modified Sims position: left lateral recumbent, with the anterior thorax resting on the table and arms hanging over the side of the table **(Fig. 10.142)**.

2. The physician stands behind the patient, grasps the patient's right leg with the caudad (right) hand, and places the hypothenar eminence of the cephalad hand on the patient's right PSIS.

3. The physician's caudad hand passively extends the patient's right hip (*white arrow*, **Fig. 10.143**), bringing the innominate into anterior rotation, until the edge of the restrictive barrier is reached.

4. The physician instructs the patient to pull the right leg forward (*black arrow*, **Fig. 10.144**) while the physician applies an equal counterforce (*white arrow*).

5. This isometric contraction is maintained for 3 to 5 seconds, and then the patient is instructed to *relax*.

6. Once the patient has completely relaxed, the physician extends the patient's right hip (*white arrow*, **Fig. 10.145**) to the edge of the new restrictive barrier.

7. Steps 4 to 6 are repeated three to five times.

8. The diagnostic parameters of the dysfunction (TART) are reevaluated to determine the effectiveness of the technique.

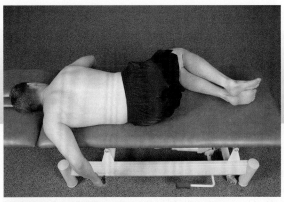

Figure 10.142. Step 1.

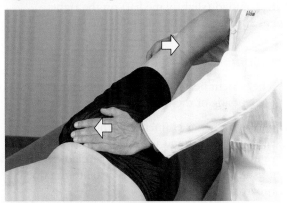

Figure 10.143. Steps 2 and 3.

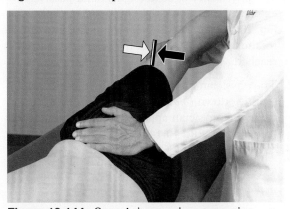

Figure 10.144. Step 4, isometric contraction.

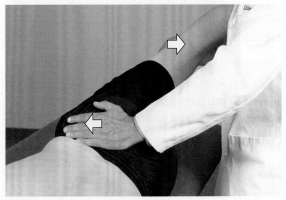

Figure 10.145. Step 6.

Pelvic Region

Iliosacral (Innominate) Dysfunction
Ex: Right Posterior Innominate Rotation
Prone, Combined Mechanisms of Action

 See Video 10.32

Diagnosis

Standing flexion test: Positive (right PSIS rises)
Loss of passively induced right sacroiliac motion
ASIS: Cephalad (slightly lateral) on the right
PSIS: Caudad (slightly medial) on the right
Sacral sulcus: Anterior, deep on the right

Technique

1. The patient lies prone, and the physician stands on the left side of the table.

2. The hypothenar eminence of the physician's cephalad (left) hand is placed on the patient's right PSIS and the physician's caudad (right) hand grasps the patient's right leg distal to the tibial tuberosity **(Fig. 10.146)**.

3. The physician's caudad (right) hand passively extends the patient's right hip (*white arrow*, **Fig. 10.147**), bringing the innominate into anterior rotation, until the edge of the restrictive barrier is reached.

4. The physician instructs the patient to pull the right leg down (*black arrow*) toward the table while the physician applies an equal counterforce (*white arrow*, **Fig. 10.148**).

5. This isometric contraction is maintained for 3 to 5 seconds, and then the patient is instructed to *stop and relax*.

6. Once the patient has completely relaxed, the physician extends the patient's right hip (*white arrow*, **Fig. 10.149**) to the edge of the new restrictive barrier.

7. Steps 4 to 6 are repeated three to five times.

8. The diagnostic parameters of the dysfunction (TART) are reevaluated to determine the effectiveness of the technique.

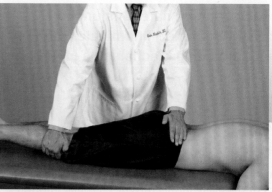

Figure 10.146. Steps 1 and 2.

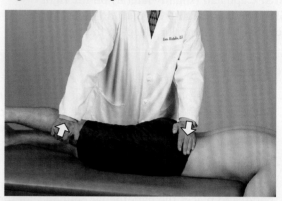

Figure 10.147. Step 3.

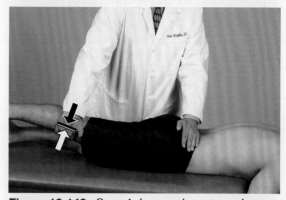

Figure 10.148. Step 4, isometric contraction.

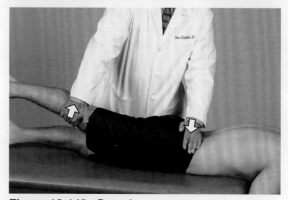

Figure 10.149. Step 6.

Pelvic Region

Iliosacral (Innominate) Dysfunction
Ex: Right Anterior Innominate Rotation
Supine, Combined Mechanisms of Action

 See Video 10.33

Diagnosis

Standing flexion test: Positive (right PSIS rises)
Loss of passively induced right sacroiliac motion
ASIS: Caudad (slightly medial) on the right
PSIS: Cephalad (slightly lateral) on the right
Sacral sulcus: Posterior, shallow on the right

Technique

1. The patient lies supine, and the physician is seated on the table facing the patient.

2. The physician places the patient's right heel on the right shoulder and passively flexes the patient's right hip and knee (*white arrow*, **Fig. 10.150**) until the edge of the restrictive barrier is reached.

3. An acceptable modification is to have the patient's right knee locked in full extension and the leg flexed at the hip with the patient's right leg on the physician's right shoulder (**Fig. 10.151**).

4. The physician instructs the patient to push the knee into the physician's hands, extending the right hip (*black arrow*, **Fig. 10.152**), while the physician applies an equal counterforce (*white arrow*).

5. This isometric contraction is maintained for 3 to 5 seconds, and then the patient is instructed to *stop and relax.*

6. Once the patient has completely relaxed, the physician flexes the patient's right hip (*white arrow*, **Fig. 10.153**) to the edge of the new restrictive barrier.

7. Steps 4 to 6 are repeated three to five times.

8. The diagnostic parameters of the dysfunction (TART) are reevaluated to determine the effectiveness of the technique.

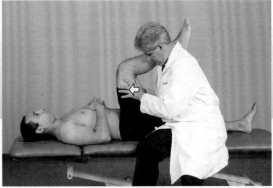
Figure 10.150. Steps 1 and 2.

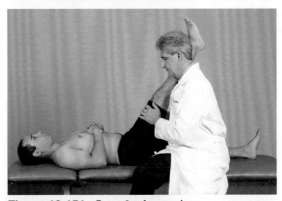
Figure 10.151. Step 3, alternative.

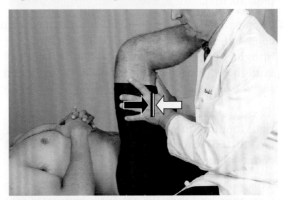
Figure 10.152. Step 4, isometric contraction.

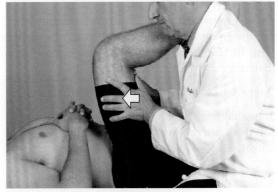
Figure 10.153. Step 6.

Pelvic Region

Iliosacral (Innominate) Dysfunction
Ex: Right Anterior Innominate Rotation
Lateral Recumbent, Combined Mechanisms

Diagnosis

Standing flexion test: Positive (right PSIS rises)
Loss of passively induced right sacroiliac motion
ASIS: Caudad (slightly medial) on the right
PSIS: Cephalad (slightly lateral) on the right
Sacral sulcus: Posterior on the right

Technique

1. The patient lies in the left lateral recumbent position, and the physician stands at the side of the table facing the patient.

2. The physician's caudad (left) hand palpates the right sacroiliac motion and stabilizes the pelvis while the physician's cephalad (right) hand places the patient's right foot against the physician's thigh **(Fig. 10.154)**.

3. Supporting the patient's right knee, the physician's cephalad hand flexes the patient's right hip, bringing the innominate into posterior rotation until the edge of the restrictive barrier is reached (*white arrow*, **Fig. 10.155**).

4. The physician instructs the patient to push the right foot into the physician's thigh (*black arrow*, **Fig. 10.156**) while the physician applies an equal counterforce (*white arrow*).

5. This isometric contraction is maintained for 3 to 5 seconds, and then the patient is instructed to *stop and relax*.

6. Once the patient has completely relaxed, the physician flexes the patient's right hip (*white arrow*, **Fig. 10.157**) to the edge of the new restrictive barrier.

7. Steps 4 to 6 are repeated three to five times.

8. The diagnostic parameters of the dysfunction (TART) are reevaluated to determine the effectiveness of the technique.

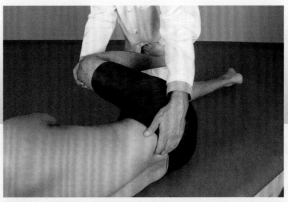

Figure 10.154. Steps 1 and 2.

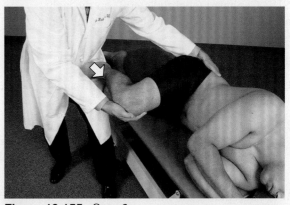

Figure 10.155. Step 3.

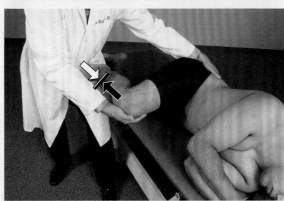

Figure 10.156. Step 4, isometric contraction.

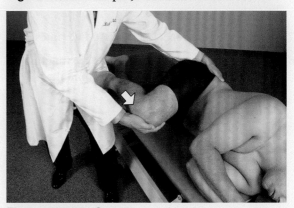

Figure 10.157. Step 6.

Pelvic Region

Iliosacral (Innominate) Dysfunction
Ex: Right Anterior Innominate Rotation
Prone, Combined Mechanisms of Action

 See Video 10.34

Diagnosis

Standing flexion test: Positive (right PSIS rises)
Loss of passively induced right sacroiliac motion
ASIS: Caudad (slightly medial) on the right
PSIS: Cephalad (slightly lateral) on the right
Sacral sulcus: Posterior on the right

Technique

1. The patient lies prone on a diagonal, so the right innominate is off the edge of the table. The physician stands at the right side of the table facing the patient's pelvis.

2. The physician's left hand stabilizes the patient's pelvis and sacrum, and the physician's right hand, supporting the patient's right leg, places the patient's right foot against the physician's right thigh or tibia **(Fig. 10.158)**.

3. The physician flexes the patient's right hip (*white arrow*, **Fig. 10.159**), bringing the right innominate into posterior rotation, until the edge of the restrictive barrier is reached.

4. The physician instructs the patient to push the right foot (*black arrow*, **Fig. 10.160**) into the physician's leg while the physician applies an equal counterforce (*white arrow*).

5. This isometric contraction is maintained for 3 to 5 seconds, and then the patient is instructed to *stop and relax*.

6. Once the patient has completely relaxed, the physician flexes the patient's right hip (*white arrow*, **Fig. 10.161**) to the edge of the new restrictive barrier.

7. Steps 4 to 6 are repeated three to five times.

8. The diagnostic parameters of the dysfunction (TART) are reevaluated to determine the effectiveness of the technique.

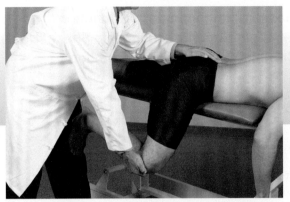

Figure 10.158. Steps 1 and 2.

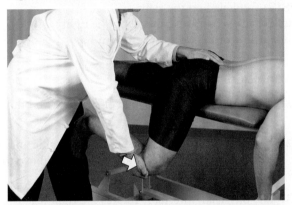

Figure 10.159. Step 3.

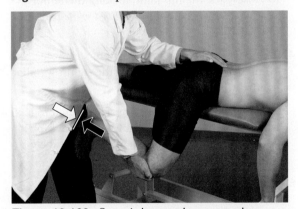

Figure 10.160. Step 4, isometric contraction.

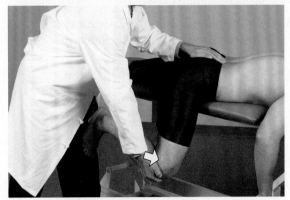

Figure 10.161. Step 6.

Pelvic Region

Iliosacral (Innominate) Dysfunction
Ex: Right Superior Innominate Shear "Upslip"
Combined Mechanisms of Action

 See Video 10.35

Diagnosis

Standing flexion test: Positive (right PSIS rises)
Loss of passively induced right sacroiliac motion
ASIS: Cephalad on the right
PSIS: Cephalad on the right
Ischial tuberosity: Cephalad on the right
Sacrotuberous ligament tension: Lax

Technique

1. The patient lies either prone or supine with both feet off the end of the table.

2. The physician stands at the foot of the table and grasps the patient's right tibia and fibula above the ankle **(Fig. 10.162)**.

3. The physician internally rotates the right leg to close-pack the hip joint, locking the femoral head into the acetabulum (*curved white arrow,* **Fig. 10.163**).

4. The physician abducts the patient's right leg 5 to 10 degrees to take tension off the right sacroiliac ligament **(Fig. 10.164)**.

5. The physician gently leans back, maintaining axial traction on the patient's right leg (*white arrow*), and instructs the patient to inhale and exhale **(Fig. 10.165)**.

6. With each exhalation, the tractional force is increased.

7. Steps 5 to 6 are repeated five to seven times.

8. With the last exhalation, the patient may be instructed to cough as the physician simultaneously tugs on the leg.

9. The diagnostic parameters of the dysfunction (TART) are reevaluated to determine the effectiveness of the technique.

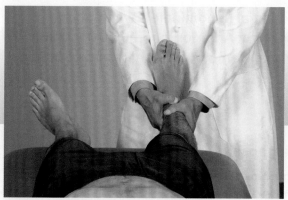

Figure 10.162. Steps 1 and 2.

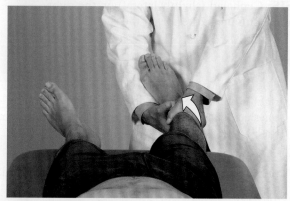

Figure 10.163. Step 3.

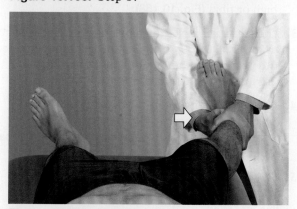

Figure 10.164. Step 4.

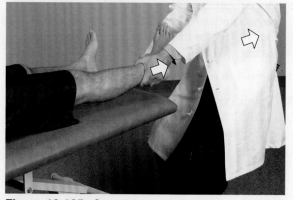

Figure 10.165. Step 5.

Pelvic Region

Iliosacral (Innominate) Dysfunction
Ex: Right Outflared Innominate
Post-Isometric Relaxation

 See Video 10.36

Diagnosis

Standing flexion test: Positive (right PSIS rises)
Loss of passively induced right sacroiliac motion
ASIS: Laterally displaced on the right
Sacral sulcus: Narrow on the right

Technique

1. The patient lies supine, and the physician stands at the left side of the table.

2. The patient's right hip and knee are flexed to about 90 degrees, and the right foot is lateral to the left knee.

3. The physician's right hand is placed under the patient's right innominate, grasping the medial aspect of the right PSIS **(Fig. 10.166)**.

4. The physician's left hand adducts the patient's right knee (*white arrow*, **Fig. 10.167**) until the edge of the restrictive barrier is reached.

5. The physician instructs the patient to abduct the flexed hip (*black arrow*, **Fig. 10.168**) while the physician applies an equal counterforce (*white arrow*).

6. This isometric contraction is maintained for 3 to 5 seconds, and then the patient is instructed to *stop and relax*.

7. Once the patient has completely relaxed, the physician further adducts the patient's right knee (*white arrow*, **Fig. 10.169**) to the edge of the new restrictive barrier and draws traction laterally on the right PSIS.

8. Steps 5 to 7 are repeated three to five times.

9. The diagnostic parameters of the dysfunction (TART) are reevaluated to determine the effectiveness of the technique.

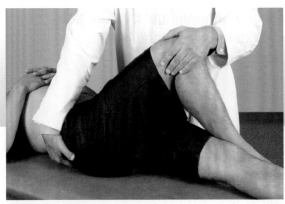
Figure 10.166. Steps 1 to 3.

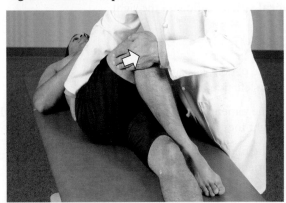
Figure 10.167. Step 4.

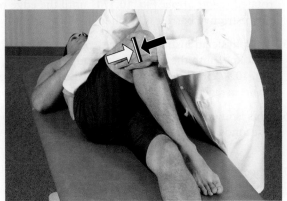
Figure 10.168. Step 5, isometric contraction.

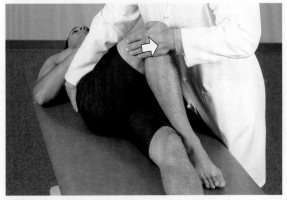
Figure 10.169. Step 7.

Pelvic Region

Iliosacral (Innominate) Dysfunction
Ex: Right Inflared Innominate
Post-Isometric Relaxation

 See Video 10.37

Diagnosis

Standing flexion test: Positive (right PSIS rises)
Loss of passively induced right sacroiliac motion
ASIS: Medially displaced on the right
Sacral sulcus: Wide on the right

Technique

1. The patient lies supine, and the physician stands at the left side of the table.

2. The patient's right hip and knee are flexed, and the right foot is on the lateral aspect of the left knee.

3. The physician's cephalad hand is placed on the patient's left ASIS (**Fig. 10.170**).

4. The physician's caudad hand is placed on the patient's right knee and the right hip is externally rotated (*white arrow*, **Fig. 10.171**) until the edge of the restrictive barrier is reached.

5. The physician instructs the patient to push the right knee into the physician's hand (*black arrow*, **Fig. 10.172**), which applies an equal counterforce (*white arrow*).

6. This isometric contraction is maintained for 3 to 5 seconds, and then the patient is instructed to *relax*.

7. Once the patient has completely relaxed, the physician further externally rotates the hip (*white arrow*, **Fig. 10.173**) to the edge of the new restrictive barrier.

8. Steps 5 to 7 are repeated three to five times.

9. The diagnostic parameters of the dysfunction (TART) are reevaluated to determine the effectiveness of the technique.

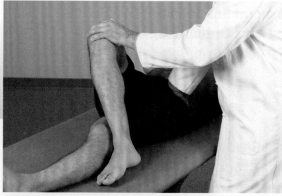

Figure 10.170. Steps 1 to 3.

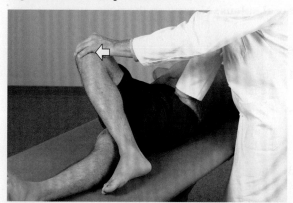

Figure 10.171. Step 4.

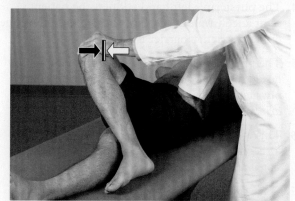

Figure 10.172. Step 5, isometric contraction.

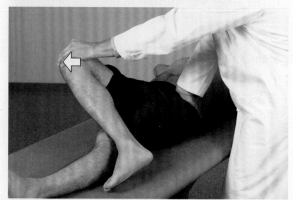

Figure 10.173. Step 7.

Pelvic Region

Superior Pubic Shear Dysfunction
Joint Mobilization Using Muscle Force
Ex: Right Superior Pubic Shear

 See Video 10.38

Diagnosis

Standing flexion test: Positive (right PSIS rises)
Loss of passively induced right sacroiliac motion
Pubic tubercle: Cephalad on the right **(Fig. 10.174)**

Technique

1. The patient lies supine, right side close to the edge of the table, and the physician stands at the right side facing the patient.

2. The physician's left hand is placed on the patient's left ASIS to stabilize the pelvis, and the right hand abducts the patient's right leg, allowing it to drop off the edge of the table.

3. The physician places the right hand just proximal to the patient's right knee and gently presses down (*white arrow*, **Fig. 10.175**) on the right knee until the edge of the restrictive barrier is reached.

4. The physician instructs the patient to lift the right knee toward the ceiling and slightly medially (*black arrow*, **Fig. 10.176**) while the physician applies an equal counterforce (*white arrow*).

5. This isometric contraction is maintained for 3 to 5 seconds after which the patient is instructed to *stop and relax.*

6. Once the patient has completely relaxed, the physician repositions the patient's leg further toward the floor (*white arrow*, **Fig. 10.177**) to the edge of the new restrictive barrier.

7. Steps 4 to 6 are repeated three to five times.

8. The diagnostic parameters of the dysfunction (TART) are reevaluated to determine the effectiveness of the technique.

Note: A left inferior shear looks statically similar to a right superior shear but will display loss of sacroiliac motion on the left side and show a positive standing flexion test on the left.

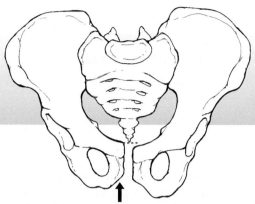

Figure 10.174. Right superior pubic shear dysfunction.

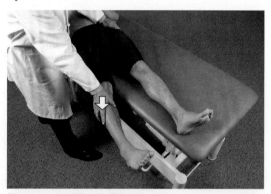

Figure 10.175. Steps 1 to 3.

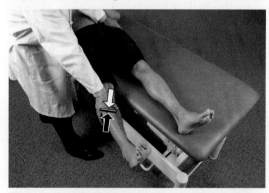

Figure 10.176. Step 4, isometric contraction.

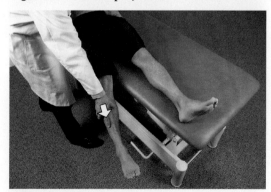

Figure 10.177. Step 6.

Pelvic Region

Inferior Pubic Shear Dysfunction
Joint Mobilization Using Muscle Force
Ex: Right Inferior Pubic Shear

 See Video 10.39

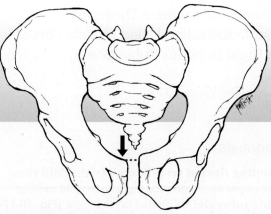

Figure 10.178. Right inferior pubic shear dysfunction.

Diagnosis

Standing flexion test: Positive (right PSIS rises)
Loss of passively induced right sacroiliac motion
Pubic tubercle: Caudad on the right **(Fig. 10.178)**

Technique

1. The patient lies supine close to the left edge of the table, and the physician stands on the left facing the patient.

2. The physician's right hand flexes and internally rotates the patient's right hip as the physician places the left thenar eminence beneath the patient's right ischial tuberosity to create a fulcrum **(Fig. 10.179)**.

3. The physician's right hand flexes the patient's right hip (*white arrow*, **Fig. 10.180**) until the edge of the restrictive barrier is engaged, positions the patient's knee under the right axilla, and then grasps the side of the treatment table.

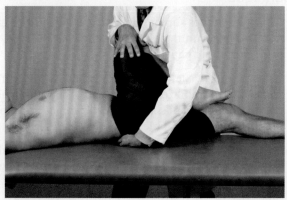

Figure 10.179. Steps 1 and 2.

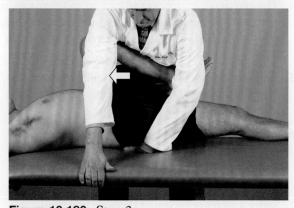

Figure 10.180. Step 3.

4. The physician instructs the patient to push the right knee up into the physician's axilla (*black arrow*, **Fig. 10.181**) while the physician applies an equal counterforce (*white arrow*).

5. This isometric contraction is maintained for 3 to 5 seconds, after which the patient is instructed to *stop and relax*.

6. Once the patient has completely relaxed, the physician flexes the right hip (*white arrow*) to the edge of the new restrictive barrier **(Fig. 10.182)**. The hand beneath the ischial tuberosity may have to be repositioned more cephalad to maintain an effective fulcrum.

7. Steps 4 to 6 are repeated three to five times.

8. The diagnostic parameters of the dysfunction (TART) are reevaluated to determine the effectiveness of the technique.

Note: A left superior shear looks statically similar to a right inferior shear but will display loss of sacroiliac motion on the left side and show a positive standing flexion test on the left.

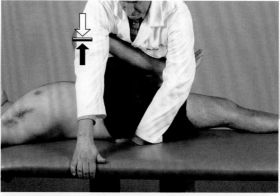

Figure 10.181. Step 4, isometric contraction.

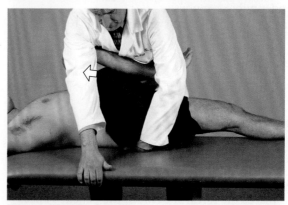

Figure 10.182. Step 6.

Pelvic Region

Pubic Compression Dysfunction
Joint Mobilization Using Muscle Force
Ex: Compressed/*AD*ducted Pubic Symphysis

 See Video 10.40

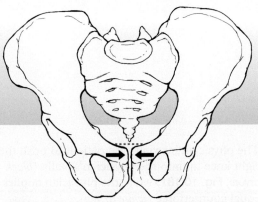

Figure 10.183. Fixed compression of the pubic symphysis.

Diagnosis

Suspicion of dysfunction by history (trauma, pregnancy, delivery)
Palpable bulging of the symphyseal cartilage
Tender pubic symphysis
May have urinary tract symptoms **(Fig. 10.183)**

Technique

1. The patient lies supine, and the physician stands at either side of the table.

2. The patient's hips are flexed to approximately 45 degrees and the knees are flexed to 90 degrees, with the feet flat on the table.

3. The physician separates the patient's knees and places the forearm between the patient's knees **(Fig. 10.184)**.

4. The physician instructs the patient to pull both knees medially (adduction shown by *black arrows*, **Fig. 10.185**) against the physician's palm and elbow (*white arrows*) while the physician applies an equal counterforce.

5. This isometric contraction is maintained for 3 to 5 seconds, and then the patient is instructed to *stop and relax*.

6. Once the patient has completely relaxed, the patient's knees are separated slightly farther from the midline (*white arrows*, **Fig. 10.186**).

7. Steps 4 to 6 are repeated three to seven times.

8. The diagnostic parameters of the dysfunction (TART) are reevaluated to determine the effectiveness of the technique.

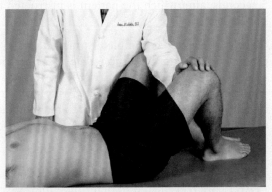

Figure 10.184. Steps 1 to 3.

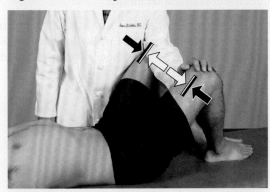

Figure 10.185. Step 4, isometric contraction.

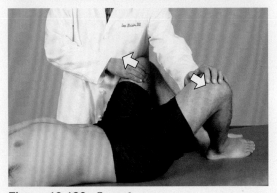

Figure 10.186. Step 6.

Pelvic Region

Pubic Gapping Dysfunction
Joint Mobilization Using Muscle Force
Ex: Gapped (*AB*ducted) Pubic Symphysis

 See Video 10.40

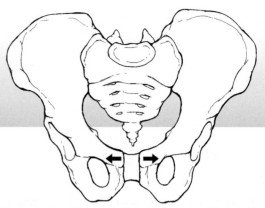

Figure 10.187. Fixed gapping of the pubic symphysis.

Diagnosis

Suspicion of dysfunction by history (trauma, pregnancy, delivery)
Sulcus deeper than normal at the pubic symphysis
Tender pubic symphysis
May have urinary tract symptoms **(Fig. 10.187)**

Technique

1. The patient lies supine, and the physician stands beside the table.

2. The patient's hips are flexed to approximately 45 degrees and the knees are flexed to about 90 degrees, with the feet flat on the table.

3. The patient's knees are separated by approximately 18 inches.

4. The knee closer to the physician is placed against the physician's abdomen, and the physician grasps the lateral aspect of the other knee with both hands **(Fig. 10.188)**.

5. The physician instructs the patient to pull both knees laterally (abduction shown by *black arrows*, **Fig. 10.189**) against the physician's abdomen and hands while the physician applies an equal counterforce (*white arrows*).

6. This isometric contraction is maintained for 3 to 5 seconds, and then the patient is instructed to *stop and relax.*

7. Once the patient has completely relaxed, the physician approximates the patient's knees 3 to 4 inches (*white arrows*, **Fig. 10.190**).

8. Steps 5 to 7 are repeated three to seven times.

9. The diagnostic parameters of the dysfunction (TART) are reevaluated to determine the effectiveness of the technique.

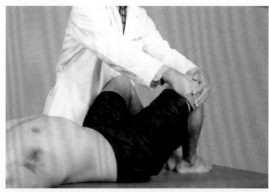

Figure 10.188. Steps 1 to 4.

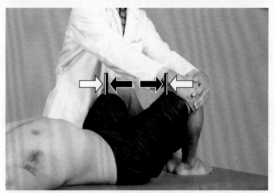

Figure 10.189. Step 5, isometric contractions.

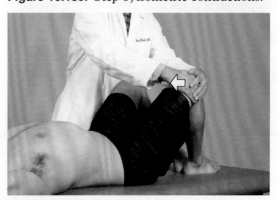

Figure 10.190. Step 7.

Pelvic Region

Psoas Major/Minor Muscles

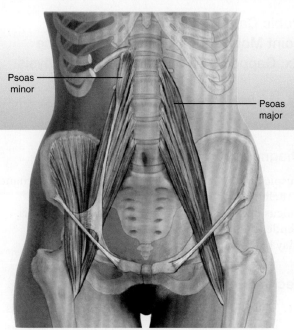

Figure 10.191. Psoas major and psoas minor muscles. (Modified with permission from Ref. (8).)

Psoas Major

Origin

The origin of the psoas major is at the lateral aspect of the T12–L4 vertebral bodies and associated intervertebral disks, and the transverse processes of L1–L5 **(Fig. 10.191).**

Insertion

The insertion of the psoas major is at the lesser trochanter of the femur.

Action

The psoas major flexes the hip and flexes and side bends (ipsilateral) the lumbar spine.

Innervation

The ventral rami of lumbar nerves (L1–L3) innervate the psoas major.

Psoas Minor

Origin

The origin of the psoas major is at the lateral aspect of the T12 and L1 vertebral bodies and associated intervertebral disks.

Insertion

The insertion of the psoas minor is at the iliac fascia and the iliopectineal eminence.

Action

The psoas minor helps the psoas major flex the pelvis and lumbar region of the vertebral column.

Innervation

The ventral rami of lumbar nerves (L1 and L2) innervate the psoas minor.

Pelvic Region

Iliacus Muscle

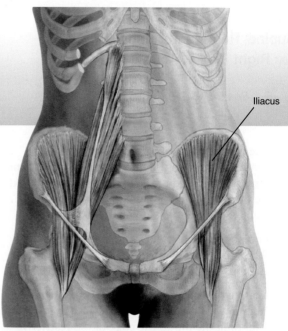

Origin

The origin of the iliacus muscle is at the iliac fossa (inner surface of iliac bone) and the lateral aspect of the sacrum **(Fig. 10.192)**.

Insertion

The insertion of the iliacus muscle is at the lesser trochanter of the femur.

Action

The iliacus muscle flexes the thigh at the hip and stabilizes the joint in conjunction with the iliopsoas.

Innervation

The femoral nerve (L2 and L3) innervates the iliacus muscle.

Figure 10.192. Iliacus muscle. (Modified with permission from Ref. (8).)

Pelvic Region

Psoas Muscle Dysfunction
Supine, Reciprocal Inhibition
Ex: Right Psoas, Acute

 See Video 10.41

1. The patient lies supine near the end of the treatment table so that the dysfunctional leg may hang over the end of the table. The patient flexes the other hip, bringing the knee to the chest. This keeps the lumbar lordosis flattened.

2. The physician, standing at the end of the table, places the hands on the patient's dysfunctional thigh just proximal to the knee **(Fig. 10.193)**.

3. The physician gently positions the patient's thigh toward the floor (*white arrow*, **Fig. 10.194**), extending the hip to the edge of the restrictive barrier.

4. The physician instructs the patient to push the leg *very gently* down toward the floor (*black arrow*, **Fig. 10.195**) while the physician applies an unyielding counterforce (*white arrow*).

5. This isometric contraction is held for 3 to 5 seconds, and then the patient is instructed to *stop and relax*.

6. Once the patient has completely relaxed, the physician gently repositions the patient's thigh toward the floor, extending the hip to the edge of the new restrictive barrier (*white arrow*, **Fig. 10.196**).

7. Steps 4 to 6 are repeated three to five times or until motion is maximally improved at the dysfunctional hip and psoas.

8. The diagnostic parameters of the dysfunction (TART) are reevaluated to determine the effectiveness of the technique.

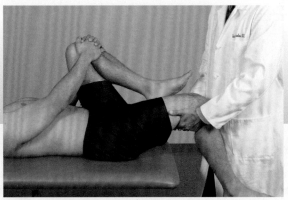

Figure 10.193. Steps 1 and 2.

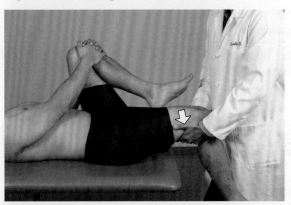

Figure 10.194. Step 3.

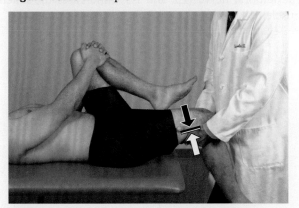

Figure 10.195. Step 4, isometric contraction.

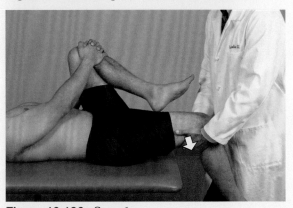

Figure 10.196. Step 6.

Pelvic Region

Psoas Muscle Dysfunction
Prone, Post-Isometric Relaxation
Ex: Right Psoas, Subacute/Chronic

 See Video 10.42

1. The patient lies prone, and the physician stands beside the table.

2. The physician flexes the patient's knee on the side to be treated 90 degrees and then grasps the patient's thigh just above the knee.

3. The physician's cephalad hand is placed over the patient's sacrum to stabilize the pelvis **(Fig. 10.197)**.

4. The physician's caudad hand gently lifts the patient's thigh upward (*white arrow*, **Fig. 10.198**) until the psoas muscle begins to stretch, engaging the edge of the restrictive barrier.

5. The physician instructs the patient to pull the thigh and knee down (*black arrow*, **Fig. 10.199**) into the physician's caudad hand, which applies an unyielding counterforce (*white arrow*).

6. This isometric contraction is held for 3 to 5 seconds, and then the patient is instructed to *stop and relax*.

7. Once the patient has completely relaxed, the physician extends the patient's hip to the edge of the new restrictive barrier (*white arrow*, **Fig. 10.200**).

8. Steps 5 to 7 are repeated three to five times or until motion is maximally improved at the dysfunctional hip and psoas.

9. Success of the technique is determined by reevaluating passive hip extension.

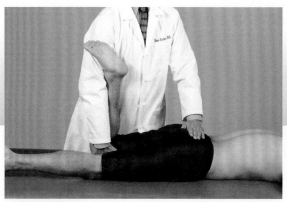
Figure 10.197. Steps 1 to 3.

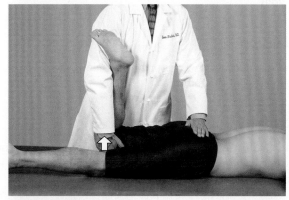
Figure 10.198. Step 4.

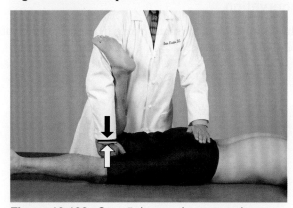
Figure 10.199. Step 5, isometric contraction.

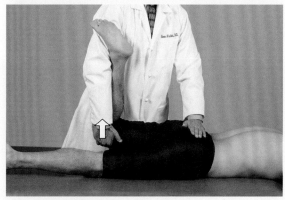
Figure 10.200. Step 7.

Pelvic Region

Piriformis Muscle

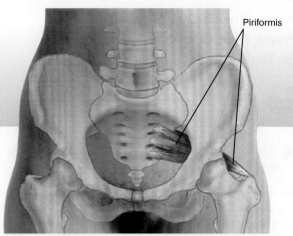

Figure 10.201. Anterior view of piriformis muscle. (Modified with permission from Ref. (8).)

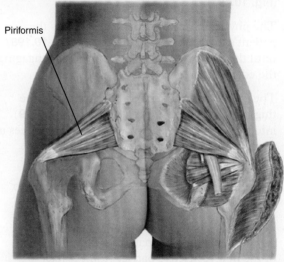

Figure 10.202. Posterior view of piriformis muscle. (Modified with permission from Ref. (8).)

Origin

The origin of the piriformis muscle is at the anterior surface of the sacrum and the superior margin of the greater ischiadic (sciatic) notch **(Figs. 10.201 and 10.202).**

Insertion

The insertion of the piriformis muscle is at the greater trochanter of the femur.

Action

The piriformis muscle rotates the thigh laterally and abducts it, and it assists in holding the femoral head in the acetabulum.

Innervation

The ventral rami of the sacral plexus (S1 and S2) innervate the piriformis muscle.

Pelvic Region

**Piriformis Muscle Dysfunction
Prone, Reciprocal Inhibition
Ex: Right Piriformis, Acute**

1. The patient lies prone, and the physician stands beside the table.

2. The physician palpates the dysfunctional piriformis muscle with the cephalad hand, grasps the patient's ankle with the caudad hand, and flexes the patient's knee 90 degrees **(Fig. 10.203)**.

3. The physician slowly moves the patient's ankle away (*white arrow*, **Fig. 10.204**) from the midline until the edge of the restrictive barrier is reached.

4. The physician, contacting the lateral aspect of the patient's ankle, instructs the patient to *very gently* push the ankle away from the midline (*black arrow*, **Fig. 10.205**) against the physician's caudad hand, which applies an unyielding counterforce (*white arrow*).

5. This isometric contraction is held for 3 to 5 seconds and then the patient is instructed to *stop and relax.*

6. Once the patient has completely relaxed, the physician repositions the ankle farther from the midline, internally rotating the hip to the edge of the new restrictive barrier (*white arrow*, **Fig. 10.206**).

7. Steps 4 to 6 are repeated three to five times or until motion is maximally improved at the dysfunctional hip and piriformis.

8. The diagnostic parameters of the dysfunction (TART) are reevaluated to determine the effectiveness of the technique.

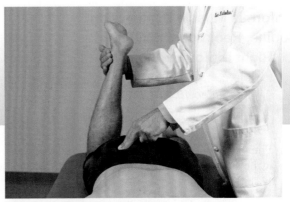

Figure 10.203. Steps 1 and 2.

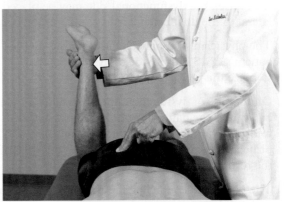

Figure 10.204. Step 3.

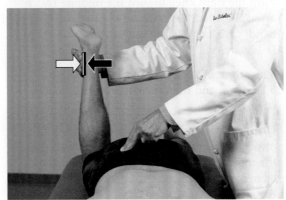

Figure 10.205. Step 4, isometric contraction.

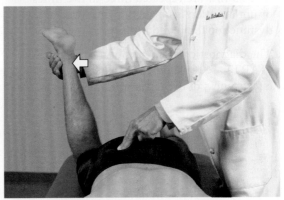

Figure 10.206. Step 6.

Pelvic Region

Piriformis Muscle Dysfunction
Supine, Reciprocal Inhibition
Ex: Right Piriformis, Acute

 See Video 10.43

1. The patient lies supine, and the physician stands at the side of the patient opposite to the side to be treated.

2. The patient's right hip and knee are flexed so that the foot on the dysfunctional side may be placed lateral to the unaffected knee.

3. The physician's cephalad hand is placed on the patient's ASIS on the side of dysfunction to stabilize the pelvis **(Fig. 10.207)**.

4. On the side of dysfunction, the physician's caudad hand pulls the patient's right knee toward the midline, internally rotating the hip, until the piriformis begins to stretch, engaging the edge of the restrictive barrier **(Fig. 10.208)**.

5. The physician, contacting the medial aspect of the patient's knee, instructs the patient to *very gently* push the right knee toward the midline (*black arrow*, **Fig. 10.209**) against the physician's caudad hand, which applies an unyielding counterforce (*white arrow*).

6. This isometric contraction is held for 3 to 5 seconds, and then the patient is instructed to *stop and relax*.

7. Once the patient has completely relaxed, the physician repositions the knee farther across the midline, internally rotating the hip to the edge of the new restrictive barrier (*white arrow*, **Fig. 10.210**).

8. Steps 5 to 7 are repeated three to five times or until motion is maximally improved at the dysfunctional hip and piriformis.

9. The diagnostic parameters of the dysfunction (TART) are reevaluated to determine the effectiveness of the technique.

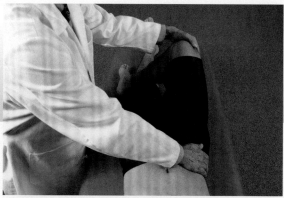

Figure 10.207. Steps 1 to 3.

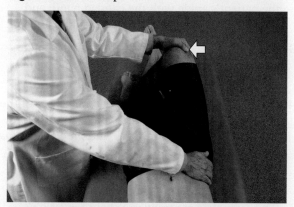

Figure 10.208. Step 4.

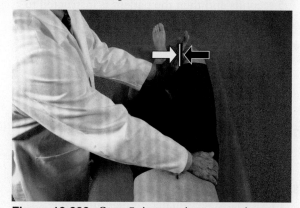

Figure 10.209. Step 5, isometric contraction.

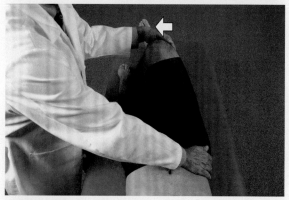

Figure 10.210. Step 7.

Pelvic Region

Piriformis Muscle Dysfunction
Prone, Post-Isometric Relaxation
Ex: Right Piriformis, Subacute/Chronic

1. The patient lies prone on the treatment table, and the physician stands beside the table.

2. The physician palpates the dysfunctional piriformis muscle with the cephalad hand and grasps the patient's ankle with the caudad hand **(Fig. 10.211)**.

3. The physician's caudad hand flexes the patient's knee 90 degrees and slowly moves the patient's ankle away from the midline, internally rotating the dysfunctional hip until the piriformis muscle begins to stretch, engaging the edge of the restrictive barrier **(Fig. 10.212)**.

4. The physician instructs the patient to push the right ankle toward the midline (*black arrow,* **Fig. 10.213**) against the physician's caudad hand, which applies an unyielding counterforce (*white arrow*).

5. This isometric contraction is held for 3 to 5 seconds, and then the patient is instructed to *stop and relax*.

6. Once the patient has completely relaxed, the physician repositions the ankle farther away from the midline, internally rotating the hip to the edge of the new restrictive barrier (*white arrow,* **Fig. 10.214**).

7. Steps 4 to 6 are repeated three to five times or until motion is maximally improved at the dysfunctional hip and piriformis.

8. The diagnostic parameters of the dysfunction (TART) are reevaluated to determine the effectiveness of the technique.

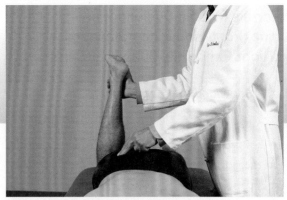
Figure 10.211. Steps 1 and 2.

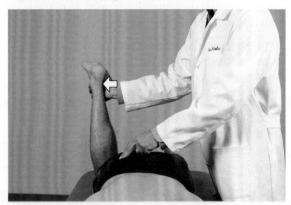
Figure 10.212. Step 3.

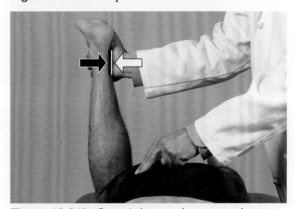
Figure 10.213. Step 4, isometric contraction.

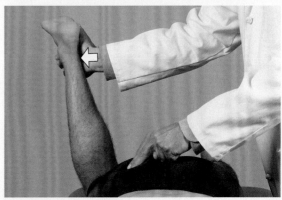
Figure 10.214. Step 6.

Pelvic Region

**Piriformis Muscle Dysfunction
Supine, Post-Isometric Relaxation
Ex: Right Piriformis, Subacute/Chronic**

 See Video 10.43

1. The patient lies supine, and the physician stands at the side of the patient opposite the side to be treated.

2. The patient's hip and knee are flexed so that the foot on the dysfunctional side may be placed lateral to the unaffected knee.

3. The physician's cephalad hand is placed on the patient's ASIS on the side of dysfunction to stabilize the pelvis **(Fig. 10.215)**.

4. On the side of dysfunction, the physician's caudad hand gently pulls the patient's knee toward the midline (*white arrow*, **Fig. 10.216**), internally rotating the hip until the piriformis begins to stretch engaging the edge of the restrictive barrier.

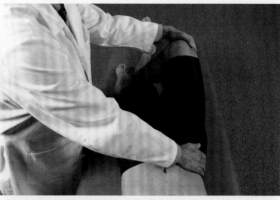

Figure 10.215. Steps 1 to 3.

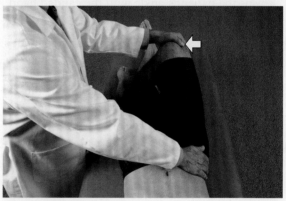

Figure 10.216. Step 4.

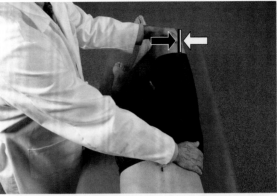

Figure 10.217. Step 5, isometric contraction.

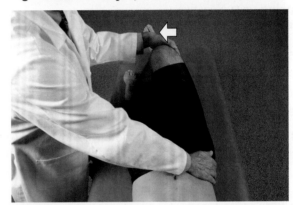

Figure 10.218. Step 7.

5. The physician instructs the patient to pull the knee away from the midline (*black arrow*, **Fig. 10.217**) against the physician's caudad hand, which applies an unyielding counterforce (*white arrow*).

6. This isometric contraction is held for 3 to 5 seconds, and then the patient is instructed to *stop and relax.*

7. Once the patient has completely relaxed, the physician repositions the knee farther across the midline, internally rotating the hip to the edge of the new restrictive barrier (*white arrow*, **Fig. 10.218**).

8. Steps 5 to 7 are repeated three to five times or until motion is maximally improved at the dysfunctional hip and piriformis.

9. The diagnostic parameters of the dysfunction (TART) are reevaluated to determine the effectiveness of the technique.

Sacral Region

Forward Torsion Around an Oblique Axis
Combined Mechanisms of Action
Ex: Left-on-Left (Forward) Sacral Torsion

 See Video 10.44

Diagnosis

Seated flexion test: Positive right
Right sacral sulcus: Anterior (ventral), deep
Left ILA: Posterior (dorsal), shallow
Spring test: Negative
Backward bending/sphinx test: Less asymmetry of sacral sulci
L5 NSLRR
Left-on-left sacral torsion **(Fig. 10.219)**

Technique

1. The patient lies in the left modified Sims position (on the side of the engaged left oblique axis) with the chest down on the table as much as possible and the right arm hanging over the table edge.

2. The physician sits on a stool at the side of the table, facing the patient.

3. The physician gently lifts the patient's knees and rests them on the anterior thigh. The physician's foot closest to the patient should be on a low stool or the rung of a chair, which enables the physician to raise the patient's knees, allowing for greater rotation of the spine for L5 to derotate.

4. The physician's cephalad hand palpates the L5–S1 interspinous space, and the caudad hand grasps the patient's heels and passively flexes and extends the patient's hips until L5 is neutral relative to S1 **(Fig. 10.220)**.

5. The patient inhales and exhales deeply three times, reaching with the right hand toward the floor after each exhalation **(Fig. 10.221)**.

6. The physician's caudad hand gently lowers the

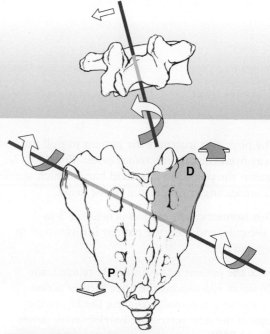

Figure 10.219. Left-on-left sacral torsion.

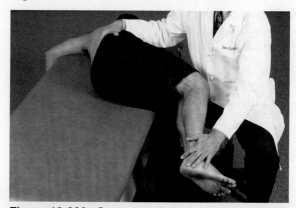

Figure 10.220. Steps 1 to 4.

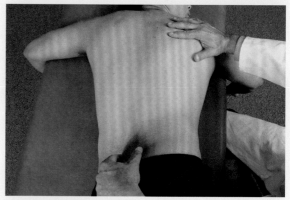

Figure 10.221. Step 5.

patient's feet (*white arrow*, **Fig. 10.222**) to the edge of the restrictive barrier.

7. The physician instructs the patient to lift both feet straight up toward the ceiling with a gentle but sustained force (*black arrow*) against the physician's caudad hand, which applies an unyielding counterforce (*white arrow*, **Fig. 10.223**). This contracts the right hip internal rotators and the left hip external rotators, which are antagonists of the right piriformis muscle (6).

8. This isometric contraction is maintained for 3 to 5 seconds, and then the patient is instructed to *stop and relax*.

9. Once the patient has completely relaxed, the physician lowers both legs toward the floor (*white arrow*, **Fig. 10.224**) to the edge of the new restrictive barrier.

10. Steps 7 to 9 are repeated three to five times.

11. The diagnostic parameters of the dysfunction (TART) are reevaluated to determine the effectiveness of the technique.

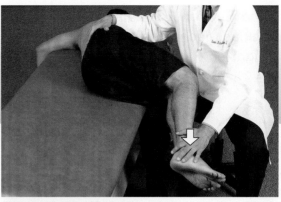

Figure 10.222. Step 6.

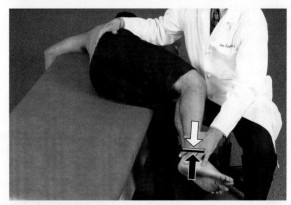

Figure 10.223. Step 7, isometric contraction.

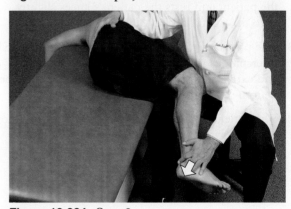

Figure 10.224. Step 9.

Sacral Region

Forward Torsion Around an Oblique Axis
Combined Mechanisms of Action
Ex: Right-on-Right (Forward) Sacral Torsion

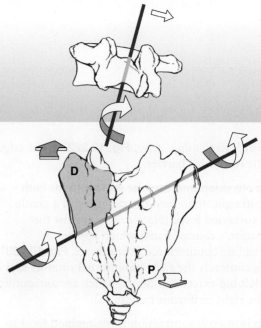

Diagnosis

Seated flexion test: Positive left
Left sacral sulcus: Anterior (ventral), deep
Right ILA: Posterior (dorsal), shallow
Spring test: Negative
Backward bending/sphinx test: Less asymmetry of sacral sulci
L5 NSRRL
Right-on-right sacral torsion **(Fig. 10.225)**

Figure 10.225. Right-on-right sacral torsion.

Technique

1. The patient lies in the right modified Sims position (on the side of the engaged right oblique axis) with the chest down on the table as much as possible and the left arm hanging over the edge of the table.

2. The physician sits on the edge of the table behind the patient and rests the patient's knees slightly onto the right anterior thigh.

3. The physician's cephalad hand palpates the L5–S1 interspinous space while the caudad hand flexes and extends the patient's hips until L5 is felt to be neutral relative to S1 **(Fig. 10.226)**.

4. The patient inhales and exhales deeply three times, reaching with the left hand toward the floor after each exhalation **(Fig. 10.227)**.

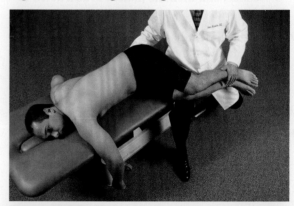

Figure 10.226. Steps 1 to 3.

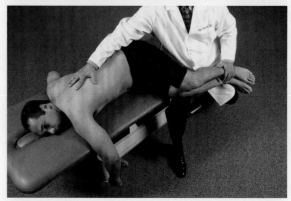

Figure 10.227. Step 4.

5. The physician's caudad hand gently lowers the patient's feet (*white arrow*, **Fig. 10.228**) until the edge of the restrictive barrier is reached.

6. The physician instructs the patient to lift both feet straight up toward the ceiling with a gentle but sustained force (*black arrow*, **Fig. 10.229**) against the physician's caudad hand, which applies an unyielding counterforce (*white arrow*). This contracts the left hip internal rotators and the right hip external rotators, which are both antagonists to the left piriformis muscle (6).

7. This isometric contraction is maintained for 3 to 5 seconds, and then the patient is instructed to *stop and relax.*

8. Once the patient is completely relaxed, the physician gently lowers both feet toward the floor (*white arrow*, **Fig. 10.230**) to the edge of the new restrictive barrier.

9. Steps 6 to 8 are repeated three to five times.

10. The diagnostic parameters of the dysfunction (TART) are reevaluated to determine the effectiveness of the technique.

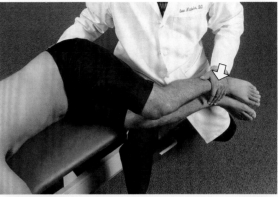

Figure 10.228. Step 5.

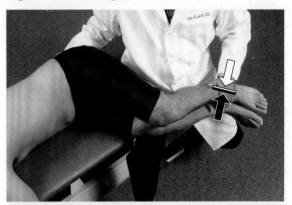

Figure 10.229. Step 6, isometric contraction.

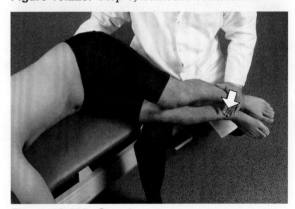

Figure 10.230. Step 8.

Sacral Region

Backward Torsion Around an Oblique Axis
Combined Mechanisms of Action
Ex: Right-on-Left (Backward) Sacral Torsion

 See Video 10.45

Diagnosis

Seated flexion test: Positive right
Right sacral sulcus: Posterior (dorsal), shallow
Left ILA: Anterior (ventral), deep
Spring test: Positive
Backward bending/sphinx test: More asymmetry
of sacral sulci
L5 E/FSLRL
Right-on-left sacral torsion **(Fig. 10.231)**

Technique

1. The patient lies in the left lateral recumbent position with the hips and knees slightly flexed.

2. The physician stands facing the patient's pelvis, and the cephalad hand palpates the L5–S1 interspinous space while the caudad hand gently moves the left leg posteriorly, extending the hip until motion is felt at the L5–S1 interspace.

3. The physician's caudad hand and forearm stabilize the patient's pelvis as the patient gently rotates the trunk to the right **(Fig. 10.232)**.

4. The patient inhales and exhales deeply three times. After each exhalation, the patient reaches back with the right arm and shoulder (*white arrow,* **Fig. 10.233**), rotating the trunk to the right to derotate L5.

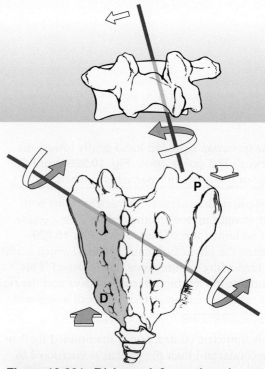

Figure 10.231. Right-on-left sacral torsion.

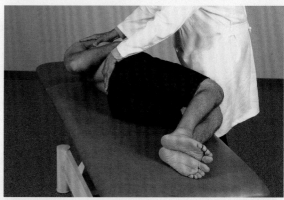

Figure 10.232. Steps 1 to 3.

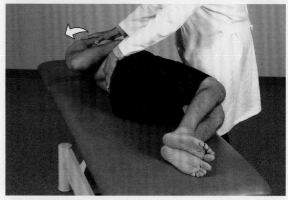

Figure 10.233. Step 4.

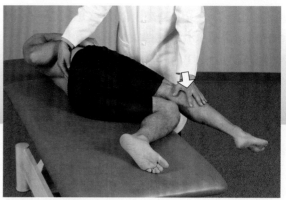

Figure 10.234. Step 5.

5. The physician's caudad hand moves the patient's right leg off the table in front of the left knee and applies gentle pressure on the patient's right knee (*white arrow*, **Fig. 10.234**) to the edge of the restrictive barrier.

6. The physician instructs the patient to lift the right knee straight up toward the ceiling with gentle but sustained force (*black arrow*, **Fig. 10.235**) against the physician's caudad hand, which applies an unyielding counterforce (*white arrow*).

7. This isometric contraction is maintained for 3 to 5 seconds, and then the patient is instructed to *stop and relax*.

8. Once the patient has completely relaxed, the physician gently lowers the right foot toward the floor until a new restrictive barrier is reached (*white arrow*, **Fig. 10.236**).

9. Steps 6 to 8 are repeated three to five times.

10. The diagnostic parameters of the dysfunction (TART) are reevaluated to determine the effectiveness of the technique.

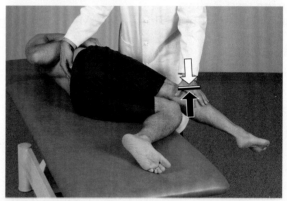

Figure 10.235. Step 6, isometric contraction.

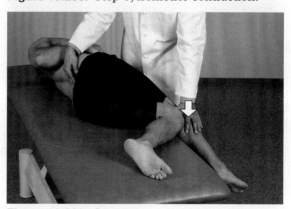

Figure 10.236. Step 8.

Sacral Region

Backward Torsion Around an Oblique Axis
Combined Mechanisms of Action
Ex: Left on Right (Backward) Sacral Torsion

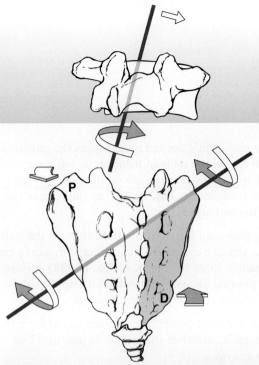

Diagnosis

Seated flexion test: Positive left
Left sacral sulcus: Posterior (dorsal), shallow
Right ILA: Anterior (ventral), deep
Spring test: Positive
Backward bending/sphinx test: More asymmetry
of sacral sulci
L5 E/FSRRR
Left-on-right sacral torsion **(Fig. 10.237)**

Technique

1. The patient lies in the right lateral recumbent
   position with the hips and knees slightly flexed.

2. The physician stands facing the patient's pelvis,
   and the cephalad hand palpates the L5–S1.
   interspinous space while the caudad hand gently
   moves the patient's right leg posteriorly, extending
   the hip until motion is felt at the L5–S1 interspace.

3. The physician's caudad hand and forearm stabilize
   the patient's pelvis as the patient gently rotates the
   trunk to the left **(Fig. 10.238)**.

4. The patient inhales and exhales deeply three times.
   After each exhalation, the patient reaches back
   with the left arm and shoulder, rotating the trunk
   to the left to derotate L5 (*white arrow*, **Fig. 10.239**).

Figure 10.237. Left-on-right sacral torsion.

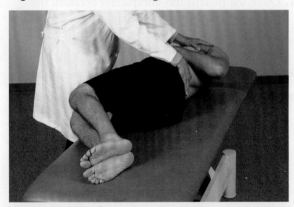

Figure 10.238. Steps 1 to 3.

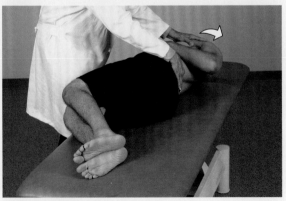

Figure 10.239. Step 4.

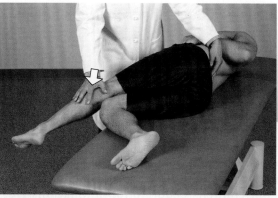

Figure 10.240. Step 5.

5. The physician's caudad hand moves the patient's left leg off the table in front of the right knee and applies gentle pressure on the patient's left knee (*white arrow*, **Fig. 10.240**) to the edge of the restrictive barrier.

6. The physician instructs the patient to lift the left leg straight up toward the ceiling with gentle but sustained force (*black arrow*, **Fig. 10.241**) against the physician's caudad hand, which applies an unyielding counterforce (*white arrow*).

7. This isometric contraction is maintained for 3 to 5 seconds, and then the patient is instructed to *stop and relax*.

8. Once the patient has completely relaxed, the physician gently lowers the left foot toward the floor (*white arrow*, **Fig. 10.242**) to the edge of the new restrictive barrier.

9. Steps 6 to 8 are repeated three to five times.

10. The diagnostic parameters of the dysfunction (TART) are reevaluated to determine the effectiveness of the technique.

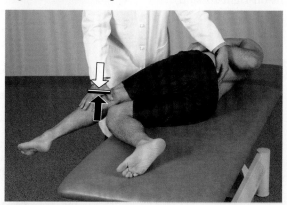

Figure 10.241. Step 6, isometric contraction.

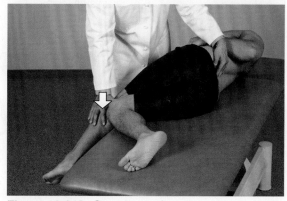

Figure 10.242. Step 8.

Sacral Region

Overview of Sacral Torsion Dysfunctions

See the American Association of Colleges of Osteopathic Medicine website for a video demonstrating right-on-right torsion (http://www.aacom.org/ome/councils/aacom-councils/ecop/motion-animations/Detail/right-on-right-torsion).

Table 10.1 outlines sacral torsion dysfunctions about an oblique axis.

Table 10.1 Sacral Torsion Dysfunctions Around an Oblique Axis

	Standing and Seated Flexion Test Positive Right	Standing and Seated Flexion Test Positive Left
L5 transverse process posterior	Right	Left
L5 dysfunction	L5NSLRR	L5NSRRL
Sacral axis	Left oblique	Right oblique
Sacral sulcus	Right deep anterior inferior	Left deep anterior inferior
Inferior lateral sacral angle	Left shallow posterior inferior	Right shallow posterior inferior
Lumbar spring test	Negative	Negative
Sphinx test (asymmetry of sacral sulcus)	Decreases (less asymmetry)	Decreases (less asymmetry)
Diagnosis	Forward torsion around a left oblique axis. Left-on-left sacral torsion	Forward torsion around a right oblique axis. Right-on-right sacral torsion

Table 10.1 Sacral Torsion Dysfunctions Around an Oblique Axis (Continued)

	Standing and Seated Flexion Test Positive Right	Standing and Seated Flexion Test Positive Left
	Positive	Positive
	Increases (more asymmetry)	Increases (more asymmetry)
	Backward torsion around a left oblique axis. Right-on-left sacral torsion	Backward torsion around a right oblique axis. Left-on-right sacral torsion

Sacral Region

Unilateral Sacral Flexion (Inferior Shear) Respiratory Assist
Ex: Left, Unilateral Sacral Flexion

 See Video 10.46

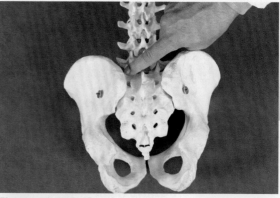

Figure 10.243. Steps 1 and 2.

Diagnosis

Seated flexion test: Positive left
Left sacral sulcus: Anterior (ventral), deep
Left ILA: Posterior (dorsal), shallow
Spring test: Negative
Backward bending/sphinx test: Less asymmetry of sacral sulci

Technique

1. The patient lies prone, and the physician stands at the right side of the table.

2. The index finger of the physician's cephalad hand palpates the patient's left sacral sulcus **(Fig. 10.243)** while the caudad hand abducts and adducts the patient's left leg to find the loosest packed position for the left sacroiliac joint (usually about 15 degrees of abduction).

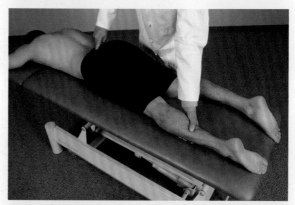

Figure 10.244. Steps 1 to 3.

3. The physician internally rotates the patient's left hip, and the patient maintains this abducted, internally rotated position throughout the treatment **(Fig. 10.244)**.

4. The heel of the physician's caudad hand is placed on the patient's left ILA of the sacrum **(Fig. 10.245)** and is reinforced by the cephalad hand **(Fig. 10.246)**.

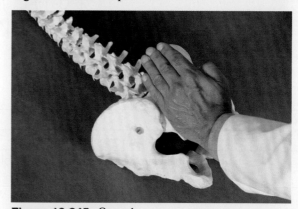

Figure 10.245. Step 4.

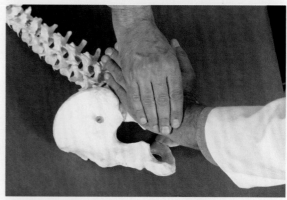

Figure 10.246. Step 4.

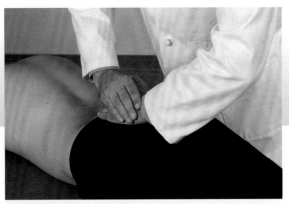

Figure 10.247. Step 5.

5. The physician's caudad hand exerts a sustained force downward on the left ILA of the sacrum. The direction of force may be altered either medial to lateral or cephalad to caudad to find the freest plane of sacral motion **(Fig. 10.247)**.

6. The patient inhales maximally while the physician's caudad hand maintains constant ventral pressure on the left ILA of the sacrum (*white arrow*, **Fig. 10.248**) to encourage sacral extension.

7. The patient exhales slowly. During exhalation, the physician's caudad hand increases the ventral pressure on the left ILA of the sacrum (*white arrow*, **Fig. 10.249**) to prevent sacral flexion.

8. Steps 5 to 7 are repeated five to seven times.

9. The diagnostic parameters of the dysfunction (TART) are reevaluated to determine the effectiveness of the technique.

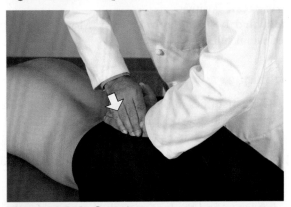

Figure 10.248. Step 6.

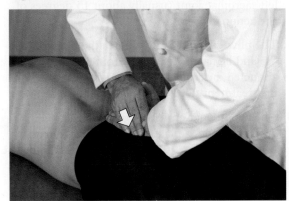

Figure 10.249. Step 7.

Sacral Region

Unilateral Sacral Extension (Superior Shear) Respiratory Assist
Ex: Left Unilateral Sacral Extension

 See Video 10.47

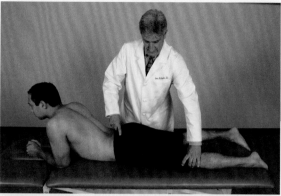

Figure 10.250. Steps 1 to 3.

Diagnosis

Seated flexion test: Positive left
Left sacral sulcus: Posterior (dorsal), shallow
Left ILA: Anterior (ventral), deep
Spring test: Positive
Backward bending/sphinx test: More asymmetry of sacral sulci

Technique

1. The patient lies in the sphinx position (propped up with the elbows supporting the upper body), and the physician stands at the right side of the table.

2. The index finger of the physician's cephalad hand palpates the patient's left sacral sulcus while the caudad hand abducts and adducts the patient's left leg to find the loosest packed position for the left sacroiliac joint (usually about 15 degrees of abduction).

3. The physician internally rotates the patient's left hip and instructs the patient to maintain this abducted, internally rotated position throughout the treatment **(Fig. 10.250)**.

4. The hypothenar eminence of the physician's cephalad hand is placed on the patient's left sacral sulcus **(Fig. 10.251)** and is reinforced by the caudad hand **(Fig. 10.252)**.

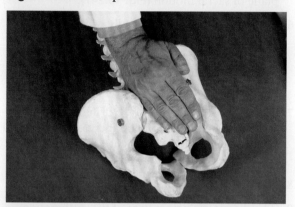

Figure 10.251. Step 4.

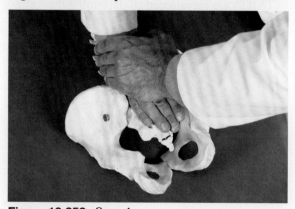

Figure 10.252. Step 4.

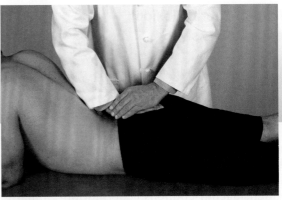

Figure 10.253. Step 5.

5. The physician's hands exert a sustained anterior (downward) force on the patient's left sacral sulcus to rotate the sacrum anteriorly and to disengage the lumbosacral joint caudally **(Fig. 10.253)**.

6. The patient inhales and then exhales forcefully. During exhalation, the physician's hands encourage sacral flexion (*white arrow*, **Fig. 10.254**).

7. The patient inhales slowly. During inhalation, the physician's hands increase the anterior force on the sacral sulcus to prevent sacral extension (*white arrow*, **Fig. 10.254**).

8. Steps 5 to 7 are repeated five to seven times.

9. The diagnostic parameters of the dysfunction (TART) are reevaluated to determine the effectiveness of the technique.

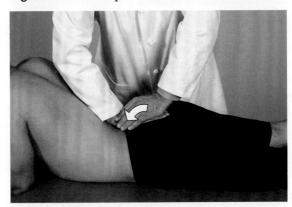

Figure 10.254. Steps 6 and 7.

Sacral Region

Bilateral Sacral Flexion Respiratory Assist

 See Video 10.48

See also the American Association of Colleges of Osteopathic Medicine website for a video demonstrating bilateral sacral flexion (http://www.aacom.org/ome/councils/aacom-councils/ecop/motion-animations/Detail/bilateral-sacral-flexion).

Diagnosis

Sacral rock test: Positive
Both sacral sulci: Anterior (ventral), deep
Both ILAs: Posterior (dorsal), shallow
Spring test: Negative
Bilateral sacral flexion **(Fig. 10.255)**

Technique

1. The patient lies prone, and the physician stands beside the patient.
2. The physician places the thenar and hypothenar eminences of the caudad hand on the ILAs of the patient's sacrum **(Fig. 10.256)**.
3. The physician's cephalad hand reinforces the caudad hand **(Figs. 10.257 and 10.258)**.
4. The physician applies a continuous anterior (downward) force on the ILAs of the patient's sacrum.
5. The patient inhales deeply.
6. The physician exaggerates sacral extension during inhalation (*white arrow*, **Fig. 10.259**) and attempts to resist sacral flexion during exhalation.
7. Steps 4 to 6 are repeated 7 to 10 times.
8. The diagnostic parameters of the dysfunction (TART) are reevaluated to determine the effectiveness of the technique.

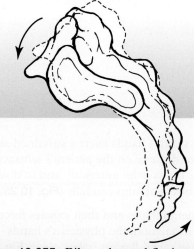

Figure 10.255. Bilateral sacral flexion.

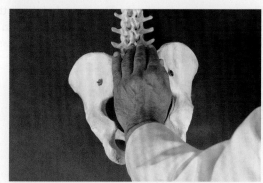

Figure 10.256. Step 2.

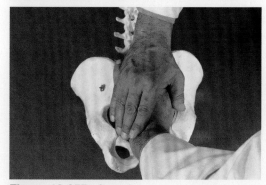

Figure 10.257. Step 3.

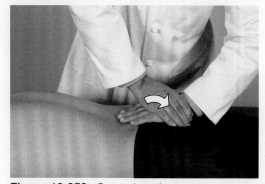

Figure 10.259. Steps 4 to 6.

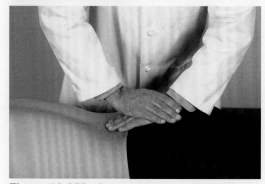

Figure 10.258. Step 3.

Sacral Region

Bilateral Sacral Extension Respiratory Assist

 See Video 10.49

Diagnosis

Both sacral sulci: Posterior (dorsal), shallow
Both ILAs: Anterior (ventral), deep
Spring test: Positive
Bilateral sacral extension **(Fig. 10.260)**

Technique

1. The patient lies prone, in the sphinx position if tolerable, and the physician stands beside the patient.

2. The physician places the index finger on the patient's left sacral sulcus and the long finger on the right sacral sulcus **(Fig. 10.261)**.

3. The physician's other hand reinforces the first hand **(Fig. 10.262)**.

4. A continuous anterior (downward) force (*white arrow*, **Fig. 10.263**) is placed on the sacral sulci.

5. The patient inhales and then exhales deeply.

6. The physician exaggerates flexion during exhalation and attempts to resist extension during inhalation.

7. Steps 4 to 6 are repeated 7 to 10 times.

8. The diagnostic parameters of the dysfunction (TART) are reevaluated to determine the effectiveness of the technique.

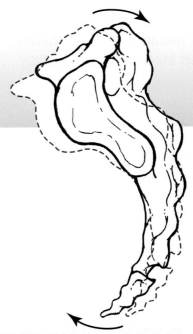
Figure 10.260. Bilateral sacral extension.

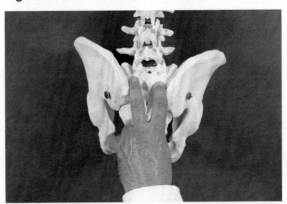
Figure 10.261. Step 2.

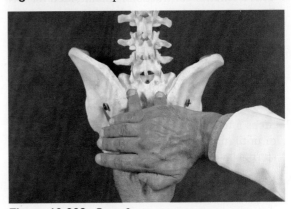
Figure 10.262. Step 3.

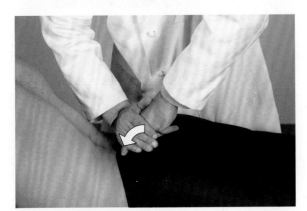
Figure 10.263. Steps 4 to 6.

Upper Extremity

Sternoclavicular Dysfunction
Ex: Right Medial Clavicle, Anterior
Combined Mechanisms of Action

Diagnosis

The sternal end of the clavicle is anteriorly rotated and restricted in posterior rotation, and the shoulder is restricted in abduction and external rotation.

Technique

1. The patient is seated, and the physician stands behind the patient.

2. The physician's left thenar eminence is placed over the superior aspect of the medial end of the dysfunctional clavicle. The physician's right hand grasps the patient's wrist.

3. The physician flexes the patient's elbow to 90 degrees and abducts the shoulder to 90 degrees. The physician then externally rotates the shoulder until the edge of the restrictive barrier is reached (*white arrow*, **Fig. 10.264**).

4. The physician instructs the patient to gently press the wrist forward and downward (*black arrow*, **Fig. 10.265**) into the physician's right hand, which applies an equal counterforce (*white arrow*). This motion produces adduction and internal rotation.

5. This isometric contraction is maintained for 3 to 5 seconds, and then the patient is instructed to *stop and relax.*

6. Once the patient has completely relaxed, the physician repositions the patient to the edge of the new abduction and external rotation barrier (*white arrow*, **Fig. 10.266**).

7. Steps 3 to 6 are repeated three to five times or until motion is maximally improved at the sternoclavicular joint.

8. Range of motion of the shoulder and sternoclavicular joint is reevaluated to determine the effectiveness of the technique.

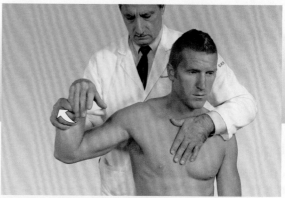

Figure 10.264. Steps 1 to 3.

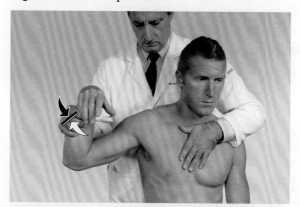

Figure 10.265. Step 4, isometric contraction.

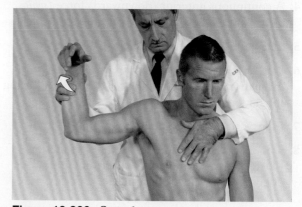

Figure 10.266. Step 6.

Upper Extremity

**Sternoclavicular Dysfunction
Ex: Right Medial Clavicle, Superior
Combined Mechanisms of Action**

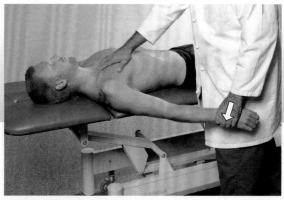

Figure 10.267. Steps 1 to 3.

Diagnosis

The sternal end of the clavicle is superior (cephalad) and the shoulder is restricted in extension and internal rotation.

Technique

1. The patient lies supine with the dysfunctional upper extremity at the edge of the table.

2. The physician stands on the side of the dysfunction and contacts the superior and medial end of the clavicle with the second, third, and fourth fingers of one hand and controls the patient's wrist/forearm with the other hand.

3. The physician internally rotates (*white arrow*) and extends (*white arrow*) the upper extremity to the edge of the restrictive barriers **(Fig. 10.267)**.

4. The physician instructs the patient to lift the arm up toward the ceiling (*black arrow*, **Fig. 10.268**) while the physician applies an equal counterforce (*white arrow*).

5. This isometric contraction is maintained for 3 to 5 seconds, and then the patient is instructed to *stop and relax*.

6. Once the patient has completely relaxed, the physician extends the upper extremity to the edge of the new restrictive barrier (*white arrow*, **Fig. 10.269**).

7. Steps 3 to 6 are repeated three to five times or until motion is maximally improved at the sternoclavicular joint.

8. Range of motion of the shoulder and sternoclavicular joint is reevaluated to determine the effectiveness of the technique.

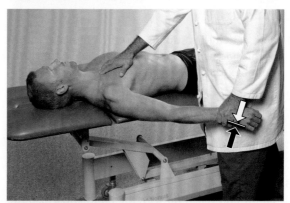

Figure 10.268. Step 4, isometric contraction.

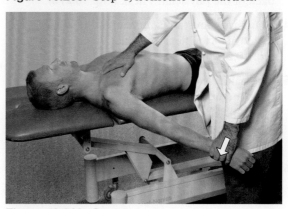

Figure 10.269. Step 6.

Upper Extremity

Sternoclavicular Dysfunction
Ex: Right Medial Clavicle, Inferior
Combined Mechanisms of Action

Diagnosis

The sternal end of the clavicle is inferior (caudad) and the shoulder is restricted in horizontal flexion.

Technique

1. The patient lies supine, and the physician stands at the side of the table opposite the dysfunctional upper extremity.

2. The physician places the thenar eminence of the cephalad hand over the sternal end of the dysfunctional clavicle and with the caudad hand contacts the patient's posterior shoulder region near the vertebral border of the scapula.

3. The physician instructs the patient to extend the elbow and reach up with the hand and grasp the back of the physician's neck **(Fig. 10.270)**.

4. The physician stands more erect to engage the edge of the flexion barrier (*whiter arrow*, **Fig. 10.271**).

5. The patient is instructed to pull down with the hand on the physician's neck (*black arrow*, **Fig. 10.272**) while the physician applies an equal counterforce over the sternal end of the dysfunctional clavicle (*white arrow*).

6. This isometric contraction is maintained for 3 to 5 seconds, and then the patient is instructed to *stop and relax*.

7. Once the patient has completely relaxed, the physician flexes the upper extremity to the edge of the new restrictive barrier by standing more erect while maintaining compression over the sternal end of the dysfunctional clavicle (*white arrow*, **Fig. 10.273**).

8. Steps 3 to 6 are repeated three to five times or until motion is maximally improved at the sternoclavicular joint.

9. Range of motion of the shoulder and sternoclavicular joint is reevaluated to determine the effectiveness of the technique.

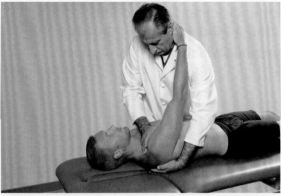

Figure 10.270. Steps 1 to 3.

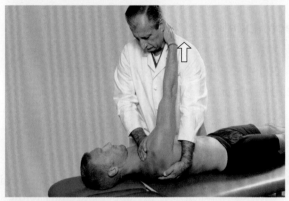

Figure 10.271. Step 4.

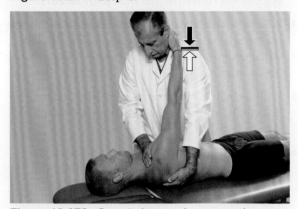

Figure 10.272. Step 5, isometric contraction.

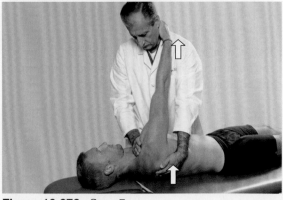

Figure 10.273. Step 7.

Upper Extremity

Acromioclavicular Dysfunction
Ex: Right Adduction
Post-Isometric Relaxation

1. The patient is seated, and the physician stands behind the patient.

2. The physician places the left hand on the distal end of the clavicle just medial to the acromioclavicular joint and the right hand grasps the patient's right elbow (**Fig. 10.274**).

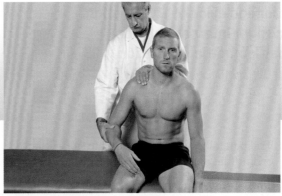

Figure 10.274. Steps 1 and 2.

3. The physician's left hand exerts a gentle compressive force to stabilize the clavicle/AC joint, as the right hand abducts the patient's shoulder to the edge of the restrictive barrier (*white arrow*, **Fig. 10.275**).

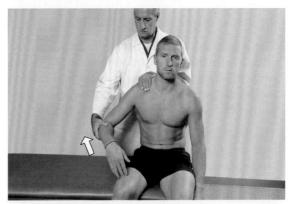

Figure 10.275. Step 3.

4. The physician instructs the patient to push the right elbow "down to the side" (*black arrow*, **Fig. 10.276**) while the physician applies an unyielding counterforce (*white arrow*).

5. This isometric contraction is held for 3 to 5 seconds, and then the patient is instructed to *stop and relax*.

6. Once the patient has completely relaxed, the physician abducts the patient's shoulder to the edge of the new restrictive barrier (*white arrow*, **Fig. 10.277**).

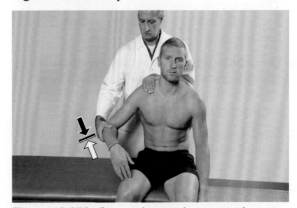

Figure 10.276. Step 4, isometric contraction.

7. Steps 4 to 6 are repeated three to five times or until motion is maximally improved at the dysfunctional acromioclavicular joint.

8. Range of motion of the shoulder and acromioclavicular joint is reevaluated to determine the effectiveness of the technique.

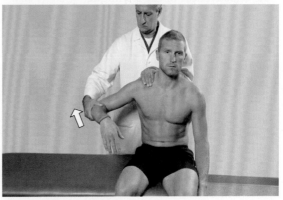

Figure 10.277. Step 6.

Upper Extremity

Acromioclavicular Dysfunction
Ex: Right Internal Rotation
Post-Isometric Relaxation

1. The patient is seated, and the physician stands behind the patient.

2. The physician places the left hand on the distal end of the clavicle just medial to the acromioclavicular joint and the right hand grasps the patient's right wrist **(Fig. 10.278)**.

3. The physician's left hand exerts a gentle compressive force to stabilize the clavicle/AC joint, while the right hand flexes, abducts, and externally rotates the patient's shoulder to the edge of the restrictive barriers (*white arrow*, **Fig. 10.279**).

4. The physician instructs the patient to push the right wrist forward and down toward the floor (*black arrow*, **Fig. 10.280**) to internally rotate the shoulder while the physician's hand (*white arrow*) applies an unyielding counterforce.

5. This isometric contraction is held for 3 to 5 seconds, and then the patient is instructed to *stop and relax.*

6. Once the patient has completely relaxed, the physician externally rotates the patient's arm/shoulder (*white arrow*, **Fig. 10.281**) to the edge of the new restrictive barrier.

7. Steps 4 to 6 are repeated three to five times or until motion is maximally improved at the dysfunctional acromioclavicular joint.

8. Range of motion of the shoulder and acromioclavicular joint is reevaluated to determine the effectiveness of the technique.

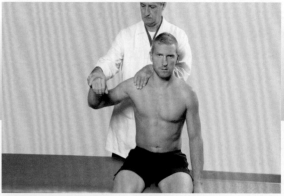

Figure 10.278. Steps 1 and 2.

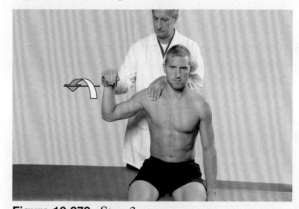

Figure 10.279. Step 3.

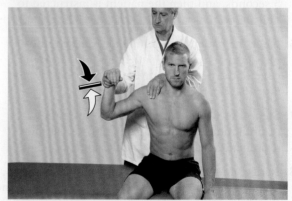

Figure 10.280. Step 4, isometric contraction.

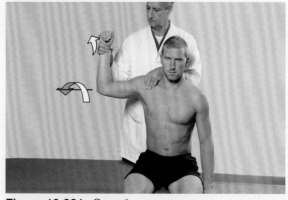

Figure 10.281. Step 6.

Upper Extremity

Acromioclavicular Dysfunction
Ex: Right External Rotation
Post-Isometric Relaxation

1. The patient is seated, and the physician stands behind the patient.

2. The physician places the left hand on the distal end of the clavicle just medial to the acromioclavicular joint and the right hand reaches under the patient's humerus and grasps the right forearm **(Fig. 10.282)**.

3. The physician's left hand exerts a gentle compressive force to stabilize the clavicle/AC joint, while the right hand flexes, abducts, and internally rotates the patient's shoulder to the edge of the restrictive barriers (*white arrow*, **Fig. 10.283**).

4. The physician instructs the patient to lift the right wrist up toward the ceiling (*black arrow*, **Fig. 10.284**) to externally rotate the shoulder while the physician's hand (*white arrow*) applies an unyielding counterforce.

5. This isometric contraction is held for 3 to 5 seconds, and then the patient is instructed to *stop and relax*.

6. Once the patient has completely relaxed, the physician internally rotates the patient's arm/shoulder (*white arrow*, **Fig. 10.285**) to the edge of the new restrictive barrier.

7. Steps 4 to 6 are repeated three to five times or until motion is maximally improved at the dysfunctional acromioclavicular joint.

8. Range of motion of the shoulder and acromioclavicular joint is reevaluated to determine the effectiveness of the technique.

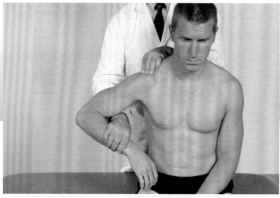
Figure 10.282. Steps 1 and 2.

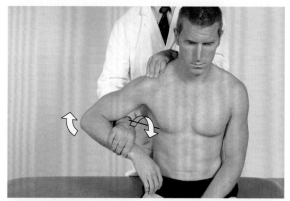
Figure 10.283. Step 3.

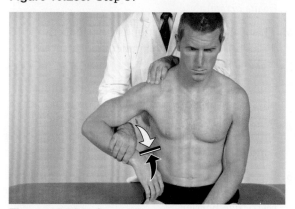
Figure 10.284. Step 4, isometric contraction.

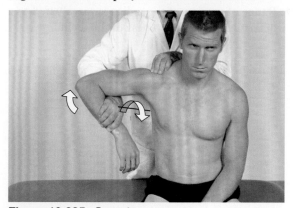
Figure 10.285. Step 6.

Upper Extremity

Elbow: Radioulnar Pronation Dysfunction
Post-Isometric Relaxation
Ex: Right Radial Head, Posterior (Pronation)

 See Video 10.50

1. The patient is seated, and the physician stands in front of and to the side of the patient's dysfunctional arm.

2. The physician grasps the patient's hand on the side of dysfunction (handshake position), contacting the palmar aspect of the distal radius with the index finger.

3. The physician's other hand is palm up with the thumb resting against the posterolateral aspect of the radial head **(Fig. 10.286)**.

4. The physician supinates the patient's forearm until the edge of the restriction barrier is reached (*white arrow*, **Fig. 10.287**) at the radial head.

5. The physician instructs the patient to attempt pronation (*black arrow*, **Fig. 10.288**) while the physician applies an unyielding counterforce (*white arrow*).

6. This isometric contraction is held for 3 to 5 seconds, and then the patient is instructed to *stop and relax*.

7. Once the patient has completely relaxed, the physician supinates the patient's forearm to the new restrictive barrier while exaggerating the anterior rotation of the radial head with the other hand **(Fig. 10.289)**.

8. Steps 5 to 7 are repeated three to five times or until there is no further improvement in the restrictive barrier.

9. Range of motion of the radius is reevaluated to determine the effectiveness of the technique.

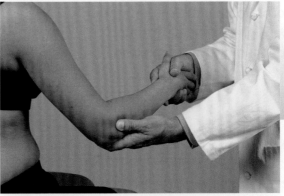
Figure 10.286. Steps 1 to 3.

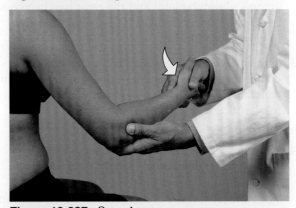
Figure 10.287. Step 4.

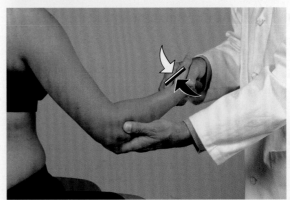
Figure 10.288. Step 5, isometric contraction.

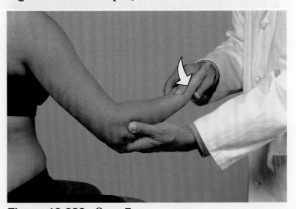
Figure 10.289. Step 7.

Upper Extremity

Elbow: Radioulnar Supination Dysfunction
Post-Isometric Relaxation
Ex: Right Radial Head, Anterior (Supination)

 See Video 10.51

1. The patient is seated, and the physician stands facing the patient.

2. The physician grasps the patient's hand on the side of dysfunction, contacting the dorsal aspect of the distal radius with the thumb.

3. The physician's other hand is palm up with the thumb resting against the anterior and medial aspect of the radial head **(Fig. 10.290)**.

4. The physician pronates the patient's forearm (*white arrow*, **Fig. 10.291**) to the edge of the restrictive barrier.

5. The physician instructs the patient to attempt supination (*black arrow*, **Fig. 10.292**) while the physician applies an unyielding counterforce (*white arrow*).

6. This isometric contraction is held for 3 to 5 seconds, and then the patient is instructed to *stop and relax*.

7. Once the patient has completely relaxed, the physician pronates the patient's forearm to the edge of the new restrictive barrier (*white arrow*, **Fig. 10.293**) while exaggerating the posterior rotation of the radial head with the left hand (*white arrow*).

8. Steps 5 to 7 are repeated three to five times or until there is no further improvement in the restrictive barrier.

9. Range of motion of the radial head is reevaluated to determine the effectiveness of the technique.

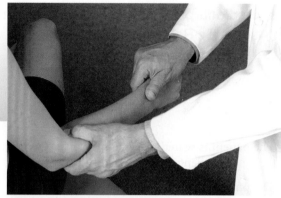
Figure 10.290. Steps 1 to 3.

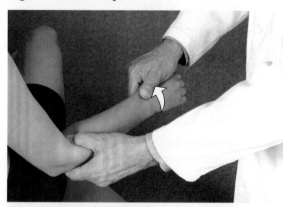
Figure 10.291. Step 4.

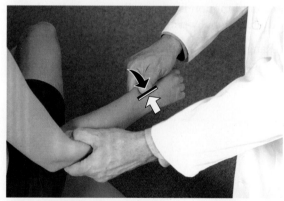
Figure 10.292. Step 5, isometric contraction.

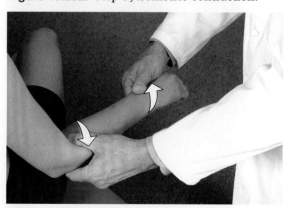
Figure 10.293. Step 7.

Upper Extremity

Wrist: Radiocarpal (Adduction) Dysfunction
Post-Isometric Relaxation
Ex: Left Wrist, Adduction/Ulnar Deviation

1. The patient is seated with the physician standing facing the patient.

2. The physician abducts the patient's wrist (radial deviation) to the edge of the restrictive barrier (*white arrow*, **Fig. 10.294**).

3. The physician instructs the patient to adduct the wrist (*black arrow*) while the physician applies an unyielding counterforce (*white arrow*, **Fig. 10.295**).

4. This isometric contraction is maintained for 3 to 5 seconds, and then the patient is instructed to *stop and relax*.

5. Once the patient has completely relaxed, the physician abducts (radially deviates) the patient's wrist to the edge of the new restrictive barrier (*white arrow*, **Fig. 10.296**).

6. Steps 3 to 5 are repeated three to five times or until motion is maximally improved at the dysfunctional wrist.

7. Range of motion of the wrist is reevaluated to determine the effectiveness of the technique.

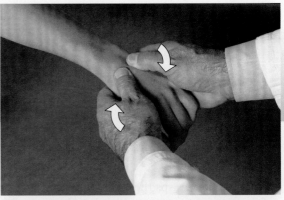

Figure 10.294. Steps 1 and 2.

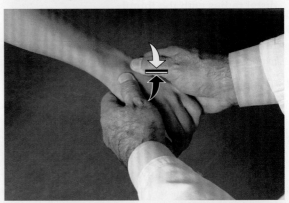

Figure 10.295. Step 3, isometric contraction.

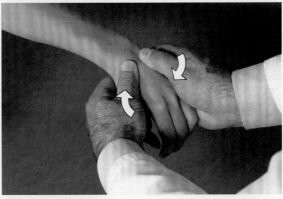

Figure 10.296. Step 4.

Upper Extremity

Wrist: Radiocarpal (Abduction) Dysfunction
Post-Isometric Relaxation
Ex: Left Wrist, Abduction/Radial Deviation

1. The patient is seated with the physician standing facing the patient.

2. The physician adducts the patient's wrist (ulnar deviation) to the edge of the restrictive barrier (*white arrow*, **Fig. 10.297**).

3. The physician instructs the patient to abduct the wrist (*black arrow*) while the physician applies an unyielding counterforce (*white arrow*, **Fig. 10.298**).

4. This isometric contraction is maintained for 3 to 5 seconds, and then the patient is instructed to *stop and relax*.

5. Once the patient has completely relaxed, the physician adducts (ulnar deviation) the patient's wrist to the edge of the new restrictive barrier (*white arrow*, **Fig. 10.299**).

6. Steps 3 to 5 are repeated three to five times or until motion is maximally improved at the dysfunctional wrist.

7. Range of motion of the wrist is reevaluated to determine the effectiveness of the technique.

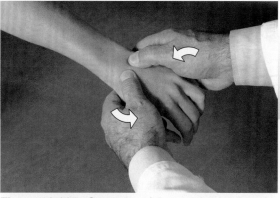

Figure 10.297. Steps 1 and 2.

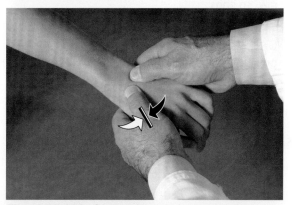

Figure 10.298. Step 3, isometric contraction.

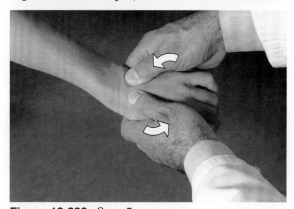

Figure 10.299. Step 5.

Upper Extremity

Wrist: Radiocarpal Flexion Dysfunction Post-Isometric Relaxation

1. The patient is seated with the physician standing facing the patient.

2. The physician extends the patient's wrist to the edge of the restrictive barrier (*white arrow*, **Fig. 10.300**).

3. The physician instructs the patient to flex the wrist (*black arrow*) while the physician applies an unyielding counterforce (*white arrow*, **Fig. 10.301**).

4. This isometric contraction is maintained for 3 to 5 seconds, and then the patient is instructed to *stop and relax.*

5. Once the patient has completely relaxed, the physician extends the patient's wrist to the edge of the new restrictive barrier (*white arrow*, **Fig. 10.302**).

6. Steps 3 to 5 are repeated three to five times or until motion is maximally improved at the dysfunctional wrist.

7. Range of motion of the wrist is reevaluated to determine the effectiveness of the technique.

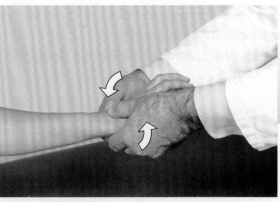

Figure 10.300. Steps 1 and 2.

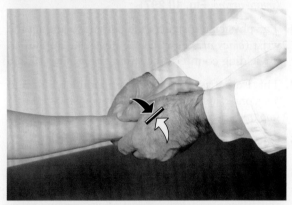

Figure 10.301. Step 3, isometric contraction.

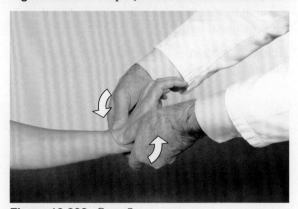

Figure 10.302. Step 5.

Upper Extremity

Wrist: Radiocarpal Extension Dysfunction Post-Isometric Relaxation

1. The patient is seated with the physician standing facing the patient.

2. The physician flexes the patient's wrist to the edge of the restrictive barrier (*white arrow*, **Fig. 10.303**).

3. The physician instructs the patient to extend the wrist (*black arrow*) while the physician applies an unyielding counterforce (*white arrow*, **Fig. 10.304**).

4. This isometric contraction is maintained for 3 to 5 seconds, and then the patient is instructed to *stop and relax*.

5. Once the patient has completely relaxed, the physician flexes the patient's wrist to the edge of the new restrictive barrier (*white arrow*, **Fig. 10.305**).

6. Steps 3 to 5 are repeated three to five times or until motion is maximally improved at the dysfunctional wrist.

7. Range of motion of the wrist is reevaluated to determine the effectiveness of the technique.

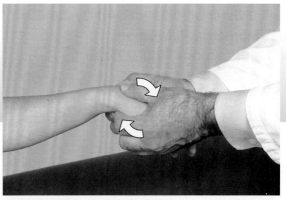

Figure 10.303. Steps 1 and 2.

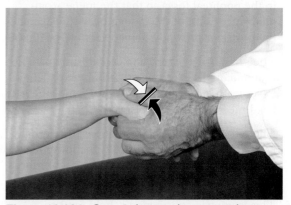

Figure 10.304. Step 3, isometric contraction.

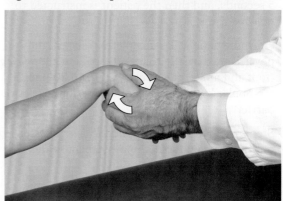

Figure 10.305. Step 5.

Lower Extremity

Knee: Posterior Fibular Head Dysfunction
Post-Isometric Relaxation
Ex: Left Posterior Fibular Head

1. The patient lies supine (or sits with the lower legs off the table), and the physician stands or sits at the side of dysfunction.

2. The physician places the hand closest to the knee in the popliteal fossa so that the metacarpal-phalangeal joint of the index finger approximates the posterior proximal fibula (head) **(Fig. 10.306)**.

3. The physician's other hand controls the patient's foot and ankle, externally rotating the patient's lower leg (*white arrow*, **Fig. 10.307**) until the fibular head meets its anterior restrictive barrier.

4. The physician instructs the patient to internally rotate (*black arrow*, **Fig. 10.308**) the lower leg while the physician applies an unyielding counterforce (*white arrow*).

5. This isometric contraction is held for 3 to 5 seconds, and then the patient is instructed to *stop and relax*.

6. Once the patient has completely relaxed, the physician externally rotates the patient's lower leg (foot and ankle) (*white arrow*, **Fig. 10.309**) until the fibular head meets its new anterior restrictive barrier.

7. Steps 4 to 6 are repeated three to five times or until there is no further improvement in the restrictive barrier.

8. Motion of the fibula is reevaluated to determine the effectiveness of the technique.

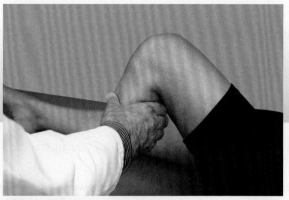
Figure 10.306. Steps 1 and 2.

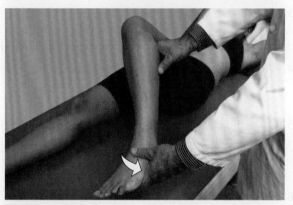
Figure 10.307. Step 3.

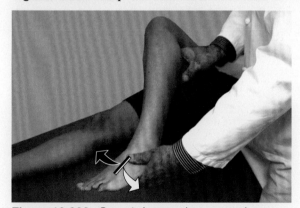
Figure 10.308. Step 4, isometric contraction.

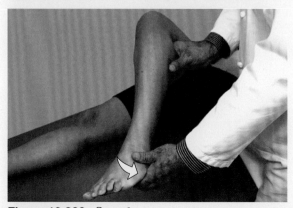
Figure 10.309. Step 6.

Lower Extremity

Knee: Anterior Fibular Head Dysfunction
Post-Isometric Relaxation
Ex: Left Anterior Fibular Head

1. The patient lies supine (or sits with the lower legs off the table), and the physician stands or sits at the side of dysfunction.

2. The physician contacts the anterolateral aspect of the fibular head with the thumb of the hand closest to the patient's knee **(Fig. 10.310)**.

3. The physician's other hand controls the patient's foot and ankle and internally rotates the patient's lower leg (*white arrow*, **Fig. 10.311**) until the fibular head meets its posterior restrictive barrier.

4. The physician instructs the patient to externally rotate (*black arrow*, **Fig. 10.312**) the lower leg as the physician applies an unyielding counterforce (*white arrow*).

5. This isometric contraction is held for 3 to 5 seconds, and then the patient is instructed to *stop and relax*.

6. Once the patient has completely relaxed, the physician internally rotates the patient's lower leg (*white arrow*, **Fig. 10.313**) until the fibular head meets its new posterior restrictive barrier.

7. Steps 4 to 6 are repeated three to five times or until there is no further improvement in the restrictive barrier.

8. Motion of the fibula is reevaluated to determine the effectiveness of the technique.

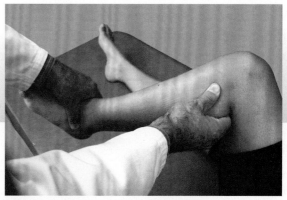

Figure 10.310. Steps 1 and 2.

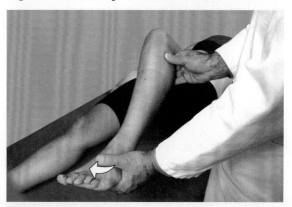

Figure 10.311. Step 3.

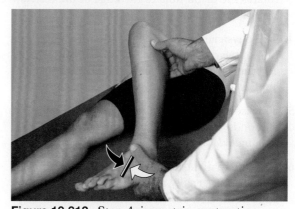

Figure 10.312. Step 4, isometric contraction.

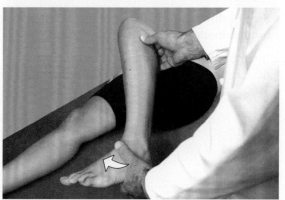

Figure 10.313. Step 6.

Lower Extremity

Tibia: External Rotation Dysfunction
Prone, Post-Isometric Relaxation
Ex: Left, External Rotation/Anteromedial Glide

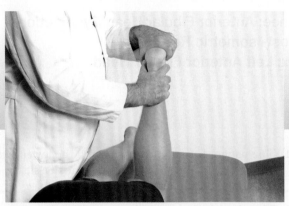

Figure 10.314. Steps 1 and 2.

Diagnosis

External rotation: Free
Internal rotation: Restricted
Anteromedial glide: Free
Posterolateral glide: Restricted
Palpation: Tenderness over the anteromedial joint space

Prone Technique

1. The patient lies prone with the knee flexed 90 degrees, and the physician stands at the edge of the table.

2. The physician grasps the patient's foot with one hand and the distal tibia and fibula with the other hand **(Fig. 10.314)**.

3. The physician dorsiflexes the ankle and internally rotates the distal tibia to the edge of the restrictive barrier (*white arrow*, **Fig. 10.315**).

4. The physician instructs the patient to "turn your foot outward" (*black arrow*, **Fig. 10.316**), which externally rotates the tibia, while the physician applies an unyielding counterforce (*white arrow*).

5. This isometric contraction is maintained for 3 to 5 seconds, and then the patient is instructed to *stop and relax.*

6. Once the patient has completely relaxed, the physician internally rotates the distal tibia to the edge of the new restrictive barrier (*white arrow*, **Fig. 10.317**).

7. Steps 4 through 6 are repeated three to five times or until motion is maximally improved.

8. Internal rotation of the tibia is reevaluated to determine the effectiveness of the technique.

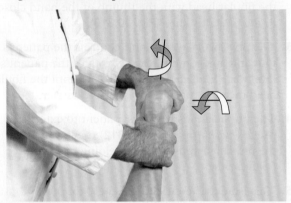

Figure 10.315. Step 3, dorsiflex ankle; internally rotate tibia.

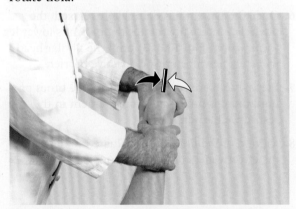

Figure 10.316. Step 4, isometric contraction.

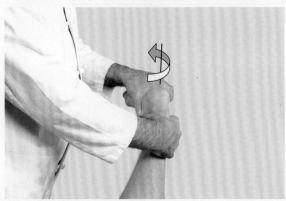

Figure 10.317. Step 6.

Lower Extremity

Tibia: External Rotation Dysfunction
Seated, Post-Isometric Relaxation
Ex: Left, External Rotation/Anteromedial Glide

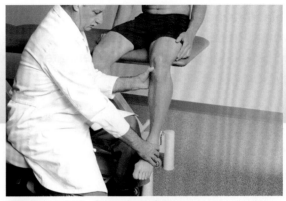

Figure 10.318. Steps 1 and 2.

Diagnosis

External rotation: Free
Internal rotation: Restricted
Anteromedial glide: Free
Posterolateral glide: Restricted
Palpation: Tenderness over the anteromedial joint space

Seated Technique

1. The patient sits with the legs hanging off the table and the physician facing the patient.

2. The physician grasps the lateral aspect of the patient's foot and ankle with one hand and the other hand contacts the medial tibial plateau to monitor motion (anteromedial and posterolateral glide) **(Fig. 10.318)**.

3. The physician dorsiflexes the ankle and internally rotates the distal tibia to the edge of the restrictive barrier (*white arrow*, **Fig. 10.319**).

4. The physician instructs the patient to "turn your foot outward" (*black arrow*, **Fig. 10.320**), which externally rotates the tibia, while the physician applies an unyielding counterforce (*white arrow*).

5. This isometric contraction is maintained for 3 to 5 seconds, and then the patient is instructed to *stop and relax.*

6. Once the patient has completely relaxed, the physician internally rotates the distal tibia to the edge of the new restrictive barrier (*white arrow*, **Fig. 10.321**).

7. Steps 4 through 6 are repeated three to five times or until motion is maximally improved.

8. Internal rotation of the tibia is reevaluated to determine the effectiveness of the technique.

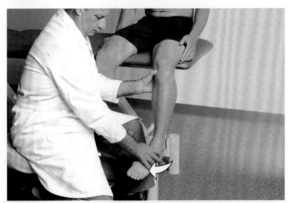

Figure 10.319. Step 3.

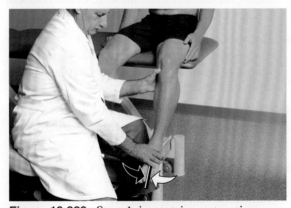

Figure 10.320. Step 4, isometric contraction.

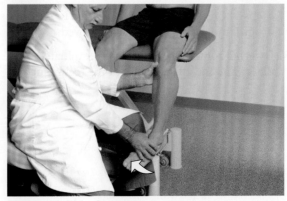

Figure 10.321. Step 6.

Lower Extremity

Tibia: Internal Rotation Dysfunction
Prone, Post-Isometric Relaxation
Ex: Left, Internal Rotation/Posterolateral Glide

Diagnosis

Internal rotation: Free
External rotation: Restricted
Posterolateral glide: Free
Anteromedial glide: Restricted
Palpation: Tenderness over the posterolateral joint space

Prone Technique

1. The patient lies prone with the knee flexed 90 degrees, and the physician stands at the edge of the table.

2. The physician grasps the medial aspect of the patient's foot with one hand and controls the calcaneous with the other hand **(Fig. 10.322)**.

3. The physician dorsiflexes the ankle and externally rotates the distal tibia to the edge of the restrictive barrier (*white arrow*, **Fig. 10.323**).

4. The physician instructs the patient to "turn your foot inward" (*black arrow*, **Fig. 10.324**), which internally rotates the tibia, while the physician applies an unyielding counterforce (*white arrow*).

5. This isometric contraction is maintained for 3 to 5 seconds, and then the patient is instructed to *stop and relax*.

6. Once the patient has completely relaxed, the physician externally rotates the distal tibia to the edge of the new restrictive barrier (*white arrow*, **Fig. 10.325**).

7. Steps 4 through 6 are repeated three to five times or until motion is maximally improved.

8. External rotation of the tibia is reevaluated to determine the effectiveness of the technique.

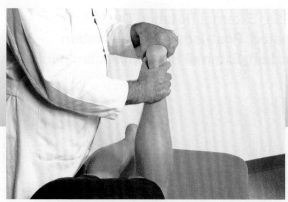

Figure 10.322. Steps 1 and 2.

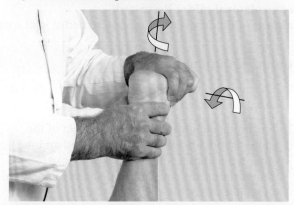

Figure 10.323. Step 3, dorsiflex ankle; externally rotate tibia.

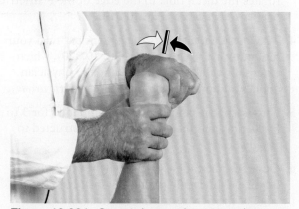

Figure 10.324. Step 4, isometric contraction.

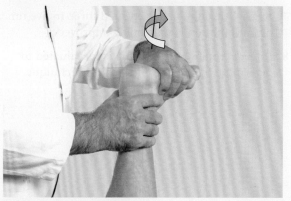

Figure 10.325. Step 6.

Lower Extremity

Tibia: Internal Rotation Dysfunction
Seated, Post-Isometric Relaxation
Ex: Left, Internal Rotation/Posterolateral Glide

Diagnosis

Internal rotation: Free
External rotation: Restricted
Posterolateral glide: Free
Anteromedial glide: Restricted
Palpation: Tenderness over the posterolateral joint space

Seated Technique

1. The patient sits with the legs hanging off the table and the physician facing the patient.

2. The physician grasps the medial aspect of the patient's foot and ankle with one hand and the other hand contacts the medial tibial plateau to monitor motion (anteromedial and posterolateral glide) **(Fig. 10.326)**.

3. The physician dorsiflexes the ankle and externally rotates the distal tibia to the edge of the restrictive barrier (*white arrow*, **Fig. 10.327**).

4. The physician instructs the patient to "turn your foot inward" (*black arrow*, **Fig. 10.328**), which internally rotates the tibia, while the physician applies an unyielding counterforce (*white arrow*).

5. This isometric contraction is maintained for 3 to 5 seconds, and then the patient is instructed to *stop and relax*.

6. Once the patient has completely relaxed, the physician externally rotates the distal tibia to the edge of the new restrictive barrier (*white arrow*, **Fig. 10.329**).

7. Steps 4 through 6 are repeated three to five times or until motion is maximally improved.

8. External rotation of the tibia is reevaluated to determine the effectiveness of the technique.

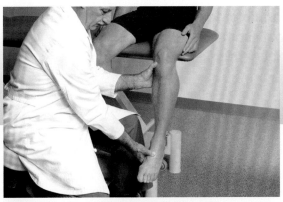

Figure 10.326. Steps 1 and 2.

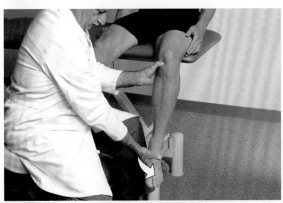

Figure 10.327. Step 3.

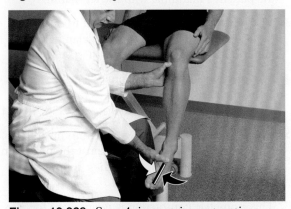

Figure 10.328. Step 4, isometric contraction.

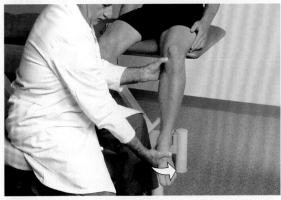

Figure 10.329. Step 6.

Temporomandibular Joint

Mandible/Jaw Deviation Dysfunction
Post-Isometric Relaxation
Ex: Left Mandibular Deviation

Diagnosis

1. The physician places the hands on either side of the patient's head with the index fingers anterior to the external auditory meatus (area of the TMJs).

2. The patient is instructed to open his or her mouth slowly as the physician, palpating the TMJs, observes the chin for deviation from the midline. If the deviation occurs to the left, that is the side of the restricted TMJ.

Technique

1. The patient lies supine, and the physician sits at the head of the table.

2. The physician's right hand supports the right side of the patient's head and contacts the left side of the patient's mandible with the left hand.

3. The physician instructs the patient to open the mouth and STOP when the physician palpates mandibular deviation to the left **(Fig. 10.330)**.

4. The physician's left hand applies a gentle force along the left side of the patient's mandible to direct it toward the right (*white arrow*, **Fig. 10.331**).

5. The physician instructs the patient to push the chin to the left (*black arrow*) against the physician's hand, which applies an unyielding counterforce (*white arrow*, **Fig. 10.332**).

6. This isometric contraction is maintained for 3 to 5 seconds, and then the patient is instructed to *stop and relax*.

7. Once the patient has completely relaxed, the physician passively repositions the patient's jaw further to the right (*white arrow*), to the edge of the new restrictive barrier **(Fig. 10.333)**.

8. Steps 5, 6, and 7 are repeated three to five times or until motion is maximally improved.

9. Reevaluate the motion of the jaw. Symmetry of temporomandibular motion is reevaluated to determine the effectiveness of the technique.

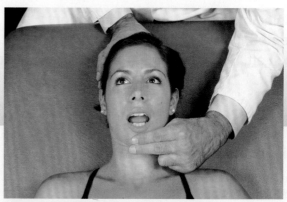

Figure 10.330. Steps 1 to 3.

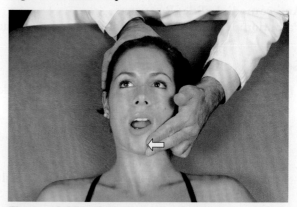

Figure 10.331. Step 4.

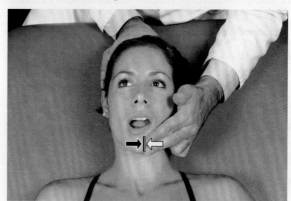

Figure 10.332. Step 5, isometric contraction.

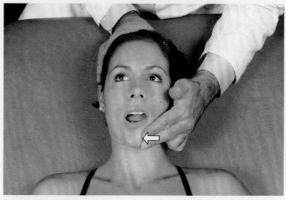

Figure 10.333. Step 7.

Temporomandibular Joint

Hypertonic Muscles of Jaw Elevation
Post-Isometric Relaxation
Ex: Masseter/Medial Pterygoid/Temporalis

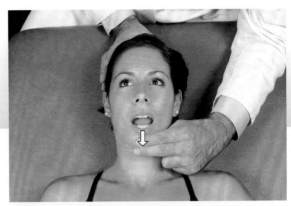

Figure 10.334. Steps 1 and 2.

Indications for Treatment

To relax the various muscles of mastication that close the mouth/jaw and elevate the mandible (medial pterygoid, temporalis, and masseter).

Post-Isometric Relaxation

1. The patient lies supine, and the physician sits at the head of the table.

2. The physician places two fingers or the thumb on the anterior surface of the patient's chin (symphysis menti) and, with the patient relaxed, gently opens the patient's mouth (depress the mandible) to the edge of the restrictive barrier (*white arrow*, **Fig. 10.334**).

3. The physician instructs the patient to close his or her mouth (*black arrow*) while the physician's fingers apply an equal counterforce (*white arrow*, **Fig. 10.335**).

4. This isometric contraction is maintained for 3 to 5 seconds, and then the patient is instructed to *stop and relax*.

5. Once the patient has completely relaxed, the physician passively opens the patient's mouth (depress the mandible) to the edge of the new restrictive barrier (*white arrow*, **Fig. 10.336**).

6. Steps 3, 4, and 5 are repeated three to five times or until motion is maximally improved.

7. Motion of the jaw/mandible is reevaluated to determine the effectiveness of the technique.

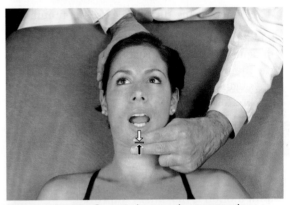

Figure 10.335. Step 3, isometric contraction.

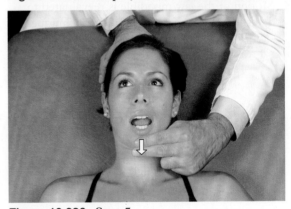

Figure 10.336. Step 5.

Temporomandibular Joint

Hypertonic Muscles of Jaw Depression
Post-Isometric Relaxation
Ex: Lateral Pterygoid/Suprahyoid/Infrahyoid

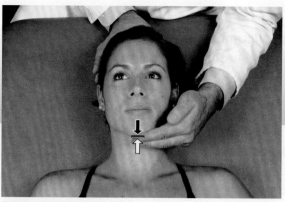

Figure 10.337. Step 2.

Indications for Treatment

To relax the various muscles of mastication that open the mouth/jaw and depress the mandible (lateral pterygoid, digastrics, mylohyoid, and geniohyoid).

1. The patient is instructed to close the mouth.

2. The physician places two fingers under the patient's chin and instructs the patient to open the mouth (*black arrow*, **Fig. 10.337**) against the physician's fingers, which apply an unyielding counterforce (*white arrow*).

3. This isometric contraction is maintained for 3 to 5 seconds, and then the patient is instructed to *stop and relax*.

4. Steps 2 and 3 are repeated three to five times or until motion is maximally improved.

5. Motion of the jaw/mandible is reevaluated to determine the effectiveness of the technique.

References

1. Ward R, exec. ed. Foundations for Osteopathic Medicine. 2nd ed. Philadelphia, PA: Lippincott Williams & Wilkins, 2003.
2. Greenman P. Principles of Manual Medicine. 2nd ed. Baltimore, MD: Williams & Wilkins, 1996.
3. Mitchell FL Jr. The Muscle Energy Manual, Vol 1. East Lansing, MI: MET, 1995.
4. Neumann HD. Introduction to Manual Medicine. Berlin, Germany: Springer-Verlag, 1989.
5. Mitchell FL Jr. The Muscle Energy Manual, Vol 2. East Lansing, MI: MET, 1998.
6. Mitchell FL Jr. The Muscle Energy Manual, Vol 3. East Lansing, MI: MET, 1998.
7. Simons DG, Travell SG, Simon LS. Myofascial Pain and Dysfunction: The Trigger Point Manual. Baltimore, MD: Lippincott Williams & Wilkins, 1999.
8. Clay JH, Pounds DM. Basic Clinical Massage Therapy: Integrating Anatomy and Treatment. Baltimore, MD: Lippincott Williams & Wilkins, 2003.

High-Velocity, Low-Amplitude Techniques

Technique Principles

High-velocity, low-amplitude technique (HVLA) is defined by the Educational Council on Osteopathic Principles (ECOP) as "an osteopathic technique employing a rapid, therapeutic force of brief duration that travels a short distance within the anatomic range of motion of a joint and that engages the restrictive barrier in one or more planes of motion to elicit release of restriction (1)." HVLA is also listed as *thrust treatment* in the ECOP glossary. The authors have an affinity for the term mobilization with impulse, since it more accurately describes this type of manipulation.

In an attempt to help osteopathic medical students understand the success and safety factors involved with this technique, as well as the forces at play in its process of treating musculoskeletal dysfunctions, we began to use the term *high-acceleration, low-distance technique (HALD)* to describe the technique parameters more accurately. We use this term to describe the forces at play because we believe that *velocity*, which is constant, does not truly define the nature of the initiating force. We believe it is more accurate to define the initiating force by *acceleration* (dv/dt, a rapid increase in velocity with respect to time, accelerating toward and then minimally through the restrictive barrier). As we taught the novice students to use this technique, it also became apparent that their ability to understand the basis of this technique was being undermined by the term *velocity*. Commonly, their idea of this force was a straight, constant thrust by the physician, which is not accurate.

We believed that the term *distance* was more easily understandable than *amplitude*. Therefore, for teaching purposes, we began to define HVLA as *HALD*; yet, for national terminological integrity, we continued to promote the name of the technique as *HVLA*, using HALD as the explanation of its forces. For use of this variety of osteopathic manipulative treatment (as with other techniques), it is important to understand the relative success and morbidity factors related to its performance. As we are most interested in performing a safe technique with a successful outcome, it is important

to remember the following relationships based on the HALD definition:

Low distance = safety

High acceleration = success

It is appropriate to think of osteopathic manipulation as a form of *work*. Using this as a basis, we can use the formula *work* = force × *distance* ($W = fd$). Knowing that *force* = mass × *acceleration* ($f = ma$), we can substitute mass and acceleration for force in the work formula and conclude that

Work = mass × acceleration × distance, or W = mad

In this formula, acceleration is the success factor and distance is the safety factor. Thus, for teaching purposes, we can denote the HALD (HVLA) formula for success and safety as

$$W = mad$$

Therefore, to perform a successful and safe HVLA technique (work), the physician must combine a rapid acceleration force with only minimal movement of the articular landmark (segment) that is being treated. With high accelerating forces, the tissue's elastic abilities (stretch) may be limited, so they act more like a solid. This is theorized to occur because of the ability of the colloidal (viscoelastic) elements reacting with non-Newtonian behavior, whereas slowly imparted forces permit stretch, creep, or a passage through the tissues and will not immediately carry the segment with the imparted force vector (2). This can be seen when a cornstarch solution is mixed and rapid versus slow forces are applied to it, reacting more solid (rapid) and liquid (slow), respectively. Therefore, when positioned at the restrictive barrier, a highly accelerated force will carry the soft tissues and the dysfunctional segment together immediately, effectively reducing the distance needed to mobilize the restrictive barrier. Because of this, the physician, in identifying the restrictive barrier(s), may be better able to determine the distance needed to mobilize the segment, knowing that the segment will move synchronously with the corrective force. Rapid acceleration also makes it difficult for the patient to resist or guard against the corrective force.

The distance in this formula should be only enough to move the dysfunctional articular segment through the restrictive barrier, not to carry it through the barrier and beyond the physiologic barrier. If, for example, a segment that normally has 7 degrees of motion is restricted at its 2-degree motion mark, the corrective technique is to use only enough force to move the segment an additional 1 degree, not the remaining 5 degrees. In the early stage of learning this technique, it is more important to use short distance for safety rather than high acceleration for success. David Heilig, DO, referred to this as giving the segment a *nudge*, because it is difficult to limit the motion when you are highly accelerating (3). As the student becomes more accomplished and masters the ability to stop at the precise point needed (immediately past the restrictive barrier in millimeters of distance), it is appropriate to increase the acceleration to more successful mobilizing levels.

Most practitioners know that when they attempt to improve and/or restore motion loss at the joint level by using this technique, an *articular pop* can occur. There have been many theories as to the cause of this sound, including cavitation (change in synovial fluid to a gaseous state) and a vacuum phenomenon (3). However, an articular pop does not mean that the correct articulation was mobilized, just that an acute movement was directed to a joint. The lack of an audible sound does not mean that the correction was unsuccessful. Therefore, the physician should be most intent on the palpatory quality and quantity of the dysfunctional articulation as it goes through the corrective process.

Technique Classification

Direct Technique

In American osteopathic circles, HVLA is mostly frequently described as a direct technique. That is, the mobilizing force used to correct the somatic dysfunction is directed toward the restrictive barrier. In accomplishing this correction, the physician should attempt to move the segment as little as possible through this barrier. In somatic dysfunction, including the articular abnormalities, the dysfunction is described for its motion freedom and position in the x-, y-, and z-axes. Therefore, the restrictive barrier that is encountered with direct technique is opposite the freedom by which the dysfunction is named.

To safely and successfully treat a dysfunction with this direct method, it is probably wise to focus on one or two axes and keep some freedom available in the remaining axis. Meeting all three axis barriers makes the joint very restricted, and it becomes more difficult to manipulate safely. Also, the patient has a greater tendency to guard against the thrust, and this can cause pain and stiffness posttreatment. For example, to treat a spinal dysfunction that has been determined to be flexed, rotated right, and side bent right, the physician would flex to the level of the dysfunction, then extend slightly to include this barrier, rotate to the restrictive barrier (left), but produce only slight side bending to the barrier to keep that axis slightly freer (similar to the *feather's edge* described in Chapter 10 in reference to muscle energy techniques). A corrective force that is vectored through only one or two of the axes often produces success with minimal side effects.

Indirect Technique

To treat the patient with indirect technique, the physician must take the area of dysfunction away from the most restrictive barrier and in the direction by which its biomechanical parameters are described. Indirect HVLA was not part of the classic, approved American osteopathic curriculum, as it was difficult to understand how mobilizing a segment through it freedom could improve the restrictive barrier. It was also thought to be potentially traumatic with greater chance of morbidity. More recently, it has been promoted by our German physician colleagues causing us to rethink this approach. Previously, some American academic (osteopathic) authorities had used the term *exaggeration method* to describe indirect technique.

If using HVLA in an indirect manner, the indirect barrier *cannot* be the normal physiologic barrier opposite the restriction. This ease barrier must be an additional (restrictive) component of the dysfunction (see Fig. 6.2). This is in itself a restriction, but it is not the most restricted barrier. If this barrier were the physiologic barrier, indirect technique would be contraindicated as a form of manipulation. In this method, treating the *least* restrictive barrier may be reversing the principle proposed by Nelson (third principle of physiologic motion), that restriction in one plane of motion causes restriction in other planes; therefore, improving motion in one plane will improve motion in all other planes.

Motion enhancement at a joint may be produced in a manner similar to removing a suction cup from a piece of glass. In performing a "direct" style of removing the suction cup from the glass pane, one would simply pull it off the glass directly toward the restriction (barrier). However, if the cup is compressed into the glass, it can be moved easily perpendicular to the most restricted direction and then simply lifted off the glass with little to no resistance. Similarly, as one vectors force to and through the articulation, causing some compression at the facet and synovium, motion in any direction perpendicular to its major restriction can facilitate increased motion in the joint, producing the "indirect" suction cup effect.

Technique Styles

In HVLA technique, the standard for setting the biomechanical force vectors is determined by how the segmental level of the dysfunction is termed. In some dysfunctions, the physician may choose to use a technique whose primary motion is rotation to affect the dysfunctional motion components. In other dysfunctions, the physician may choose to use side bending as the direction of choice and vector the force in that plane. In still other dysfunctions, flexion or extension is used.

Most HVLA techniques are performed by directing the forces from above. Some techniques set the forces from below. However, for the technique to be direct, when the forces come from below, the inferior segment must be carried toward the named free motion parameters of the dysfunction, and the superior segment must be carried toward the restrictive barrier. For example, if the dysfunction is at L1, by definition, L1 is restricted on L2; L2 is not dysfunctional under L1. Also, L1 is not dysfunctional as it relates to T12. To treat a dysfunction of L1 on L2, L1 must move through its restrictive barrier (bind), while L2 is either held stable in neutral or carried through the described ease of L1. Taking the segment below to the dysfunctional segment's described ease augments the technique. Simply put, if L1 is rotated right, by direct method, it must move to the left. This left rotation can be achieved by rotating L1 to the left over L2 or by rotating L2 to the right under L1. Rotating L2 to the left under a stabilized L1 would be considered an indirect HVLA technique. This is a common misconception with the lateral recumbent lumbar technique. If the side of the rotational component is placed off the table and the thrust is made from below, carrying it toward its barrier, the technique does not follow the definition of the dysfunction and at best was successful because of unintended side bending effects, not rotation. If the upper segment is rotated in the opposing direction, the technique may be effective because of indirect, not direct, measures.

Another way HVLA techniques can be described is to delineate them by the method in which the thrust/impulse is directed into the dysfunctional segment. If the force vector is applied directly at the level of the dysfunction and onto the bony landmark utilized as the focal point, this is considered to be a "short lever" technique. However, if the force vector is directed from a distance to the level of the dysfunction utilizing traction forces through the myofascial components to elicit a mobilization, it is considered a "long lever" technique.

Indications

HVLA in general is used to restore motion to a previously mobile articulation that is exhibiting restriction in all or part of its intersegmental range of motion.

Greenman (4) describes a number of possible etiologies for joint restriction. These include alteration of opposing joint surfaces, articular capsule changes or meniscoids, short restrictor muscle tension, and nociceptors. Diagnostic signs that are attributable to an articular dysfunction are loss of or reduction of intersegmental joint motion and/or qualitative changes in joint play or joint end feel. Palpable tissue texture changes may be present over the articular area involved or distal to it, but they do not necessarily mean that the dysfunction is articular. Pain is another finding that may be present but again does not definitively mean that an articular dysfunction is present. Motion asymmetries associated with motion loss are the definitive signs of an articular dysfunction.

If a myofascial-induced dysfunction is causing the joint restriction, a myofascial-based technique may be more appropriate.

Contraindications

Relative Contraindications

1. Mild-to-moderate strain or sprain in the area to be treated
2. Mild osteopenia or osteoporosis in the area that will be receiving compression, torsion, or another such force from the positioning and/or thrust
3. Osteoarthritic joints with moderate motion loss
4. Rheumatoid disease other than in the spine
5. Minimal disc bulge and/or herniation with radicular symptoms
6. Atypical joint or facet and other conditions with associated congenital anomalies
7. Some hypermobile states

Absolute Contraindications

1. Joint instability
2. Severe osteoporosis
3. Metastasis in the area that will be receiving compression, torsion, or other such force from the positioning and/or thrust
4. Osteoarthritic joint with ankylosis
5. Severe discogenic spondylosis with ankylosis
6. Osteomyelitis in the area that will be receiving compression, torsion, or other such force from the positioning and/or thrust
7. Infection of the tissues in the area that will be receiving compression from the positioning and/or thrust
8. Joint replacement in the area that will be receiving compression, torsion, or other such force and/or thrust
9. Severe herniated disc with radiculopathy

10. Congenital anomalies such as Klippel-Feil syndrome, blocked vertebra, Chiari malformation, and so on
11. Conditions such as Down syndrome (especially cervical spine)
12. Rheumatoid arthritis of the cervical (especially at C1–C2) region
13. Achondroplastic dwarfism (cervical spine)
14. Vertebrobasilar insufficiency

General Considerations and Rules

HVLA technique is one of the oldest forms of manual medicine and is one that has been studied most in terms of clinical response. It is the technique that is least time-consuming. It does have, on the other hand, a relatively long learning curve for competence and user confidence.

Shorthand Rules

1. Diagnose.
2. Localize the segment to be treated.
3. Control the area so the patient is comfortable and relaxed.
4. Position to the restrictive barrier (the edge, not the wall).
5. Use release-enhancing maneuvers if necessary (e.g., patient's breathing, isometric contraction, jaw clenching, and then relaxing).
6. When confident that the patient is relaxed and not guarded, add a rapid acceleration (mobilizing force) thrust within the articulatory plane or planes of the joint with total joint movement kept to the absolute minimum.
7. Reassess the components of the dysfunction (tissue texture abnormality, asymmetry of position, restriction of motion, tenderness [TART], especially intersegmental joint motion).

Cervical Region

Occipitoatlantal (OA, C0–C1) Dysfunction
Ex: OA, F/E or N-SLRRR

 See Video 11.1

1. The patient lies supine, and the physician sits or stands at the head of the table to the patient's right.
2. The physician rotates the patient's head to the left.
3. The physician places the left forearm under the patient's left rotated head and with the left hand cups the patient's chin **(Fig. 11.1)**.
4. The head resting on the forearm creates a minimal side bending into the right side bending barrier.
5. The physician's right hand (metacarpophalangeal joint [MCP] of the index finger, hypothenar eminence, or thumb) is placed just posterior to the mastoid process **(Figs. 11.2 to 11.4)**.
6. The physician uses both hands to exert continuous traction (*white arrows*, **Fig. 11.5**). This is key to a successful mobilization.
7. With the patient relaxed and not guarding, the physician delivers a thrust (*white arrow*, **Fig. 11.6**) toward the patient's left orbit. This thrust is not linear but an arc.
8. Effectiveness of the technique is determined by reassessing motion at the occipitoatlantal articulations.

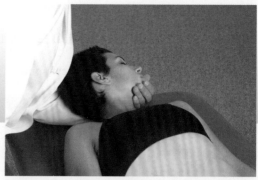

Figure 11.1. Steps 1 to 3.

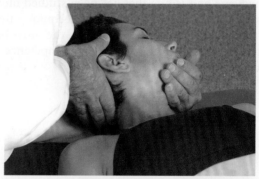

Figure 11.2. Step 5, MCP position.

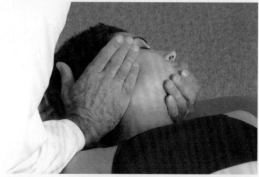

Figure 11.3. Step 5, hypothenar eminence variation.

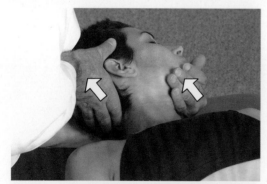

Figure 11.5. Step 6, cephalad traction.

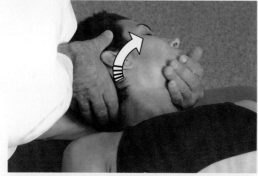

Figure 11.6. Step 7.

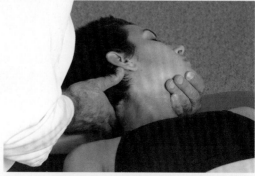

Figure 11.4. Step 5, thumb variation.

Cervical Region

Atlantoaxial (AA, C1–C2) Dysfunction
Ex: C1 RL

 See Video 11.2

1. The patient lies supine, and the physician sits or stands at the head of the table.

2. The physician's hands sandwich the patient's head, cradling both temporoparietal regions **(Fig. 11.7)**.

3. The physician rotates the patient's head to the right, engaging the restrictive barrier **(Fig. 11.8)**. There is no side bending, flexion, or extension with this rotation.

4. The patient can be asked to breathe slowly, and at exhalation, further slack may be taken out of the soft tissues.

5. With the patient relaxed and totally unguarded (may use end exhalation as point of relaxation), a thrust is delivered exaggerating rotation (minimally) through the restrictive barrier (*white arrow*, **Fig. 11.9**). This may be only a few degrees of motion.

6. Effectiveness of the technique is determined by reassessing motion at the atlantoaxial articulations.

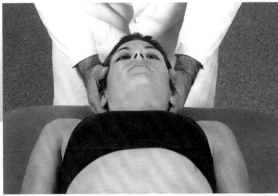

Figure 11.7. Step 2.

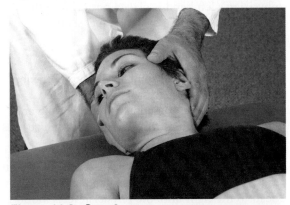

Figure 11.8. Step 3.

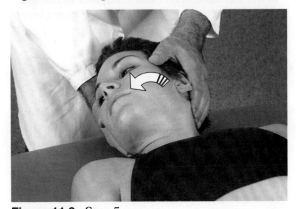

Figure 11.9. Step 5.

Cervical Region

C2–C7 Dysfunctions
Short-Lever, Rotational Emphasis
Ex: C4 FSLRL

 See Video 11.3

1. The patient is supine, and the physician stands or sits at the head of the table on the patient's left side.

2. The MCP joint of the index finger of the physician's left hand is placed posterior to the articular pillar of the dysfunctional segment.

3. Side bending to the left is introduced until the physician elicits the movement of C4, which segments the cervical spine to this level. Flexion or extension is not necessary as a separated motion, as the combination of side bending and subsequent rotation will effectively neutralize these components **(Fig. 11.10)**.

4. With the side bending held in place, the physician grasps the chin with the right hand and rotates the head to the right until the physician feels motion in the left hand. The head is allowed to rest on the physician's right forearm, which may elevate slightly to effect further isolation of the C4 on C5 articulation **(Fig. 11.11)**.

5. Slight axial traction may be applied (*white arrows*, **Fig. 11.12**) with both hands.

6. With the patient relaxed and not guarding, the physician's left MCP directs an arc-like thrust in the plane of the oblique facet of C4 (*white arrow*, **Fig. 11.13**).

7. Effectiveness of the technique is determined by reassessing intersegmental motion at the level of the dysfunctional segment.

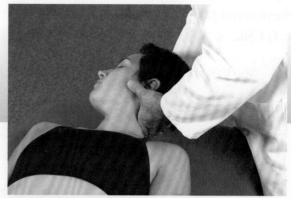

Figure 11.10. Steps 1 to 3.

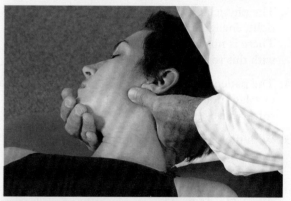

Figure 11.11. Step 4.

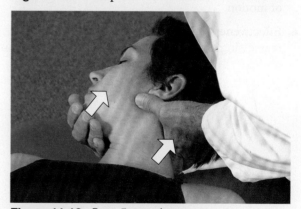

Figure 11.12. Step 5, traction.

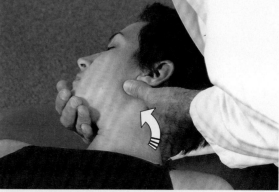

Figure 11.13. Step 6.

Cervical Region

C2–C7 Dysfunctions
Long-Lever, Rotational Emphasis
Ex: C5 ESRRR

 See Video 11.4

1. The patient lies supine, and the physician is seated at the head of the table.

2. The physician's right index finger pad or MCP is placed behind the right articular pillar of C6 to restrict motion at that segment.

3. The patient's head is supported by the physician's left hand **(Fig. 11.14)**.

4. The head is side bent right (*white arrow*, **Fig. 11.15**) until C5 begins to move. This takes tension off the paravertebral muscles at the level of the dysfunction. Flexion should be added until C5 again begins to move.

5. The physician carefully rotates the head to the left until the restrictive barrier engages, being mindful to maintain the original right side bending **(Fig. 11.16)**.

6. With the patient relaxed and not guarding, the physician, using rapid acceleration, supinates the left hand and wrist, which directs a left rotational arc-like thrust in the plane of the oblique facet (*white arrow*, **Fig. 11.17**). This produces side bending left and rotation left.

7. The physician's right hand remains rigid as a fulcrum against which to move the cervical column.

8. Effectiveness of the technique is determined by reassessing intersegmental motion at the level of the dysfunctional segment.

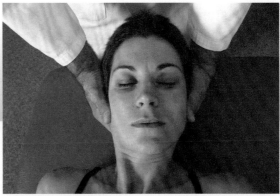

Figure 11.14. Steps 1 to 3.

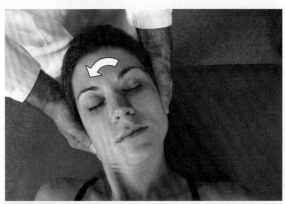

Figure 11.15. Step 4.

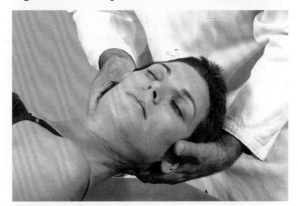

Figure 11.16. Step 5.

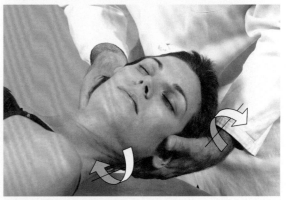

Figure 11.17. Step 6.

Cervical Region

C2–C7 Dysfunctions
Short-Lever, Side Bending Emphasis
Ex: C5 NSLRL

 See Video 11.5

1. The patient lies supine, and the physician stands or sits at the head of the table.

2. The physician supports the patient's head with the pads of the index fingers on the articular pillars of the dysfunctional vertebra (C5).

3. The physician gently flexes the patient's head and neck until C5 begins to move over C6 **(Fig. 11.18)**.

4. The physician, while monitoring the posterior articular pillars of C5, gently rotates the patient's head and neck to the left until motion at C5 is felt.

5. The physician gently side bends the patient's head and neck to the right, engaging the side bending barrier of C5 on C6 **(Fig. 11.19)**.

6. The physician places the MCP of the right index finger posterior to the right articular pillar of C5 **(Fig. 11.20)**.

7. The physician adjusts flexion or extension as needed to localize all three planes of motion at the dysfunctional segment.

8. With the patient relaxed and not guarding, the physician's right hand (second MCP) directs an arc-like thrust caudally (*white arrow*, **Fig. 11.21**), across the midline in the oblique plane of the C5 facet, engaging the right side bending and right rotational barriers.

9. Effectiveness of the technique is determined by reassessing intersegmental motion at the level of the dysfunctional segment.

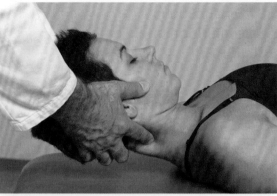
Figure 11.18. Steps 1 to 3.

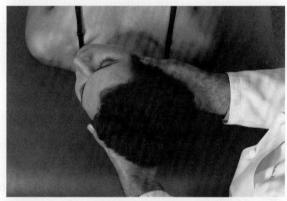
Figure 11.19. Steps 4 and 5.

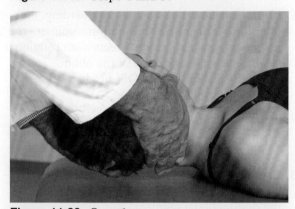
Figure 11.20. Step 6.

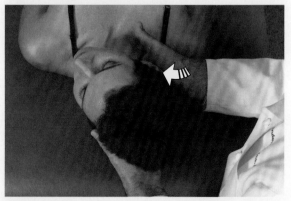
Figure 11.21. Step 8, right side bending impulse.

Thoracic Region

T1–T12 "Neutral" Dysfunctions
Short-Lever, Rotational Emphasis
Ex: T5 NSRRL

 See Video 11.6

1. The patient lies supine with the physician standing at the patient's right side (opposite the rotational component).

2. The physician draws the patient's left arm across the patient's chest and places the right arm below it. This should form a V. The patient grasps the opposite shoulders with the hands **(Fig. 11.22)**.

3. The physician carefully and minimally rolls the patient toward the physician by grasping and lifting the patient's left posterior shoulder girdle.

4. The physician places the right thenar eminence posterior to the upper of the two vertebra of the dysfunctional spinal unit at the left transverse process of T5 **(Fig. 11.23)**.

5. The patient's elbows are directed to the physician's upper abdomen just inferior to the costal arch and xiphoid process.

6. The physician's left hand and arm are placed under the patient's head, neck, and upper thoracic region to add slight tension to the dysfunctional segment (T5). Side bending left in the thoracic spine down to the dysfunction is carried out by gently moving the patient's thoracic region to the left (*white arrow*) **(Fig. 11.24)**.

7. The patient inhales and exhales, and on exhalation, the physician directs slight pressure with the abdomen toward but slightly lateral to the left transverse process of the upper of the two vertebrae involved in this dysfunctional unit (T5) (*white arrow*, **Fig. 11.25**).

8. Effectiveness of the technique is determined by reassessing intersegmental motion at the level of the dysfunctional segment.

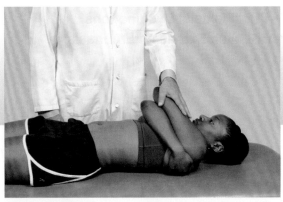

Figure 11.22. Steps 1 and 2.

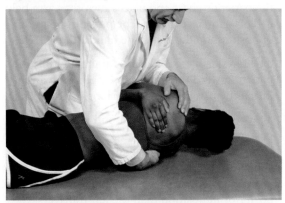

Figure 11.23. Steps 3 and 4.

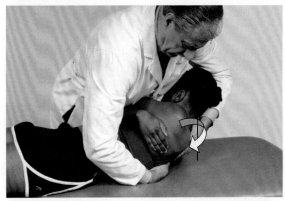

Figure 11.24. Steps 5 and 6.

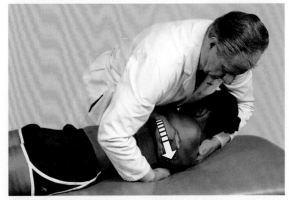

Figure 11.25. Step 7, corrective thrust to T5.

Thoracic Region

T1–T12 "Flexion" Dysfunctions
Short-Lever, Extension Emphasis
Ex: T4 FSRRR

1. The patient lies supine with the physician standing at the patient's right side (same side as the rotational component).

2. The physician draws the patient's left arm across the patient's chest and places the other arm below it. This should form a V. The patient grasps the opposite shoulders with the hands **(Fig. 11.26)**.

3. The physician carefully and minimally rolls the patient toward the physician by grasping and lifting the patient's left posterior shoulder girdle.

4. The physician's right thenar eminence is placed posterior to the left transverse process of T5 (the lower of the two vertebrae of the dysfunctional spinal unit) **(Fig. 11.27)**. *Note*: In this dysfunction, the left transverse process of T5 is relatively more posterior in position than the left transverse process of the dysfunctional segment (T4), whereas the right T4 transverse process is more posterior than the right T5 transverse process.

5. The patient's elbows are directed into the physician's upper abdomen just inferior to the costal arch and xiphoid process.

6. The physician places the left hand and arm under the patient's head and neck to add slight tension in forward bending. Side bending left in the thoracic spine down to and including T4 is carried out by gently moving the patient's thoracic area to the left (*white arrow*, **Fig. 11.28**). The patient inhales and exhales.

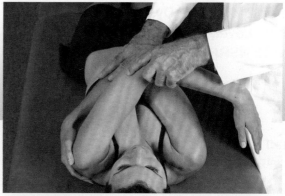

Figure 11.26. Steps 1 and 2.

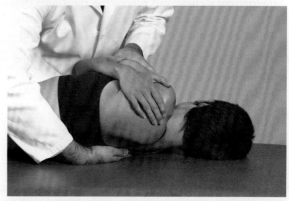

Figure 11.27. Steps 3 and 4.

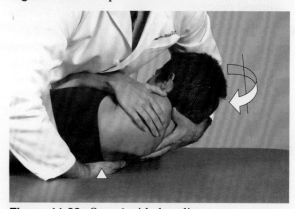

Figure 11.28. Step 6, side bending.

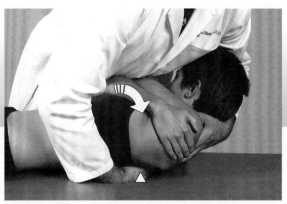

Figure 11.29. Cephalad-directed impulse.

7. On exhalation, an impulse (approximately 1 pound of pressure) is directed with the physician's abdomen toward the upper of the two vertebrae (T4) involved in this dysfunctional unit (T4–T5) (*white arrow*, **Fig. 11.29**).

8. Effectiveness of the technique is determined by reassessing intersegmental motion at the level of the dysfunctional segment.

Figure 11.30 demonstrates the fulcrum principle as used in this technique.

As the flexion and extension HVLA techniques in the supine position are initially counterintuitive to novice medical students, a number of mnemonic acronyms have been used, which we have found helpful. Below are two that are used for (1) direction of the physician's

force and (2) positioning of the physician in relation to a flexion dysfunction's rotational component.

FUEL = **F**lexion **U**pper/**E**xtension **L**ower

Flexion—force is directed to the upper of the two segments involved

Extension—force is directed to the lower of the two segments involved

FOSOB = **F**lexion, **O**pposite **S**ide-**O**ne **B**elow (Fuller D, *Personal Communication* 2014.)

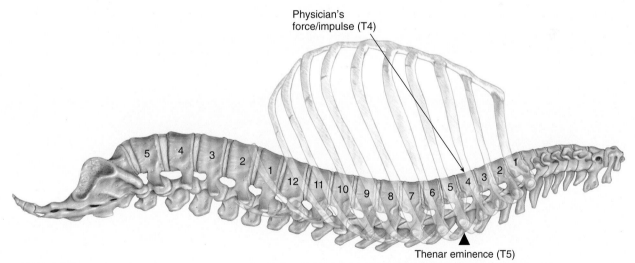

Figure 11.30. Lateral supine view of the human spine illustrating the physician-generated force vector toward T4 and thenar eminence placement at T5 transverse process as fulcrum for T4 somatic dysfunction with a flexion component. (Modified with permission from Tank PW, Gest TR. Lippincott Williams & Wilkins Atlas of Anatomy. Baltimore, MD: Lippincott Williams & Wilkins, 2009.)

Thoracic Region

T1–T12 "Extension" Dysfunctions
Short-Lever, Flexion Emphasis
Ex: T9 ESRRR

 See Video 11.7

1. The patient lies supine with the physician standing at the patient's left side (opposite the rotational component).

2. The physician draws the patient's right arm across the patient's chest and places the other arm below it. This should form a V. The patient grasps the opposite shoulders with the hands **(Fig. 11.31)**.

3. The physician carefully and minimally rolls the patient by grasping and lifting the patient's right posterior shoulder girdle.

4. The physician places the thenar eminence posterior to the upper of the two vertebrae of the dysfunctional spinal unit at the right transverse process (T9) **(Fig. 11.32)**.

5. The patient's elbows are directed to the physician's upper abdomen just inferior to the costal arch and xiphoid process.

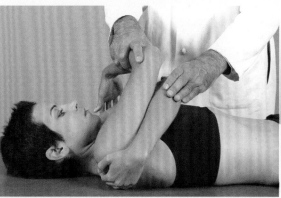

Figure 11.31. Steps 1 and 2.

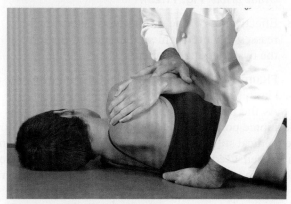

Figure 11.32. Steps 3 and 4.

6. The physician's right hand and arm are placed under the patient's head, neck, and upper thoracic region to add slight tension in forward bending. Side bending left in the thoracic spine down to the dysfunction is carried out by gently moving the patient's thoracic region to the left (*white arrow*, **Fig. 11.33**). The patient inhales and exhales.

7. On exhalation, the physician directs slight pressure with the abdomen toward the lower of the two vertebrae in this dysfunctional spinal unit (T10) (*white arrow*, **Fig. 11.34**).

8. Effectiveness of the technique is determined by reassessing intersegmental motion at the level of the dysfunctional segment.

Figure 11.35 demonstrates the fulcrum principle as used in this technique.

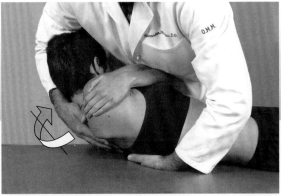

Figure 11.33. Step 6, side bending left.

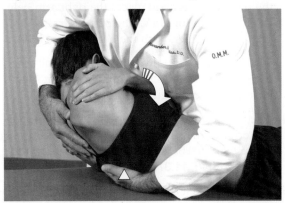

Figure 11.34. Step 7, caudad-directed impulse.

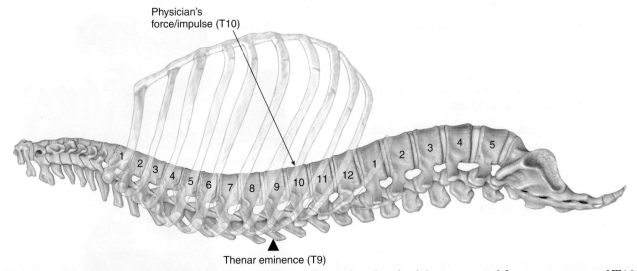

Physician's force/impulse (T10)

Thenar eminence (T9)

Figure 11.35. Lateral supine view of the human spine illustrating the physician-generated force vector toward T10 and thenar eminence placement at T9 transverse process as fulcrum for T9 somatic dysfunction with an extension component. (Modified with permission from Tank PW, Gest TR. Lippincott Williams & Wilkins Atlas of Anatomy. Baltimore, MD: Lippincott Williams & Wilkins, 2009.)

Thoracic Region

T1–T6 "Extension" Dysfunctions
Long-/Short-Lever, Flexion Emphasis
Ex: T4 ESRRR

1. The patient lies supine with the physician standing at the patient's right side (ipsilateral of the rotational component).

2. The physician draws the patient's left arm across the patient's chest and places the right arm below it. This should form a V. The patient grasps the opposite shoulders with the hands **(Fig. 11.36)**.

3. The physician carefully and minimally rolls the patient by grasping and lifting the patient's left posterior shoulder girdle.

4. The physician's right thenar eminence is placed posterior to the left transverse process of the lower of the two vertebrae of the dysfunctional spinal unit (T5) **(Fig. 11.37)**.

5. The patient's elbows are directed to the physician's upper abdomen just inferior to the costal arch and xiphoid process.

6. The physician's left hand/forearm is placed under the patient's head and neck, controlling the patient's upper thoracic spine to add slight tension in forward bending. The physician next produces side bending left by gently moving the patient's thoracic region to the left (*white arrows*) until engaging the upper of the two vertebrae of the dysfunctional unit **(Fig. 11.38)**.

7. The patient inhales and exhales, and on end exhalation, the physician adds a force toward the left transverse process of T5 while minimally flexing the upper thoracic spine by pulling upward toward the ceiling with the left arm and hand (*white arrow*) **(Fig. 11.39)**.

8. The physician's left hand and arm produce a *long-levered* flexion and side bending left effect and, with the right thenar eminence, a *short-levered* rotation left effect by rotating T5 to the right under the dysfunctional, rotated right T4.

9. Effectiveness of the technique is determined by reassessing intersegmental motion at the level of the dysfunctional segment.

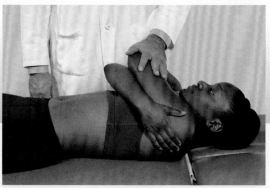

Figure 11.36. Steps 1 and 2.

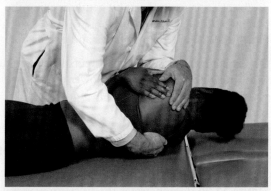

Figure 11.37. Steps 3 and 4, thenar eminence placed under T5.

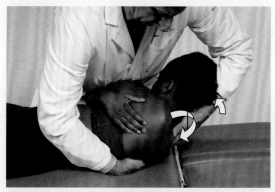

Figure 11.38. Steps 5 and 6.

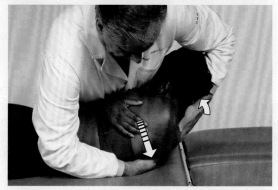

Figure 11.39. Step 7, corrective thrust to T5 with simultaneous traction on the upper thoracic spine.

Thoracic Region

T1–T8 "Flexion" Dysfunctions
Short-Lever, Extension Emphasis
Ex: T2 FSLRL

 See Video 11.8

1. The patient lies supine, and the physician stands at the head of the table.

2. The physician places the flexed left knee on the table with the patient's left T2 area resting on the physician's thigh **(Fig. 11.40)**. For flexion dysfunctions at the lower thoracic range, the physician's thigh is placed more caudally. (*Note*: The side of rotational component determines which thigh is used on which paravertebral side of the patient.)

3. The patient's hands are clasped behind the head with the elbows held outward.

4. The physician's hands pass through the space made by the patient's forearms and upper arms.

5. The physician encircles the patient's rib cage with the fingers over the rib angles posterolaterally **(Fig. 11.41)**.

6. The patient inhales and exhales.

7. At the end of exhalation, the physician quickly but gently pulls the patient's chest downward into the thigh while adding cephalad traction (*white arrow*) **(Fig. 11.42)**.

8. Effectiveness of the technique is determined by reassessing intersegmental motion at the level of the dysfunctional segment.

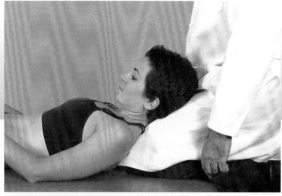

Figure 11.40. Steps 1 and 2.

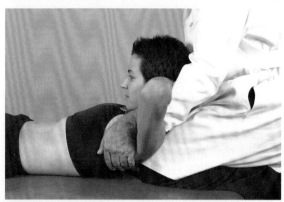

Figure 11.41. Steps 3 to 5.

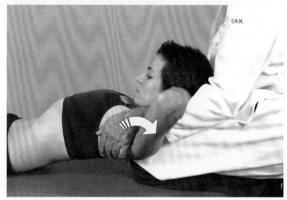

Figure 11.42. Step 7.

Thoracic Region

T3–T8 "Flexion" Dysfunctions
Short-Lever, Side Bending/Extension Emphasis
Ex: T6 FSRRR

 See Video 11.9

May be attempted in neutral dysfunctions but not indicated in extension dysfunctions.

1. The patient lies prone with the head and neck in neutral if possible. A pillow may be placed under the patient's chest and/or abdomen to increase the posterior curve and for increased comfort, especially if performing the technique with a neutral dysfunction.

2. The physician stands at the patient's left for greater efficiency; however, either side may be used **(Fig. 11.43)**.

3. The physician places the right thenar eminence on the right transverse process of T6 with the fingers pointing cephalad. The caudad or cephalad direction of the physician's hands is determined by the side bending barrier.

4. The physician places the left hypothenar eminence on the left transverse process of T6 with the fingers pointing caudally **(Fig. 11.44)**.

5. The patient inhales and exhales, and on exhalation, a thrust impulse is delivered in the direction in which the fingers (*white arrows*, **Fig. 11.45**) are pointing with slightly greater pressure on the right transverse process of T6. *Note*: In a T6 FSLRL (flexion, side bent left, rotated left) dysfunction, the left hand points cephalad and the right caudad, and the force is slightly greater on the left. In a T6 NSRRL (side bent right, rotated left) dysfunction, the hands would be as originally described.

6. Effectiveness of the technique is determined by reassessing intersegmental motion at the level of the dysfunctional segment.

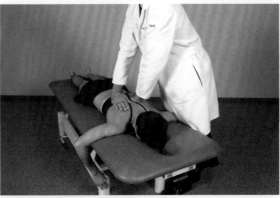

Figure 11.43. Steps 1 and 2.

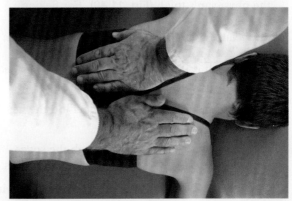

Figure 11.44. Steps 3 and 4.

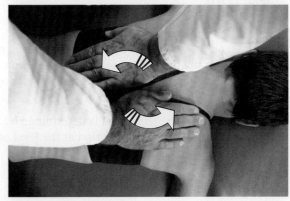

Figure 11.45. Step 5.

Thoracic Region

T1–T4 "Flexion" Dysfunctions
Long-Lever, Rotational Emphasis
Ex: T2 FSRRR

1. The patient lies prone with the head and neck rotated to the left. *Note*: A pillow may be placed under the patient's chest and/or abdomen to increase the posterior curve.

2. The physician stands at the head of the treatment table and side bends the patient's head to the left until palpating motion at the T2–T3 articulation **(Fig. 11.46)**.

3. The physician's left thenar eminence is placed over the left transverse process of T3 as a restrictor and anchor **(Fig. 11.47)**.

4. The physician's right hand is cupped and placed over the left parietooccipital region of the patient's head **(Fig. 11.48)**.

5. The patient inhales and exhales, and on exhalation, a thrust is made by the hand on the head. This is done in a rapidly accelerating manner, creating rotation to the left (*white arrow*, **Fig. 11.49**).

6. Effectiveness of this technique is determined by reassessing intersegmental motion at the level of the dysfunctional segment.

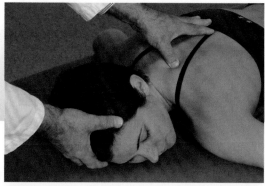

Figure 11.46. Step 2.

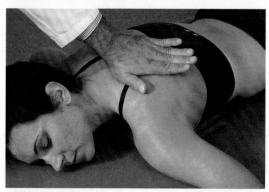

Figure 11.47. Step 3.

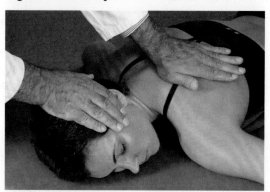

Figure 11.48. Step 4.

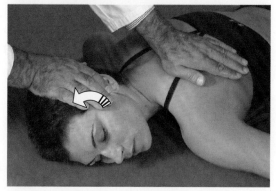

Figure 11.49. Step 5, long-lever rotation left impulse.

Thoracic Region

T1–T4 "Flexion" Dysfunctions
Short-Lever, Side Bending/Rotational Emphasis
Ex: T3 NSRRL

1. The patient lies prone with the head and neck side bent left and rotated right. A pillow should be placed under the patient's chest to enhance the thoracic curve and permit some *freeplay* along the anteroposterior axis **(Fig. 11.50)**.

2. The physician stands at the head of the table and, using the right hand, palpates the right transverse processes of T3 and T4 and places the palm of the left hand over the right parietooccipital region of the patient's head **(Fig. 11.51)**.

3. Using the left hand, the physician carefully rotates the patient's head to the right until the physician's right hand senses this motion over the patient's right T3 transverse process (*white curved arrow*) and stops just before engaging T4 (*white straight arrow*) **(Fig. 11.52)**.

4. The patient inhales and exhales, and on exhalation, a thrust is made by the physician's right thenar eminence onto the patient's right T4 transverse process in an anterior and caudad direction (*white arrow*, **Fig. 11.53**) while holding the head and the tethered T1–T3 segments in a side bending left, rotation right (SLRR) coupled position.

5. The correction is done in a rapidly accelerating manner, creating a side bending left and rotation right (SLRR) effect on the dysfunctional T3, by the relative movement of T4's right transverse process inferior and anterior in its relation to the T3 above.

6. Effectiveness of the technique is determined by reassessing intersegmental motion at the level of the dysfunctional segment.

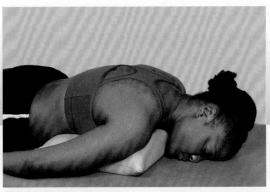

Figure 11.50. Step 1.

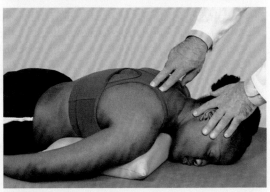

Figure 11.51. Step 2.

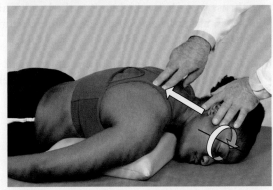

Figure 11.52. Step 3, rotate the head/neck to the right to engage T3.

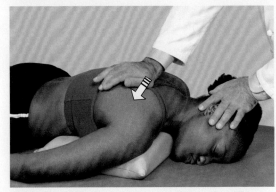

Figure 11.53. Step 4, thrust directed to T4.

Thoracic Region

T8–T12 "Extension" Dysfunctions
Short-Lever, Rotational Emphasis
Ex: T9 ESRRR

 See Video 11.10

1. The patient is seated straddling the table with the posterior aspect of the pelvis at one end so that the patient is facing the length of the table.

2. The physician stands behind the patient on the side opposite the rotational component of the dysfunction (left side in this RR case).

3. The patient places the right hand behind the neck and the left hand on the right elbow **(Fig. 11.54)**. (*Note*: Both hands can be placed behind the neck if this is more comfortable.)

4. The physician places the left hand under the patient's left axilla and on top of the patient's right upper arm.

5. The physician places the right thenar eminence paravertebrally over the right T9 transverse process **(Fig. 11.55)**.

6. The patient is told to relax, and the physician carries the patient into slight forward bending and left side bending until T9 begins to move.

7. The patient inhales deeply and on exhalation is carried into left rotation while slight flexion and left side bending are maintained.

8. The patient again inhales, and on exhalation, the physician quickly and minimally pulls the patient through the left rotational barrier **(Fig. 11.56)** while the right hand imparts an impulse on T9 (*white arrow*, **Fig. 11.57**) causing an HVLA effect in left rotation.

9. Effectiveness of the technique is determined by reassessing intersegmental motion at the level of the dysfunctional segment.

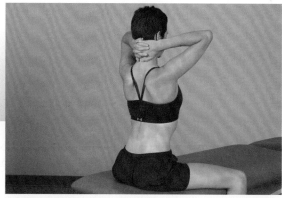

Figure 11.54. Steps 1 to 3.

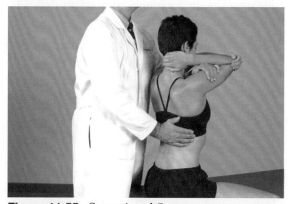

Figure 11.55. Steps 4 and 5.

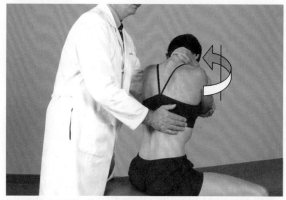

Figure 11.56. Step 8, barrier.

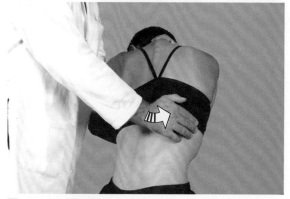

Figure 11.57. Step 8, impulse.

Thoracic Region

T8–T12 "Extension" Dysfunctions
Long-Lever, Rotational Emphasis
Ex: T10 ESRRR

 See Video 11.10

1. The patient is seated straddling the table with the posterior aspect of the pelvis at one end, facing the length of the table.

2. The physician stands behind the patient on the side opposite the rotational component (left side in this RR case).

3. The patient places the right hand behind the neck and the left hand on the right elbow **(Fig. 11.58)**. (*Note*: Both hands can be placed behind the neck if this is more comfortable.)

4. The physician places the left hand under the patient's left axilla and on top of the patient's right upper arm.

5. The physician places the heel of the right hand midline and supraspinously on the lower of the two dysfunctional segments (T11) **(Fig. 11.59)**.

6. The patient is told to relax, and the physician carries the patient into slight forward bending and left side bending until T10 begins to move.

7. The patient inhales deeply and on exhalation is carried into left rotation (*white arrow*, **Fig. 11.60**) while slight flexion and left side bending are maintained.

8. At the restrictive barrier, the patient inhales and exhales. On exhalation, the physician pulls the patient through the left rotational barrier (*white arrow*, **Fig. 11.61**), maintaining pressure on T11 with the right hand to allow T10 to rotate through its barrier while preventing motion at T11.

9. Effectiveness of the technique is determined by reassessing intersegmental motion at the level of the dysfunctional segment.

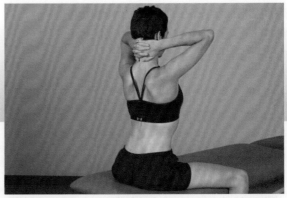
Figure 11.58. Steps 1 to 3.

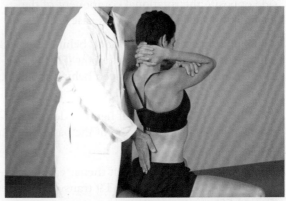
Figure 11.59. Steps 4 and 5.

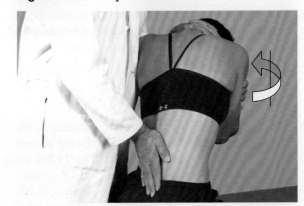
Figure 11.60. Step 7, barrier.

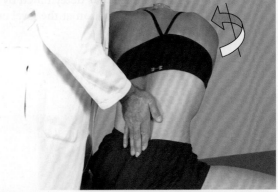
Figure 11.61. Step 8, long-lever direction of force.

Thoracic Region

T4–T12 "Flexion" Dysfunctions
Short-Lever, Extension/Rotational Emphasis
Ex: T6 FSRRR

1. The patient sits, and the physician stands behind the patient.

2. The patient's right arm is crossed over the left (they should form a V) in order to move the right scapula more laterally, and the physician's foot is placed on the table behind the patient **(Fig. 11.62)**.

3. The physician's knee is placed over the left side of the lower of the two segments involved in the dysfunction (T7) with a pillow or rolled up towel between the knee and the patient's thoracic spine **(Fig. 11.63)**.

4. The physician's hands are cupped under the patient's olecranon processes, and controlling the patient's trunk, the physician side bends the patient to the left while pulling backward and slightly superior **(Fig. 11.64)**. Pressure is maintained with the knee.

5. The patient inhales and exhales.

6. At the end of exhalation, the physician quickly but gently directs a force superior and posterior through the patient's elbows (*white dashed arrow*) **(Fig. 11.65)** while maintaining pressure with the knee (*arrow*) on the left transverse process of T7. This causes an extension of T6 on T7 while rotating and side bending T6 to the left.

7. Effectiveness of this technique is determined by reassessing intersegmental motion at the level of the dysfunctional segment.

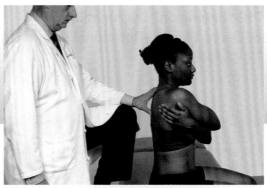

Figure 11.62. Steps 1 and 2.

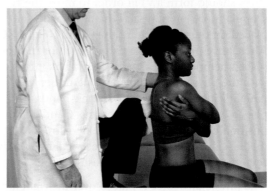

Figure 11.63. Step 3.

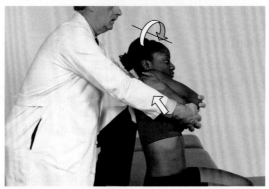

Figure 11.64. Step 4, side bending left with slight extension.

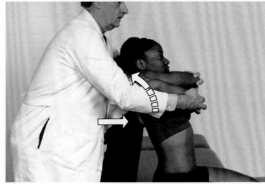

Figure 11.65. Step 6, T6, extended, rotated, and side bent to the left.

Thoracic Region

T4–T12 "Extension" Dysfunctions
Short-Lever, Flexion/Rotational Emphasis
Ex: T7 ESRRR

1. The patient sits, and the physician stands behind the patient.

2. The patient's right arm is crossed over the left (they should form a V) in order to move the right scapula more laterally, and the physician's foot is placed on the table behind the patient **(Fig. 11.66)**. Alternative position: The patient's hands may be placed behind the neck with the fingers interlocked with the physician's arms reaching under the patient's axillae and the physician's hands placed over the patient's forearms. Caution! This position can cause increased flexion stress on the myofascial components of the cervical and thoracic region and the intervertebral discs (5).

3. The physician's knee is placed over the right side of the upper of the two segments involved in the dysfunction (T7) with a pillow or rolled up towel between the knee and the patient's thoracic spine **(Fig. 11.67)**.

4. The physician's hands are cupped under the patient's olecranon processes and, controlling the patient's trunk, side bends the patient to the left while pulling backward and slightly superior **(Fig. 11.68)**. Pressure is maintained with the knee.

5. The patient inhales and exhales.

6. At the end of exhalation, the physician quickly but gently directs a force inferior and posterior through the patient's elbows toward T8 (*white dashed arrow*) **(Fig. 11.69)** while maintaining pressure with the knee (*arrow*) on the right transverse process of T6. This causes a flexion of T7 on T8 while rotating and side bending T7 to the left.

7. Effectiveness of this technique is determined by reassessing intersegmental motion at the level of the dysfunctional segment.

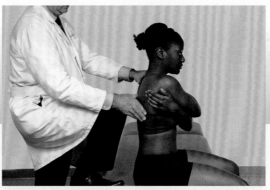

Figure 11.66. Steps 1 and 2.

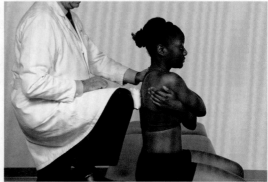

Figure 11.67. Step 3, knee contacts T6 right transverse process.

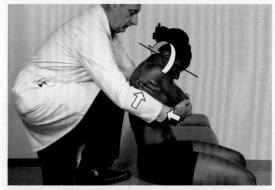

Figure 11.68. Step 4, side bending left with slight extension.

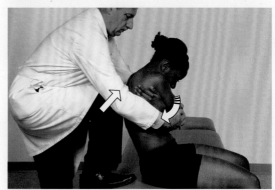

Figure 11.69. Step 6, the physician's force directed to T7 resulting in flexion of T6 on T7.

Costal Region

Rib 1, Rib 2 Inhalation Dysfunctions
Seated Short-Lever, Exhalation Emphasis
Ex: Right Rib 1 Inhaled/Elevated

 See Video 11.11

1. The patient sits on the table with the physician standing behind the patient.

2. The physician places the shoeless left foot on the table at the patient's left, so that the patient's left axilla is supported by the physician's left thigh **(Fig. 11.70)**.

3. The physician places the left hand on top of the patient's head with the forearm alongside of the patient's face.

4. The physician places the thumb or second MCP of the right hand superior and posterior to the angle of the dysfunctional right first rib.

5. The physician side bends the patient's head and neck to the right and rotates to the left until the motion barrier is met **(Fig. 11.71)**. (In some patients, rotation right may be appropriate.)

6. The patient inhales and exhales. During exhalation, further side bending and rotational slack are taken up.

7. At the end of exhalation, a force is directed with the physician's thumb (or second MCP) downward and forward toward the patient's left nipple (*white arrow*, **Fig. 11.72**).

8. Effectiveness of the technique is determined by reassessing motion of the dysfunctional rib.

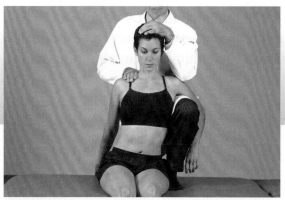
Figure 11.70. Steps 1 and 2.

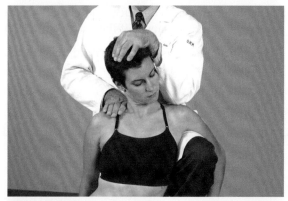
Figure 11.71. Steps 3 to 5.

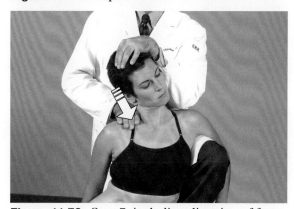
Figure 11.72. Step 7, including direction of force.

Costal Region

Rib 1, Rib 2 Inhalation Dysfunctions
Supine Short-Lever, Exhalation Emphasis
Ex: Left Rib 1 Inhaled/Elevated

1. The patient is supine, and the physician sits or stands at the patient's head.

2. The physician places the right hand along the patient's right temporoparietal area **(Fig. 11.73)**.

3. The physician places the left second MCP superior and posterior to the angle of the dysfunctional rib.

4. The patient's head is slightly forward bent, rotated right, and side bent left with the control of the physician's right hand **(Fig. 11.74)**.

5. The patient inhales and exhales.

6. At the end of exhalation, the physician's left hand directs a caudal and medial thrust (*white arrow*, **Fig. 11.75**) toward the patient's right nipple.

7. Effectiveness of the technique is determined by reassessing motion of the dysfunctional rib.

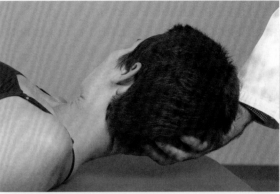

Figure 11.73. Steps 1 and 2.

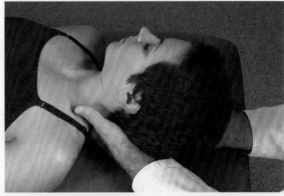

Figure 11.74. Steps 3 and 4.

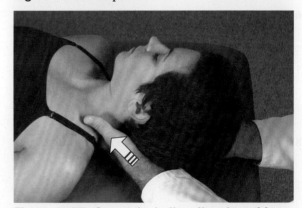

Figure 11.75. Step 6, including direction of force.

Costal Region

Rib 3–Rib 10 Inhalation Dysfunctions
Short-Lever, Exhalation Emphasis
Ex: Left Rib 6 Inhaled/Elevated

 See Video 11.12

1. The patient is supine, and the physician stands at the side of the table opposite the side of the rib dysfunction.

2. The physician draws the patient's arm on the side of the rib dysfunction across the patient's rib cage with the patient's other arm below it. The patient's arms should form a V **(Fig. 11.76)**.

3. The physician slightly rolls the patient toward the physician by gently pulling the left posterior shoulder girdle forward.

4. The physician places the thenar eminence of the right hand posterior and superior to the angle of the dysfunctional rib **(Fig. 11.77)**.

5. The patient is rolled back over the physician's hand, and the surface created by the patient's crossed arms rests against the physician's chest or abdomen.

6. Pressure is directed through the patient's chest wall, localizing at the thenar eminence.

7. The patient inhales and exhales, and at the end of exhalation, a thrust impulse (*white arrows*, **Figs. 11.78 and 11.79**) is delivered through the patient's chest wall slightly cephalad to the thenar eminence.

8. Effectiveness of the technique is determined by reassessing motion of the dysfunctional rib.

Note: This technique is vectoring through the bucket-handle axis, not the pump-handle axis!

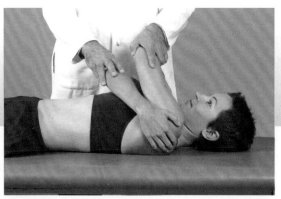

Figure 11.76. Steps 1 and 2.

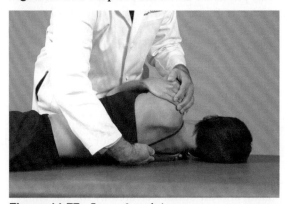

Figure 11.77. Steps 3 and 4.

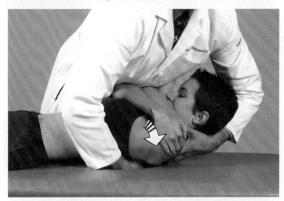

Figure 11.78. Steps 5 to 7, including direction of force.

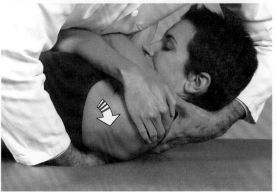

Figure 11.79. Steps 5 to 7, including direction of force.

Costal Region

Rib 3–Rib 10 Exhalation Dysfunctions
Short-Lever, Inhalation Emphasis
Ex: Left Rib 8 Exhaled/Depressed

See Video 11.13

1. The patient lies supine, and the physician stands at the side of the table opposite the side of the rib dysfunction.

2. The physician draws the patient's arm on the side of the dysfunction across the patient's rib cage with the patient's other arm below it. The patient's arms should form a V **(Fig. 11.80)**.

3. The physician slightly rolls the patient toward the physician by gently pulling the left posterior shoulder girdle forward.

4. The physician places the thenar eminence of the right hand posterior and inferior to the angle of the dysfunctional rib **(Fig. 11.81)**.

5. The patient is rolled back over the physician's hand, and the surface created by the patient's crossed arms rests against the physician's chest or abdomen.

6. Gentle pressure is directed through the patient's chest wall, localizing at the physician's thenar eminence.

7. The patient inhales and exhales, and at the end of exhalation, a thrust impulse (*white arrows*, **Figs. 11.82 and 11.83**) is delivered through the patient's chest wall slightly caudad to the physician's thenar eminence.

8. Effectiveness of the technique is determined by reassessing motion of the dysfunctional rib.

Note: This technique is vectoring through the bucket-handle axis, not the pump-handle axis!

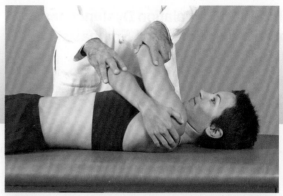

Figure 11.80. Steps 1 and 2.

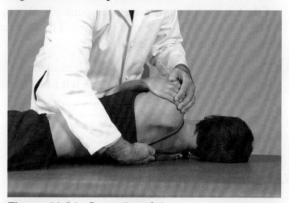

Figure 11.81. Steps 3 and 4.

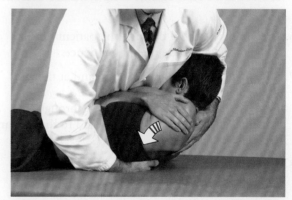

Figure 11.82. Steps 5 to 7, including direction of force.

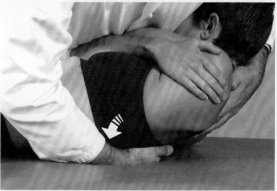

Figure 11.83. Steps 5 to 7, including direction of force.

Costal Region

Rib 11, Rib 12 Inhalation Dysfunctions
Short-Lever, Exhalation Emphasis
Ex: Right Rib 12 Inhaled/Dorsal

 See Video 11.14

1. The patient lies prone on the table.

2. The physician stands at the left side of the table and positions the patient's legs 15 to 20 degrees to the right to take tension off the quadratus lumborum, which attaches to the inferior medial aspect of rib 12 **(Fig. 11.84)**.

3. The physician places the left hypothenar eminence medial and inferior to the angle of the dysfunctional rib and exerts gentle sustained lateral and cephalad traction.

4. The physician's right hand may grasp the patient's right anterior superior iliac spine to stabilize the pelvis **(Fig. 11.85)**.

5. The patient inhales and exhales deeply.

6. During exhalation, the physician's left hand applies a cephalad and lateral HVLA thrust impulse (*white arrow*, **Fig. 11.86**).

7. Success of the technique is determined by reassessing motion of the dysfunctional rib.

Note: This technique is commonly done after performing the muscle energy respiratory assist technique for ribs 11 and 12 held in inhalation.

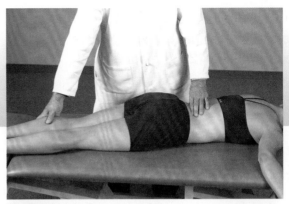

Figure 11.84. Steps 1 and 2.

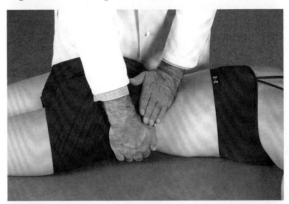

Figure 11.85. Steps 3 and 4.

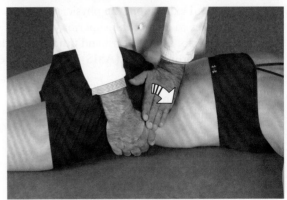

Figure 11.86. Steps 5 to 6, including direction of force.

Costal Region

**Rib 11, Rib 12 Exhalation Dysfunctions
Long-Lever, Inhalation Emphasis
Ex: Right Rib 12 Exhaled/Ventral**

 See Video 11.14

1. The patient lies prone on the table.

2. The physician stands at the left side of the table and positions the patient's legs 15 to 20 degrees to the left to put tension on the quadratus lumborum, which attaches to the inferior medial aspect of rib 12 **(Fig. 11.87)**.

3. The physician places the left thenar (or hypothenar) eminence on the rib immediately superior and lateral to the angle of the dysfunctional rib exerting a gentle downward force in order to anchor it and prevent it from moving with the mobilizing force.

4. The physician's right hand grasps the patient's right anterior superior iliac spine and gently lifts toward the ceiling **(Fig. 11.88)**.

5. The patient inhales and exhales deeply.

6. During the end exhalation, the physician's left hand continues to anchor the superior, non-dysfunctional rib, as the right hand quickly lifts the anterior superior iliac spine (ASIS) up toward the ceiling **(Fig. 11.89)**.

7. Success of the technique is determined by reassessing motion of the dysfunctional rib.

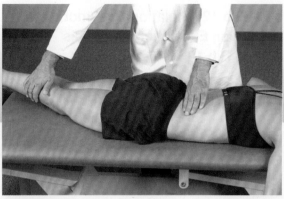
Figure 11.87. Steps 1 and 2.

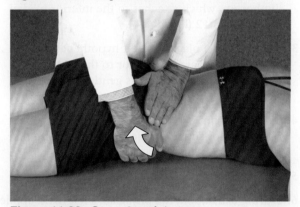
Figure 11.88. Steps 3 and 4.

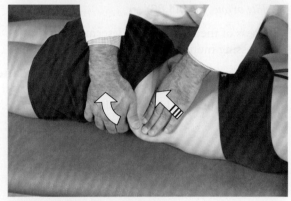
Figure 11.89. Steps 5 and 6.

Lumbar Region

L1–L5 "Type I/Neutral" Dysfunctions
Long-Lever, Rotational/Side bending Emphasis
Ex: L5 NSLRR

 See Video 11.15

1. The patient lies in the right lateral recumbent (side lying) position with the physician standing at the side of the table facing the patient.

2. The physician palpates between the spinous processes of L5 and S1 and flexes the patient's knees and hips until L5 is in a neutral position relative to S1 **(Fig. 11.90)**.

3. The physician further positions the patient's left leg so that it drops over the side of the table cephalad to the right leg. The patient's foot must not touch the floor **(Fig. 11.91)**.

4. While continuing to palpate L5, the physician places the cephalad hand in the patient's left antecubital fossa while resting the forearm gently on the patient's anterior pectoral and shoulder region.

5. The physician places the caudad forearm along a line between the patient's left posterior superior iliac spine (PSIS) and greater trochanter **(Fig. 11.92)**.

6. The patient's pelvis is rotated anteriorly to the edge of the restrictive barrier, and the patient's shoulder and thoracic spine are rotated posteriorly to the edge of the restrictive barrier. The patient inhales and exhales, and during exhalation, further rotational slack is taken up.

7. If the rotational slack or motion barrier is not effectively met, the physician can grasp the patient's right arm, drawing the shoulder forward until rotational movement is palpated between L5 and S1.

8. With the patient relaxed and not guarded, the physician delivers an impulse thrust with the caudad forearm directed at right angles to the patient's spine while simultaneously moving the shoulder slightly cephalad and the pelvis and sacrum caudad (*white arrows*, **Fig. 11.93**) to impart side bending right and rotation left movement.

9. Effectiveness of the technique is determined by reassessing intersegmental motion at the level of the dysfunctional segment.

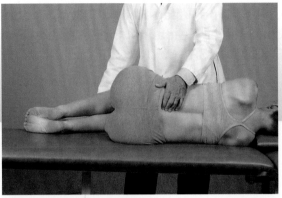
Figure 11.90. Steps 1 and 2.

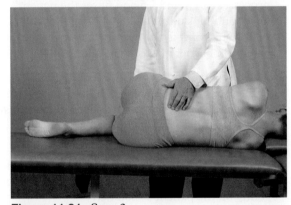
Figure 11.91. Step 3.

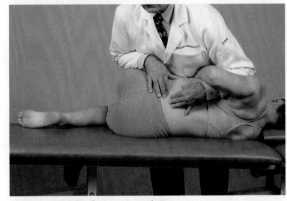
Figure 11.92. Steps 4 and 5.

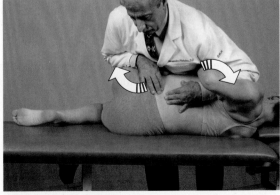
Figure 11.93. Step 8.

Lumbar Region

L1–L5 "Type II/Non-Neutral" Dysfunctions
Long-Lever, Rotational/Side Bending Emphasis
Ex: L4 FRRSR

 See Video 11.16

1. The patient lies in the right lateral recumbent position with the physician standing at the side of the table facing the patient.

2. The physician palpates between the spinous processes of L4 and L5 and flexes the patient's knees and hips until L4 is in a neutral position relative to L5. It is not necessary to meet the extension barrier at this point **(Fig. 11.94)**.

3. The physician further positions the patient's left leg so that it drops over the side of the table cephalad to the right leg. The patient's foot must not touch the floor **(Fig. 11.95)**.

4. While continuing to palpate L4, the physician places the cephalad hand in the antecubital fossa of the patient's left arm while resting the forearm gently on the patient's shoulder.

5. The physician's caudad hand stabilizes L5 **(Fig. 11.96)**.

6. The patient's shoulder and pelvis are axially rotated in opposite directions. The patient inhales and exhales, and during exhalation, further rotational slack is taken up.

7. If the rotational slack or motion barrier is not effectively met, the physician can grasp the patient's right arm, drawing the shoulder forward until rotational movement is palpated between L4 and L5.

8. With the patient relaxed and not guarded, the physician delivers an impulse with the forearms (*white arrows*, **Fig. 11.97**), simultaneously moving the shoulder slightly caudad and the pelvis and sacrum cephalad.

9. Effectiveness of the technique is determined by reassessing intersegmental motion at the level of the dysfunctional segment.

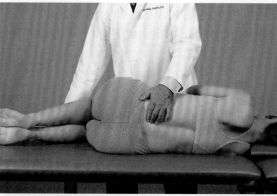

Figure 11.94. Steps 1 and 2.

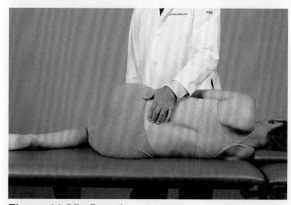

Figure 11.95. Step 3.

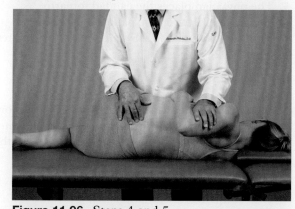

Figure 11.96. Steps 4 and 5.

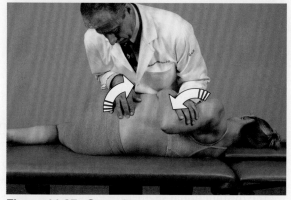

Figure 11.97. Steps 8.

Lumbar Region

L1–L5 Dysfunction with Radicular Symptoms
Long-Lever, Traction/Gapping Emphasis
Ex: Left, L5/S1 Radiculitis

 See Video 11.17

Clinical presentation as to the severity of symptoms or a particular neurologic deficit may contraindicate this technique.

1. The patient is in the right lateral recumbent position with the physician standing at the side of the table facing the patient.

2. The physician palpates between the patient's spinous processes of L5–S1 and flexes the patient's hips and knees until L5 is fully flexed in relation to S1 **(Fig. 11.98)**.

3. The physician positions the patient's left leg so that it drops over the side of the table cephalad to the right leg. The patient's leg should not touch the floor **(Fig. 11.99)**.

4. While continuing to palpate L5, the physician places the cephalad hand in the patient's antecubital fossa of the left arm while resting the forearm gently on the patient's shoulder.

5. The physician places the caudad forearm in a line between the patient's PSIS and greater trochanter **(Fig. 11.100)**.

6. The physician's arms move apart to introduce a separation of L5 and S1 on the left side. This causes distraction, or joint gapping, of L5 and S1.

7. The patient, relaxed and not guarding, inhales and exhales. During exhalation, the physician delivers an impulse that separates L5 from S1 (*white arrows*, **Fig. 11.101**) without permitting rotation or torsion.

8. Effectiveness of the technique is determined by reassessing the severity of radicular symptoms.

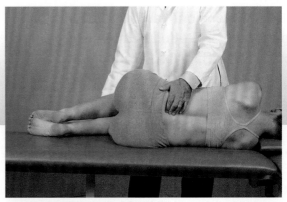
Figure 11.98. Steps 1 and 2.

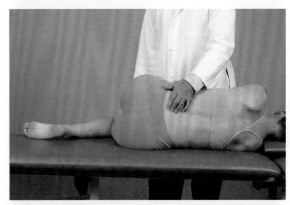
Figure 11.99. Step 3.

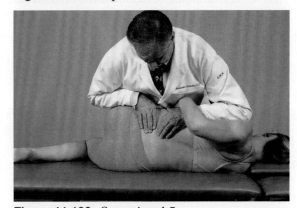
Figure 11.100. Steps 4 and 5.

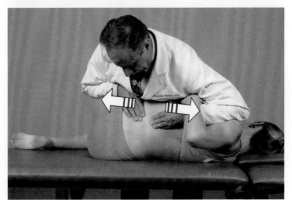
Figure 11.101. Steps 6 and 7.

Lumbar Region

L1–L5 "Extension/Neutral" Dysfunctions
Long-Lever, Rotational Emphasis
Ex: L4 NSLRR, "Walk-Around"

 See Video 11.18

1. The patient lies supine with both hands behind the neck and the fingers interlaced.

2. The physician stands at the head of the table to the patient's right and slides the right forearm through the space created by the patient's flexed right arm and shoulder.

3. The dorsal aspect of the physician's hand is carefully placed at midsternum on the patient's chest wall **(Fig. 11.102)**.

4. The physician then walks around the head of the table to the left side of the patient.

5. The physician, while palpating posteriorly with the caudad hand, side bends the patient's trunk to the right until L4 begins to move.

6. The physician begins to rotate the patient to the left while continuing to maintain the original side bending **(Fig. 11.103)**.

7. The physician's caudad hand anchors the patient's pelvis by placing the palm on the patient's right ASIS.

8. With the patient relaxed and not guarding, the physician directs an impulse that pulls the patient minimally into further left rotation (*white arrows*, **Fig. 11.104**).

9. Effectiveness of the technique is determined by reassessing intersegmental motion at the level of the dysfunctional segment.

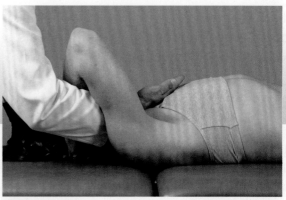
Figure 11.102. Steps 1 to 3.

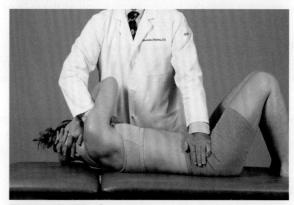
Figure 11.103. Steps 4 to 6.

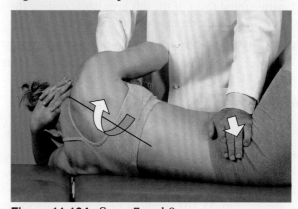
Figure 11.104. Steps 7 and 8.

Lumbar Region

L1–L5 Dysfunctions
Short-Lever, Rotational Emphasis
Ex: L2 ESRRR

 See Video 11.19

1. The patient sits, preferably straddling and facing the length of the table, to restrict the sacrum and pelvis.

2. The physician stands behind and to the left of the patient.

3. The patient places the right hand behind the neck and the left hand on the right elbow (both hands can be placed behind the neck if this is more comfortable) **(Fig. 11.105)**.

4. The physician passes the left hand under the patient's left axilla and on top of the patient's right upper arm.

5. The physician places the right thenar eminence or palm on the paravertebral muscles over the L2 right transverse process **(Fig. 11.106)**.

6. The patient is instructed to relax as the physician positions the patient into slight forward bending and then left side bending until motion is palpated at L2.

7. The patient inhales deeply, and on exhalation, the patient is positioned into left rotation (while the slight flexion and left side bending are maintained) **(Fig. 11.107)**.

8. With the patient relaxed and not guarding, the physician directs an impulse force, pulling the patient minimally through further left rotation while directing a short lever thrust on L2 with the right hand (*white arrows*, **Fig. 11.108**).

9. Effectiveness of the technique is determined by reassessing intersegmental motion at the level of the dysfunctional segment.

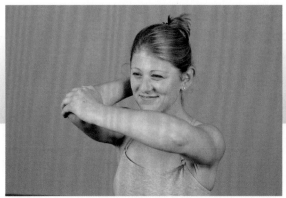

Figure 11.105. Steps 1 to 3.

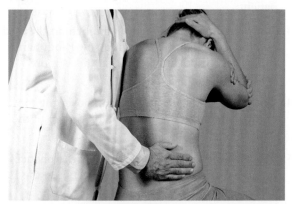

Figure 11.106. Steps 4 and 5.

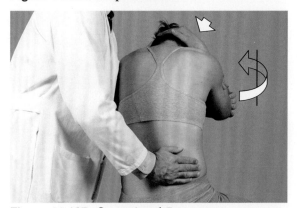

Figure 11.107. Steps 6 and 7.

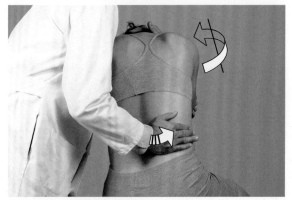

Figure 11.108. Step 8.

Lumbar Region

L1–L5 Dysfunctions
Long-Lever, Rotational Emphasis
Ex: L2 ESRRR

 See Video 11.19

1. The patient sits, preferably straddling and facing the length of the table, to restrict the sacrum and pelvis.

2. The physician stands behind and to the left of the patient.

3. The patient places the right hand behind the neck and the left hand on the right elbow (both hands can be placed behind the neck if this is more comfortable) **(Fig. 11.109)**.

4. The physician passes the left hand over the top of the patient's left upper arm and on top of the patient's right upper arm.

5. The physician places the right thenar eminence or palm midline at the interspace between the L2 and L3 spinous processes **(Fig. 11.110)**.

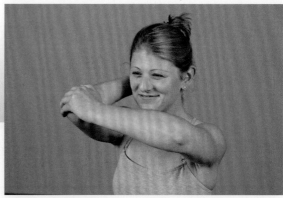

Figure 11.109. Steps 1 to 3.

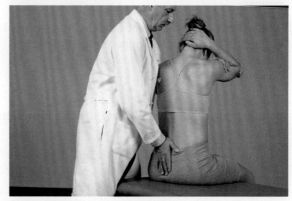

Figure 11.110. Steps 4 and 5.

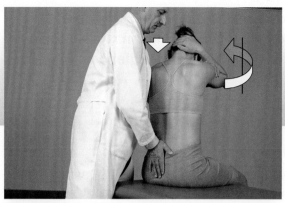

Figure 11.111. Steps 6 and 7.

6. The patient is instructed to relax, and the physician positions the patient into slight forward bending and left side bending until motion is palpated at L2.

7. The patient inhales deeply, and on exhalation, the patient is positioned into left rotation while slight flexion and left side bending are maintained **(Fig. 11.111)**.

8. With the patient relaxed and not guarding, the physician's right hand stabilizes L3 (*white arrow*), as the physician's left hand pulls the patient into further left rotation *(white pulsed arrow)* (this rotates L2 to the left in relation to L3) **(Fig. 11.112)**.

9. Effectiveness of the technique is determined by reassessing intersegmental motion at the level of the dysfunctional segment.

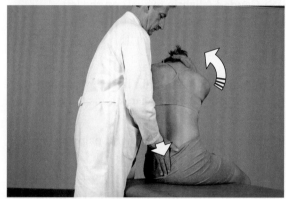

Figure 11.112. Step 8.

Pelvic Region

Iliosacral (Innominate) Dysfunction
Ex: Left, Posterior Innominate Rotation
Short-Lever, Anterior Rotational Emphasis

 See Video 11.20

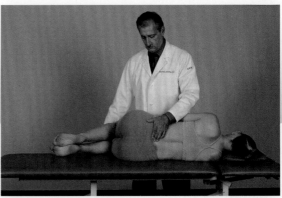

Figure 11.113. Steps 1 to 3.

Diagnosis

Standing flexion test: Positive (left PSIS rises)
Loss of passively induced left sacroiliac motion
ASIS: Cephalad (slightly lateral) on the left
PSIS: Caudad (slightly medial) on the left
Sacral sulcus: Deep, anterior on the left

Technique

1. The patient is in the right lateral recumbent position, and the physician stands facing the patient.

2. The physician's cephalad hand palpates between the patient's spinous processes of L5 and S1.

3. The physician's caudad hand flexes the patient's knees and hips until the L5 and S1 spinous processes separate **(Fig. 11.113)**.

4. The physician maintains the left leg in this position and instructs the patient to straighten the right leg, placing the left foot just distal to the right popliteal fossa.

5. The physician places the cephalad hand on the patient's left antecubital fossa with the forearm resting on the patient's left anterior shoulder **(Fig. 11.114)**.

6. Use one of the following techniques:
   a. Using the caudad hand, the physician places the palmar aspect of the hypothenar eminence on the left PSIS with the fourth and fifth digits encompassing the left posterior iliac crest **(Fig. 11.115)**.

or

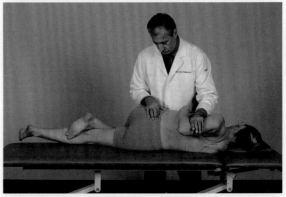

Figure 11.114. Steps 4 and 5.

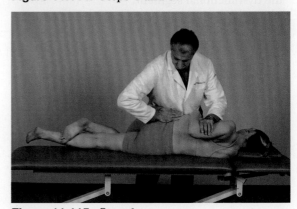

Figure 11.115. Step 6a.

b. Using the caudad arm, the physician places the ventral aspect of the forearm on the left PSIS and left posterior iliac crest **(Fig. 11.116)**.

or

c. The physician, standing at the level of the patient's shoulder and facing the patient's pelvis, places the forearm of the caudad arm on the left PSIS and left posterior iliac crest **(Fig. 11.117)**.

7. The physician introduces axial rotation in the opposing direction by gently pushing the patient's left shoulder posterior and rolling the pelvis anterior. These motions should be continued until movement of the left sacrum is palpated at the left SI joint.

8. With the patient relaxed and not guarding, the physician delivers an impulse with the right hand or forearm (*white arrow*, **Fig. 11.118**) toward the patient's umbilicus.

9. Effectiveness of the technique is determined by reassessing left sacroiliac joint motion.

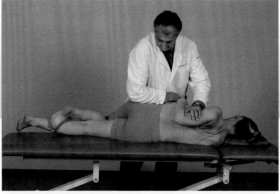

Figure 11.116. Step 6b.

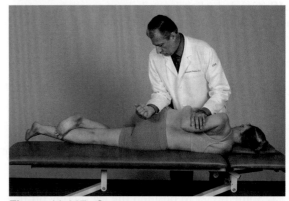

Figure 11.117. Step 6c.

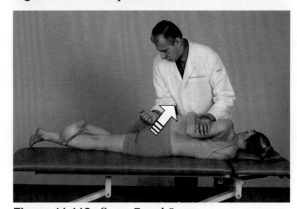

Figure 11.118. Steps 7 and 8.

Pelvic Region

Iliosacral (Innominate) Dysfunction
Ex: Right, Posterior Innominate Rotation
Traction, Anterior Rotational Emphasis

 See Video 11.21

Diagnosis

Standing flexion test: Positive (right PSIS rises)
Loss of passively induced right sacroiliac motion
ASIS: Cephalad (slightly lateral) on the right
PSIS: Caudad (slightly medial) on the right
Sacral sulcus: Deep, anterior on the right

Technique

1. The patient is supine, and the physician stands at the foot of the table.

2. The physician grasps the patient's right ankle.

3. The physician raises the patient's right leg no more than 30 degrees and applies traction down the shaft of the leg (*white arrow*, **Fig. 11.119**).
   a. Some prefer to position the leg slightly off the side of the table approximately 10 to 20 degrees (**Fig. 11.120**).

4. This traction is maintained as the patient is asked to take three to five slow breaths.

5. At the end of the last breath, the physician delivers a thrust in the direction of the traction (*white arrow*, **Fig. 11.121**).

6. Effectiveness of the technique is determined by reassessing right sacroiliac joint motion.

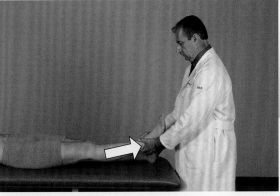

Figure 11.119. Steps 1 to 3.

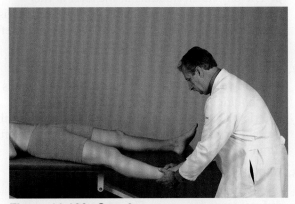

Figure 11.120. Step 3a.

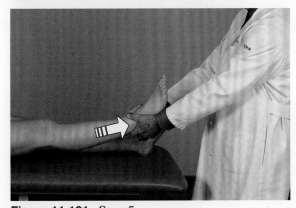

Figure 11.121. Step 5.

Pelvic Region

Iliosacral (Innominate) Dysfunction
Ex: Left, Posterior Innominate Rotation
Long-Lever with Fulcrum, Rotational Emphasis

 See Video 11.22

Diagnosis

Standing flexion test: Positive (left PSIS rises)
Loss of passively induced left sacroiliac motion
ASIS: Cephalad (slightly lateral) on the left
PSIS: Caudad (slightly medial) on the left
Sacral sulcus: Deep, anterior on the left

Technique

1. The patient is supine, and the physician stands to the patient's right.

2. The physician flexes the patient's knees and hips.

3. The physician rolls the patient's legs toward the physician.

4. The physician places the thenar eminence of the cephalad hand under the patient's left PSIS to serve as a fulcrum against which to move the innominate **(Fig. 11.122)**.

5. The physician rolls the patient onto the left PSIS with the patient's weight directly over the fulcrum (*white arrow*, **Fig. 11.123**).

6. The patient extends the left knee and then slowly lowers the leg toward the table (*white arrows*, **Figs. 11.124 and 11.125**), causing a short and long levering of the left innominate.

7. Effectiveness of the technique is determined by reassessing left sacroiliac joint motion.

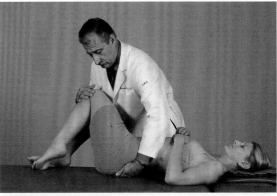
Figure 11.122. Steps 1 to 4.

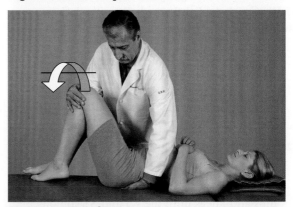
Figure 11.123. Step 5.

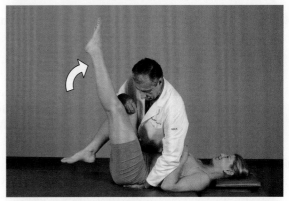
Figure 11.124. Steps 5 and 6.

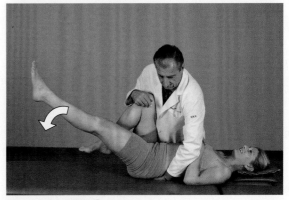
Figure 11.125. Step 6.

Pelvic Region

Iliosacral (Innominate) Dysfunction
Ex: Left, Anterior Innominate Rotation
Short-Lever, Rotational Emphasis

 See Video 11.23

Diagnosis

Standing flexion test: Positive (left PSIS rises)
Loss of passively induced left sacroiliac motion
PSIS: Cephalad (slightly lateral) on the left
ASIS: Caudad (slightly medial) on the left
Sacral sulcus: Posterior on the left

Technique

1. The patient is in the right lateral recumbent position, and the physician stands at the side of the table facing the patient **(Fig. 11.126)**.

2. The physician palpates between the spinous processes of L5 and S1 with the cephalad hand.

3. The physician's caudad hand flexes the patient's hips and knees until the L5 and S1 spinous processes separate.

4. The physician positions the patient's left leg so that it drops off the side of the table, over and slightly more flexed than the right leg. The patient's foot should not touch the floor.

5. The physician places the caudad forearm in a line between the patient's left PSIS and trochanter and the cephalad hand or forearm on the patient's left shoulder **(Fig. 11.127)**.

6. The physician introduces axial rotation in opposing directions by gently pushing the patient's left shoulder dorsally (posteriorly) and rolling the pelvis ventrally (anteriorly) (*white arrow*, **Fig. 11.128**). These motions should be continued until movement of the sacrum is palpated at the left sacroiliac joint.

7. If no motion is felt, the physician grasps the patient's right arm and draws the shoulder forward until rotational movement is elicited at the left sacroiliac joint.

8. With the patient relaxed and not guarding, the physician delivers an impulse along the shaft of the femur (*white arrows*, **Fig. 11.129**).

9. Effectiveness of the technique is determined by reassessing left sacroiliac joint motion.

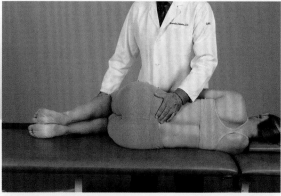

Figure 11.126. Step 1.

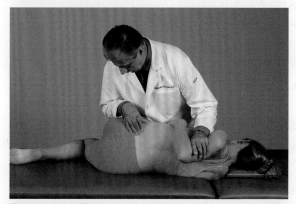

Figure 11.127. Steps 2 to 5.

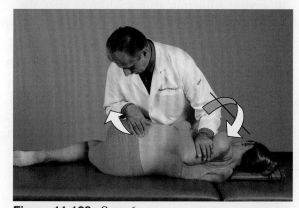

Figure 11.128. Step 6.

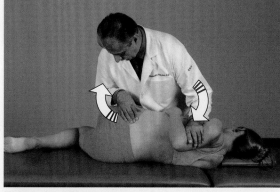

Figure 11.129. Steps 7 and 8.

Pelvic Region

Iliosacral (Innominate) Dysfunction
Ex: Right, Anterior Innominate Rotation
Traction/Posterior Rotational Emphasis

 See Video 11.24

Diagnosis

Standing flexion test: Positive (right PSIS rises)
Loss of passively induced right sacroiliac motion
PSIS: Cephalad (slightly lateral) on the right
ASIS: Caudad (slightly medial) on the right
Sacral sulcus: Posterior on the right

Technique

1. The patient is supine, and the physician stands at the foot of the table.

2. The physician grasps the patient's right ankle.

3. The patient's right leg is raised 45 degrees or more, and traction is applied down the shaft of the leg (*white arrow*, **Fig. 11.130**).

4. This traction is maintained, and the patient is asked to take three to five slow breaths. At the end of each exhalation, traction is increased (**Fig. 11.131**).

5. At the end of the last breath, the physician delivers an impulse thrust in the direction of the traction (*white arrow*, **Fig. 11.132**).

6. Effectiveness of the technique is determined by reassessing right sacroiliac joint motion.

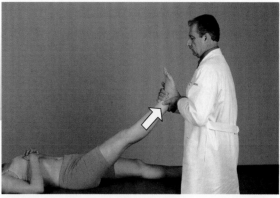

Figure 11.130. Steps 1 to 3.

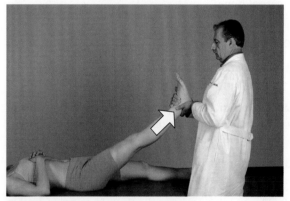

Figure 11.131. Step 4.

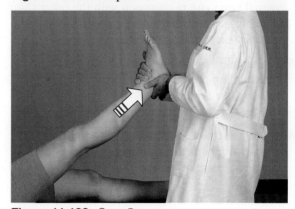

Figure 11.132. Step 5.

Upper Extremity Region

Wrist: Carpal Flexion Dysfunctions
Short-Lever, Extension Emphasis
Ex: Distal Carpal, Flexed (Dorsal)

 See Video 11.25

Diagnosis

Symptoms: Wrist discomfort with inability to fully extend the wrist

Palpation: Dorsal prominence and/or pain of a single carpal bone

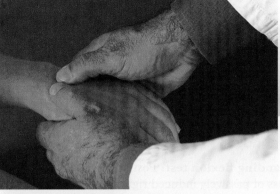

Figure 11.133. Steps 1 and 2.

Technique

1. The patient is seated on the table, and the physician stands facing the patient.

2. The physician grasps the patient's wrist with the physician's thumbs on the dorsal aspect of the wrist **(Fig. 11.133)**.

3. The dorsally dysfunctional carpal bone is identified with the physician's thumbs.

4. The physician places the thumb over the displaced carpal bone and reinforces it with the other thumb. The physician's other fingers wrap around the palmar surface **(Fig. 11.134)**.

5. A simple *whipping motion* is carried out, maintaining pressure over the displaced carpal bone (*white arrow*, **Fig. 11.135**). (No traction is needed for this technique.)

6. Effectiveness of the technique is determined by reassessing both the prominent carpal bone and the wrist range of motion.

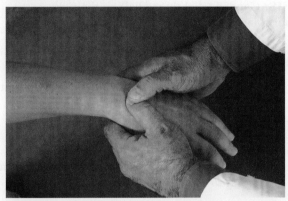

Figure 11.134. Steps 3 and 4.

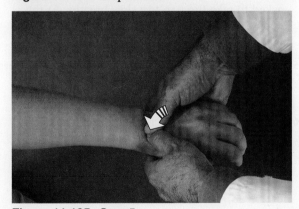

Figure 11.135. Step 5.

Upper Extremity Region

Elbow: Ulnohumeral Flexion Dysfunction
Short-Lever, Extension Emphasis
Ex: Right, Ulnohumeral Flexion

 See Video 11.26

Diagnosis

Symptom: Elbow discomfort
Motion: Inability to fully extend the elbow
Palpation: Olecranon fossa palpable even when the elbow is fully extended

Technique

1. The patient is seated on the table, and the physician stands in front of the patient.

2. The wrist of the arm to be treated is held against the physician's waist using the elbow **(Fig. 11.136)**.

3. The physician places the thumbs on top of the forearm in the area of the antecubital fossa.

4. Traction is down toward the floor; the elbow is carried into further flexion (*white arrow*, **Fig. 11.137**).

5. Pressure is placed under the elbow up toward the shoulder (*white arrow*, **Fig. 11.138**). This pressure is maintained as the elbow is carried into full extension (*white arrow*, **Fig. 11.139**).

6. Effectiveness of the technique is determined by reassessing the elbow range of motion.

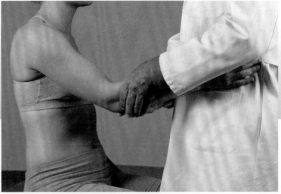

Figure 11.136. Steps 1 and 2.

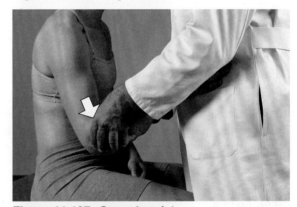

Figure 11.137. Steps 3 and 4.

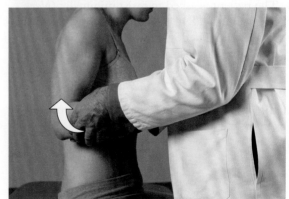

Figure 11.138. Step 5.

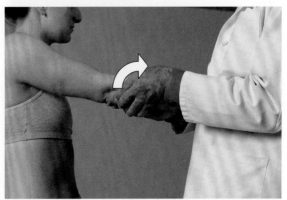

Figure 11.139. Step 5.

Upper Extremity Region

Elbow: Ulnohumeral Extension Dysfunction
Short-Lever, Flexion Emphasis
Ex: Right, Ulnohumeral Extension

 See Video 11.27

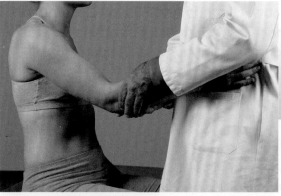

Figure 11.140. Steps 1 to 3.

Diagnosis

Symptom: Elbow discomfort
Motion: Inability to fully flex the elbow
Palpation: No palpable olecranon fossa with the elbow
fully extended

Technique

1. The patient is seated on the table, and the physician stands facing the patient.

2. The patient's arm to be treated is held against the physician's waist with the physician's elbow against the patient's hand.

3. The physician places the thumbs on top of the forearm in the region of the antecubital fossa **(Fig. 11.140)**.

4. The patient is asked to resist minimally (*black arrows*, **Figs. 11.141 to 11.143**) as the physician applies traction down toward the floor (*white arrow*, **Fig. 11.141**). Maintaining this traction, the patient's elbow is carried into full extension (*white arrows*, **Figs. 11.142 and 11.143**).

5. Effectiveness of the technique is determined by reassessing the elbow extension.

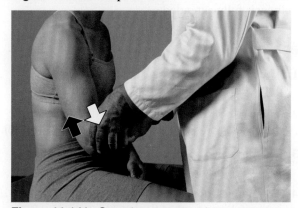

Figure 11.141. Step 4.

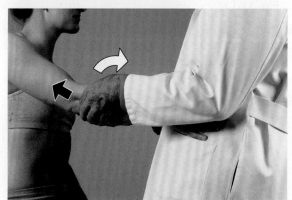

Figure 11.142. Step 4.

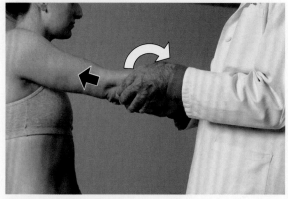

Figure 11.143. Step 4.

Upper Extremity Region

Elbow: Anterior Radial Head Dysfunction
Long-Lever/Fulcrum, Pronation Emphasis
Ex: Right Radial Head, Anterior (Supination)

 See Video 11.28

Diagnosis

Symptoms: Discomfort at the radial head
Motion: Loss of passive pronation of the forearm
Palpation: Anterior prominence and tenderness of the radial head

Technique

1. The patient is seated on the table, and the physician stands facing the patient.

2. The physician holds the hand of the dysfunctional arm as if shaking hands with the patient. The physician places the thumb of the opposite hand anterior to the radial head **(Fig. 11.144)**.

3. The physician rotates the forearm into pronation until the restrictive barrier is reached.

4. With the patient completely relaxed, the physician carries the forearm into slight flexion and pronation while maintaining thumb pressure over the anterior radial head **(Fig. 11.145)**.

5. Effectiveness of the technique is determined by retesting pronation of the forearm and palpating for reduced prominence of the radial head.

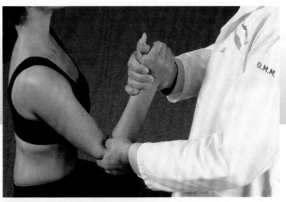
Figure 11.144. Steps 1 and 2.

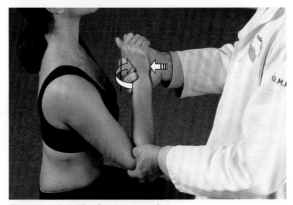
Figure 11.145. Steps 3 and 4.

Upper Extremity Region

Elbow: Posterior Radial Head Dysfunction
Long-Lever/Fulcrum, Supination Emphasis
Ex: Right, Radial Head Posterior, (Pronation)

 See Video 11.29

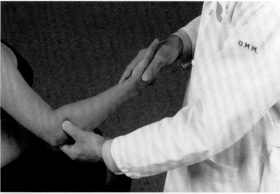

Figure 11.146. Steps 1 and 2.

Diagnosis

Symptoms: Discomfort at the radial head
Motion: Loss of passive supination of the forearm
Palpation: Posterior prominence and tenderness of the radial head

Technique

1. The patient is seated on the table, and the physician stands facing the patient.

2. The physician holds the hand of the dysfunctional arm as if shaking hands with the patient. The physician places the thumb of the opposite hand posterior to the radial head **(Fig. 11.146)**.

3. The physician rotates the forearm into supination until the restrictive barrier is reached.

4. With the patient completely relaxed, the physician carries the forearm into extension and supination while maintaining thumb pressure over the posterior radial head **(Fig. 11.147)**.

5. Effectiveness of the technique is determined by retesting pronation of the forearm and palpating for reduced prominence of the radial head.

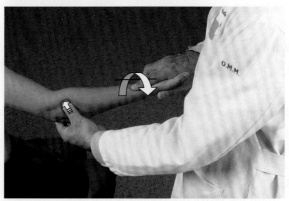

Figure 11.147. Steps 3 and 4.

Upper Extremity Region

Elbow: Ulnohumeral "Abduction" Dysfunction
Long/Short-Lever, Adduction/Lateral Emphasis
Ex: Right Ulna, Abduction with Medial Glide

Diagnosis

Symptoms: Discomfort at the medial or lateral (radial head) elbow
Observation: Increased carrying angle
Motion: Proximal ulna restricted in lateral glide during adduction
Palpation: Distal ulna lateral, olecranon medial

Technique

1. The patient is seated, and the physician stands in front of the patient. (May be performed supine.)

2. The patient's distal right forearm is held in the anatomic position by the physician's left hand.

3. The physician's right "cupped" palm/hand is placed under the patient's right olecranon with the physician's thenar eminence placed on the medial aspect **(Fig. 11.148)**.

4. The physician slowly carries the patient's elbow to the *feather's edge* of the extension barrier and then, holding the medial elbow in place, brings the distal forearm medially to the "feather's edge" of the distal ulna's adduction barrier (*white arrows*, **Fig. 11.149**).

5. With the patient completely relaxed, the physician's left hand quickly moves the elbow (forearm) minimally into extension (*white short curved arrow*) and adduction (*white arrow*) on the distal aspect of the ulna (wrist). Simultaneously, the physician's right hand directs a medial to lateral impulse on the medial aspect of the olecranon (*white pulsed arrow*, **Fig. 11.150**).

6. Effectiveness of the technique is determined by retesting humeral-ulnar motion and reassessing the carrying angle of the elbow.

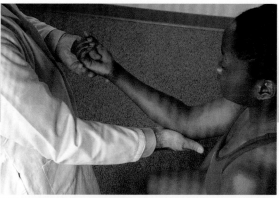
Figure 11.148. Step 3.

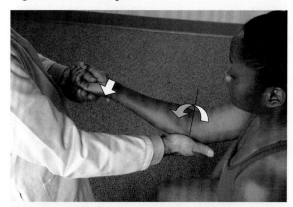
Figure 11.149. Step 4, adduction barrier.

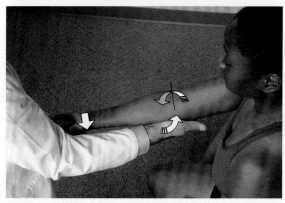
Figure 11.150. Step 5, lateral force to medial olecranon.

Upper Extremity Region

Elbow: Ulnohumeral "Adduction" Dysfunction
Long-/Short-Lever, Abduction/Medial Emphasis
Ex: Right, Ulnar Adduction with Lateral Glide

Diagnosis

Symptoms: Discomfort at the medial or lateral (radial head) elbow

Observation: Decreased carrying angle

Motion: Proximal ulna restricted in medial glide during abduction

Palpation: Distal ulna medial, olecranon lateral

Technique

1. The patient is seated, and the physician stands in front of the patient. (May be performed supine.)

2. The patient's distal right forearm is held in the anatomic position by the physician's right hand.

3. The physician's left "cupped" palm/hand is placed under the patient's right olecranon with the physician's thenar eminence placed on the lateral aspect **(Fig. 11.151)**.

4. The physician slowly carries the patient's elbow to the *feather's edge* of the extension barrier and then, holding the medial elbow in place, brings the distal forearm lateral to the "feather's edge" of the distal ulna's abduction barrier (*white arrows,* **Fig. 11.152**).

5. With the patient completely relaxed, the physician quickly moves the forearm minimally into slight increased extension *(white curved axis arrow)* with a simultaneous medially directed force on the lateral olecranon *(white pulsed arrow)* and laterally directed force on the distal ulna (wrist) *(white short curved arrows,* **Fig. 11.153**).

6. Effectiveness of the technique is determined by retesting humeral-ulnar motion and reassessing the carrying angle of the elbow.

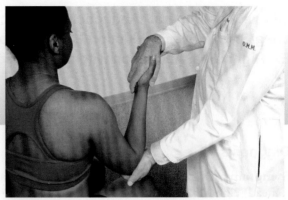

Figure 11.151. Steps 1 to 3.

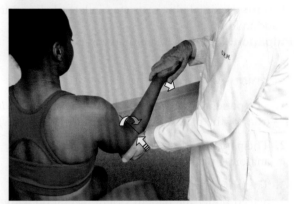

Figure 11.152. Step 4, abduction barrier.

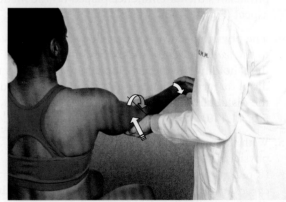

Figure 11.153. Step 5, medial force on lateral olecranon.

Lower Extremity Region

Anterior, Proximal Tibial Dysfunctions
Short-Lever, Posterior Tibial Emphasis
Ex: Right Tibia, Anterior (Femur Posterior)

 See Video 11.30

Diagnosis

Symptoms: Knee discomfort, inability to comfortably extend the knee
Motion: Restricted posterior spring (drawer-like test) with loss of anterior freeplay motion
Palpation: Prominence of the tibial tuberosity

Technique

1. The patient is supine with the dysfunctional knee flexed to 90 degrees with the foot flat on the table.

2. The physician sits on the patient's foot anchoring it to the table.

3. The physician places the thenar eminences over the anterior aspect of the tibial plateau with the fingers wrapping around the leg **(Fig. 11.154)**.

4. After all of the posterior freeplay motion is taken out of the knee joint, a thrust (*arrow*, **Fig. 11.155**) is delivered posteriorly parallel to the long axis of the femur.

5. Effectiveness of the technique is determined by reassessing anterior freeplay glide as well as range of motion of the knee.

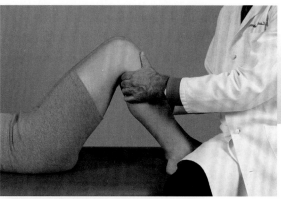

Figure 11.154. Steps 1 to 3.

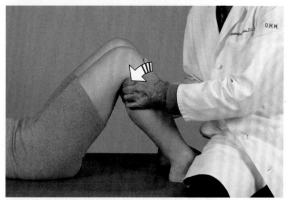

Figure 11.155. Step 4.

Lower Extremity Region

Anterior, Proximal Tibial Dysfunctions
Short-Lever/Traction, Posterior Emphasis
Ex: Right Tibia Anterior (Femur Posterior)

 See Video 11.31

Diagnosis

Symptoms: Knee discomfort, inability to comfortably extend the knee

Motion: Restricted posterior spring (drawer-like test) with loss of anterior freeplay motion

Palpation: Prominence of the tibial tuberosity

Technique

1. The patient is seated on the side of the table with a small pillow beneath the thigh as a cushion.

2. The physician places the thumbs on the anterior tibial plateau with the fingers wrapping around the leg **(Fig. 11.156)**.

3. The thigh is sprung up and down to ensure total relaxation of the thigh musculature (*white arrows*, **Fig. 11.157**).

4. A thrust is delivered straight down toward the floor, simultaneous with a posterior pressure impulse with the thumbs (*white arrows*, **Fig. 11.158**).

5. Effectiveness of the technique is determined by reassessing anterior freeplay glide as well as range of motion of the knee.

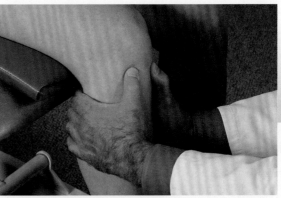

Figure 11.156. Steps 1 and 2.

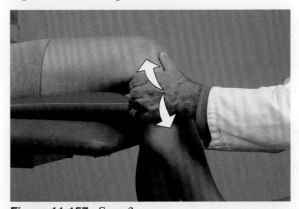

Figure 11.157. Step 3.

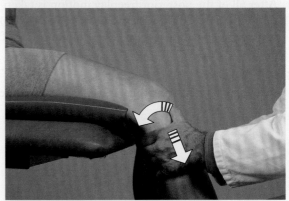

Figure 11.158. Step 4.

Lower Extremity Region

Posterior, Proximal Tibial Dysfunctions
Short-Lever, Anterior Tibial Emphasis
Ex: Left Tibia, Posterior (Femur Anterior)

 See Video 11.32

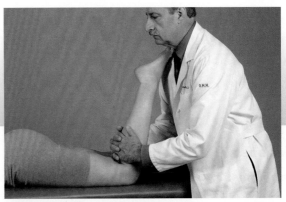

Figure 11.159. Steps 1 to 3.

Diagnosis

Symptoms: Knee discomfort, inability to comfortably flex the knee

Motion: Restricted anterior spring (drawer-like test) with loss of posterior freeplay motion

Technique

1. The patient lies prone with the dysfunctional knee flexed to approximately 90 degrees if possible.

2. The physician stands or sits at the end of the table with the dorsum of the patient's foot on the anteromedial aspect of the physician's shoulder. Placement of the patient's foot on the physician's shoulder will plantar flex the foot, taking tension off the gastrocnemius muscle.

3. The physician's fingers are interlaced and wrapped around the proximal tibia just distal to the popliteal region **(Fig. 11.159)**.

4. A thrust impulse is delivered with both hands toward the physician and parallel to the table (*white arrow*, **Fig. 11.160**).

5. Effectiveness of the technique is determined by reassessing posterior freeplay glide at the knee and by rechecking the knee range of motion.

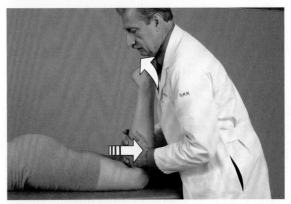

Figure 11.160. Step 4.

Lower Extremity Region

Posterior, Proximal Tibial Dysfunctions
Short-Lever, Anterior Tibial Emphasis
Ex: Right Tibia, Posterior (Femur Anterior)

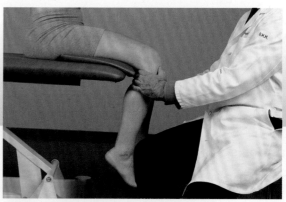

Figure 11.161. Steps 1 and 2.

Diagnosis

Symptoms: Knee discomfort, inability to comfortably flex the knee

Motion: Restricted posterior spring (drawer-like test) with loss of anterior freeplay motion

Technique

1. The patient is seated on the side of the table with a small pillow beneath the thigh as a cushion.

2. The physician places the thumbs on the anterior tibial plateau with the fingers wrapping around the leg contacting the popliteal fossa and adding a slight flexion to the knee so the foot may go under the edge of the table **(Fig. 11.161)**.

3. The thigh is then sprung up and down to ensure total relaxation of the thigh musculature.

4. A thrust is delivered down toward the floor (*white arrow*, **Fig. 11.162**), simultaneous with an anterior pressure impulse with the popliteal contacting fingers.

5. Effectiveness of the technique is determined by reassessing anterior freeplay glide and range of motion of the knee.

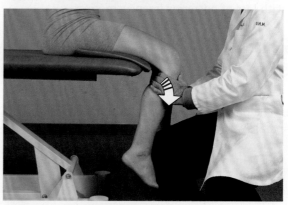

Figure 11.162. Steps 3 and 4.

Lower Extremity Region

Anterior, Proximal Fibular Dysfunction
Short-Lever, Posterior with Inversion Emphasis
Ex: Right, Fibula Anterior

 See Video 11.33

Diagnosis

Symptoms: Lateral leg soreness and muscle cramping with tenderness over the proximal fibula

Motion: Increased anterior glide with restricted motion of the proximal fibula posterior the glide

History: Common following a medial ankle sprain, forced dorsiflexion of the ankle, and genu recurvatum deformity

Technique

1. The patient lies supine with a small pillow under the dysfunctional knee to maintain the knee in slight flexion.

2. The physician's caudad hand internally rotates the patient's ankle to bring the proximal fibula more anterior.

3. The physician places the heel of the cephalad hand over the anterior surface of the proximal fibula **(Fig. 11.163)**.

4. A thrust is delivered through the fibular head straight back toward the table (*pulsed white arrow*, **Fig. 11.164**).

5. Simultaneously, an internal rotation counterforce is introduced from the ankle (*curved white arrow*, **Fig. 11.164**).

6. Effectiveness of the technique is determined by reassessing the anterior glide motion of the proximal fibula.

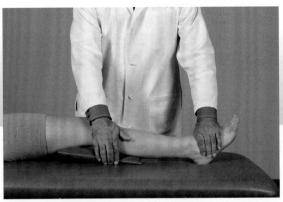

Figure 11.163. Steps 1 to 3.

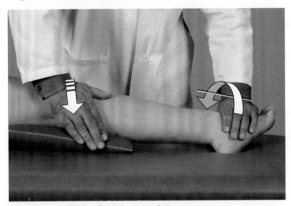

Figure 11.164. Steps 4 and 5.

Lower Extremity Region

Knee: Fibular Head Dysfunctions
Long-Lever, Fulcrum/Eversion Emphasis
Ex: Left, Posterior Fibular Head

 See Video 11.34

Diagnosis

Symptoms: Pain at the lateral knee and persistent ankle pain beyond that expected for normal ankle recovery

Motion: Increased posterior glide and decreased anterior glide

Palpation: Tenderness at the fibular head; fibular head prominent posteriorly

History: Common following inversion sprains of the ankle

Technique

1. The patient lies prone with the dysfunctional knee flexed at 90 degrees.

2. The physician stands at the side of the table opposite the side of the dysfunction.

3. The physician places the MCP of the cephalad index finger behind the dysfunctional fibular head, and the hypothenar eminence is angled down into the hamstring musculature to form a wedge behind the knee.

4. The physician's caudad hand grasps the ankle on the side of dysfunction and gently flexes the knee until the restrictive barrier is reached **(Fig. 11.165)**.

5. The patient's foot and leg are gently externally rotated to carry the fibular head back against the fulcrum formed by the physician's cephalad hand (*white arrow,* **Fig. 11.166**).

6. The physician's caudad hand, controlling the patient's foot and ankle, delivers a thrust toward the patient's buttock in a manner that would normally result in further flexion of the knee (*white arrow,* **Fig. 11.167**). However, the wedge fulcrum formed by the physician's cephalad hand prevents any such motion.

7. Effectiveness of the technique is determined by reassessing motion of the fibular head and by palpating for restoration of normal position of the fibula.

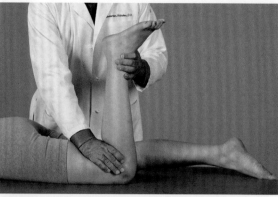

Figure 11.165. Steps 1 to 4.

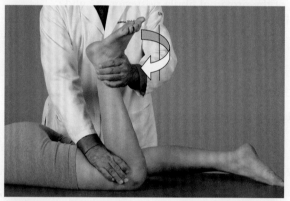

Figure 11.166. Step 5.

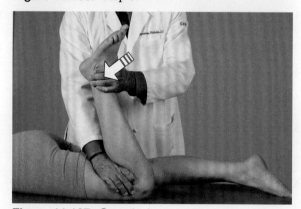

Figure 11.167. Step 6.

Lower Extremity Region

Knee: Medial Meniscus Dysfunction
Long-Lever, Traction Emphasis
Ex: Right, Anteromedial Medial Meniscus

 See Video 11.35

Diagnosis

Symptoms: Medial knee discomfort and locking of the knee short of full extension

Physical findings: Palpable bulging of the meniscus just medial to the patellar tendon, positive McMurray test, and positive Apley compression test

Technique

1. The patient lies supine with the hip and knee flexed.

2. The physician stands at the side of the table on the side of the dysfunction.

3. The physician places the ankle of the dysfunctional leg under the physician's axilla and against the lateral rib cage **(Fig. 11.168)**.

4. The physician places the thumb of the medial hand over the bulging meniscus. The fingers of the lateral hand lie over the thumb of the medial hand reinforcing it. The physician may use the palmar aspect of the fingers to reinforce thumbs, but they must be distal to the patella **(Fig. 11.169)**.

5. The physician places a valgus stress on the knee and externally rotates the foot (*white arrows*, **Fig. 11.170**).

6. This position is maintained, and moderate to heavy pressure is exerted with the thumbs over the medial meniscus. This pressure is maintained as the knee is carried into full extension **(Fig. 11.171)**.

7. Effectiveness of the technique is determined by reassessment of the knee range of motion.

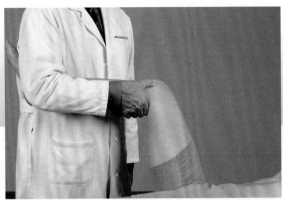

Figure 11.168. Steps 1 to 3.

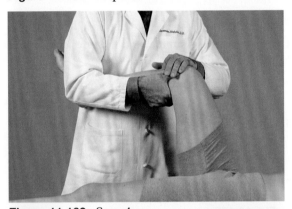

Figure 11.169. Step 4.

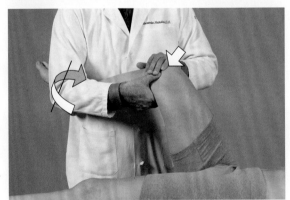

Figure 11.170. Step 5.

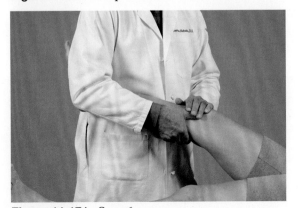

Figure 11.171. Step 6.

Lower Extremity Region

Anterior, Distal Tibial Dysfunction
Short-Lever, Posterior Emphasis
Ex: Left, Anterior Tibia on Talus

 See Video 11.36

Diagnosis

Drawer test: Loss of anterior glide (freeplay motion) with decreased posterior drawer test

Technique

1. The patient lies supine, and the physician stands at the foot of the table.

2. The physician's one hand cups the calcaneus anchoring the foot (slight traction may be applied).

3. The physician places the other hand on the anterior tibia proximal to the ankle mortise **(Fig. 11.172)**.

4. A thrust is delivered with the hand on the tibia straight down toward the table (*white arrow*, **Fig. 11.173**).

5. Effectiveness of the technique is determined by reassessing ankle range of motion.

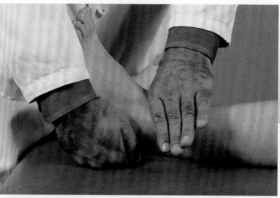
Figure 11.172. Steps 1 to 3.

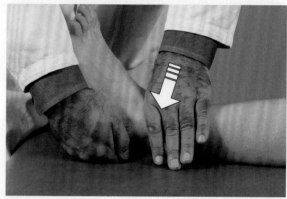
Figure 11.173. Step 4.

Lower Extremity Region

Posterior Distal Tibial Dysfunction
Short-Lever Traction Emphasis
Ex: Left, Posterior Tibia on Talus

 See Videos 11.36, 11.37, and 11.38

Diagnosis

Drawer test: Loss of posterior glide (freeplay motion) with decreased anterior drawer test

Technique

1. The patient lies supine, and the physician stands at the foot of the table.

2. The physician's hands are wrapped around the foot with the fingers interlaced on the dorsum.

3. The foot is dorsiflexed to the motion barrier using pressure from the physician's thumbs on the ball of the foot **(Fig. 11.174)**.

4. Traction is placed on the leg at the same time dorsiflexion of the foot is increased (*white arrows*, **Fig. 11.175**).

5. The physician delivers a tractional thrust foot while increasing the degree of dorsiflexion (*white arrows*, **Fig. 11.176**).

6. Effectiveness of the technique is determined by reassessing the ankle range of motion.

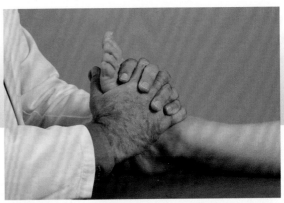

Figure 11.174. Steps 1 to 3.

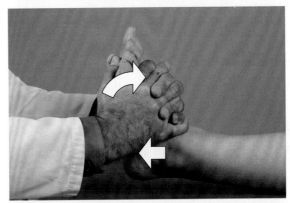

Figure 11.175. Step 4.

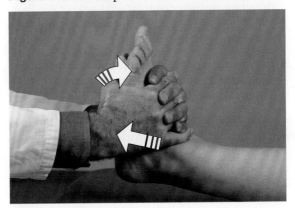

Figure 11.176. Step 5.

Lower Extremity Region

Cuneiform, Plantar Dysfunctions
Short-Lever (Hiss Whip), Dorsal Emphasis
Ex: Right, Plantar First Cuneiform

 See Video 11.39

Diagnosis

Symptom: Plantar discomfort

Motion: Longitudinal arch and forefoot will not readily spring toward supination.

Palpation: Tender prominence on the plantar surface of the foot overlying the dysfunctional cuneiform

Technique

1. The patient lies prone with the leg off the table flexed at the knee.

2. The physician stands at the foot of the table.

3. The physician's hands are wrapped around the foot with the thumbs placed over the dropped cuneiform **(Fig. 11.177)**.

4. A *whipping motion* is carried out with the thumbs thrusting straight down into the sole of the foot at the level of the dysfunctional cuneiform (*white arrow*, **Fig. 11.178**).

5. Effectiveness of the technique is determined by reassessing motion of the forefoot and palpating for the dropped cuneiform.

This technique may also be applied to plantar dysfunction of the proximal metatarsals.

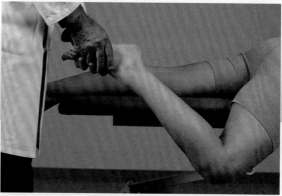

Figure 11.177. Steps 1 to 3.

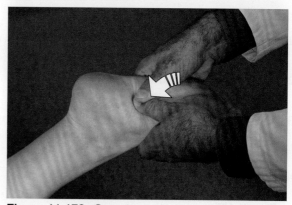

Figure 11.178. Step 4.

Lower Extremity Region

Metatarsal, Plantar Dysfunctions
Long-Lever with Fulcrum, Dorsal Emphasis
Ex: Left, Plantar Fifth Metatarsal

 See Video 11.40

Diagnosis

History: Common following inversion sprain of the ankle

Technique

1. The patient lies supine.

2. The physician sits at the foot of the table and stabilizes the patient's ankle.

3. The physician places the thumb over the dorsal aspect and distal end of the fifth metatarsal.

4. The physician places the MCP of the index finger beneath the styloid process **(Fig. 11.179)**.

5. A thrust is delivered by both fingers simultaneously. The thumb exerts pressure toward the sole, and the index finger exerts a force toward the dorsum of the foot (*white arrows*, **Fig. 11.180**).

6. Effectiveness of the technique is determined by reassessing the position and tenderness of the styloid process of the fifth metatarsal.

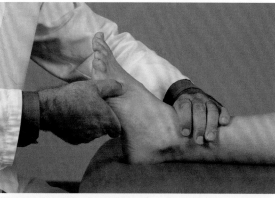

Figure 11.179. Steps 1 to 4.

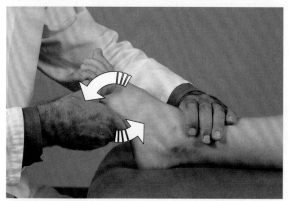

Figure 11.180. Step 5.

Lower Extremity Region

Cuboid, Plantar Dysfunction
Short-Lever (Whip), Dorsal Emphasis
Ex: Right, Plantar Rotation

 See Video 11.39

Diagnosis

Tenderness: Lateral plantar aspect of the foot just proximal to the styloid process of the fifth metatarsal and overlying the tendon of the peroneus longus muscle

Palpation: Groove distal to the styloid process of the fifth metatarsal deeper than normal; cuboid prominent on the plantar aspect of the lateral foot

History: Common following inversion sprain of the ankle

Technique

1. The patient lies prone with the leg flexed 30 degrees at the knee.

2. The physician stands at the foot of the table.

3. The physician places the thumb on the medial side of the foot over the plantar prominence of the cuboid.

4. The physician's thumb on the lateral side of the foot reinforces the medial thumb **(Fig. 11.181)**.

5. The lateral aspect of the foot is opened by adducting the forefoot **(Fig. 11.182)**.

6. The thrust is delivered in a whipping motion toward the lateral aspect of the foot (*white arrows*, **Figs. 11.183 and 11.184**).

7. Effectiveness of the technique is determined by reassessing the position and tenderness of the cuboid.

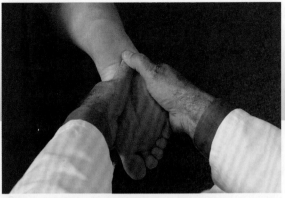
Figure 11.181. Steps 1 to 4.

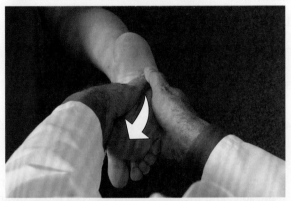
Figure 11.182. Step 5.

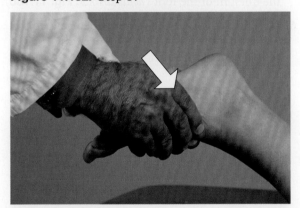
Figure 11.183. Step 6.

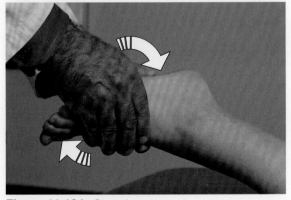
Figure 11.184. Step 6.

References

1. Chila AG, exec.ed. Foundations of Osteopathic Medicine. 3rd ed. Baltimore, MD: Lippincott Williams & Wilkins, 2011.
2. Iatridis JC, Weidenbaum M, Selton LA, et al. Is the nucleus pulposus a solid or fluid? Mechanical behavior of the nucleus pulposus of the human intervertebral disc. Spine 1996;21(10):1174–1184.
3. Heilig D. The thrust technique. J Am Osteopath Assoc 1981;81:244–248.
4. Greenman P. Principles of Manual Medicine. 2nd ed. Baltimore, MD: Williams & Wilkins, 1996.
5. Kimberly P. Outline of Osteopathic Procedures: The Kimberly Manual. Marceline, MO: Walsworth Publishing Co., 2006.

12

Facilitated Positional Release Techniques

Technique Principles

Facilitated positional release (FPR) technique is a patient-passive, indirect technique, and as such, it shares principles with the other indirect osteopathic techniques, especially myofascial release, balanced ligamentous tension, and ligamentous articular strain. Its positioning is very similar to counterstrain and the initial indirect positioning for Still technique. The Education Council on Osteopathic Principles (ECOP) defines FPR as "a system of indirect myofascial release treatment developed by Stanley Schiowitz, DO. The component region of the body is placed into a neutral position, diminishing tissue and joint tension in all planes, and an activating force (compression or torsion) is added" (1). The primary goal of this technique is to reduce abnormal muscle hypertonicity (superficial and deep) and restore lost motion to a restricted articulation.

As with counterstrain technique, the primary neurophysiologic mechanism affected by FPR is thought to be the relationship between Iα-afferent and γ-efferent activity (1–3). If the dysfunctional region is positioned appropriately, the intrafusal fibers may return to normal length, which in return decreases tension in the extrafusal fibers. This reduced tension in the area of the muscle spindle further decreases the Iα-afferent impulses, which in turn continues this beneficial interaction, eventually allowing the muscles to achieve their normal length and tone (4). Other beneficial aspects of this form of treatment may be related to the treatment position's secondary effects of improving lymphatic and venous drainage and other bioelectric phenomena affecting fluid dynamics and local metabolic processes.

The principles of positioning in this technique are basic to indirect treatments, and therefore, the physician will attempt to place the dysfunctional segment, muscle, or other structure toward its position of motion ease or reduced tension. This is done by first attempting to place the myofascial or articular dysfunction in a neutral position, which Schiowitz describes as *flattening* the anteroposterior spinal curve (facets are in a position between the beginning of flexion and the beginning of

extension) (3). With a flexed or extended dysfunction, the initial positioning is to flatten the anteroposterior spinal curve and find the neutral position within the dysfunction. This example is common to type II dysfunctions. With type I dysfunctions, less anterior and/or posterior positioning are necessary.

If the primary focus is the treatment of muscle hypertonicity and tension (when there is no predominant x-axis, y-axis, and z-axis diagnosis), the hypertonic muscle is placed in a position of ease of tension. This is based on palpating the abnormal tissue textures and their response to positioning (3). If a dysfunctional muscle is causing thoracic tension anteriorly, flexion is the most probable position of ease. Posterior thoracic muscle hypertonicity commonly is associated with an extended position of ease (2).

The major discriminating factor we see in this technique when comparing it to the other indirect techniques is its *release-enhancing mechanism*. DiGiovanna and Schiowitz describe this as a facilitating muscle force (1,3). This may be a compression force, but it can accommodate all directions of motion ease or directions in which the muscle tension is reduced. Because of side bending and rotational components in most dysfunctions (spinal and extremity), it is generally necessary for the physician to add some form of torsion (side bending combined with rotation) force during the positional component of the technique. On achieving the proper position of ease with the facilitating forces, the physician holds the treatment position for 3 to 5 seconds, returns the patient to neutral (pretreatment position), and follows by reassessing the dysfunction using the palpatory parameters for tissue texture changes, motion restriction, asymmetry, and tenderness (sensitivity). After holding the patient in the position of ease for 3 to 5 seconds, the physician may choose to add a very rapid articulatory (on and off) springing force. This is implemented by introducing quick, indirect/direct impulses moving through extremely small distances. This was not included in Dr. Schiowitz's original descriptions, but was later described by him as his "secret ingredient" during his Heilig Symposium presentations at PCOM (Schiowitz S. *Personal communication.* Heilig Symposium, 2007. Philadelphia, PA: Philadelphia College of Osteopathic Medicine.).

Technique Classification

Indirect

As with all indirect techniques, the physician attempts to position the patient in the direction that reduces the myofascial tissue tension or in the direction of the motion freedom.

Technique Styles

Myofascial (Muscle Hypertonicity)

To treat a hypertonic muscle with FPR, the physician flattens the spinal curve in the region or segment to be treated or in the extremities, adding compression toward the joint. Then the physician assesses for tissue texture changes (e.g., tension, inelasticity, bogginess) and positions the patient until these dysfunctional parameters are optimally reduced. Next, the physician adds the appropriate facilitating forces (additional compression and torsion) and holds for 3 to 5 seconds and then returns the affected area to a neutral position and reassesses. It is recommended to use this style initially when the physician has difficulty determining the primary component of the dysfunction (myofascial vs. articular). This may be similar to the effects of indirect myofascial release and counterstrain techniques.

Articular (Intervertebral and Intersegmental *x*-Axis, *y*-Axis, *z*-Axis) Dysfunction

In articular technique, the physician uses the palpatory clues for primary intersegmental (joint) dysfunctions. These clues are generally tissue texture changes, restriction of motion, asymmetric motion (may exhibit symmetrically reduced motion), end feel or joint free-play qualitative changes, and pain. Intersegmental motion restriction and asymmetry are the salient qualities. The physician starts by flattening the anteroposterior spinal curve of the region being treated. By flattening the curve, we are not attempting to regionally reduce the lordotic or kyphotic nature of that spinal region, but rather to help develop a long lever tethering effect in order to localize a force vector at the specified dysfunctional level, as seen in other technique styles (i.e., HVLA, ME, etc.) so that the ensuing facilitating forces will be vectored appropriately through the dysfunctional barrier(s). The dysfunctional segment should then be positioned toward the ease of motion in all affected planes. Next, the physician adds the appropriate axial

facilitating forces (compression and torsion) and holds statically for 3 to 5 seconds.

Indication

Myofascial or articular somatic dysfunction

Contraindications

1. Moderate to severe joint instability
2. Herniated disc where the positioning could exacerbate the condition
3. Moderate to severe intervertebral foraminal stenosis, especially in the presence of radicular symptoms at the level to be treated if the positioning could cause exacerbation of the symptoms by further narrowing the foramen
4. Severe sprains and strains where the positioning may exacerbate the injury
5. Certain congenital anomalies or conditions in which the position needed to treat the dysfunction is not possible (e.g., ankylosis)
6. Vertebrobasilar insufficiency

General Considerations and Rules

The physician must be able to make an accurate diagnosis and, when possible, to distinguish between a myofascial and an articular dysfunction. The anteroposterior spinal curve is flattened, and then a position of ease or a position that maximally reduces myofascial tension is approached. A facilitating force of compression combined with side bending and/or rotation (torsion) is applied for 3 to 5 seconds. A springing force may also be used.

Shorthand Rules

Primary Myofascial Dysfunction

1. Make diagnosis (tissue texture abnormality).
2. Flatten the anteroposterior spinal curve to reduce myofascial tension.
3. Add a compression or torsional facilitating force (Note: This may be performed at this point or after step #4.) (1).
4. Place the dysfunctional myofascial structure into its ease (shortened, relaxed) position.
5. Hold for 3 to 5 seconds, and then slowly release pressure while returning to neutral.
6. The physician reassesses the dysfunctional components (tissue texture abnormality, asymmetry of position, restriction of motion, tenderness [TART]).

Primary Articular (x-axis, y-axis, z-axis) Type I and II Dysfunctions

1. Make a diagnosis (e.g., type I or II).
2. Flatten (flex or extend) the anteroposterior curve in the spinal region of treatment.
3. Add the facilitating force (compression or torsion).
4. Move the dysfunctional segment toward its flexion or extension ease.

5. Move the dysfunctional segment toward its side bending and rotational ease.
6. Hold for 3-5 seconds (may introduce a few quick, on/off impulses) and slowly release pressure while returning to neutral.
7. Reassess the dysfunctional components (TART).

Cervical Region

Right Suboccipital Muscle Hypertonicity

 See Video 12.1

1. The patient lies supine, and the physician sits at the head of the table.

2. The physician gently supports the occipital and upper cervical regions of the patient's head with the right hand.

3. With the left hand on the patient's head, the physician neutralizes the cervical spine by gently flattening the anteroposterior curve (slight flexion).

4. An activating force in the form of a gentle (1 pound or less) axial compression is added with the left hand.

5. While maintaining compression, the physician gently positions the patient's head and cervical region toward extension and right side bending and rotation (*arrows*, **Figs. 12.1 and 12.2**) until maximal reduction of tissue and muscle tension is achieved.

6. The physician holds this position for 3 to 5 seconds and then slowly releases the compression while returning to neutral.

7. If a release is not palpated within a few seconds, axial compression should be released, and steps 3 to 6 can be repeated.

8. The physician reassesses the components of the dysfunction (TART).

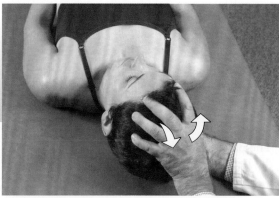

Figure 12.1. Steps 1 to 5.

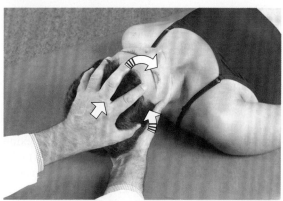

Figure 12.2. Steps 1 to 5.

Cervical Region

C2–C7 Dysfunctions
Ex: C4 FSRRR

 See Video 12.2

1. The patient lies supine, and the physician sits at the head of the table.

2. The physician gently supports the cervical region with the right hand.

3. With the left hand on the patient's head, the physician neutralizes the cervical spine by gently flattening the anteroposterior curve (slight flexion).

4. An activating force (*arrow*) in the form of a gentle (1 pound or less) axial compression is added with the left hand.

5. While maintaining compression, the physician gently positions the patient's head toward flexion and right side bending and rotation (*arrows*) until maximal reduction of tissue and muscle tension is achieved (**Figs. 12.3 and 12.4**).

6. The physician holds this position for 3 to 5 seconds and then slowly releases the compression while returning to neutral.

7. If a release is not palpated within a few seconds, axial compression should be released, and steps 3 to 6 can be repeated.

8. The physician reassesses the components of the dysfunction (TART).

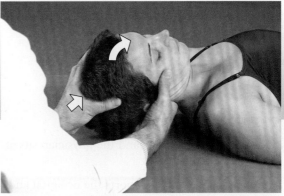

Figure 12.3. Steps 1 to 5.

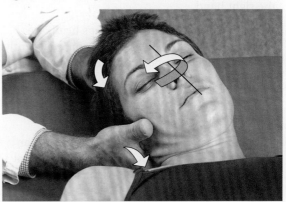

Figure 12.4. Steps 1 to 5.

Thoracic Region

T4–T12 "Extension" Dysfunctions
Ex: T6 ESRRR

1. The patient sits at the edge of the table with the physician standing at the right side and slightly posterior to the patient.

2. The physician's left hand monitors the patient's dysfunction at the spinous processes of T6 and T7 and the right transverse process of T6.

3. The physician places the right forearm on the patient's upper right trapezius (shoulder girdle) with the remainder of the physician's right forearm and hand resting across the patient's upper back just behind the patient's neck **(Fig. 12.5)**.

4. The patient sits up straight until the normal thoracic curvature is straightened and flattened, so that extension is palpated at the level of T6.

5. The physician's right forearm applies an activating force in the form of gentle (1 pound or less) compression.

6. While maintaining compression, the physician places a caudad and posterior force with the right forearm (*white arrow*, **Fig. 12.6**) to position T6 into further extension and right side bending and rotation. This should be carried to a point of balance and minimum muscle tone.

7. The physician holds this position for 3 to 5 seconds and then slowly releases the compression while returning to neutral.

8. If a release is not palpated within a few seconds, compression should be released, and steps 3 to 6 can be repeated.

9. The physician reassesses the components of the dysfunction (TART).

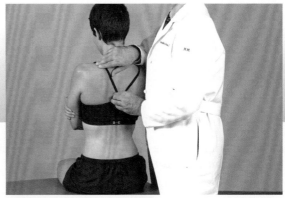

Figure 12.5. Steps 1 to 3.

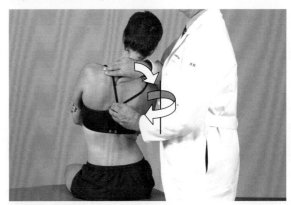

Figure 12.6. Steps 4 to 6.

Thoracic Region

Right, Trapezius Muscle Hypertonicity

1. The patient lies prone on the treatment table with the head and neck rotated to the right.

2. The physician stands at the left side, facing the patient.

3. The physician's left hand palpates the right, hypertonic trapezius muscle **(Fig. 12.7)**.

4. The physician's right hand reaches across the body of the patient and grasps the patient's right shoulder at the anterior deltoid and acromioclavicular region **(Fig. 12.8)**.

5. The physician places a caudad and posterior force (*white arrow*, **Fig. 12.9**) to achieve a point of balance and minimal muscle tension in the right trapezius muscle.

6. On achieving the proper position, the physician's right hand applies an activating force (*white arrow*, **Fig. 12.10**) in the form of a gentle (1 pound or less) compression for 3 to 5 seconds.

7. If a release is not palpated within a few seconds, compression should be released, and steps 3 to 6 can be repeated.

8. The physician reassesses the components of the dysfunction (TART).

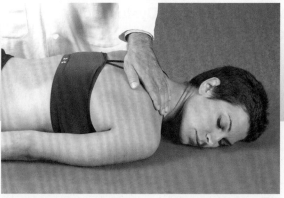

Figure 12.7. Steps 1 to 3.

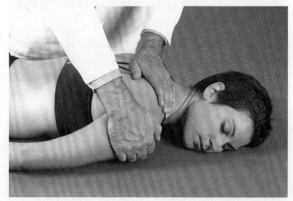

Figure 12.8. Step 4.

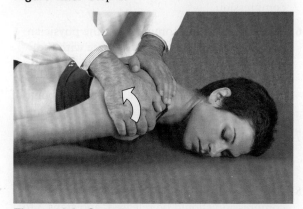

Figure 12.9. Step 5.

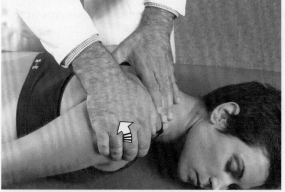

Figure 12.10. Step 6.

Costal Region

First Rib "Elevated" Dysfunction
Nonphysiologic Model, Myofascial Emphasis
Ex: Left, First Rib Elevated (Posterior)

1. The patient lies supine, and the physician stands facing the patient on the dysfunctional side.

2. The patient's left arm is flexed at the elbow, and a pillow or rolled towel is placed under the patient's upper arm.

3. The physician's left hand controls the olecranon process while the index and third fingers of the right hand palpate the posterior aspect of the first rib, monitoring for tissue texture changes **(Fig. 12.11)**.

4. The physician's left hand flexes the patient's shoulder to approximately 90 degrees and then abducts slightly and internally rotates the shoulder to the position that produces the most laxity and softening of the tissues **(Fig. 12.12)**.

5. The physician adducts the arm and simultaneously applies a compression through the patient's left upper arm toward the monitoring fingers at the first rib (*straight arrow*, **Fig. 12.13**) while pushing the patient's elbow down toward the chest (*curved arrow*) over the pillow.

6. This position is held for 3 to 5 seconds, and a slight on-and-off pressure can be applied.

7. After 3 to 5 seconds, the arm is brought through further adduction and then inferiorly swung back to the lateral bodyline.

8. The physician reassesses the components of the dysfunction (TART).

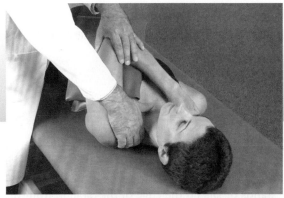
Figure 12.11. Steps 1 to 3.

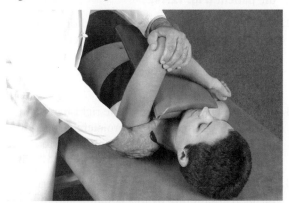
Figure 12.12. Step 4.

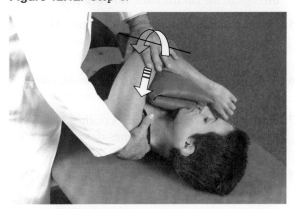
Figure 12.13. Step 5.

Costal Region

Rib 3–Rib 10 Inhalation Dysfunctions
Ex: Left Seventh Rib, Inhaled/Elevated

1. The patient lies in the right lateral recumbent (side lying) position with the arm flexed and abducted to approximately 90 degrees, and the physician stands or sits on the edge of the table in front of the patient **(Fig. 12.14)**.

2. The physician places the index and/or third finger pads of the right hand over the posterior aspect of the seventh rib at the costotransverse articulation. The thumb is placed over the inferior edge of the lateral aspect of the same rib.

3. The physician's webbing of the right hand (thumb abducted) contours the anterolateral aspect of the seventh rib, being careful not to put too much pressure over the chondral portion **(Fig. 12.15)**.

4. The physician gently pushes the rib posterior (*arrow*), attempting by this compression to disengage the rib from the vertebra **(Fig. 12.16)**.

5. The physician adds a cephalad-vectored force (bucket handle) toward the inhalation ease (*arrow*, **Fig. 12.17**), through the bucket-handle vector.

6. This position is held for 3 to 5 seconds, and a slight on-and-off pressure can be applied.

7. After 3 to 5 seconds, the rib is pushed slowly back to neutral as the patient brings the arm down to the lateral bodyline.

8. The physician reassesses the components of the dysfunction (TART).

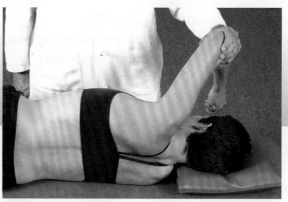

Figure 12.14. Step 1.

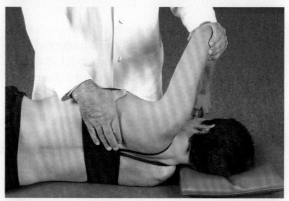

Figure 12.15. Steps 2 and 3.

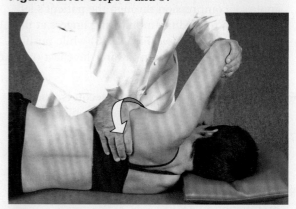

Figure 12.16. Step 4.

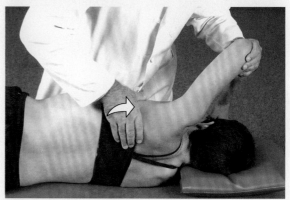

Figure 12.17. Step 5.

Lumbar Region

L1–L5 "Neutral/Extension" Dysfunctions
Ex: L3 NSLRR

1. The patient lies prone on the table. A pillow may be placed under the abdomen to decrease the normal lumbar curvature.

2. The physician stands at the left side of the patient, facing the patient.

3. The physician's left hand monitors the patient's L3 and L4 spinous processes and the right transverse process of L3 (**Fig. 12.18**).

4. The physician rests the left knee on the table against the patient's left ilium.

5. The physician crosses the patient's right ankle over the left and grasps the patient's right knee while sliding the patient's legs to the patient's left (**Fig. 12.19**).

6. The physician repositions the right hand to grasp the patient's right thigh and directs a force dorsally and toward external rotation (*white arrow*, **Fig. 12.20**). This combined movement is carried to a point of balance and minimum muscle tension as perceived by the physician's left hand at the level of L3–L4.

7. On achieving the proper position, the physician's left hand (*arrow*, **Fig. 12.21**) applies an activating force over the right transverse process of L4 in the form of a gentle (1 pound or less) axial compression for 3 to 5 seconds.

8. If a release is not palpated within a few seconds, compression should be released and steps 3 to 7 can be repeated.

9. The physician reassesses the components of the dysfunction (TART).

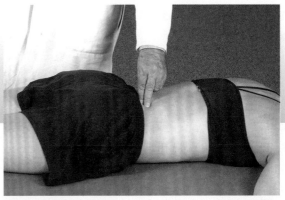

Figure 12.18. Steps 1 to 3.

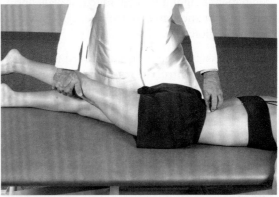

Figure 12.19. Steps 4 and 5.

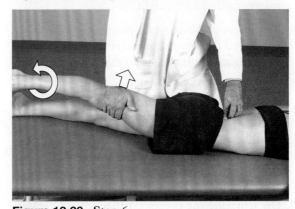

Figure 12.20. Step 6.

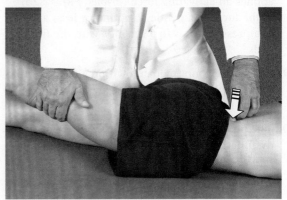

Figure 12.21. Step 7.

Lumbar Region

L1–L5 Dysfunctions
Ex: L4 FSRRR

1. The patient lies in the left lateral recumbent position, and the physician stands at the side of the table facing the patient.

2. The physician's right forearm and hand control the patient's right anterolateral chest wall, and the left forearm and hand control the right pelvic and lumbar region **(Fig. 12.22)**.

3. The physician's right index and third finger pads monitor and control the transverse processes of L4 while the left index and third finger pads monitor and control the transverse processes of L5 **(Fig. 12.23)**.

4. The physician gently flexes the patient's hips until L4 is fully flexed on L5.

5. The physician carefully pushes the patient's right shoulder posteriorly until L4 is engaged and rotates farther to the right on L5.

6. The physician then gently pushes the patient's pelvic and lumbar region anteriorly until L5 is fully engaged and rotated to the left under L4.

7. The patient inhales and exhales fully. On exhalation, the physician, with both the forearms and fingers on the transverse processes, increases the force through the same set of rotational vectors (*curved arrows*, **Fig. 12.24**), simultaneously approximating the forearms (*straight arrows*), thereby producing increased side bending right.

8. On achieving the proper position, the physician applies an activating force (*arrows*, **Fig. 12.25**) in the form of a gentle (1 pound or less) axial compression for 3 to 5 seconds with the finger pads.

9. If a release is not palpated within a few seconds, compression should be released, and steps 3 to 8 can be repeated.

10. The physician reassesses the components of the dysfunction (TART).

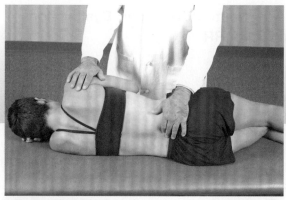

Figure 12.22. Steps 1 and 2.

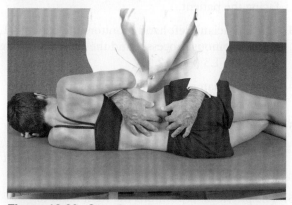

Figure 12.23. Step 3.

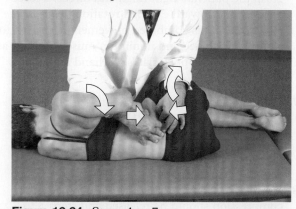

Figure 12.24. Steps 4 to 7.

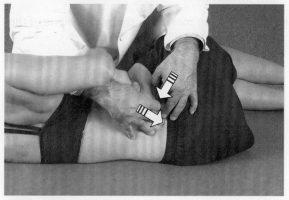

Figure 12.25. Step 8.

Lumbar Region

Left Erector Spinae Muscle Hypertonicity

1. The patient lies prone on the treatment table. A pillow may be placed under the abdomen to decrease the normal lumbar curvature. The physician faces the patient on the left.

2. Using the left hand, the physician monitors the patient's dysfunctional erector spinae hypertonicity **(Fig. 12.26)**.

3. The physician's left knee is placed on the table against the patient's left ilium.

4. The physician crosses the patient's right ankle over the patient's left ankle and grasps the patient's right knee, sliding both of the patient's legs to the left **(Fig. 12.27)**.

5. The physician repositions the right hand to grasp the patient's right thigh and directs a force dorsally and toward external rotation (*white arrows*, **Fig. 12.28**). This combined movement should be carried to a point of balance and minimum muscle tone as perceived by the physician's left hand.

6. On achieving the proper positioning, the physician's left hand applies an activating force (*white arrow*, **Fig. 12.29**) in the form of a gentle (1 pound or less) axial compression for 3 to 5 seconds.

7. If a release is not palpated within a few seconds, compression should be released, and steps 3 to 6 can be repeated.

8. The physician reassesses the components of the dysfunction (TART).

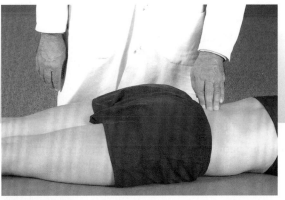

Figure 12.26. Steps 1 and 2.

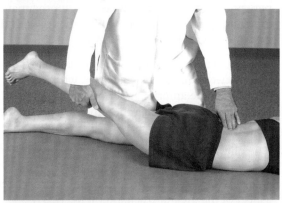

Figure 12.27. Steps 3 and 4.

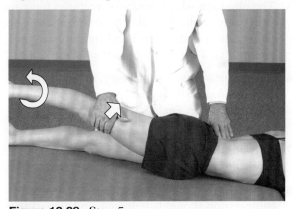

Figure 12.28. Step 5.

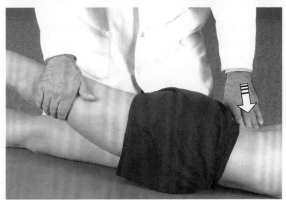

Figure 12.29. Step 6.

Pelvic Region

Iliosacral (Innominate) Dysfunction
Ex: Left, Posterior Innominate Rotation

1. The patient lies in the right lateral recumbent position, and the physician stands in front of the patient at the side of the table.

2. The physician's right arm reaches under the patient's left thigh and abducts it to approximately 30 degrees. The physician controls the leg with this arm and the shoulder **(Fig. 12.30)**.

3. The physician's left hand is placed palm down over the superior edge of the iliac crest, with the thumb controlling the anterior superior iliac spine (ASIS) and the hand controlling the superior edge of the iliac crest.

4. The physician's right hand is placed over the posterior iliac crest and posterior superior iliac spine (PSIS) with the forearm on the posterolateral aspect of the greater trochanter **(Fig. 12.31)**.

5. The physician adds a posterior-vectored force with a slight arc (right-turn direction) with the left hand (*down arrow*) as the right hand and forearm pull inferiorly and anteriorly (*up arrow*) **(Fig. 12.32)**.

6. As the pelvis rotates posteriorly, the physician adds a compressive force (1 pound or less) toward the table (*arrow*, **Fig. 12.33**) to approximate the sacroiliac joint surfaces.

7. This position is held for 3 to 5 seconds, and a gentle on-and-off pressure can be applied.

8. If a release is not palpated within a few seconds, compression should be released, and steps 3 to 8 can be repeated.

9. The physician reassesses the components of the dysfunction (TART).

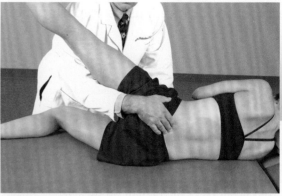

Figure 12.30. Steps 1 and 2.

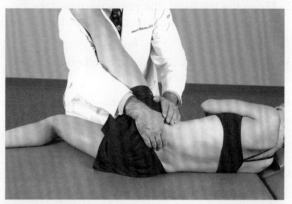

Figure 12.31. Steps 3 and 4.

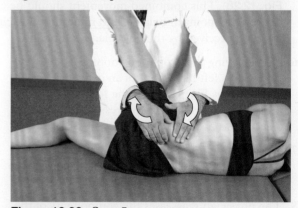

Figure 12.32. Step 5.

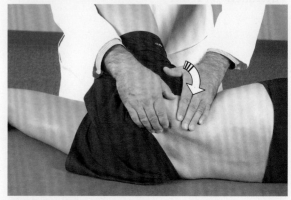

Figure 12.33. Step 6.

Pelvic Region

Iliosacral (Innominate) Dysfunction
Ex: Left, Anterior Innominate Rotation

1. The patient lies in the right lateral recumbent position, and the physician stands in front of the patient at the side of the table.

2. The physician's right arm reaches under the patient's left thigh and abducts it to approximately 30 to 40 degrees. The physician controls the leg with this arm and the shoulder (**Fig. 12.34**).

3. The physician places the left hand palm down over the superior edge of the iliac crest with the thumb controlling the ASIS and the hand controlling the superior edge of the iliac crest.

4. The pad of physician's right index finger is placed over the posterior iliac crest at the level of the PSIS with the heel of the right hand at the level of the ischial tuberosity (**Fig. 12.35**).

5. The physician adds an anterior-vectored force (*arrow*, **Fig. 12.36**) with a slight arc (left-turn direction) with the right hand as the left hand pulls superiorly and anteriorly.

6. As the pelvis rotates anteriorly, the physician adds a compressive force (1 pound or less) toward the table (*arrow*, **Fig. 12.37**) to approximate the sacroiliac joint surfaces.

7. This position is held for 3 to 5 seconds, and a gentle on-and-off pressure can be applied.

8. If a release is not palpated within a few seconds, compression should be released, and steps 3 to 7 can be repeated.

9. The physician reassesses the components of the dysfunction (TART).

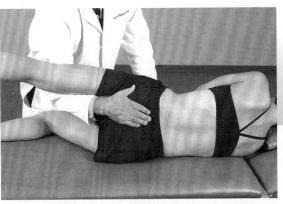

Figure 12.34. Steps 1 and 2.

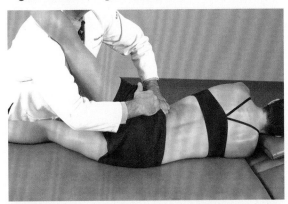

Figure 12.35. Steps 3 and 4.

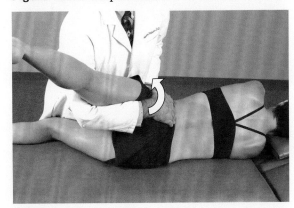

Figure 12.36. Step 5.

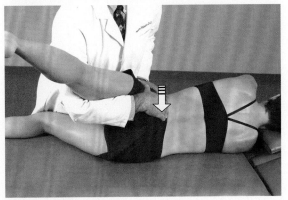

Figure 12.37. Step 6.

References

1. Chila AG, ed. Foundations of Osteopathic Medicine. 3rd ed. Baltimore, MD: Lippincott Williams & Wilkins, 2011.
2. Jones L, Kusunose R, Goering E. Jones Strain-Counterstrain. Boise, ID: Jones Strain-Counterstrain, Inc., 1995.
3. DiGiovanna E, Schiowitz S. An Osteopathic Approach to Diagnosis and Treatment. 3rd ed. Philadelphia, PA: Lippincott Williams & Wilkins, 2005.
4. Carew TJ. The Control of Reflex Action: Principles of Neural Science. 2nd ed. New York: Elsevier, 1985.

Techniques of Still

Technique Principles

As noted earlier in this book, many osteopathic techniques have gross similarities but fall into different categories. The technique of Still is no exception; it may be a classic example of how a number of other techniques combine and undergo a metamorphosis to become yet another technique, in this case, the Still technique. Basically, Still technique is a combination of some of the components of indirect, articulatory, and long-levered high-velocity, low-amplitude (HVLA) techniques. At Philadelphia College of Osteopathic Medicine (PCOM), a number of these techniques were included in these other categories (HVLA, articulatory) for years and were used commonly for costal, lumbar, innominate, and extremity dysfunctions (i.e., *Atlas of Osteopathic Techniques*, 1974). In 2000, with publication of *The Still Technique Manual*, by Richard L. Van Buskirk, DO, PhD, FAAO, many of these techniques became more formally structured and classified. Therefore, we have reclassified those previously taught as HVLA techniques into this category. However, as these techniques were taught previous to Van Buskirk's work, some do not include the aspects of compression or traction throughout the technique process. Yet, these older techniques do rely on proper localization and force vectoring through the dysfunctional segment's restrictive barrier in an indirect, then direct motion arc. It may be appropriate to remember that Still himself did not routinely describe, in writing, most of his techniques; but rather left it up to the osteopathic physician to consider the *principles of osteopathy* and utilize anatomy and physiology to develop a treatment plan specific to the patient's presentation. Historically, it has been common to see slight variations of osteopathic techniques over time, and this remains true with the development of Van Buskirk's contemporary style of "Still" technique.

Technique Classification

Indirect, Then Direct

The diagnostic components for Still technique are the same for all osteopathic techniques (tissue texture abnormality, asymmetry of position, restriction of motion, tenderness [TART]). The range of motion and ease-bind (tight-loose) barrier asymmetries must be noted, as the starting point of this technique is in indirect positioning similar to that of facilitated positional release (FPR) and other indirect techniques. For example, if the dysfunction is documented as L4, flexed, rotated right, and side bent right (L4 FRRSR), the initial (indirect) positioning would be to move L4 into flexion, rotation right, and side bending right, which is the ease or most free motion available in the cardinal (x, y, z) planes of motion.

Continuing this principle of indirect positioning, a slight compressive force may be added similar to FPR technique. Then, using a part of the patient's anatomy (e.g., trunk, extremity) to cause a long-levered force vector, the dysfunctional segment is carried through a motion arc or path of least resistance toward the *bind-tight* restrictive barrier. Carrying the segment through a path of least resistance is important, as the articular surfaces and other elements (e.g., bony, ligamentous) should not be compromised and stressed; otherwise, untoward side effects, such as pain, can result. This motion at the terminal phase may be similar to a long-levered HVLA; however, the dysfunctional segment does not necessarily have to be moved through the restrictive bind barrier, as the dysfunctional pattern may be eliminated during the movement within the range between ease and bind limits. This is different from HVLA, wherein the restrictive barrier is met and then passed through (albeit minimally). Therefore, in its simplest description, this technique is defined as "a specific nonrepetitive articulatory method that is indirect then direct (1,2)."

Technique Styles

Compression

When positioning the patient at the indirect barrier, the physician may attempt a slight compression of the articulatory surfaces before beginning the transfer of the segment toward the restrictive barrier.

This compression may help in producing a slight disengagement of the dysfunction and should be <5 pounds (<2 kg) of pressure (3). However, depending on the patient's health and functional capacity at the area, it may not be prudent to hold this compression at the outset of movement toward the restrictive barrier, as a shear effect can be produced and the articular cartilage may be injured. Also, if the patient has any foraminal narrowing, nerve root irritation may be an unwanted side effect. We have found that continuation of the compression throughout the technique may be uncomfortable for some of our patients with degenerative joint disease, etc., and therefore, we typically release the compression in these patients immediately after the start of the articular movement. As stated previously, this may differ slightly from how Van Buskirk described the technique, but the control of the dysfunctional segment is not lost if the correct long-levered tethering is maintained at the level of the dysfunction and we have found it to be a safe and effective variation. Otherwise, a compression (or traction) force may be added and continued throughout the indirect to direct motion arc, and even though this may not be included in each step-by-step description, it may be considered as inherent to the technique depending on the patient's condition.

Traction

When positioning the patient at the indirect barrier, the physician may attempt a slight traction of the articulatory surfaces before beginning the transfer of the segment toward the restrictive barrier. This distraction may help in producing a slight disengagement of the dysfunction. We have found that this is more comfortable in many patients than the compression style.

Indications

1. Articular somatic dysfunctions associated with intersegmental motion restriction
2. Myofascial somatic dysfunctions associated with muscle hypertonicity or fascial bind

Contraindications

1. Severe loss of intersegmental motion secondary to spondylosis, osteoarthritis, or rheumatoid arthritis in the area to be treated
2. Moderate to severe joint instability in the area to be treated
3. Acute strain or sprain in the area to be treated if the tissues may be further compromised by the motion introduced in the technique

Cervical Region

Occipitoatlantal (C0–C1, OA) Dysfunction
Ex: C0 ESRRL

1. The patient sits on the table (if preferred, this may be performed with the patient supine and physician sitting at head of table).

2. The physician stands behind the patient and places the left hand on top of patient's head.

3. The physician places the right index finger pad (or thumb pad) at the right basiocciput to monitor motion **(Fig. 13.1)**.

4. The physician may minimally extend the occiput and then add a slight compression on the head (*straight arrow*, **Fig. 13.2**) and side bends the head to the right (*curved arrow*) enough to engage the occiput on the atlas, approximately 5 to 7 degrees.

5. The physician then rotates head to the left (*arrow*, **Fig. 13.3**) only enough to engage the occiput on the atlas 5 to 7 degrees.

6. The physician increases the head compression minimally and then with moderate speed flexes the head minimally (10 to 15 degrees) **(Fig. 13.4)** and adds side bending left and rotation right (*arrows*, **Fig. 13.5**) while monitoring the right basiocciput to insure that the motion does not engage the segments below C1.

7. The physician re-evaluates the dysfunctional (TART) components.

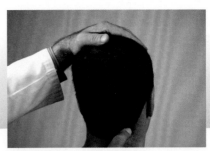
Figure 13.1. Steps 1 to 3, setup.

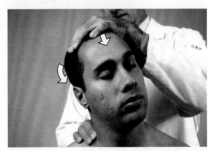
Figure 13.2. Step 4, compression and side bending to right.

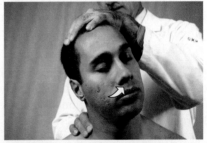
Figure 13.3. Step 5, rotation to left.

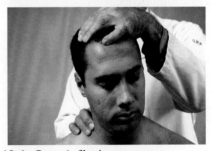
Figure 13.4. Step 6, flexion.

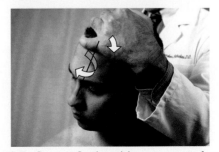
Figure 13.5. Step 6, final position to engage barrier.

Cervical Region

Atlantoaxial (C1–C2) Dysfunction
Ex: C1 RL

1. The patient lies supine on the treatment table, and the physician sits or stands at the head of the table. This may also be performed with the patient seated.

2. The physician places the hands over the parietotemporal regions, and the left index finger pad palpates the left transverse process of C1 **(Fig. 13.6)**.

3. The physician rotates the patient's head to the left ease barrier (*arrow*, **Fig. 13.7**).

4. The physician introduces gentle compression through the head directed toward C1 **(Fig. 13.8)** and then with moderate acceleration begins to rotate the head toward the right restrictive barrier (*arrow*, **Fig. 13.9**).

5. The release should occur before the restrictive barrier is engaged. If not, the physician should not carry the head and dysfunctional C1 more than a few degrees through the barrier.

6. The physician re-evaluates the dysfunctional (TART) components.

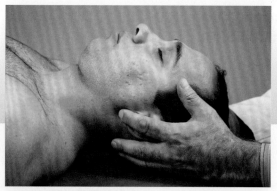

Figure 13.6. Step 2, hand placement.

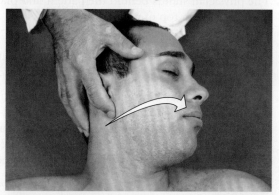

Figure 13.7. Step 3, rotate to ease.

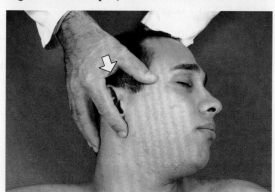

Figure 13.8. Step 4, compression.

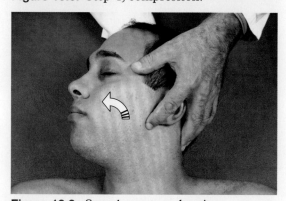

Figure 13.9. Step 4, rotate to barrier.

Cervical Region

C2–C7 Dysfunctions
Ex: C4 ESRRR

1. The patient lies supine on the treatment table.

2. The physician's right index finger pad palpates the patient's right C4 articular process.

3. The physician places the left hand over the patient's head so that the physician can control its movement **(Fig. 13.10)**.

4. The physician extends the head (*arrow*, **Fig. 13.11**) until C4 is engaged.

5. The physician then rotates and side bends the head so that C4 is still engaged **(Fig. 13.12)**.

6. The physician introduces a compression force (*straight arrow*, **Fig. 13.13**) through the head directed toward C4 and then with moderate acceleration begins to rotate and side bend the head to the left (*curved arrows*), simultaneously adding graduated flexion.

7. The release should normally occur before the restrictive barrier is engaged. If not, the physician should not carry the head and dysfunctional C4 more than a few degrees through the barrier.

8. The physician reevaluates the dysfunctional (TART) components.

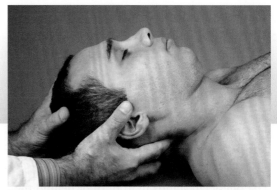

Figure 13.10. Steps 1 to 3, hand placement.

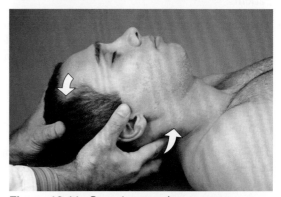

Figure 13.11. Step 4, extension to ease.

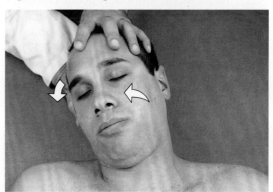

Figure 13.12. Step 5, side bend and rotate to ease.

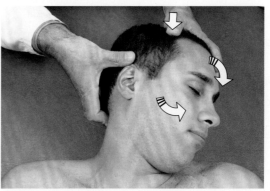

Figure 13.13. Step 6, compression, side bending left and rotation left (SLRL) to barrier.

Thoracic Region

T1, T2 Dysfunctions (Seated)
Ex: T1 ESRRR

1. The patient is seated (may be performed with patient supine).

2. The physician stands in front of or behind the patient.

3. The physician palpates the dysfunctional segment (T1) with the index finger pad of one hand while controlling the patient's head with the other hand (**Fig. 13.14**).

4. The physician, with the head-controlling hand, extends the head slightly until this motion is palpated at T1 (*arrow*, **Fig. 13.15**).

5. The physician then introduces right side bending and rotation (*arrows*, **Fig. 13.16**) until this occurs at T1.

6. Next, the physician introduces gentle compression force through the head toward T1 and with moderate acceleration begins to rotate and side bend the head to the left (*arrows*, **Fig. 13.17**), simultaneously adding graduated flexion.

7. This motion is carried toward the restrictive barrier. The release may occur before the barrier is met. If not, the head must not be carried more than a few degrees beyond.

8. The physician reevaluates the dysfunctional (TART) components.

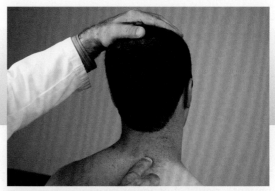

Figure 13.14. Step 3, setup.

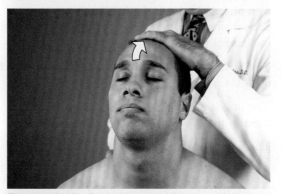

Figure 13.15. Step 4, extend to ease.

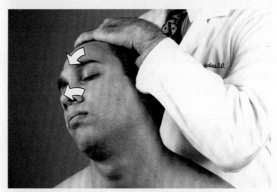

Figure 13.16. Step 5, side bend and rotate to ease.

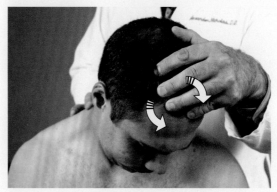

Figure 13.17. Step 6, compression, engage barrier.

Thoracic Region

T1, T2 Dysfunctions (Supine)
Ex: T2 FSLRL

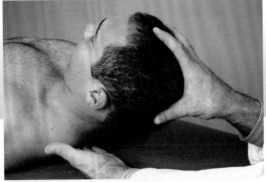

Figure 13.18. Step 3, setup.

1. The patient is supine on the treatment table (may be performed with patient seated).

2. The physician sits or stands at the head of the table.

3. The physician palpates the dysfunctional segment (T2) with the index finger pad of the left hand, controlling the patient's head with the other hand **(Fig. 13.18)**.

4. The physician, with the head-controlling hand, flexes the patient's neck slightly (*arrow*, **Fig. 13.19**) until this motion is palpated at T2.

5. The physician introduces left rotation and side bending (*arrows*, **Fig. 13.20**) until this motion occurs at T2.

6. The physician introduces gentle compression force through the head (*straight arrow*, **Fig. 13.21**) toward T2 and then with moderate acceleration begins to rotate and side bend the head to the right (*curved arrows*, **Fig. 13.21**) with a simultaneous graduated extension **(Fig. 13.22)**.

7. This motion is carried toward the restrictive barrier, and the release may occur before the barrier is met. If not, the head must not be carried more than a few degrees beyond.

8. The physician reevaluates the dysfunctional (TART) components.

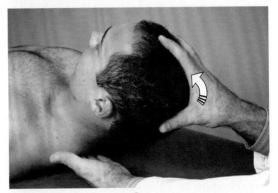

Figure 13.19. Step 4, flex to ease.

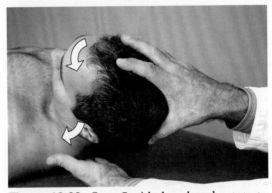

Figure 13.20. Step 5, side bend and rotate to ease.

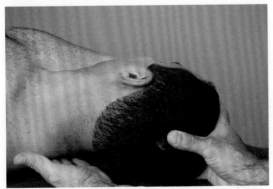

Figure 13.22. Step 6, engaging extension, rotation right, side bend right (ERRSR) barrier.

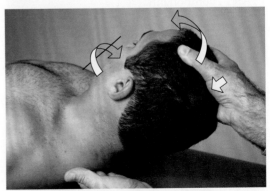

Figure 13.21. Step 6, compression, rotate right and side bend right (RRSR).

Thoracic Region

T3–T12 (Seated)
Ex: T5 NSLRR

1. The patient is seated on the treatment table.

2. The physician stands or sits to the left of the patient.

3. The physician instructs the patient to place the right hand behind the neck and the left hand palm down over the right antecubital fossa.

4. The physician's left hand reaches under the patient's left arm or lies palm down over the patient's right humerus **(Fig. 13.23)**.

5. The physician places the right thenar eminence over the T6 left transverse process and the thumb and index finger over the left and right transverse processes of T5, respectively **(Fig. 13.24)**.

6. The physician gently positions the patient's thoracic spine to T5 in side bending left and rotation right (*arrows*, **Fig. 13.25**).

7. The physician, while maintaining the spine in neutral position relative to T5–T6, adds a compression force through the spine to T5 (*arrow*, **Fig. 13.26**) by gently pulling or leaning down on the patient. The physician simultaneously introduces side bending right (*curved sweep arrow*) and rotation left (*curved arrow*, **Fig. 13.27**).

8. This motion is carried toward the restrictive barrier, and the release may occur before the barrier is met. If not, the head must not be carried more than a few degrees beyond.

9. The physician reevaluates the dysfunctional (TART) components.

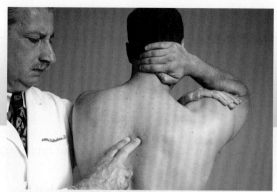

Figure 13.23. Steps 1 to 4, positioning.

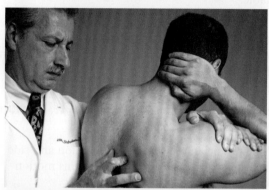

Figure 13.24. Step 5, monitoring T5–T6.

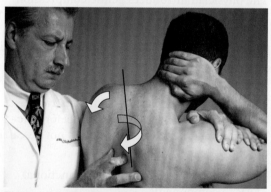

Figure 13.25. Step 6, side bend left, rotate right (SLRR).

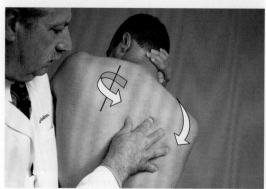

Figure 13.27. Step 7, accelerating to side bend right, rotate left (SRRL) barrier.

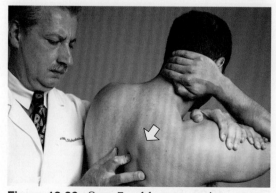

Figure 13.26. Step 7, add compression.

Coastal Region

Rib 1 Elevated Dysfunction
Nonphysiologic, Depressed Emphasis
Ex: Right Posterior Rib 1 Elevated

1. The patient is seated, and the physician stands behind the patient.

2. The physician's cupped left hand reaches over the patient's left shoulder and across the patient's chest to lie palm down over the patient's right shoulder with the second and third finger pads anchoring the first rib **(Fig. 13.28)**. An alternative position similar to an HVLA technique may be preferred **(Fig. 13.29)**.

3. The physician's right hand side bends the patient's head to the left (*arrow*, **Fig. 13.30**) while the left arm keeps the patient's trunk from following.

4. The physician's right hand adds a gentle compression force (*arrow*, **Fig. 13.31**) toward the right first rib.

5. The physician instructs the patient to inhale and exhale.

6. On exhalation, the physician pushes the patient's head to the right (*arrow*, **Fig. 13.32**) while maintaining compression on the head and on the rib with the finger.

7. This motion is carried toward the restrictive barrier, and the release may occur before the barrier is met. If not, the head must not be carried more than a few degrees beyond.

8. The physician reevaluates the dysfunctional (TART) components.

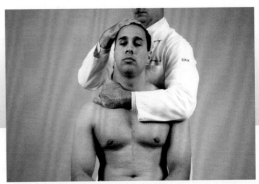

Figure 13.28. Steps 1 and 2, positioning.

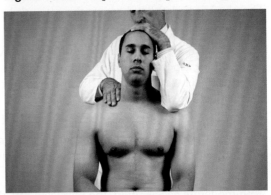

Figure 13.29. Steps 1 and 2, alternative technique position.

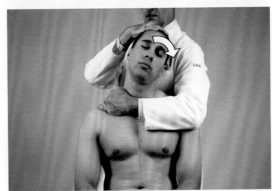

Figure 13.30. Step 3, side bending left.

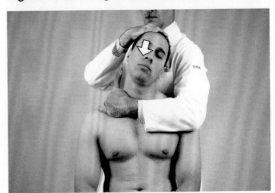

Figure 13.31. Step 4, compressive force.

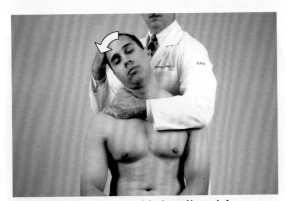

Figure 13.32. Step 6, side bending right.

Coastal Region

Rib 1, Rib 2 Exhalation Dysfunctions
Shoulder Circumduction, Inhalation Emphasis
Ex: Left Rib 1 Exhaled/Depressed

1. The patient is seated, and the physician stands behind the patient on the side of the dysfunctional rib.

2. The physician's left hand grasps the patient's left forearm.

3. The physician places the other hand (thumb) over the posterior aspect of the dysfunctional left first rib immediately lateral to the T1 transverse costal articulation **(Fig. 13.33)**.

4. The physician draws the patient's left arm anteriorly, adducts it across the patient's chest, and pulls (*arrow*, **Fig. 13.34**) the adducted arm toward the floor.

5. With moderate acceleration, the physician lifts the arm, simultaneously flexing and abducting with a circumduction motion **(Fig. 13.35)**.

6. The acceleration is continued posteriorly and then back to the side of the patient **(Fig. 13.36)**.

7. The physician reevaluates the dysfunctional (TART) components.

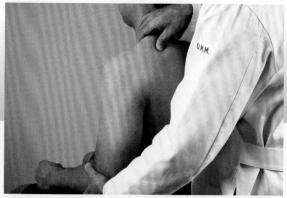

Figure 13.33. Steps 1 to 3, positioning.

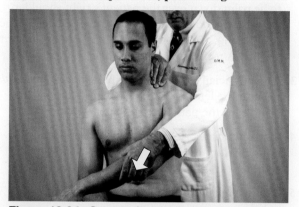

Figure 13.34. Step 4, drawing patient's arm.

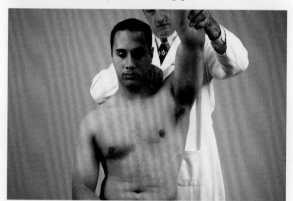

Figure 13.35. Step 5, accelerate to barrier.

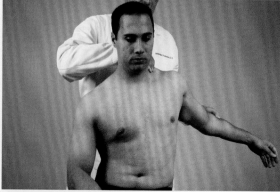

Figure 13.36. Step 6, accelerate posteriorly.

Coastal Region

Rib 1 Exhalation Dysfunction
Head/Neck Leverage, Inhalation Emphasis
Ex: Right Rib 1 Exhaled/Depressed

1. The patient is seated, and the physician stands behind the patient.

2. The physician's right hand palpates the posterior aspect of the first rib at the attachment at its costotransverse articulation.

3. The physician places the left hand over the patient's head.

4. The physician's left hand slowly flexes the patient's head (*curved arrow*, **Fig. 13.37**) until the T1 segment and first rib are engaged.

5. The patient's head is then side bent and rotated right (*curved arrows*, **Fig. 13.38**) until these motion vectors engage T1 and the first rib, exaggerating its exhalation dysfunction position.

6. The patient is instructed to inhale and exhale, and on repeated inhalation, the patient's head is carried (*curved arrows*, **Fig. 13.39**) toward left-side bending and rotation.

7. As the dysfunctional rib is engaged, a slight extension of the head is introduced, carrying the rib through a pump-handle (slight bucket-handle) axis of motion **(Fig. 13.40)**.

8. This motion is carried toward the inhalation restrictive barrier, and the release may occur before the barrier is met. If not, the head must not be carried more than a few degrees beyond.

9. The physician reevaluates the dysfunctional (TART) components.

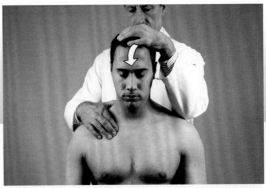

Figure 13.37. Steps 1 to 4, setup, engage T1 and first rib.

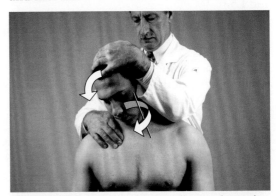

Figure 13.38. Step 5, side bending and rotation to right.

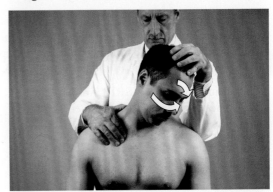

Figure 13.39. Step 6, head carried toward SLRL.

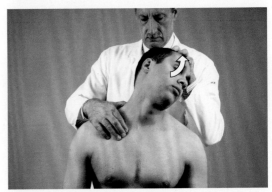

Figure 13.40. Step 7, add slight extension.

Lumbar Region

L1–L5 Dysfunctions
Pelvic/Hip Circumduction Emphasis
Ex: L4 NSRRL

1. The patient lies supine, and the physician stands on the side of the rotational component (left).

2. The physician places the right hand under the patient to monitor the transverse processes of L4 and L5.

3. The physician instructs the patient to flex the right hip and knee.

4. The physician's other hand controls the patient's flexed right leg at the tibial tuberosity and flexes the hip until the L5 segment is engaged and rotated to the right under L4 **(Fig. 13.41)**.

5. The physician externally rotates and abducts the hip while the other hand monitors motion at L4–L5. This position should place the L4 segment indirectly (side bent right, rotated left [SRRL]) as it relates to its dysfunctional position on L5, while L5 has been rotated to the right **(Fig. 13.42)**.

6. The physician, with moderate acceleration, pulls the patient's right leg to the left in adduction and internal rotation **(Fig. 13.43)** and then fully extends the leg across the midline to the left **(Fig. 13.44)**.

7. This motion carries L5 (SRRL) under L4 (SLRR) toward the L4–L5 restrictive barriers, and the release may occur before the barrier is met.

8. The physician reevaluates the dysfunctional (TART) components.

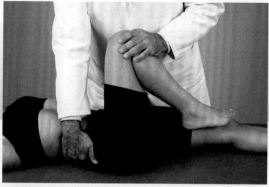

Figure 13.41. Steps 1 to 4, setup toward rotational ease.

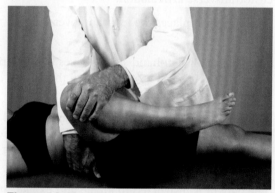

Figure 13.42. Step 5, externally rotate hip.

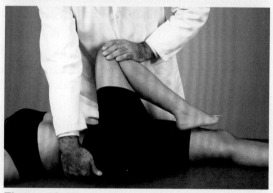

Figure 13.43. Step 6, accelerate into internal rotation and adduction.

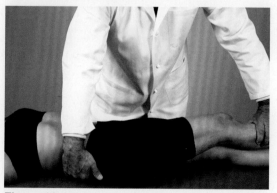

Figure 13.44. Step 6, extension across midline.

Lumbar Region

L1–L5 Dysfunctions
Lateral Recumbent, Side Bending/Rotation
Ex: L3 ESRRR

1. The patient lies in the right lateral recumbent (side lying) position.

2. The physician stands at the side of the table in front of the patient.

3. The physician's caudad hand controls the patient's legs and flexes the hips while the cephalad hand monitors motion at L3–L4.

4. The patient's legs are flexed until L3 is engaged **(Fig. 13.45)**.

5. The physician's forearm pulls the patient's left shoulder girdle forward (*arrow*, **Fig. 13.46**) and the caudal arm pushes the patient's ilium posteriorly (*arrow*) while the fingers continue to monitor the L3–L4 vertebral unit.

6. The physician adds slight traction (*arrows*, **Fig. 13.47**) between the shoulder girdle and the pelvis and then, with a moderate acceleration, reverses this traction (*straight arrows*, **Fig. 13.48**) and simultaneously pushes the shoulder posteriorly (*pulsed arrow at right*, **Fig. 13.48**) and the pelvis anteriorly (*pulsed arrow at left*, **Fig. 13.48**) to achieve side bending left and rotation left.

7. The release may occur before the barrier is met. If not, the segment should be carried only minimally through it.

8. The physician re-evaluates the dysfunctional (TART) components.

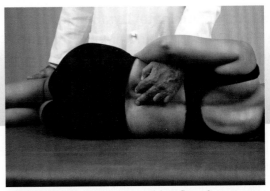

Figure 13.45. Steps 1 to 4, hips flexed to engage segment.

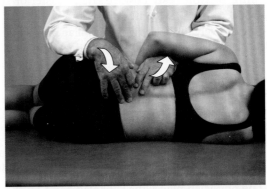

Figure 13.46. Step 5, position into rotational ease.

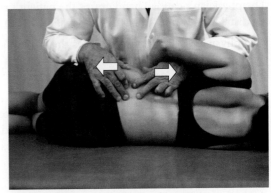

Figure 13.47. Step 6.

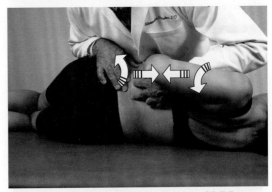

Figure 13.48. Step 6, accelerate to SLRL.

Pelvic Region

Iliosacral (Innominate) Dysfunction
Ex: Right, Anterior Innominate Rotation
Modified Sims, Posterior Rotation Emphasis

 See Video 13.1

Note: This technique was originally identified as *Indirect/ Direct Long-Lever HVLA.*

Diagnosis

Standing flexion test: Positive (right posterior superior iliac spine [PSIS] rises)
Loss of passively induced right sacroiliac motion
PSIS: Cephalad (slightly lateral) on the right
Anterior superior iliac spine (ASIS): Caudad (slightly medial) on the right
Sacral sulcus: Posterior on the right

Technique

1. The patient is in the left modified Sims position, and the physician stands behind the patient (**Fig. 13.49**).

2. The physician places the cephalad hand on the patient's sacrum to resist sacral movement.

3. The physician's caudad hand grasps the patient's right leg distal to the knee (tibial tuberosity) (**Fig. 13.50**).

4. The physician's caudad hand flexes the patient's right hip and knee (**Fig. 13.51**) and then returns them to an extended position (**Fig. 13.52**).

5. This motion is repeated three times, and at the end of the third flexion, the patient's hip is accelerated into flexion (*curved white arrow*) with a cephalad impulse (thrust) while the left hand immobilizes to sacrum (*straight white arrow*, **Fig. 13.53**).

6. The right leg and hip are then extended, and right sacroiliac motion is retested to assess the effectiveness of the technique.

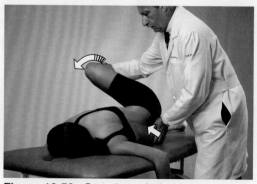

Figure 13.53. Step 5, cephalad impulse.

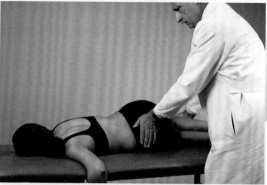

Figure 13.49. Step 1, positioning.

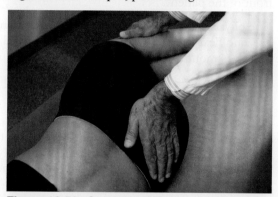

Figure 13.50. Steps 2 and 3, hand placement.

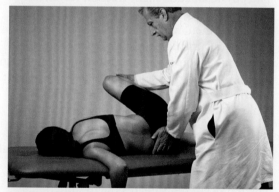

Figure 13.51. Step 4, flex hip and knee.

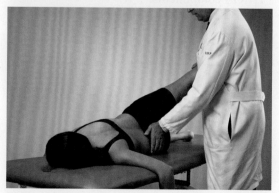

Figure 13.52. Step 4, return to extension.

Pelvic Region

Iliosacral (Innominate) Dysfunction
Ex: Right, Posterior Innominate Rotation
Modified Sims, Anterior Rotation Emphasis

 See Video 13.2

Note: This technique was originally identified as *Indirect/Direct Long-Lever HVLA.*

Diagnosis

Standing flexion test: Positive (right PSIS rises)
Loss of passively induced right sacroiliac motion
ASIS: Cephalad (slightly lateral) on the right
PSIS: Caudad (slightly medial) on the right
Sacral sulcus: Deep, anterior on the right

Technique

1. The patient is in the left modified Sims position, and the physician stands behind the patient.

2. The physician places the left hand on the patient's right PSIS while the right hand grasps the patient's right leg just distal to the knee (tibial tuberosity) **(Fig. 13.54)**.

3. The patient's right leg is moved in an upward, outward circular motion (*white arrows*, **Fig. 13.55**) as the hip is flexed, abducted, externally rotated, and carried into extension **(Fig. 13.56)** to check hip range of motion.

4. This circular motion is applied for three cycles, and at the end of the third cycle, the patient is instructed to kick the leg straight, positioning the hip and knee into extension.

5. While this kick is taking place (*arrow at left*, **Fig. 13.57**), the physician's left hand on the patient's right PSIS delivers an impulse (*arrow at right*) toward the patient's umbilicus.

6. Right sacroiliac motion is retested to assess the effectiveness of the technique.

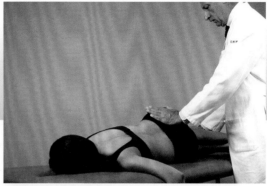
Figure 13.54. Steps 1 and 2, setup.

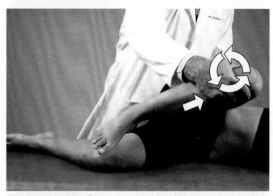
Figure 13.55. Step 3, circular hip motion.

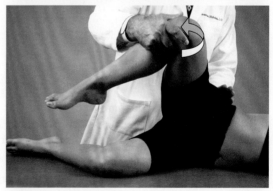
Figure 13.56. Step 3, abduction, external rotation, and extension.

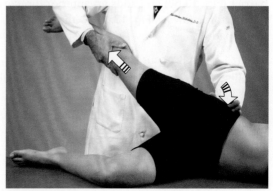
Figure 13.57. Steps 4 and 5, kick leg straight with impulse on PSIS.

Upper Extremity Region

Elbow: Radioulnar Pronation Dysfunction
Radial Head, Supination Emphasis
Ex: Left Radial Head, Pronation

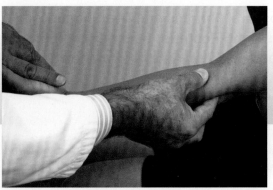

Figure 13.58. Steps 1 to 3, setup, hand placement.

Note: This technique was originally identified as *Indirect/ Direct Long-Lever HVLA.*

Diagnosis

Symptoms: Elbow discomfort with inability to fully supinate the forearm
Motion: Restricted supination of the forearm
Palpation: Tenderness at the radial head with posterior prominence of the radial head

Technique

1. The patient is seated on the table, and the physician stands in front of the patient.

2. The physician holds the patient's hand on the dysfunctional arm as if shaking hands with the patient.

3. The physician places the index finger pad and thumb of the other hand so that the thumb is anterior and the index finger pad is posterior to the radial head **(Fig. 13.58).**

4. The physician rotates the hand into the indirect pronation position and pushes the radial head posteriorly with the thumb until the ease barrier is engaged **(Fig. 13.59).**

5. Finally, the physician, with a moderate acceleration through an arc-like path of least resistance, supinates the forearm toward the restrictive bind barrier **(Fig. 13.60)** and adds an anterior directed counterforce (*arrow,* **Fig. 13.61**) with the index finger pad.

6. The release may occur before the barrier is met. If not, the radial head must not be carried more than a few degrees beyond.

7. The physician reevaluates the dysfunctional (TART) components.

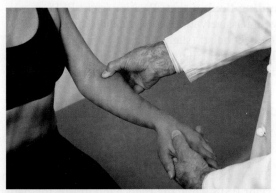

Figure 13.59. Step 4, engage pronation and radial head ease.

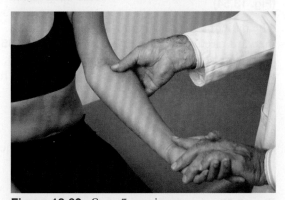

Figure 13.60. Step 5, supinate.

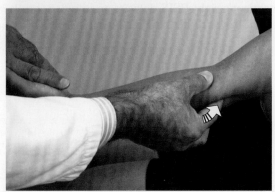

Figure 13.61. Step 5, anterior counterforce.

CHAPTER **13** | TECHNIQUES OF STILL **451**

Upper Extremity Region

Elbow: Radioulnar Supination Dysfunction
Radial Head, Pronation Emphasis
Ex: Left Radial Head, Supination

Note: This technique was originally identified as *Indirect/Direct Long-Lever HVLA*.

Diagnosis

Symptoms: Elbow discomfort with inability to fully pronate the forearm

Motion: Restricted pronation of the forearm

Palpation: Tenderness at the radial head with anterior (ventral) prominence of the radial head

Technique

1. The patient is seated on the table, and the physician stands in front of the patient.

2. The physician holds the patient's hand on the dysfunctional arm as if shaking hands with the patient.

3. The physician places the index finger pad and thumb of the other hand so that the thumb is anterior and the index finger pad is posterior to the radial head **(Fig. 13.62)**.

4. The physician rotates the hand into the indirect supination position **(Fig. 13.63)** and pushes the radial head anteriorly (*arrow*, **Fig. 13.64**) with the index finger pad until the ease barrier is engaged.

5. Finally, the physician, with moderate acceleration through an arc-like path of least resistance, pronates the forearm toward the restrictive bind barrier and adds a posterior directed counterforce (*arrow*, **Fig. 13.65**) with the thumb.

6. The release may occur before the barrier is met. If not, the radial head must not be carried more than a few degrees beyond.

7. The physician reevaluates the dysfunctional (TART) components.

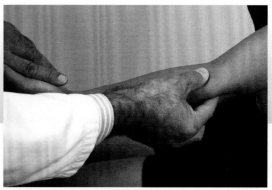

Figure 13.62. Steps 1 to 3, setup: hand placement.

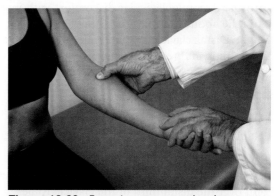

Figure 13.63. Step 4, engage supination.

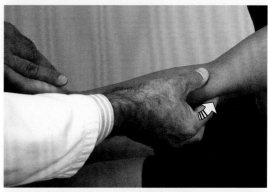

Figure 13.64. Step 4, engage radial head ease.

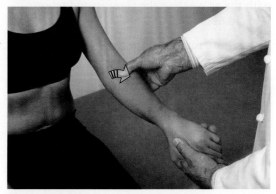

Figure 13.65. Step 5, pronate with posterior counterforce.

Upper Extremity Region

Acromioclavicular Joint Dysfunction
Ex: Right Distal Clavicle, Elevated

 See Video 13.3

Note: This technique was originally identified as *Indirect/ Direct Long-Lever HVLA.*

Diagnosis

Symptoms: Acromioclavicular discomfort with inability to fully abduct and flex the shoulder

Findings: Distal clavicle palpably elevated relative to the acromion and resists caudad pressure

Technique

1. The patient is seated, and the physician stands behind the patient toward the side to be treated.

2. The physician, using the hand closest to the patient, places the second metacarpal-phalangeal joint over the distal third of the clavicle to be treated.

3. The physician maintains constant caudad pressure over the patient's clavicle throughout the treatment sequence.

4. The physician's other hand grasps the patient's arm on the side to be treated just below the elbow **(Fig. 13.66)**.

5. The patient's arm is pulled down and then drawn backward into extension **(Fig. 13.67)** with a continuous motion similar to throwing a ball overhand, circumducting the arm **(Fig. 13.68)** until it is once again in front of the patient, finishing with the arm across the chest in adduction **(Fig. 13.69)**.

6. The release may occur before the barrier is met.

7. The physician reevaluates the dysfunctional (TART) components.

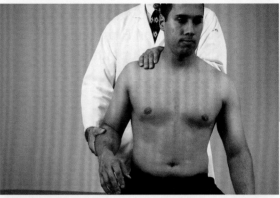

Figure 13.66. Steps 1 to 4, setup: hand placement.

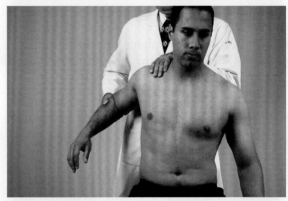

Figure 13.67. Steps 4 and 5, backward extension.

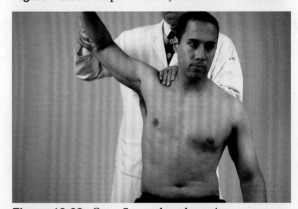

Figure 13.68. Step 5, overhand motion.

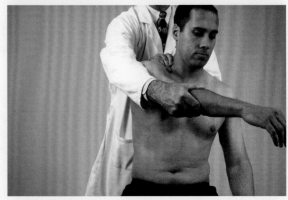

Figure 13.69. Step 5, arm across chest.

Upper Extremity Region

Sternoclavicular Joint Dysfunction
Ex: Right Proximal Clavicle, Elevated

 See Video 13.3

Note: This technique was originally identified as *Indirect/Direct Long-Lever HVLA.*

Diagnosis

Symptoms: Tenderness at the sternoclavicular joint with inability to abduct the shoulder fully without pain
Motion: Restricted abduction of the clavicle
Palpation: Prominence and elevation of the proximal end of the clavicle

Technique

1. The patient is seated with the physician standing behind the patient.

2. The physician's left hand reaches around in front of the patient and places the thumb over the proximal end of the patient's right clavicle.

3. The physician's left thumb maintains constant caudad pressure over the patient's clavicle throughout the treatment sequence.

4. The physician's right hand grasps the patient's right arm just below the elbow **(Fig. 13.70)**.

5. The patient's arm is brought toward flexion from adduction to abduction **(Fig. 13.71)**. With a continuous backstroke motion **(Fig. 13.72)**, the arm is circumducted toward extension until it is at the side of the patient **(Fig. 13.73)**. The arm can be brought forward and placed across the chest if this is comfortable to the patient.

6. The release may occur before the barrier is met.

7. The physician re-evaluates the dysfunctional (TART) components.

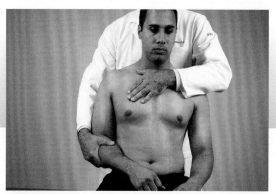
Figure 13.70. Steps 1 to 4, setup: hand placement.

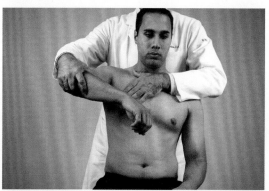
Figure 13.71. Step 5, flexion and abduction.

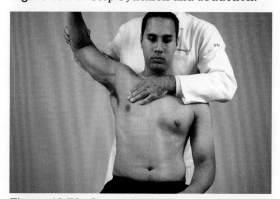
Figure 13.72. Step 5, backstroke motion.

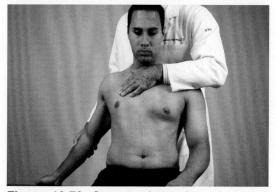
Figure 13.73. Step 5, circumducted toward extension.

References

1. Van Buskirk RL. The Still Technique Manual: Applications of a Rediscovered Technique of Andrew Taylor Still, MD. Indianapolis, IA: American Academy of Osteopathy, 2000.
2. Ward R, exec.ed. Foundations for Osteopathic Medicine. 2nd ed. Philadelphia, PA: Lippincott Williams & Wilkins, 2003.
3. Chila AG, exec.ed. Foundations of Osteopathic Medicine. 3rd ed. Baltimore, MD: Lippincott Williams & Wilkins, 2011.

14

Balanced Ligamentous Tension and Ligamentous Articular Strain Techniques

Technique Principles

Balanced ligamentous tension (BLT) and ligamentous articular strain (LAS) techniques may be considered as two separate techniques or as one. The history of the development of these techniques probably started during A. T. Still's time but developed greatly through the work of a number of osteopathic physicians including, but not limited to, W. G. Sutherland, DO; H. A. Lippincott, DO; R. Lippincott, DO; R. Becker, DO; and A. Wales, DO (1–3). It appears that a geographic separation and minimal contact between two groups may have caused the same technique to be known by two names. Those in the central United States (i.e., Texas) eventually promoted the term LAS, and those in the northeastern United States (i.e., New Jersey and New England) promoted the term BLT. As the two names suggest, some variance in the techniques developed, and the practitioners developed their own particular nuances for the application of the treatment. The term LAS seems to describe the dysfunction while the term BLT describes the process or goal of the treatment. The ECOP glossary definitions of these techniques are as follows (4):

BLT: 1. According to Sutherland's model, all the joints in the body are balanced ligamentous articular mechanisms. The ligaments provide proprioceptive information that guides the muscle response for positioning the joint, and the ligaments themselves guide the motion of the articular components (*Foundations*). 2. First described in "Osteopathic Technique of William G. Sutherland" that was published in the *1949 Year Book of Academy of Applied Osteopathy*

LAS: 1. A manipulative technique in which the goal of treatment is to balance the tension in opposing ligaments where there is abnormal tension present. 2. A set of myofascial release (MFR) techniques described by Howard Lippincott, DO, and Rebecca Lippincott, DO. 3. Title of reference work by Conrad Speece, DO, and William Thomas Crow, DO

Sutherland may have been most responsible for the technique being taught in early osteopathic study

groups. In the 1940s, he began teaching a method of treatment of the body and extremities with the principles promoted for the treatment of the cranium. He talked about the joint's relation with its ligaments, fascia, and so on (*ligamentous articular mechanism*), and we can extrapolate this to include the potential for mechanoreceptor excitation in dysfunctional states. One of Sutherland's ideas, a key concept in this area, was that normal movements of a joint or articulation do not cause asymmetric tensions in the ligaments and that the tension distributed through the ligaments in any given joint is balanced (2,5). These tensions can change when the ligament or joint is stressed (*strain* or *unit deformation*) in the presence of altered mechanical force. In this case, the term strain follows the definition of stress to an object and should not be confused with the clinical definitions of strain (musculotendinous) and sprain (ligamentous) and their respective first-, second-, and third-degree severity levels of injury. Today, this principle is similar to the architectural and biomechanical (structural) principles of tensegrity, as seen in the geodesic dome of R. Buckminster Fuller and the art of Kenneth Snelson, his student (6–8). This principle is commonly promoted in the postulate that an anterior anatomic (fascial) bowstring is present in the body. The theory is that the key dysfunction may produce both proximal and distal effects. These effects can produce symptoms both anteriorly and posteriorly (1).

One of the aspects mentioned in some osteopathic manipulative technique styles is a release-enhancing mechanism. This mechanism may be isometric contraction of a muscle; a respiratory movement of the diaphragm, eye, and tongue movements; or, in the case of BLT or LAS, the use of *inherent forces*, such as circulatory (Traube-Hering-Mayer), lymphatic, or a variety of other factors (e.g., primary respiratory mechanism) (2). The physician introduces a force to position the patient so that a fulcrum may be set. This fulcrum, paired with the subsequent lever action of the tissues (ligaments), combines with fluid dynamics and other factors to produce a change in the dysfunctional state. In some cases, the technique is used to affect the myofascial structures.

In the case of treating a myofascial structure, the differentiating factor between BLT/LAS and myofascial release (MFR) is that an inherent force (fluid model) is the release-enhancing mechanism in BLT/LAS; in MFR, the thermodynamic reaction to pressure is the primary release factor.

Technique Classification

Indirect Technique

In the case of BLT/LAS, the physician positions the patient's dysfunctional area toward the ease barrier. This indirect positioning is the classic method of treatment in this technique.

When beginning the treatment, the physician typically attempts to produce some *freeplay* in the articulation. This attempt to allow the most motion to occur without resistance is termed *disengagement*. It can be produced by compression or traction (1,3). In our practice, compression most commonly achieves this *freeplay*. *Exaggeration* is the second step described. It is produced by moving toward the ease or to what some refer as the original position of injury (1). This "exaggerated" positioning is synonymous with the ease asymmetry as documented in an articular dysfunction (e.g., C5, FRRSR). Placing the tissues in an optimal balance of tension (i.e., *balance point, still point*) at the articulation or area of dysfunction is the final positioning step of this technique (3). Some refer to this point as the *wobble point*. This is similar to the sensation of balancing an object on the fingertip. The *wobble point* is central to all radiating tensions, and those tensions feel asymmetric when not at the point. While holding this position, the physician awaits a release. This release has been described as a gentle movement toward the ease and then a slow movement backward toward the balance point (ebb and flow) and then, finally, toward and through the restrictive barrier to its normal physiologic position (3).

For example, if the dysfunction being treated is described as L4, F SL RL, the ease or direction of freedom is in the following directions: flexion, side bending left, and rotation left. Moving L4 (over a stabilized L5) in this direction is described as moving away from the restrictive barrier and therefore defines the technique as *indirect*.

Direct Technique

Some have included a direct style of technique, which follows direct myofascial release or soft tissue "inhibitory" technique (1). Others describe the technique as direct, as with some dysfunctions, the physician must "directly" penetrate hypertonic myofascial structures in order to gain access to the deeper articular and capsular structures. However, as both descriptions of this style of osteopathic treatment (BLT, LAS) include the term ligamentous, and by defining and introducing the idea of the *point of balance*, especially at the articular/capsular level, the technique must be inherently indirect.

Technique Styles

Diagnosis and Treatment with Respiration

In this method, the physician palpates the area involved and attempts to discern the pattern of dysfunction with extremely light palpatory technique. This could be described as nudging the segment through the x, y, and z axes with the movements caused by respiration. Therefore, the movements used in the attempt to diagnose and treat the dysfunction are extremely small.

Diagnosis and Treatment with Intersegmental Motion Testing (Physician Active)

In intersegmental motion testing/treatment style, slightly more motion and/or force can be used to test motion parameters in the dysfunctional site and to begin to move the site into the appropriate indirect position of balanced tensions. There may be more compression or traction in this form as well, depending on the dysfunctional state, site, or preference of the treating physician.

Indications

1. Somatic dysfunctions of articular basis
2. Areas of lymphatic congestion or local edema (note: see Lymphatic Techniques, Lower Extremity, Hip for an LAS style of technique, which is excellent in both situations)

Relative Contraindications

1. Fracture, dislocation, or gross instability in area to be treated
2. Malignancy, infection, or severe osteoporosis in area to be treated

General Considerations and Rules

The technique is specific palpatory balancing of the tissues surrounding and inherent to a joint or the myofascial structures related to it. The object is to balance the articular surfaces or tissues in the directions of physiologic motion common to that articulation. The physician is not so much causing the change as helping the body to help itself. In this respect, it is very osteopathic, as the fluid and other dynamics of the neuromusculoskeletal system find an overall normalization or balance. It is important not to put too much pressure into the technique; the tissue must not be taken beyond its elastic limits, and the physician must not produce discomfort to a level that causes guarding. It generally should be very tolerable to the patient.

General Information for All Dysfunctions

Positioning

1. The physician makes a diagnosis of somatic dysfunction in all planes of permitted motion.
2. The physician positions the superior (upper or proximal) segment over the stabilized inferior (lower or distal) segment to a point of BLT in *all planes* of permitted motion, simultaneously if possible.
   a. This typically means moving away from the barrier(s) to a loose (ease) site.
   b. All planes must be fine-tuned to the most balanced point.
3. Fine-tune: Have patient breathe slowly in and out to assess phase of respiration that feels most loose (relaxed, soft, etc.); patient holds breath at the point (it may be only partially complete inhalation or exhalation) where the balance is maximal.

Treatment

1. At the point of BLT, the physician adjusts the relative position between the superior and inferior segments to maintain balance.

   a. This typically means shifting the top segment continuously away from the direct barrier to prevent the tissues from tightening as they release.
      i. The lower or distal segment can be anchored or moved in a direction opposite the named dysfunctional segment to decrease to amount of movement needed at that level.
   b. The tissues, as they release, are often described as if they are melting or softening.
   c. Tissue texture changes should occur during the release; if they are not palpated, the position of BLT has not been set.
2. When a total release is noted, the physician reassesses the components of somatic dysfunction (tissue texture abnormality, asymmetry of position, restriction of motion, tenderness [TART]). The physician repeats if necessary.

The shorthand rules for this are as follows (1):

1. Disengagement (encourage *freeplay* or additional loosening)
2. Exaggeration (move in the direction of the documented dysfunctional pattern)
3. Balance until release occurs (achieve a point where tension in all directions is equal)

Cervical Region

Occipitoatlantal (OA, C0–C1) Dysfunction
Ex: C0 ESLRR

 See Video 14.1

1. The patient lies supine, and the physician sits at the head of the table.

2. The patient is far enough away to permit the physician's forearms and elbows to rest on the table.

3. The physician places the hands palms up under the patient's head so that the contact is made at the level of the tentorium cerebelli (1), mostly with the heel of the hands toward the hypothenar eminences.

4. The physician's index or third fingers palpate the patient's C1 transverse processes **(Figs. 14.1 and 14.2)**.

5. The physician's palpating fingers simultaneously carry the C1 transverse processes upward and cephalad (*arrows*, **Fig. 14.3**) toward the extension ease and toward side bending right, rotation left under the occiput. This should produce a relative side bending left, rotation right effect at the occiput.

6. As the physician introduces the vectored force, the head is gently side bent left and rotated right (*arrows*, **Fig. 14.4**) until a balanced point of tension is met.

7. When this balanced position is achieved, a slow rhythmic ebb and flow of pressure may present itself, and the physician will hold this position against it until a release in the direction of ease occurs.

8. The physician reassesses the components of the dysfunction (TART).

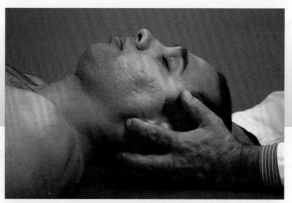

Figure 14.1. Head and vertebral contact.

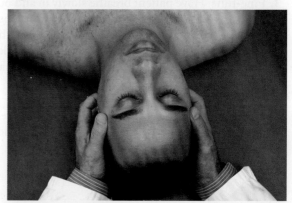

Figure 14.2. Steps 3 and 4.

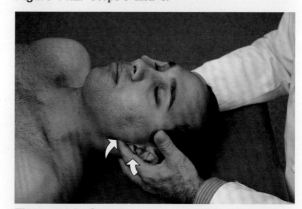

Figure 14.3. Step 5.

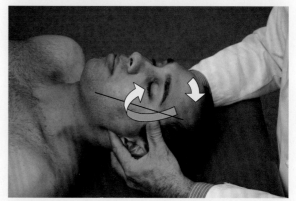

Figure 14.4. Step 6.

Cervical Region

Atlantoaxial (AA, C1–C2) Dysfunction
Ex: C1 RR

 See Video 14.2

1. The patient lies supine, and the physician sits at the head of the table.

2. The patient is far enough away to permit the physician's forearms and elbows to rest on the table.

3. The physician places the hands palms up under the patient's head so that the contact is made at the level of the tentorium cerebelli (1), mostly with the heel of the hands toward the hypothenar eminences.

4. The physician's index or third fingers palpate the patient's C2 articular processes **(Figs. 14.5 and 14.6)**.

5. The physician's palpating fingers simultaneously carry the C2 articular processes upward and cephalad to disengage C1–C2 while simultaneously rotating C2 left (*sweep arrow*) under C1 (*curved arrow*, **Fig. 14.7**). This should produce a relative C1, rotation right effect.

6. As the physician introduces the vectored force, the head with C1 may be minimally and gently rotated right (*arrow*, **Fig. 14.8**) until a balanced point of tension is met.

7. When this balanced position is achieved, a slow rhythmic ebb and flow of pressure may present itself, and the physician will hold the position against it until a release in the direction of ease occurs.

8. The physician reassesses the components of the dysfunction (TART).

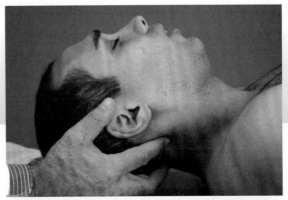

Figure 14.5. Palpation of C2 articular pillars.

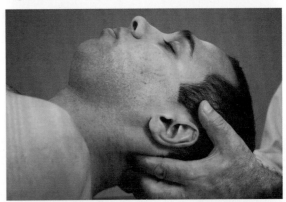

Figure 14.6. Steps 3 and 4.

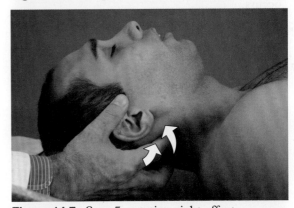

Figure 14.7. Step 5, rotation right effect.

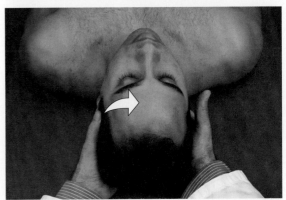

Figure 14.8. Step 6.

Cervical Region

Atlantoaxial (AA, C1–C2) Dysfunction
Ex: Right C1 Lateral Translation

1. The patient lies supine, and the physician sits at the head of the table.

2. The physician's hands cup the head by contouring over the parietotemporal regions.

3. The physician places the index finger pads over the C1 transverse processes **(Fig. 14.9)**.

4. The physician gently and slowly introduces a translational force (*arrow*, **Fig. 14.10**) that is directed from left to right toward the ease barrier. The physician may have to go back and forth between left and right to determine the balanced position **(Figs. 14.10 and 14.11)**.

5. When this balanced position is achieved, a slow rhythmic ebb and flow of pressure may present itself, and the physician will hold the position against it until a release in the direction of ease occurs.

6. This can be performed as a direct technique if preferred or indicated.

7. The physician reassesses the components of the dysfunction (TART).

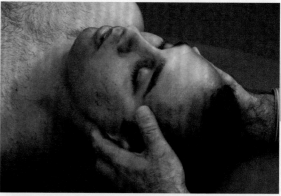
Figure 14.9. Steps 2 and 3, hand position.

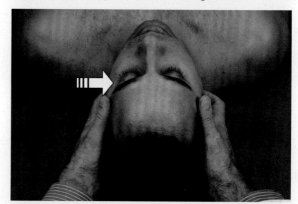
Figure 14.10. Step 4, translation left to right.

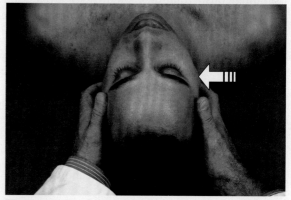
Figure 14.11. Step 4, translation right to left.

Cervical Region

C2–C7 Dysfunctions
Ex: C4 ESRRR

 See Video 14.3

1. The patient lies supine, and the physician sits at the head of the table.

2. The patient is far enough away to permit the physician's forearms and elbows to rest on the table.

3. The physician places the hands palms up under the patient's head so that the contact is made at the level of the tentorium cerebelli (1), mostly with the heel of the hands toward the hypothenar eminences (**Fig. 14.12**).

4. The physician's index or third fingers palpate the patient's C5 articular processes (*arrow*, **Fig. 14.13**).

5. The physician's palpating fingers simultaneously carry the C5 articular processes upward and cephalad to disengage C4–C5 while simultaneously rotating and side bending C5 left (*sweep arrow*) under C4 (*curved arrow*, **Fig. 14.14**). This should produce a relative effect of C4 side bending and rotation right.

6. As the physician introduces the vectored force, the head, with C1–C4 as a unit, may be minimally and gently compressed toward the cervical region to the level of the dysfunctional segment and then rotated right (*arrow*, **Fig. 14.15**) until a balanced point of tension is met.

7. When this balanced position is achieved, a slow rhythmic ebb and flow of pressure may present itself, and the physician holds the position against it until a release in the direction of ease occurs.

8. The physician reassesses the components of the dysfunction (TART).

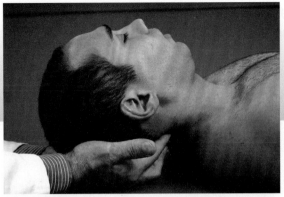

Figure 14.12. Steps 1 to 3, head contact.

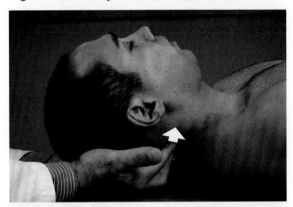

Figure 14.13. Step 4.

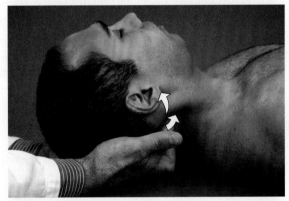

Figure 14.14. Step 5, $S_R R_R$.

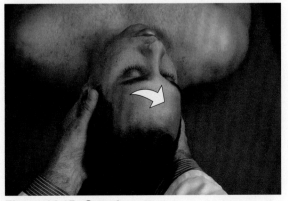

Figure 14.15. Step 6.

Thoracic Region

T1–T2 Dysfunctions
Ex: T1 FSRRR

1. The patient lies supine, and the physician sits at the head of the table.

2. The patient is far enough away to permit the physician's forearms and elbows to rest on the table.

3. The physician places the hands palms up under the patient's cervical spine at the level of C2 or C3 so that the cervical spine rests comfortably on them.

4. The physician places the index finger pads on the transverse processes of T1 and the third finger pads on the transverse processes of T2 (Figs. 14.16 and 14.17).

5. The physician's palpating fingers lift the T2 transverse processes up and down (arrows, Fig. 14.18) to find a point of disengagement between the flexion and extension barriers.

6. Using the third finger pads, the physician gently side bends (curved arrow) and rotates (sweep arrow) T2 to the left, which causes a relative side bending right and rotation right at T1 (Fig. 14.19).

7. As the physician introduces the vectored force, the index finger pads on the T1 segment may minimally and gently rotate and side bend T1 to the right until a balanced point of tension is met (Fig. 14.20).

8. When this balanced position is achieved, a slow rhythmic ebb and flow of pressure may present itself, and the physician holds the position against it until a release in the direction of ease occurs.

9. The physician reassesses the components of the dysfunction (TART).

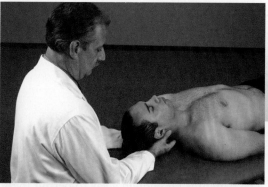

Figure 14.16. Steps 3 and 4, hand and finger positioning.

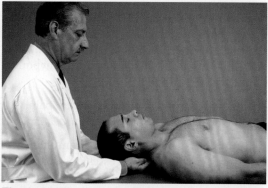

Figure 14.17. Steps 3 and 4, palpation of patient.

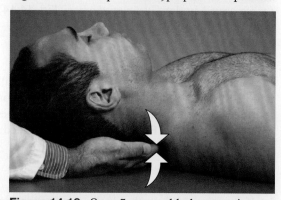

Figure 14.18. Step 5, neutral balance point.

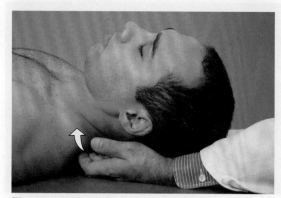

Figure 14.20. Step 7, T1, SRRR.

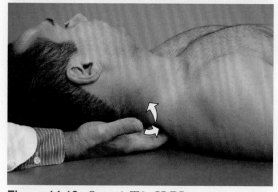

Figure 14.19. Step 6, T2, SLRL.

Thoracic Region

T4–T12 "Neutral" Dysfunctions
Ex: T6 NSRRL, Seated

1. The patient is seated, and the physician sits or stands behind the patient.

2. The physician's left thumb is placed immediately posterior to the left transverse process of T6 (upper of the two contiguous segments involved).

3. The physician's right thumb is placed immediately posterior to the right transverse process of T7 (lower of the two contiguous segments involved) **(Fig. 14.21)**.

4. The patient is instructed to lean forward until the upper of the two begins to move into flexion (*long arrow*) and then asked to stop and slightly begin extending (*short arrow*) until the physician senses the neutral or *balanced point* between flexion and extension **(Fig. 14.22)**.

5. The patient is then asked to tilt the shoulder down on the right to induce side bending right (SR) (*arrow*) and then turn to the left, to induce rotation left (RL) (*arrow*) until the physician notices the *balanced point* between the restrictive barriers in these planes **(Fig. 14.23)**. This may be difficult to hold and may be felt to "wobble" along these planes as the physician attempts to maintain the balanced point (similar to the feeling one has when balancing an object on the end of the finger).

6. The patient is instructed to inhale and exhale to the point which also maintains the balanced position and then asked to "hold your breath" as long as is comfortable. A slow rhythmic ebb and flow of pressure may present itself at the dysfunctional segment while the physician attempts to maintain the balanced position until a release in the direction of ease occurs.

7. The physician reassesses the components of the dysfunction (TART).

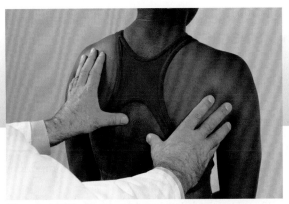

Figure 14.21. Steps 1 to 3.

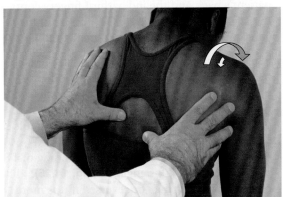

Figure 14.22. Step 4, find "neutral" between flexion and extension.

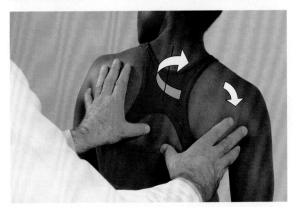

Figure 14.23. Step 5, side bending right/rotation left balancing.

Thoracic Region

T4–T12 "Neutral/Extension" Dysfunctions
Ex: T8 NSLRR, Supine

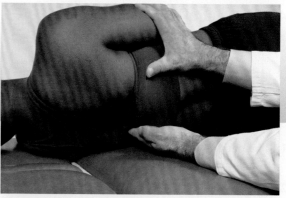

Figure 14.24. Steps 1 and 2.

1. The patient lies supine, and the physician sits at the right side of the table (rotational component side of the dysfunction).

2. The physician's left hand is placed under the patient's back and the index/third fingers contact the left transverse process of T8 (upper of the two contiguous segments involved) **(Fig. 14.24)**.

3. The physician's right arm and hand are draped over the patient's anterior chest wall, and the physician begins to pull the left chest wall to the right (*arrow*) to induce left side bending. The patient may be asked to depress the left shoulder (*arrow*) until the posterior-placed left hand palpates the beginning of left side bending of T8 and stops before T9 is engaged **(Fig. 14.25)**. (The physician's hands may be reversed if it is more comfortable!)

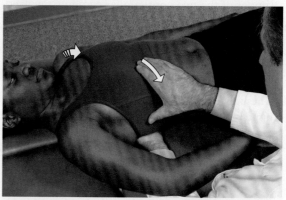

Figure 14.25. Step 3, side bending left.

4. The physician gently begins to lift upward with the posterior-contacting fingers on the T8, left transverse process to induce right rotation and flexes the fingers while pulling toward the physician to add slight left side bending **(Fig. 14.26)**.

5. The patient is instructed to inhale and exhale to the point which also maintains the balanced position and is asked to "hold your breath" as long as is comfortable. A slow rhythmic ebb and flow of pressure may present itself at the dysfunctional segment while the physician attempts to maintain the balanced position until a release in the direction of ease occurs.

6. The physician reassesses the components of the dysfunction (TART).

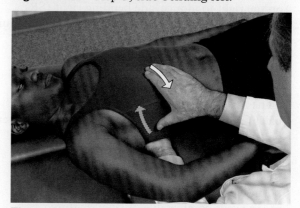

Figure 14.26. Step 4, T8, right rotation.

Thoracic and Lumbar Regions

T3–L4 "Extension" Dysfunctions
Ex: T12 ESLRL

1. The patient lies prone, and the physician stands beside the table.

2. The physician places the left thumb over the left transverse process of T12 and the index and third finger pads of the left hand over the right transverse process of T12.

3. The physician places the right thumb over the left transverse process of L1 and the index and third finger pads over the right transverse process of L1 **(Fig. 14.27)**.

4. The patient inhales and exhales, and on exhalation, the physician follows the motion of these two segments.

5. The physician adds a compression force (*long arrows*) approximating T12 and L1 and then directs a force downward (*short arrows*) toward the table to vector it to the extension barrier **(Fig. 14.28)**.

6. Next, the physician's thumbs approximate the left transverse processes of T12 and L1, which produces side bending left (*horizontal arrows*) while simultaneously rotating T12 to the left (*left index finger arrow*) and L1 to the right (*right thumb, downward arrow*) **(Fig. 14.29)**.

7. When this total balanced position is achieved, a slow rhythmic ebb and flow of pressure may present itself at the dysfunctional segment. The physician holds the position against it until a release in the direction of ease occurs.

8. The physician reassesses the components of the dysfunction (TART).

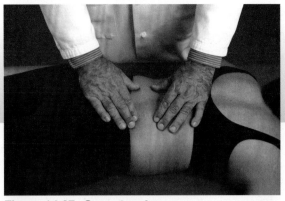

Figure 14.27. Steps 1 to 3.

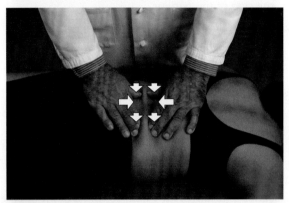

Figure 14.28. Step 5.

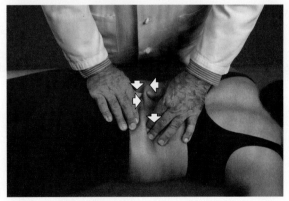

Figure 14.29. Step 6.

Thoracic and Lumbar Regions

T8–L5 Dysfunctions
Spinal-Sacral Tethering Emphasis
Ex: L5 FSRRR

If no sacral component is present, the hands may contact each segment of the vertebral unit involved in the dysfunction (e.g., L2 and L3).

1. The patient lies supine, and the physician sits at the side of the patient.

2. The physician places the caudad hand under the patient's sacrum so that the finger pads are at the sacral base and the heel is toward the sacrococcygeal region.

3. The physician places the cephalad hand across the spine at the level of the dysfunctional segment so that the heel of the hand and finger pads contact the left and right L5 transverse processes **(Figs. 14.30 and 14.31)**.

4. The sacral hand moves the sacrum cephalad and caudad (*arrows*, **Fig. 14.32**) to find a point of ease as the lumbar-contacting hand does the same.

5. The lumbar hand may need to lift upward and downward (*arrows*, **Fig. 14.33**) to balance between flexion and extension.

6. The lumbar-contacting hand then side bends and rotates L5 to the right (*arrows*) to find balanced tension in these directions **(Fig. 14.34)**.

7. When this total balanced position is achieved, a slow rhythmic ebb and flow of pressure may present itself at the dysfunctional segment. The physician holds the position against it until a release in the direction of ease occurs.

8. The physician reassesses the components of the dysfunction (TART).

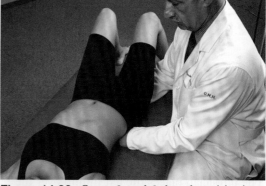

Figure 14.30. Steps 2 and 3, hand positioning.

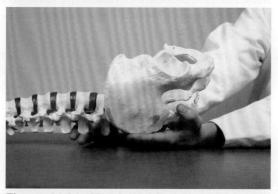

Figure 14.31. Hand positioning with sacrum and lumbar vertebra.

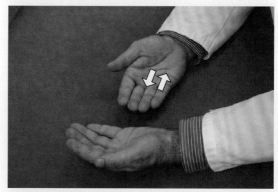

Figure 14.32. Step 4.

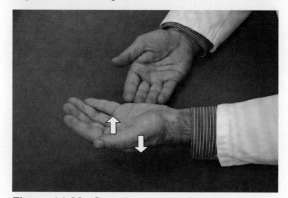

Figure 14.33. Step 5.

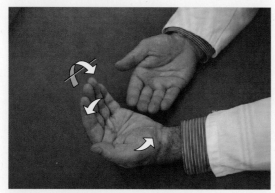

Figure 14.34. Step 6, L2, $S_R R_R$.

Costal Region

Rib 1 Nonphysiologic Dysfunction
Ex: Left Rib 1 Posterior Elevation
Nonphysiologic/Nonrespiratory Emphasis

1. The patient sits or lies supine, and the physician sits at the head of the table.

2. The physician places the left thumb over the posterior aspect of the elevated left first rib at the costotransverse articulation **(Fig. 14.35)**.

3. The physician directs a force caudally (*arrow*, **Fig. 14.36**) through the overlying tissues and into the elevated left first rib.

4. The force applied should be moderate but not severe.

5. The pressure is maintained until a release occurs as indicated by the thumb being permitted to move through the restrictive barrier.

6. The physician reassesses the components of the dysfunction (TART).

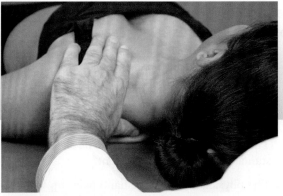

Figure 14.35. Step 2, thumb placement.

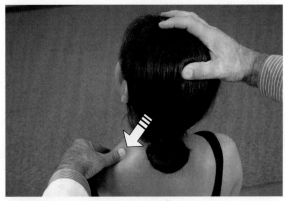

Figure 14.36. Step 3, caudal force.

Costal Region

Respiratory Diaphragm Dysfunction
Ex: Right Rib 9 Exhaled (Depressed)

1. The patient lies supine, and the physician sits or stands at the side of the patient.

2. The physician places one hand palm up with the fingers contouring the angle of the rib cage posteriorly.

3. The other hand is placed palm down with the fingers contouring the angle of the rib cage anteriorly **(Fig. 14.37)**.

4. The hands impart a moderated compression force (*arrows*, **Fig. 14.38**) that is vectored toward the xiphoid process.

5. This pressure is adjusted toward the ease of movement of the ribs and underlying tissues until a balance of tension is achieved.

6. When this total balanced position is achieved, a slow rhythmic ebb and flow of pressure may present itself at the dysfunctional segment. The physician holds the position against it until a release in the direction of ease occurs.

7. The physician reassesses the components of the dysfunction (TART).

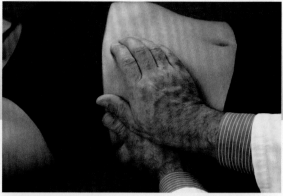

Figure 14.37. Steps 2 and 3, hand placement.

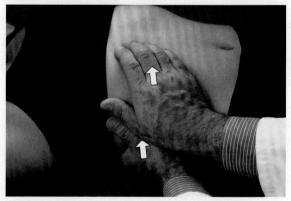

Figure 14.38. Step 4, compression force.

Costal Region

Ribs 4–12 Exhalation Dysfunctions
Ex: Right Rib 7 Exhaled (Depressed)

1. The patient is seated (or supine), and the physician sits or stands on the right side.

2. The physician's left hand is placed over the right posterior chest wall to contact the upper border of the seventh rib and, with the pads of the index/third finger, controls the rib immediately lateral to the right costotransverse articulation.

3. The physician's right hand is placed over the right, anterolateral chest wall, contouring the hand to contact the upper border of the costochondral junction associated with the seventh rib, using the thumb, webbing of the thumb, and index finger **(Figs. 14.39 and 14.40)**.

4. The physician instructs the patient to lean down on the right, toward the physician (*curved white arrow*), to produce a counterweight facilitating further "exhalation effect" while the physician adds a downward and medially directed compression force onto the seventh rib (*straight white arrow*) with both hands **(Fig. 14.41)**.

5. The patient may be asked to turn slightly to the left or right to best free the rib from its vertebral attachments.

6. The patient is then instructed to inhale and exhale deeply and hold the exhalation while the physician attempts to maintain a point of balance between the seventh rib's inhalation and exhalation barriers. A slow rhythmic ebb and flow of pressure may present itself at the dysfunctional rib while the physician attempts to maintain the balanced position until a release in the direction of ease occurs.

7. The physician reassesses the components of the dysfunction (TART).

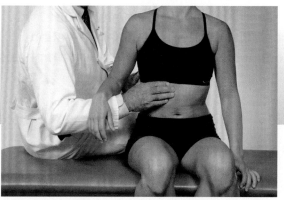

Figure 14.39. Steps 1 to 3, seated.

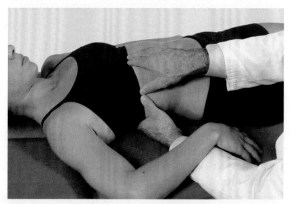

Figure 14.40. Steps 1 to 3, supine variation.

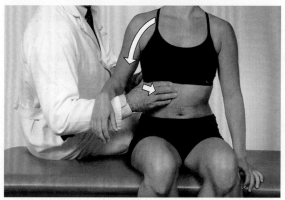

Figure 14.41. Step 4, facilitating exhalation.

Pelvic Region

Iliosacral (Innominate) Dysfunction
Ex: Left Posterior Innominate Rotation
Common Compensatory Pattern Emphasis

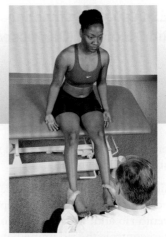

Figure 14.42. Steps 1 and 2.

1. The patient is seated, and the physician sits in front of the patient's legs.

2. The physician holds each of the patient's lower legs at the distal tibial or talotibial articulation, whichever gives the physician the most control **(Fig. 14.42)**.

3. The physician slowly pushes up (cephalad, ease direction) on the patient's left leg while simultaneously pulling down (distally, ease direction) on the right leg (*white arrows*) **(Fig. 14.43)**.

4. The physician attempts to find a point of balance between the left and right initiated movements and then instructs the patient to turn the thoracolumbar region to the left (*arrow*) until the physician senses the left leg begin to draw upward with this motion **(Fig. 14.44)**.

5. The physician finds a new point of balance with the patient in this left rotated position.

6. While holding the patient in this position, the physician may instruct the patient to inhale deeply and hold this for 5 to 10 seconds continuing to keep the balance point.

7. A slow rhythmic ebb and flow of pressure may present itself through the patient's pelvis and legs while physician attempts to maintain the balanced position until a release in the direction of ease occurs.

8. The physician reassesses the components of the dysfunction (TART).

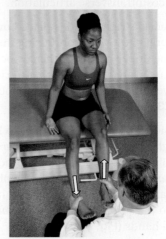

Figure 14.43. Step 3, left posterior/right anterior innominate rotations.

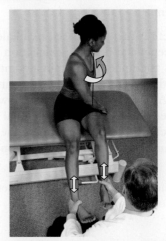

Figure 14.44. Step 4, indirect engaging of pelvic CCP.

Upper Extremity Region

Sternoclavicular Dysfunction
Ex: Left Proximal Clavicle, Compressed Direct Method

Symptom and Diagnosis

The symptom is pain at either end of the clavicle.

Technique

1. The patient sits on the side of the table.

2. The physician sits on a slightly lower stool and faces the patient.

3. The physician's left thumb is placed on the tip of the inferomedial sternal end of the clavicle immediately lateral to the sternoclavicular joint **(Fig. 14.45)**.

4. The physician places the right thumb on the lateral clavicle just medial and inferior to the acromioclavicular joint **(Fig. 14.46)**.

5. The patient may drape the forearm of the dysfunctional arm over the physician's upper arm.

6. The physician moves both thumbs (*arrows*, **Fig. 14.47**) laterally, superiorly, and slightly posteriorly while the patient retracts (*sweep arrow*) the unaffected shoulder posteriorly.

7. The physician maintains a balanced lateral, superior, and posterior pressure with both thumbs (*arrows*, **Fig. 14.48**) until a release is noted.

8. The physician reassesses the components of the dysfunction (TART).

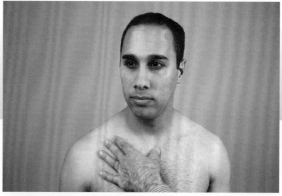

Figure 14.45. Step 3.

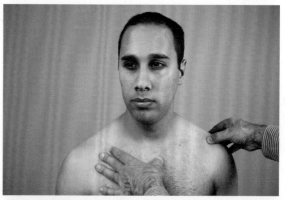

Figure 14.46. Step 4.

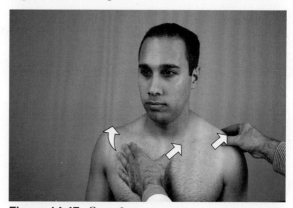

Figure 14.47. Step 6.

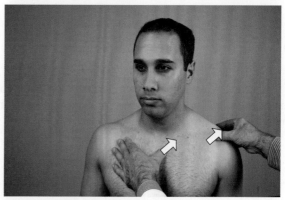

Figure 14.48. Step 7.

Upper Extremity Region

Glenohumeral Dysfunction
Regional Restriction, Lymphatic Emphasis
Ex: Right Fibrous Adhesive Capsulitis

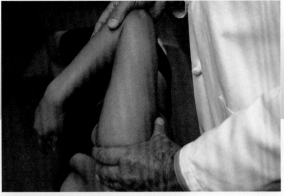

Figure 14.49. Step 3.

Symptoms and Diagnosis

The indication is subdeltoid bursitis or frozen shoulder.

Technique

1. The patient lies in the lateral recumbent position with the injured shoulder up.

2. The physician stands at the side of the table behind the patient.

3. The physician places the olecranon process of the patient's flexed and relaxed elbow in the palm of the distal hand and grasps the patient's shoulder with the opposite hand **(Fig. 14.49)**.

4. The physician controls the humerus from the patient's elbow and compresses it into the glenoid fossa (*arrow*, **Fig. 14.50**).

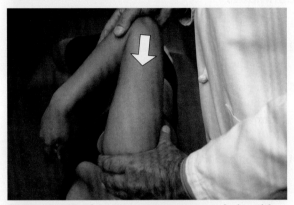

Figure 14.50. Step 4, compress toward glenoid.

5. The physician draws the elbow laterally and slightly anteriorly or posteriorly (*arrows*, **Fig. 14.51**) to bring balanced tension through the shoulder.

6. The physician draws the shoulder anteriorly or posteriorly and simultaneously compresses it inferiorly (*arrows*, **Fig. 14.52**), directing the vector into the opposite glenohumeral joint.

7. The physician holds the position of balanced tension until a release is felt.

8. When this total balanced position is achieved, a slow rhythmic ebb and flow of pressure may present itself at the dysfunctional segment. The physician holds the position against it until a release in the direction of ease occurs.

9. The physician reassesses the components of the dysfunction (TART).

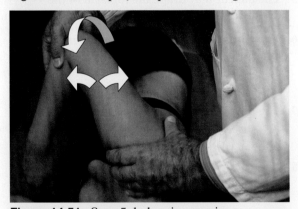

Figure 14.51. Step 5, balancing tensions.

After the release, the humerus may be carried superiorly and anteriorly, making a sweep past the ear and down in front of the face (1).

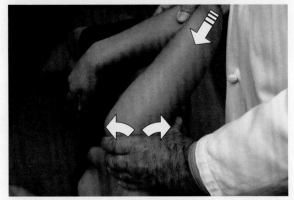

Figure 14.52. Step 6, point of balance.

Upper Extremity Region

Radioulnar and/or Ulnohumeral Dysfunctions Combined, Direct/Indirect Emphasis
Ex: Left Flexion with Posterior Radial Head

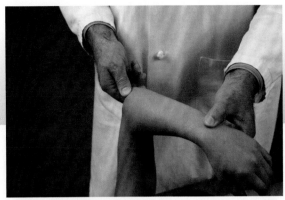

Figure 14.53. Steps 2 and 3.

Symptoms and Diagnosis

The indication is elbow pain or stiffness.

Technique

1. The patient lies supine, and the physician stands or sits at the side of the patient.

2. The physician grasps the patient's olecranon process with the thumb (lateral aspect) and index finger (medial aspect) at the proximal tip of the olecranon process at the grooves, bilaterally.

3. The physician's other hand grasps the dorsum of the patient's flexed wrist **(Fig. 14.53)**.

4. The physician rotates the patient's forearm into full pronation (*curved arrow*, **Fig. 14.54**) and the hand into full flexion (*short arrow*).

5. The physician's hands compress (*straight arrow*, **Fig. 14.55**) the patient's forearm while slowly extending (*curved arrow*) the patient's elbow.

6. Steady balanced pressure is maintained against any barriers until the elbow straightens and the physician's thumb and fingertip slide through the grooves on either side of the olecranon process.

7. This treatment resolves any torsion of the radial head and any lateral or medial deviations of the olecranon process in the olecranon fossa (i.e., lateral or medial deviation of the ulna on the humerus).

8. The physician reassesses the components of the dysfunction (TART).

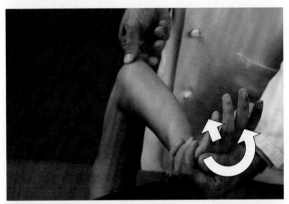

Figure 14.54. Step 4, pronation and flexion.

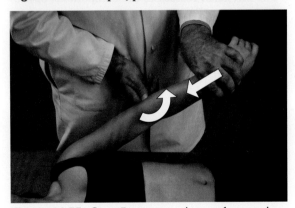

Figure 14.55. Step 5, compression and extension.

Upper Extremity Region

Carpal-Metacarpal Dysfunctions
Combined, Direct/Indirect Emphasis
Ex: Left Carpal Tunnel Syndrome

1. The patient lies supine, and the physician stands next to the outstretched arm of the dysfunctional wrist.

2. The physician's medial hand controls the patient's thumb and thenar eminence (**Fig. 14.56**).

3. The physician's other hand grasps the patient's hypothenar eminence and then supinates the forearm (*arrow*, **Fig. 14.57**).

4. At full supination, the patient's wrist is flexed to its tolerable limit (*long arrow*, **Fig. 14.58**) and the thumb is pushed dorsally (*short arrow*).

5. The physician, maintaining the forces, slowly pronates the forearm to its comfortable limit and adds a force (*arrow*, **Fig. 14.59**) vectored toward ulnar deviation.

6. The physician reassesses the components of the dysfunction (TART).

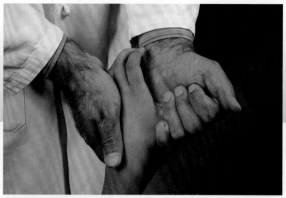

Figure 14.56. Steps 1 and 2.

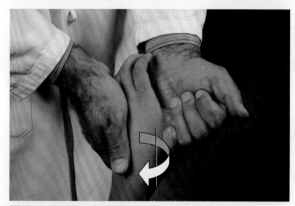

Figure 14.57. Step 3, supination.

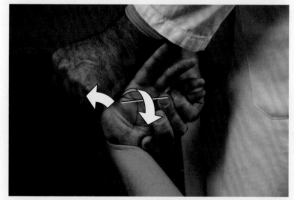

Figure 14.58. Step 4, wrist flexion.

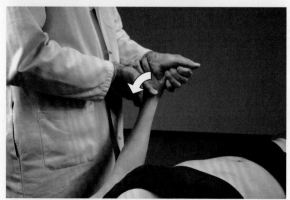

Figure 14.59. Step 5, ulnar deviation.

Lower Extremity Region

Fibular (Inversion) Dysfunction
Ex: Left Posterior Fibular Head

1. The patient lies supine, and the physician sits at the side of the dysfunctional leg.

2. The patient's hip and knee are both flexed to approximately 90 degrees.

3. The thumb of the physician's cephalad hand is placed at the superolateral aspect of the fibular head.

4. The physician's other hand controls the foot just inferior to the distal fibula **(Fig. 14.60)**.

5. The physician's thumb adds pressure on the proximal fibula in a vector straight toward the foot (*arrow at right*, **Fig. 14.61**) while the other hand (*arrows at left*) inverts the foot and ankle.

6. The physician attempts to determine a point of balanced tension at the proximal fibula and maintains this position.

7. When this total balanced position is achieved, a slow rhythmic ebb and flow of pressure may present itself at the dysfunctional segment. The physician holds the position against it until a release in the direction of ease occurs.

8. The physician reassesses the components of the dysfunction (TART).

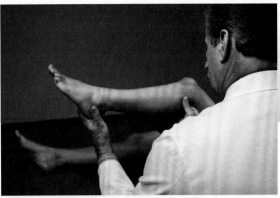

Figure 14.60. Steps 1 to 4.

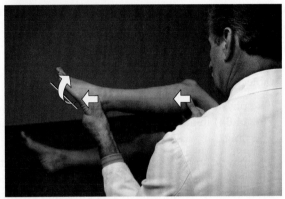

Figure 14.61. Step 5.

Lower Extremity Region

Femorotibial Dysfunctions with Sprain Rotation/Torsion Emphasis
Ex: Cruciate Ligament Sprain

1. The patient lies supine, and the physician stands at the side of the dysfunctional knee.

2. The physician places the cephalad hand palm down over the anterior distal femur.

3. The physician places the caudad hand palm down over the tibial tuberosity (**Fig. 14.62**).

4. The physician leans down onto the patient's leg (*arrows*, **Fig. 14.63**), directing a force toward the table.

5. The physician adds a compressive force (*arrows*, **Fig. 14.64**) in an attempt to approximate the femur and tibia.

6. The physician adds internal or external rotation to the tibia (*arrows*, **Fig. 14.65**) with the caudad hand to determine which is freer. The physician attempts to maintain this position.

7. When this total balanced position is achieved, a slow rhythmic ebb and flow of pressure may present itself at the dysfunctional segment. The physician holds the position against it until a release in the direction of ease occurs.

8. The physician reassesses the components of the dysfunction (TART).

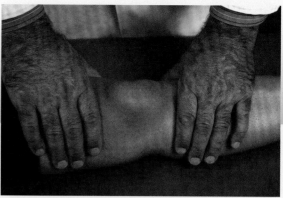

Figure 14.62. Steps 1 to 3.

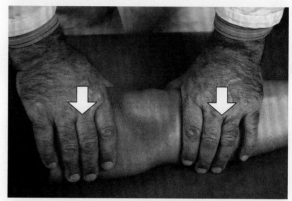

Figure 14.63. Step 4, downward force.

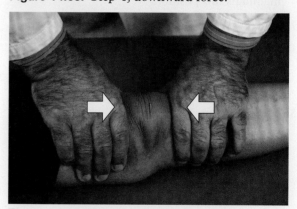

Figure 14.64. Step 5, joint compression.

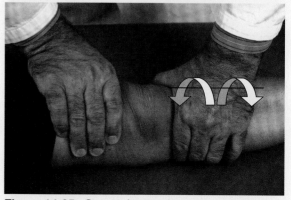

Figure 14.65. Step 6, internal or external rotation.

Lower Extremity Region

Ankle (Tibiotalar) Dysfunction
Ex: Left Tibia Posterior (Talus Anterior)

1. The patient lies supine with the heel of the foot on the table.

2. The physician stands at the foot of the table on the side of symptomatic ankle.

3. The physician places the proximal hand palm down across the distal tibia with the metacarpal-phalangeal joint of the index finger proximal to the distal tibia **(Fig. 14.66)**.

4. The physician presses directly down (*arrow*, **Fig. 14.67**) toward the table and balances the tension coming up through the heel and the tibiotalar joint.

5. The physician's other hand can be placed on top of the treating hand to create more pressure. The physician internally rotates **(Fig. 14.68)** or externally rotates **(Fig. 14.69)** the tibia slightly to bring the compression to a point of balanced tension.

6. When this total balanced position is achieved, a slow rhythmic ebb and flow of pressure may present itself at the dysfunctional segment. The physician holds the position against it until a release in the direction of ease occurs.

7. The physician reassesses the components of the dysfunction (TART).

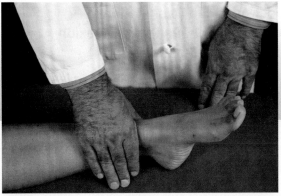

Figure 14.66. Steps 1 to 3.

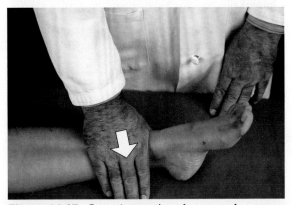

Figure 14.67. Step 4, pressing downward.

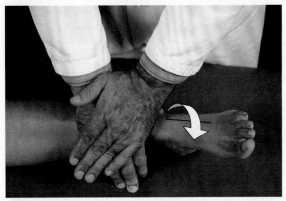

Figure 14.68. Step 5, internal rotation.

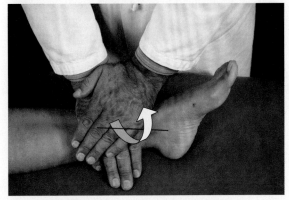

Figure 14.69. Step 5, external rotation.

Lower Extremity Region

Foot and Ankle Dysfunctions
Ex: Left Calcaneus Plantar Flexion
The "Boot-Jack" Technique

 See Video 14.4

1. The patient lies supine, and the physician stands on the left, facing the foot of the table.

2. The patient's left lower thigh and knee are placed under the physician's right axilla and against the lateral rib cage for balance and control.

3. The physician grasps the patient's left calcaneus with the right thumb and index finger **(Fig. 14.70)**.

4. The physician flexes the patient's left hip and knee approximately 90 degrees and gently externally rotates and abducts the patient's femur (*arrow*, **Fig. 14.71**).

5. The physician's right distal humerus and elbow touch the patient's distal femur just above the popliteal fossa as a fulcrum to generate proximal pressure.

6. The physician controls the patient's left foot by wrapping the fingers around the medial aspect of the foot.

7. The physician leans back, carrying the patient's left hip and knee into further flexion while maintaining tight control of the patient's left calcaneus. This exerts a distraction effect (*arrow*, **Fig. 14.72**) on the calcaneus from the talus.

8. The physician's left hand induces slight plantar flexion (*arrow*, **Fig. 14.73**) to a point of balanced tension in the metatarsals and tarsals of the patient's left foot.

9. When this total balanced position is achieved, a slow rhythmic ebb and flow of pressure may present itself at the dysfunctional segment. The physician holds the position against it until a release in the direction of ease occurs.

10. The physician reassesses the components of the dysfunction (TART).

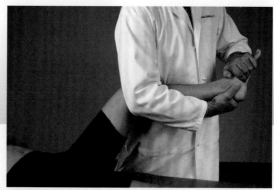

Figure 14.70. Steps 1 to 3.

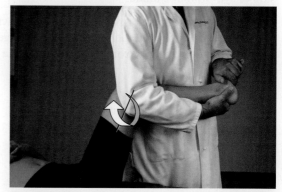

Figure 14.71. Step 4, external rotation/abduction of femur.

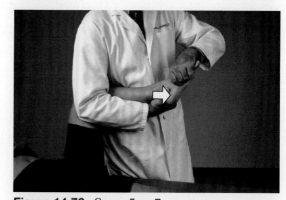

Figure 14.72. Steps 5 to 7.

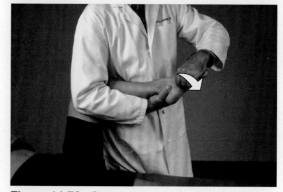

Figure 14.73. Step 8, plantar flexion to balance.

Lower Extremity Region

Cuneiform Metatarsal Dysfunctions
Ex: Right Metatarsal Flexion

1. The patient lies supine, and the physician stands or is seated at the foot of the table.

2. The physician grasps the foot with both hands, the fingers on the plantar aspect of the distal metatarsals **(Fig. 14.74)** and the thumbs on the dorsal aspect of the foot **(Fig. 14.75)**.

3. The physician flexes the distal forefoot (*arrow*, **Fig. 14.76**) slightly by contracting the fingers on the plantar aspect of the foot.

4. The physician then presses the thumbs downward into the metatarsals toward the table (*arrow*, **Fig. 14.77**).

5. The physician attempts to position the foot at a point of balanced tension.

6. When this total balanced position is achieved, a slow rhythmic ebb and flow of pressure may present itself at the dysfunctional segment. The physician holds the position against it until a release in the direction of ease occurs.

7. The physician reassesses the components of the dysfunction (TART).

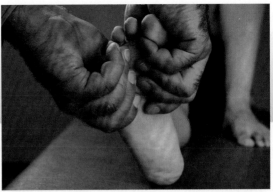

Figure 14.74. Steps 1 and 2, fingers on plantar surface.

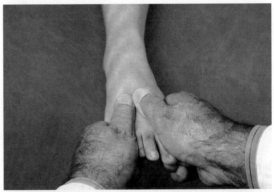

Figure 14.75. Steps 1 and 2, thumbs on dorsal surface.

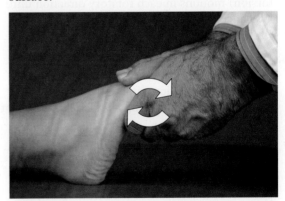

Figure 14.76. Step 3, flexion of forefoot.

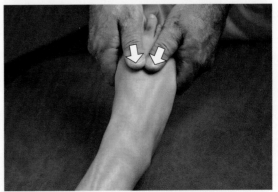

Figure 14.77. Step 4, press toward table.

Lower Extremity Region

Phalangeal Extension Dysfunction Compressed, Secondary to Sprain Ex: Right "Great" Toe, Dorsiflexed

1. The patient lies supine, and the physician is seated at the right foot of the table.

2. The physician, using the index finger and thumb of either hand, grasps the dorsal and plantar surfaces of the toe (do not grasp the medial/lateral borders and compress as the nerves may be irritated).

3. The physician's other hand encircles the plantar and dorsal aspects of the patient's right foot to control the distal first metatarsal bone **(Fig. 14.78)**.

4. The physician then adds a compression or traction force (*arrows*) and determines which best comfortably disengages (increases freeplay) to metatarsal-phalangeal joint **(Fig. 14.79)**. A minimal flexion or extension positioning may also be applied if that improves the disengagement.

5. Holding the patient's toe in this disengaged position, the physician next adds rotational (spin/torsion) motions in each rotatory direction until a balanced point is determined toward the ease (indirect) barrier **(Fig. 14.80)**.

6. Holding the patient's toe in this position, the physician then adds/"stacks" a side bending (adduction/abduction) motion to the rotational point of balance, achieving a final balanced point **(Fig. 14.81)**.

7. A slow rhythmic ebb and flow of pressure may present itself at the dysfunctional toe while the physician attempts to maintain the balanced position until a release in the direction of ease occurs.

8. The physician reassesses the components of the dysfunction (TART).

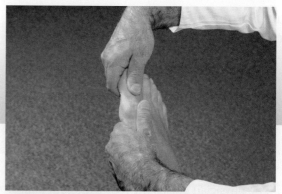

Figure 14.78. Steps 1 to 3, hand placement.

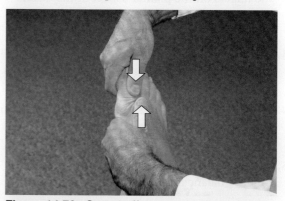

Figure 14.79. Step 4, disengagement.

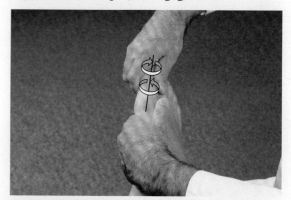

Figure 14.80. Step 5, find rotational balance.

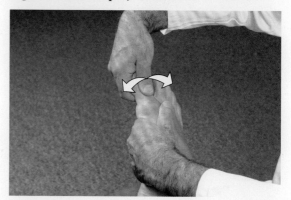

Figure 14.81. Step 6, find adduction/abduction balance.

Cranial Region

Temporomandibular Joint (TMJ) Dysfunction
Ex: Bilateral TMJs, "Closed"

Examination has revealed that the TMJs are freely closing but are not able to open normally

1. The patient lies supine, and the physician sits at the head of the table.

2. The physician's finger pads are placed under the mandible and are contoured around and under the jaw to control the movement of the mandible **(Fig. 14.82)**.

3. The physician begins to add a compressive force by flexing the fingers and drawing the teeth together (*white curved arrows*) while also adding a posterior force toward the TMJs (*white straight arrows*) **(Fig. 14.83)**.

4. The physician next assesses for a lateral ease-bind asymmetry by moving the mandible left and right (*arrows*) and attempts to find an indirect point of balance **(Fig. 14.84)**.

5. When a balance is achieved a slow rhythmic ebb and flow of pressure may present itself through the patient's jaw (TMJ). The physician attempts to maintain the balanced position until a release in the direction of ease occurs.

6. The physician reassesses the components of the dysfunction (TART).

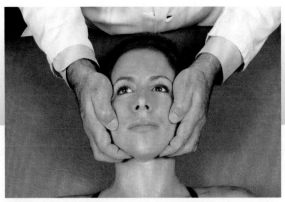

Figure 14.82. Steps 1 and 2.

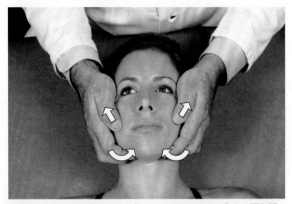

Figure 14.83. Step 3, disengagement of the TMJs.

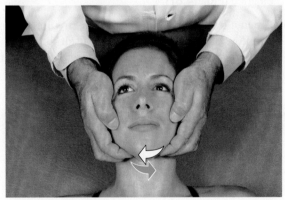

Figure 14.84. Step 4, assessing lateral asymmetry.

Cranial Region

Temporomandibular Joint (TMJ) Dysfunction
Ex: Bilateral TMJs, "Open"

Examination has revealed that the TMJs are freely opening but are not able to close normally

1. The patient lies supine, and the physician sits at the head of the table.

2. The physician's hands are placed on each side of the patient's face and jaw contacting the patient's head from the temporal region and downward to the inferior/lateral jaw line **(Fig. 14.85)**.

3. The physician next draws the jaw open and gaps the TMJs by pushing the jaw inferior by extending the fingers (*white arrows*) while the heel of the physician's hand remains locked at the temporal region as an anchor **(Fig. 14.86)**.

4. The physician next assesses for a lateral ease-bind asymmetry by moving the mandible left and right (*arrows*) and attempts to find an indirect point of balance **(Fig. 14.87)**.

5. When a balance is achieved, a slow rhythmic ebb and flow of pressure may present itself through the patient's jaw (TMJ). The physician attempts to maintain the balanced position until a release in the direction of ease occurs.

6. The physician reassesses the components of the dysfunction (TART).

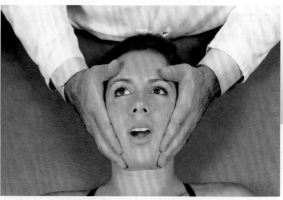

Figure 14.85. Steps 1 and 2.

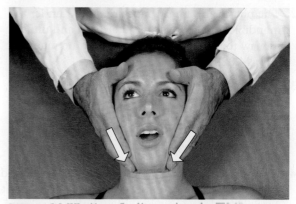

Figure 14.86. Step 3, distracting the TMJs.

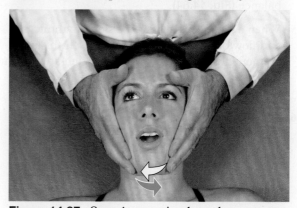

Figure 14.87. Step 4, assessing lateral asymmetry.

References

1. Speece C, Crow T. Ligamentous Articular Strain: Osteopathic Techniques for the Body. Seattle, WA: Eastland, 2001.
2. Ward R, ed. Foundations for Osteopathic Medicine. 2nd ed. Philadelphia, PA: Lippincott Williams & Wilkins, 2003.
3. Chila, AG, ed. Foundations of Osteopathic Medicine. 3rd ed. Baltimore, MD: Lippincott Williams & Wilkins, 2011.
4. Glossary of Osteopathic Terminology, Educational Council on Osteopathic Principles of the American Association of Colleges of Osteopathic Medicine. http://www.aacom.org
5. Sutherland WG. Teachings in the Science of Osteopathy. Wales A, ed. Portland, OR: Rudra, 1990.
6. Fuller RB. Synergetics. New York, NY: Macmillan, 1975.
7. Snelson K. Frequently Asked Questions (FAQ) and Structure & Tensegrity. Accessed February 4, 2007, http://www.kennethsnelson.net/
8. Ingber DE. The architecture of life. Sci Am 1998;278:48–57.

15

Visceral Techniques

Technique Principles

Osteopathic visceral (VIS) techniques are defined in the glossary of osteopathic terminology by the Educational Council on Osteopathic Principles (ECOP) as "a system of diagnosis and treatment directed to the viscera to improve physiologic function; typically the viscera are moved toward their fascial attachments to a point of fascial balance; also called ventral techniques" (1). Visceral techniques have been part of the osteopathic manipulative armamentarium since the time of Still, as he developed and promoted his system of diagnosis and the following manipulative techniques for human illness, not just musculoskeletal pain. In fact, most of Still's writing has to do with the circulatory (arterial, venous, and lymphatic), neurologic, visceral, and humeral systems. He did not write a treatise on low back pain and so on. All osteopathic intervention was based on trying to treat patients in a more benign and effective manner.

At many osteopathic medical schools, VIS techniques were reduced in favor of teaching the techniques that were more directly associated with the musculoskeletal dysfunctions that caused head, neck, low back, and extremity pain. However, many of the techniques (hepatic, splenic, gastrointestinal, pulmonary, and lymphatic) that had such positive effects on the viscera and general health status continued to be taught. In addition, the somatovisceral and viscerosomatic relations and the effects of dysautonomia continued to be important in the overall osteopathic curriculum. As there may be somatic components of disease (2), it is important to note the spinal cord levels of the visceral organs' preganglionic neurons. By knowing these levels and the fact that afferent information can move along somatic efferents causing somatic reactions in a slightly wider range, the physician can gain additional information through osteopathic layer-by-layer palpation (3) (Table 15.1). In somatovisceral conditions, these related areas, if treated with OMT, may alleviate the condition, whereas, in viscerosomatic conditions, they may be better as diagnostic criteria. Osteopathic clinical importance has largely centered on the sympathetic reactions; however, observation for and treatment of the parasympathetic (cranial-sacral) relationships are clinically important for the patient's total health care. Areas of somatic dysfunction adversely affecting the visceral systems may be treated with any of the various osteopathic manipulative treatments (OMTs) mentioned in this atlas. If OMT addresses a somatic component of disease and the effect is to improve the condition of the patient, that technique could be considered a visceral technique. Therefore, this chapter illustrates some techniques that have an indirect or distal effect on the visceral system, but in most cases, it illustrates techniques that are more directly associated with it.

Other chapters discuss osteopathic palpatory diagnosis for detection of somatic dysfunction. The same ease-bind asymmetries of tissue tension and motion used for the diagnosis and development of treatment vectors are also appropriate for the viscera. The nature of the organ's mobility should be accepted by most physicians; however, the more evolved thinking of motility expanded the thinking of osteopathic treatment in this area. With practice, the physician cannot only palpate organomegaly and restriction of mobility but can also discern fine changes in the inherent motility of the organ itself.

More recently, the works of Barral have again excited those who had lost touch with techniques affecting the viscera (4). Any osteopathic diagnostic examination should include a layer-by-layer palpatory approach, which when used in the visceral regions may determine tissue texture changes, asymmetry of structure and/or motion (mobility and motility), restriction of such motion, and tenderness (sensitivity).

Technique Classification

Direct, Indirect, or Combined

Depending on the patient's history and physical findings, the physician may choose to introduce forces in any of the above styles. The rationale for implementing these relates to the major components of the dysfunction

Table 15.1 Paraspinal *Sympathetic* Viscerosomatic/Somatovisceral Segmental Reflex Levels

Head and neck	T1–T5
Cardiac	T1–T5
Myocardial	T1–T5 (L)
Coronary artery	C3–C5
Pulmonary	T2–T5
Bronchomotor reflex	T1–T3
"Asthma reflex"	T2 (L)
Bronchial mucosa reflex	T2–T3
Lung parenchymal reflex	T3–T4
Parietal pleura	T1–T12
Upper extremity	T2–T7
Upper GI	T3–T10
Esophagus	T5–T6
Lower esophagus and stomach	T5–T10 (L)
Duodenum	T6–T8 (R)
Lower GI	T5–L3
Pancreas	T5–T9 (B/L to right)
Spleen	T7–T9 (L)
Liver and gallbladder	T5–T10 (R)
Adrenal	T8–T10
Small intestine	T8–T11 (B/L)
Ascending and transverse colon	T10–L1
Appendix and cecum	T9–T12 (R)
Descending/sigmoid colon, rectum	L1–L3 (L)
Urinary tract	T9–L3
Kidney	T9–L1, ipsilateral
Ureters (proximal)	T10–L3 (B/L)
Ureters (distal)	L1–L2
Bladder	L1–L2 (B/L)
Urethra	T11–T12 (B/L)
Genital tract	T9–L2
Ovary/testes	T9–T11, ipsilateral
Prostate and prostatic urethra	T10–L2 (B/L)
Cervix	T10–L2
External genital organs	T12 (B/L)
Uterus	T9–L2 (B/L)
Fallopian tubes	T10–L2 (B/L)
Lower extremity	T10–L3

Sources: Chila AG, exec. ed. Foundations of Osteopathic Medicine. 3rd ed. Baltimore, MD: Lippincott Williams & Wilkins, 2011; Nelson KE, Glonek T. Somatic Dysfunction in Osteopathic Family Medicine. Baltimore, MD: Lippincott Williams & Wilkins, 2007.

and the principle being utilized to attain the most significant improvement. For example

1. Diagnose connective tissue restrictions of the mesentery and use a direct myofascial-oriented technique to improve the elastic properties of the tissues.
2. Diagnose a spinal dysfunction that causes a secondary hypersympathetic reaction to the heart resulting in an arrhythmia and use an indirect BLT style technique to reduce the components of the spinal dysfunction and, therefore, reduce the secondary cardiac response.

Technique Styles

Alleviation of Somatic Dysfunction

In somatic dysfunction that appears to directly cause an organ to function abnormally, treating the area of related somatic dysfunction sometimes can reduce or ablate the visceral abnormality. This is an example of a somatovisceral reflex being quieted by the elimination of the somatic dysfunction. The abnormal somatic afferent bombardment is eliminated, causing the previously associated (abnormal) reactionary visceral efferent innervation to be normalized.

Reflex Oriented

These techniques attempt to produce a secondary reaction in an organ system by affecting the autonomic nervous system (usually sympathetic but sometimes parasympathetic). This is similar to using other autonomic reflexes, such as carotid massage, vagal induction through Valsalva maneuver, ocular pressure, ice water immersion, and so on. These treatments are in areas that can affect the autonomic nervous system in specific ways associated with either sympathetic or parasympathetic reactivity. They are an attempt either to increase or to decrease the levels of autonomic output at the area in question. Routinely, we prefer to think of reducing the area of somatic dysfunction rather than increasing or decreasing the level of autonomic activity. However, in some cases, this appears to produce the appropriate clinical response, such as a patient with asthma having the sympathetic portion of the autonomic system stimulated by thoracic pump in the upper thoracic region and exhibiting less airway reactivity.

Chapman reflex is another potential diagnostic aid in the determination of the exact diagnosis and the key dysfunction. It is defined in the glossary of osteopathic terminology by ECOP as (a) a system of reflex points that present as predictable anterior and posterior fascial tissue texture abnormalities (plaque-like changes or stringiness of the involved tissues) assumed to be reflections of visceral dysfunction or pathology (b) originally used by Frank Chapman, DO, and described by Charles Owens, DO (1). Besides Chapman and Owens, many osteopathic physicians have promoted the use of this diagnostic and therapeutic approach (i.e., Kimberly; Kuchera, W; Kuchera, M; Arbuckle; Lippincott; and Patriquin) each adding another component or theory as to their development and/or treatment (2).

Chapman's earliest writings were concerned with the endocrine system and declared the thyroid the most important gland in the body (2,5). Other areas of the body are also described as being involved or associated with an endocrine problem; Owens reported that "an innominate…[dysfunction] always indicates an endocrine disturbance" (5). As medicine developed a better understanding of viscerosomatic reflexing, those findings proposed by Chapman gained more acceptance (2). Chapman originally described these tissue texture abnormalities as *gangliform*-contracted lymphoid tissue nodules (ganglioformed) and later terms such as neurolymphatic nodules were used. But, the underlying etiology has centered on a visceral and autonomic (mostly sympathetic) reflexing that causes localized congestion and various tissue reactions at specific locations.

Various palpatory descriptions have been used to help teach students how to locate and determine their presence and over the years have included "BB shot-like," pea-shaped and pea-sized, rice-like, and tapioca pearl-like. The distinguishing factor is generally a moderate to severe pain (acute) when they are palpated, although they may be painless (chronic) (2). When trying to categorize the proper osteopathic model of care in which to place the diagnosis and treatment of these nodules, it might be best to place them in a combined category we have used—"neuroendocrine-immune"—thus blending the respiratory-circulatory and neurologic models. It is common to palpate first for an anterior point and then confirm its viscerosomatic etiology by palpating the posterior-related reflex point (5). The order of treatment of these Chapman points has generally recommended beginning anteriorly and then move to the posterior points (2,5).

As the osteopathic profession began to integrate these ideas, many drawings and charts were developed to help students and physicians remember their locations and how to properly elicit their presence (**Figs. 15.1 and 15.2**). However, as the charting helped in more easily remembering the locations of these points, it may have led to a less complete understanding of the conditions in which they are present. Past descriptions by others associated the reflex points to organs without relating to symptoms or conditions while the original work also proposed diagnosis-related presentations, for example, conjunctivitis, otitis media, bronchitis, and cystitis (2,5). Presently, the original clinical considerations by Owens have seen a revival (2). Chapman (Owens) also described treatment of other somatic areas that were believed to be linked to the reflex point itself, as well as recommending other treatment, that is, nutritional supplements, yet stated that "in no instance should a general osteopathic treatment be included where reflex treatment is being given (5)."

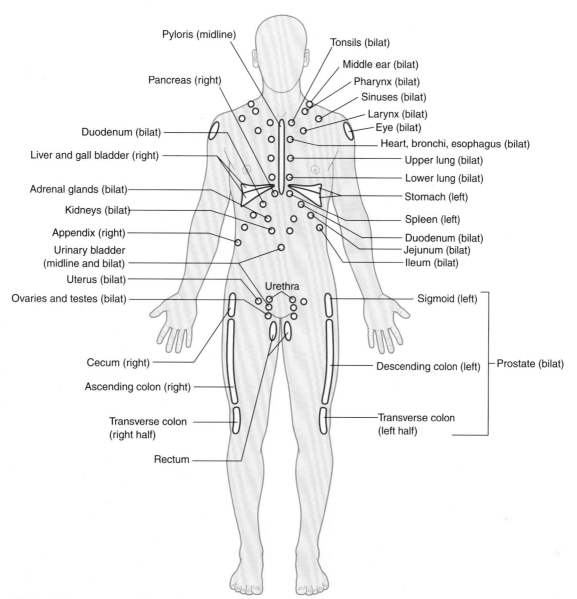

Figure 15.1. Anterior Chapman points.

While modern diagnostic methods make the differential diagnosis much easier to develop than 80 to 100 years ago when Chapman was in practice, there are still times when they can help diagnostically. A recent case in point is a female patient who presented to a local emergency department with a week-long history of abdominal bloating and pain. After physical exam, laboratory blood tests, and CT scan with contrast were performed, she was diagnosed as having an ovarian tumor. She was transferred from the general surgery service to the gynecologic surgical service, and when these surgeons visualized the area, it turned out to be a ruptured appendix (Mahon VN. *Personal Communication*, 2012). These two organs have different locations for their respective Chapman reflex, and by palpating for these reflexed tissue texture changes, the surgeons may have been able to accurately diagnose the patient presurgery.

Myofascial Oriented

The fascial component to visceral mobility is the primary aspect in diagnosis and treatment in this technique. (The style labeled balanced ligamentous tension, or ligamentous articular strain [BLT/LAS], is singled out because of its different palpatory expression of diagnosis and treatment, although it uses the same tissues to effect change that myofascial release [MFR] uses.) Using the layer-by-layer approach, the physician palpates at various levels in the region of the specific organ and determines whether any tethering is taking place in relation to ease-bind barrier concepts. Then, the physician decides whether to use a direct or indirect MFR-like technique. This can directly affect the venous and lymphatic drainage from the region (including interstitial spaces) inhabited by the visceral organ, with clinical response from the reduction in inflammatory response, nociception, and so on.

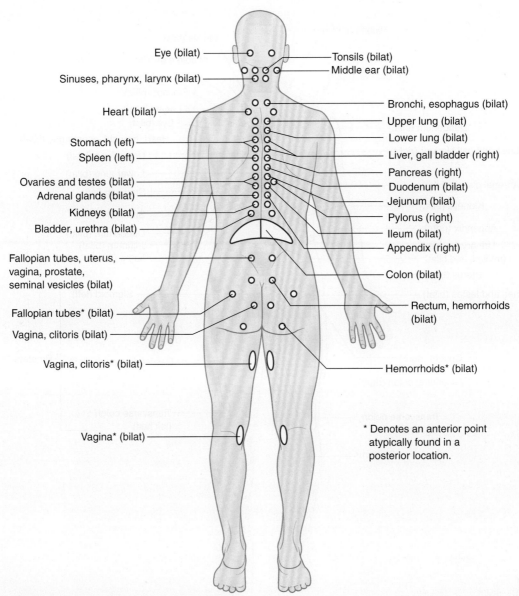

Figure 15.2. Posterior Chapman points.

Balanced Ligamentous Tension or Ligamentous Articular Strain

The BLT/LAS method of diagnosis and treatment is an attempt to discern the ease-bind asymmetry. Then, using palpatory techniques to sense the inherent motility of the organ, the physician attempts to balance the tissues through indirect (and sometimes direct) technique by disengaging the organ from its restrictive presentation (compression, traction), exaggerating its free motion pattern, and then balancing at a point that exhibits equal tension in the x, y, and z axes.

Vibratory or Stimulatory Technique

Vibratory or stimulatory technique uses a repetitive motion over the organ, gently to moderately vibrating, shaking, or percussing over the organ to facilitate fluid movement through the arterial, venous, and lymphatic

vessels and to help decongest the organ. These techniques are often used in splenic and hepatic problems when this type of force is not contraindicated.

Indications

The indications for vibratory or stimulatory treatment are organ dysfunctions expressing themselves in many clinical manifestations, including but not limited to the following (6):

1. Cardiac arrhythmia, congestive heart failure, and hypertension
2. Asthma, bronchitis, pneumonia, atelectasis, and emphysema
3. Gastroesophageal reflux, gastritis, and hiatal hernia
4. Hepatitis, cholelithiasis, cholecystitis, pancreatitis, chronic fatigue, and hormonal imbalance

5. Diverticulosis, ulcerative colitis, irritable bowel, constipation, diarrhea, and hemorrhoids
6. Pyelonephritis and renal lithiasis
7. Recurrent cystitis, interstitial cystitis, and stress incontinence
8. Dysmenorrhea, dyspareunia, and infertility

Contraindications

There are no absolute contraindications to this type of treatment; however, clinical judgment again is the rule. Pressure, compression, or traction over an inflamed, seriously infected, or bleeding organ is not appropriate.

General Considerations and Rules

The physician must determine whether there is a somatic component to the disease state. Depending on the disease and the nature of the associated dysfunction (somatovisceral, viscerosomatic, etc.), the physician must develop a treatment plan that reduces the somatic dysfunction in a safe, benign manner. The physician must also note whether there is an autonomic complication (e.g., facilitated segment) and if there is such, treat that first, if possible.

Reflex-Oriented Treatment

Occipitomastoid Suture Pressure

 See Video 15.1

Indications

The indications for occipitomastoid suture pressure release are tachycardia (hypoparasympathetic state) and bradycardia (hyperparasympathetic state).

Physiologic Goal

The goal is to use a reflex (parasympathetic) to decrease the patient's pulse by influencing cardiac rate via cranial nerve X (vagus) or by treating cranial somatic dysfunction at this area **(Fig. 15.3)** that could be causing a secondary bradycardia (somatovisceral type).

Technique

1. The patient lies supine, and the physician is seated at the head of the table.

2. The physician palpates the occipitomastoid grooves bilaterally.

3. The physician places the index fingers over each mastoid process immediately proximal to the anterior aspect of the groove.

4. The physician places the third fingers over the occiput immediately proximal to the posterior aspect of the groove **(Fig. 15.4)**.

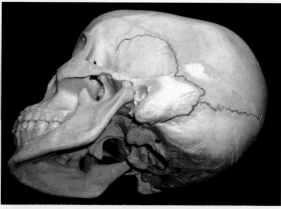

Figure 15.3. The occipitomastoid suture.

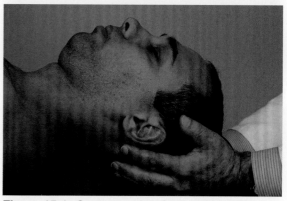

Figure 15.4. Steps 3 and 4, finger placement.

5. The pads of the physician's fingers exert gentle axial traction over the sutures combined with a lateral spreading force away from the midline (*arrows*, **Figs. 15.5 and 15.6**).

6. Gentle pressure is maintained until the desired effect is obtained or until it is determined that the technique will be ineffective.

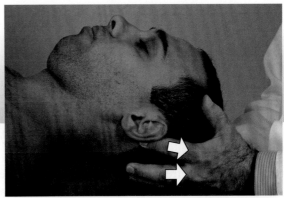

Figure 15.5. Step 5, traction with fingers.

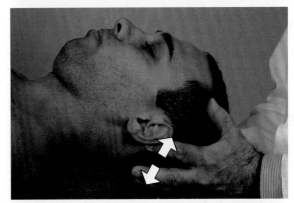

Figure 15.6. Step 5, separation of suture by fingers.

Reflex-Oriented Treatment

Alternating Pressure, Left Second Rib

 See Video 15.2

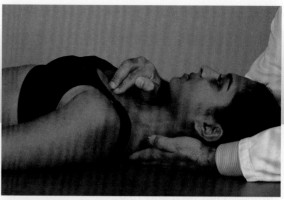

Figure 15.8. Steps 1 to 3, anterior and posterior placement of fingers.

Indications

The indications for treatment are tachycardia (hypersympathetic state) and bradycardia (hyposympathetic state).

Physiologic Goal

The goal is to use the sympathetic reflex to increase the patient's pulse by influencing cardiac rate via sympathetic chain ganglia **(Fig. 15.7)** or treating thoracocostal somatic dysfunction at this area, which may influence cardiac rate.

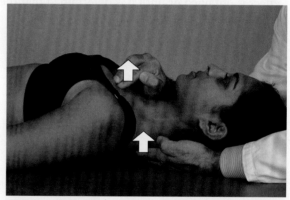

Figure 15.9. Step 4, anterior-directed pressure.

Technique

1. The patient lies supine, and the physician is seated at the head of the table.

2. The physician reaches under the patient and places the pads of the index and middle fingers on the angle of the left second rib near the costotransverse articulation.

3. The physician places the pads of the other index and middle finger on the anterior aspect of the left second rib near the costochondral junction **(Fig. 15.8)**.

4. The physician presses upward with the bottom hand while releasing pressure from the top hand **(Fig. 15.9)**.

5. The physician holds this position for several seconds, after which the bottom hand releases pressure and the top hand exerts downward pressure **(Fig. 15.10)**.

6. This pressure is likewise held for several seconds before switching again. This alternating pressure is continued until the desired effects are obtained or it is determined that the technique will be ineffective.

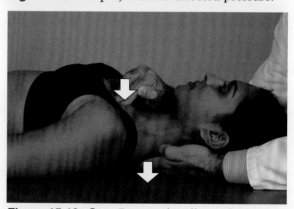

Figure 15.10. Step 5, posterior-directed pressure.

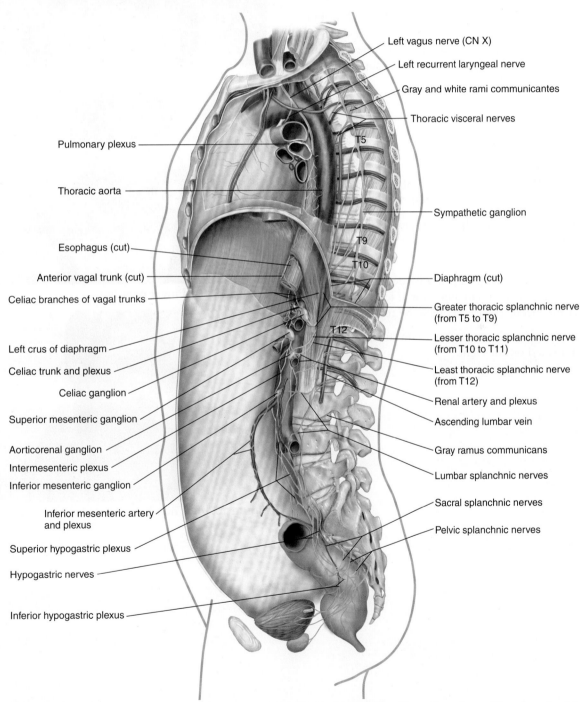

Left vagus nerve (CN X)

Left recurrent laryngeal nerve

Gray and white rami communicantes

Thoracic visceral nerves

Pulmonary plexus

T5

Thoracic aorta

Sympathetic ganglion

T9

Esophagus (cut)

T10

Anterior vagal trunk (cut)

Diaphragm (cut)

Celiac branches of vagal trunks

Greater thoracic splanchnic nerve
(from T5 to T9)

T12

Lesser thoracic splanchnic nerve
(from T10 to T11)

Left crus of diaphragm

Least thoracic splanchnic nerve
(from T12)

Celiac trunk and plexus

Renal artery and plexus

Celiac ganglion

Superior mesenteric ganglion

Ascending lumbar vein

Aorticorenal ganglion

Gray ramus communicans

Intermesenteric plexus

Lumbar splanchnic nerves

Inferior mesenteric ganglion

Sacral splanchnic nerves

Inferior mesenteric artery
and plexus

Pelvic splanchnic nerves

Superior hypogastric plexus

Hypogastric nerves

Inferior hypogastric plexus

Figure 15.7. Anatomic location of the sympathetic chain ganglia. Posterior view. (Reprinted with permission from Ref. (7)).

Reflex-Oriented Treatment

Singultus (Hiccups)

See Video 15.3

The phrenic nerve arises primarily from C4 but also receives fibers from C3 and C5. It runs deep to the omohyoid muscle and superficial to the anterior scalene muscle. It is the only motor nerve supplying the diaphragm **(Fig. 15.11)**.

Technique

1. The patient may be seated or lie supine.

2. The physician locates the triangle formed by the sternal and clavicular heads of the left sternocleidomastoid muscle **(Fig. 15.12)**.

3. The physician, using the thumb, index finger, or middle finger, presses deep into this triangle **(Figs. 15.13 and 15.14)**.

4. This pressure should elicit a mild degree of pain (to tolerance) and be maintained for at least a minute after the hiccups cease to break the reflex arc.

5. If the technique is unsuccessful on the left, it may be repeated on the right.

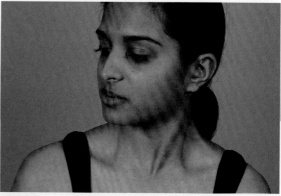

Figure 15.12. Steps 1 and 2.

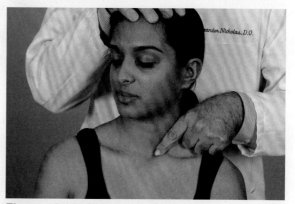

Figure 15.13. Finger pressure.

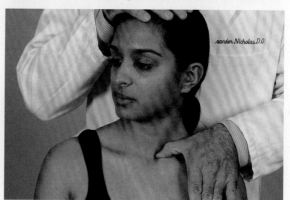

Figure 15.14. Thumb pressure variation.

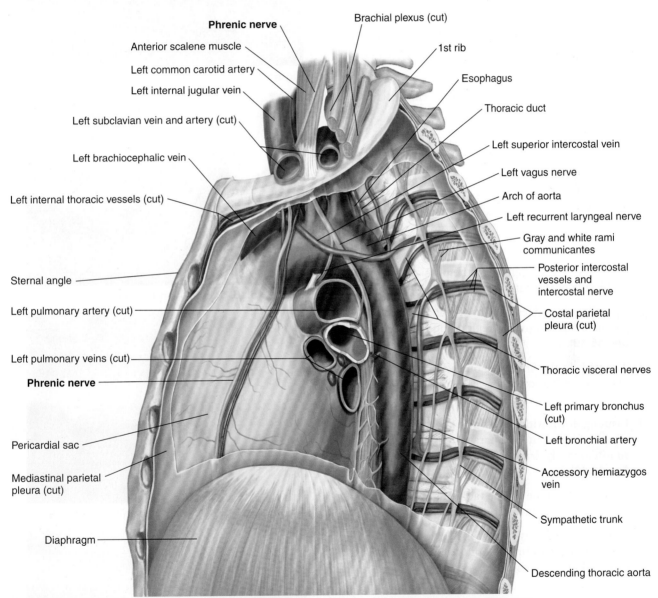

Figure 15.11. Anatomic location of phrenic nerve. (Reprinted with permission from Ref. (7)).

Reflex-Oriented Treatment

Rib Raising

 See Video 15.4

See Chapter 16.

Indications

To relieve postoperative paralytic ileus
To improve respiratory excursion of the ribs
To facilitate lymphatic drainage

Contraindications

Rib fracture
Spinal cord injury and surgery
Malignancy

Technique

1. The patient lies supine, and the physician is seated at the side of the patient.

2. The physician slides both hands under the patient's thoracolumbar region **(Figs. 15.15 and 15.16)**.

3. The pads of the fingers lie on the paravertebral tissues over the costotransverse articulation on the side near the physician **(Fig. 15.17)**.

4. Leaning down with the elbows, the physician lifts the fingers into the paravertebral tissues, simultaneously drawing the fingers (*arrows*, **Fig. 15.18**) in.

5. This lifts the spine off the table and places a lateral stretch on the paravertebral tissues.

6. This technique may be performed as an intermittent kneading technique or with sustained *deep* inhibitory pressure.

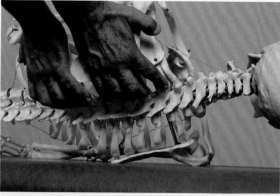

Figure 15.15. Skeletal hand contact.

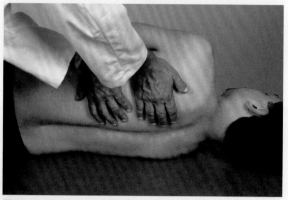

Figure 15.16. Patient hand contact.

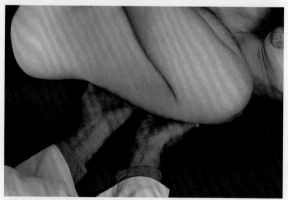

Figure 15.17. Physician and patient positioning.

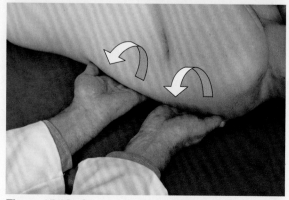

Figure 15.18. Step 4, ventral and then lateral pressure.

Reflex-Oriented Treatment

Sacral Rock

 See Video 15.5

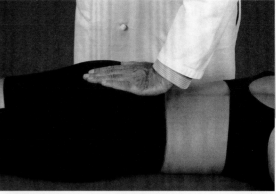

Figure 15.19. Cephalad hand.

Indications

Dysmenorrhea
Pelvic congestion syndrome
Sacroiliac dysfunction

Contraindications

Undiagnosed pelvic pain
Pelvic malignancy

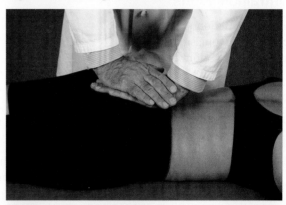

Figure 15.20. Caudad hand.

Technique

1. The patient lies prone, and the physician stands at the side of the table.

2. The physician places the cephalad hand with the heel of the hand at the sacral base, fingers pointing toward the coccyx **(Fig. 15.19)**.

3. The physician's caudad hand reinforces the cephalad hand with fingers pointing in the opposite direction **(Fig. 15.20)**.

4. The physician, keeping the elbows straight, exerts gentle pressure on the sacrum.

5. The physician introduces a rocking motion to the sacrum synchronous with the patient's respiration. Sacral extension (*arrow*, **Fig. 15.21**) occurs during inhalation. Sacral flexion (*arrow*, **Fig. 15.22**) occurs during exhalation.

6. This technique is continued for several minutes.

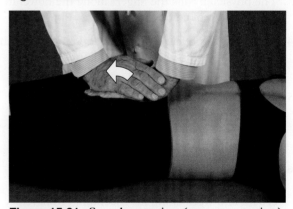

Figure 15.21. Sacral extension (counternutation).

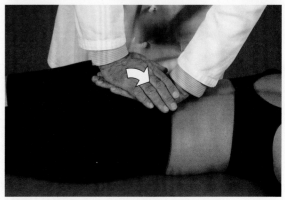

Figure 15.22. Sacral flexion (nutation).

Stimulatory/Vibratory Treatment

Colonic Stimulation

 See Video 15.6

Indication

Constipation

Contraindications

Bowel obstruction
Abdominal neoplasm
Undiagnosed abdominal pain

Technique

1. The patient lies supine, and the physician stands at the patient's side.

2. The physician places the pads of the fingers on the abdominal wall overlying the splenic flexure of the colon **(Fig. 15.23)**.

3. The physician rolls the fingers along the bowel in the direction of colonic flow (*arrows*, **Fig. 15.24**).

4. The physician releases pressure and repositions the hands one hand's-width farther along the colon toward the sigmoid region.

5. After several excursions down the descending colon, the physician repositions the hands to begin at the hepatic flexure and work along the transverse and descending colon **(Fig. 15.25)**.

6. After several of these excursions, the physician repositions the hands to begin at the region of the cecum and work along the ascending, transverse, and descending colon (*arrows*, **Fig. 15.26**).

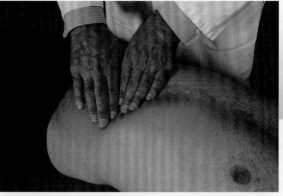

Figure 15.23. Steps 1 and 2.

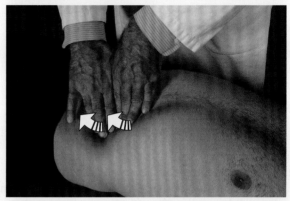

Figure 15.24. Step 3.

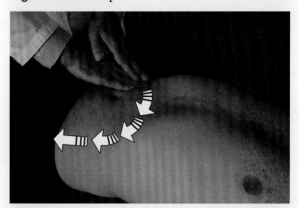

Figure 15.25. Step 5.

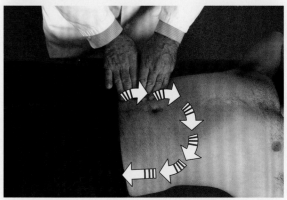

Figure 15.26. Step 6, entire length of large bowel.

Stimulatory/Vibratory Treatment

Splenic Stimulation

 See Video 15.7

Indications

Any infectious disease, also preventive

Contraindications

Infectious mononucleosis, any splenic enlargement
Neoplasm infiltrating the spleen

Technique

1. The patient lies supine, and the physician stands at the left side of the patient.

2. The physician's right hand abducts the patient's left arm 90 degrees and exerts gentle traction (*arrow*, **Fig. 15.27**).

3. The physician places the left hand on the lower costal cartilages overlying the spleen, with the fingers following the intercostal spaces **(Fig. 15.27)**.

4. The physician's left hand exerts pressure directly toward the center of the patient's body, springing the ribs inward.

5. A springing motion (*arrow*, **Fig. 15.28**) is carried out at two per second and continued for 30 seconds to several minutes.

6. One modification of this technique involves compressing the lower left rib cage slowly between the physician's hands with a sudden release (also called a chugging motion) **(Figs. 15.29 and 15.30)**.

7. A second modification has the physician place one hand over the lower costal cartilages and thump and percuss the back of the hand with a fist or forearm (*arrow*, **Fig. 15.31**).

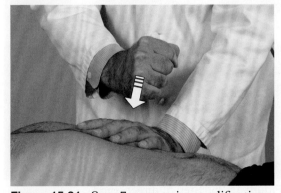

Figure 15.31. Step 7, percussive modification.

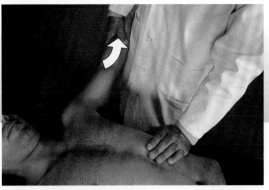

Figure 15.27. Steps 1 to 3.

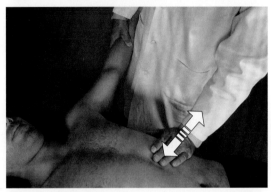

Figure 15.28. Step 5.

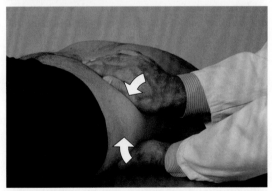

Figure 15.29. Step 6, sudden release modification (compression).

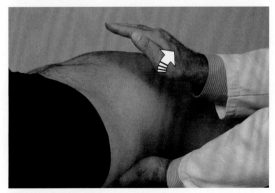

Figure 15.30. Step 6, release.

Myofascial Release/BLT Treatment

Gastric Release

 See Video 15.8

Indications

Gastroesophageal reflux
Gastric ptosis

Technique

1. The patient is seated, and the physician stands behind the patient.

2. The physician places the left and right hands over the left and right anterior subcostal and subxiphoid region, respectively **(Fig. 15.32)**.

3. The physician's hands contour the upper abdominal quadrants, and the finger pads curl slightly and press inward (*arrows*, **Fig. 15.33**).

4. The physician adds slightly more pressure inward and then tests for tissue texture changes and asymmetry in ease-bind motion freedom.

5. The physician directs a constant pressure to the ease (indirect) or bind (direct), depending on the patient's tolerance and physician's preference **(Figs. 15.34 and 15.35)**.

6. The physician holds this until a release is palpated and continues until no further improvement is produced.

7. A release-enhancing mechanism, such as deep inhalation and exhalation, can be helpful.

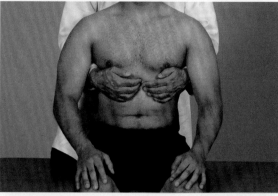

Figure 15.32. Steps 1 and 2.

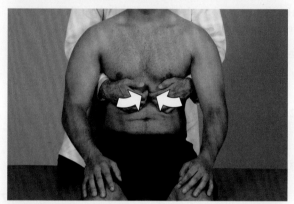

Figure 15.33. Step 3.

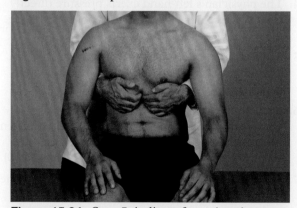

Figure 15.34. Step 5, indirect force (ease).

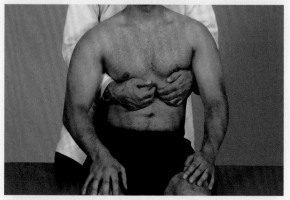

Figure 15.35. Step 5, direct (bind).

Myofascial Release/BLT Treatment

Hepatic Release

 See Video 15.9

Indications

Hepatitis
Cirrhosis
Cholelithiasis

Technique

1. The patient lies supine, and the physician sits to the right and faces the patient.

2. The physician places the left hand under the rib cage at the level of the liver.

3. The physician places the right hand immediately inferior to the subcostal angle at the patient's right upper quadrant **(Fig. 15.36)**.

4. The physician gently compresses the patient with both hands (*arrows*, **Fig. 15.37**) and attempts to palpate the liver.

5. The physician next tests for any ease-bind tissue texture and motion asymmetries.

6. On noting any asymmetry, the physician maintains a constant pressure at either the ease (indirect) or the bind (direct), depending on the patient's tolerance and physician's preference **(Fig. 15.38)**.

7. The physician holds this until a release is palpated and continues until no further improvement is produced.

8. A release-enhancing mechanism, such as deep inhalation and exhalation, can be helpful.

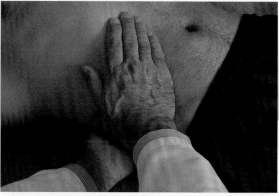
Figure 15.36. Steps 1 to 3.

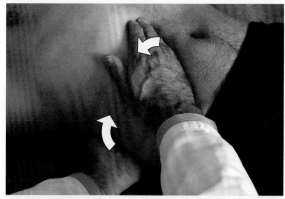
Figure 15.37. Compress to palpate liver.

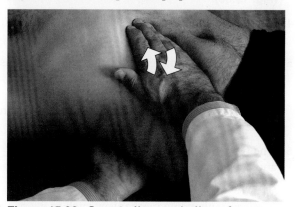
Figure 15.38. Step 6, direct or indirect force.

Myofascial Release/BLT Treatment

Gallbladder Release

 See Video 15.10

Indications

Cholecystitis
Cholestasis
Chronic upper abdominal pain

Technique

1. The patient is seated, and the physician stands behind the patient.

2. The physician places the index, third, and fourth fingers of the left hand just inferior to the xiphoid process, midline to slightly right.

3. The physician places the index, third, and fourth fingers of the right hand just inferior to the subcostal margin, just lateral of midline immediately to the right of the gallbladder **(Fig. 15.39)**.

4. The physician tests for any ease-bind tissue texture and motion asymmetries.

5. On noting any asymmetry, the physician maintains constant pressure (*arrows*, **Figs. 15.40 and 15.41**) at either the ease (indirect) or the bind (direct), depending on the patient's tolerance and physician's preference.

6. The physician holds until a release is palpated and continues until no further improvement is produced.

7. A release-enhancing mechanism, such as deep inhalation and exhalation, can be helpful.

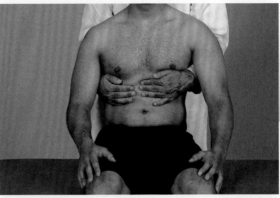

Figure 15.39. Steps 1 to 3.

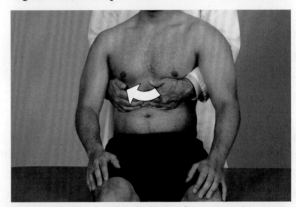

Figure 15.40. Step 5, indirect force (ease).

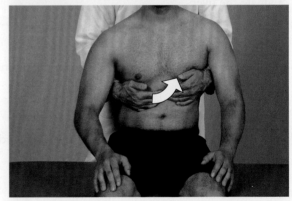

Figure 15.41. Step 5, direct force (bind).

Myofascial Release/BLT Treatment

Kidney Release

 See Video 15.11

Indications

Pyelonephritis
Renal lithiasis
Flank and inguinal pain

Technique

1. The patient lies supine with the hip and knee flexed on the affected side.

2. The physician stands on the affected side at the level of the hip.

3. The patient's knee is placed anterior to the physician's axilla at the coracoid process, and hip flexion is added to relax the anterior abdominal region **(Fig. 15.42)**.

4. The physician places the lateral hand palm up under the patient's back just below the floating ribs.

5. The physician's medial hand reaches around the patient's thigh to lie over the upper abdominal quadrant on the affected side and presses downward (posteriorly) (*top arrow*, **Fig. 15.43**) until palpating the kidney.

6. The physician's posterior hand lifts (*bottom arrow*, **Fig. 15.43**) upward (anterior) to facilitate the renal palpation.

7. The physician next tests for any ease-bind tissue texture and motion asymmetries.

8. On noting asymmetry, the physician maintains a constant pressure (*arrows*, **Fig. 15.44**) at either the ease (indirect) or the bind (direct), depending on the patient's tolerance and physician's preference.

9. The physician holds until a release is palpated and continues until no further improvement is produced.

10. A release-enhancing mechanism, such as deep inhalation and exhalation, can be helpful.

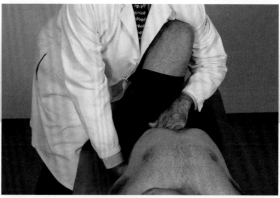
Figure 15.42. Steps 1 to 3.

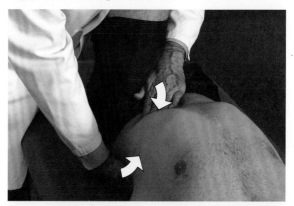
Figure 15.43. Steps 4 to 6.

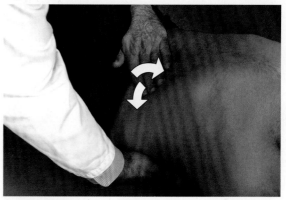
Figure 15.44. Step 8, direct or indirect force.

References

1. American Association of Colleges of Osteopathic Medicine. Glossary of Osteopathic Terminology, http://www.aacom.org, 2013.
2. Chila AG, exec. ed. Foundations of Osteopathic Medicine. 3rd ed. Baltimore, MD: Lippincott Williams & Wilkins, 2011.
3. Nelson KE, Glonek T. Somatic Dysfunction in Osteopathic Family Medicine. Baltimore, MD: Lippincott Williams & Wilkins, 2007.
4. Barral JP, Mercier P. Visceral Manipulation. Seattle, WA: Eastland, 1988.
5. Owens F. An Endocrine Interpretation of Chapman's Reflexes. Chattanooga, TN: Chattanooga Printing & Engraving Co., 1937.
6. Ward R, exec. ed. Foundations for Osteopathic Medicine. 2nd ed. Philadelphia, PA: Lippincott Williams & Wilkins, 2003.
7. Agur AMR, Dalley AF. Grant's Atlas of Anatomy. 11th ed. Baltimore, MD: Lippincott Williams & Wilkins, 2005.

16

Lymphatic Techniques

Technique Principles

Lymphatic techniques have not until recently been considered a specific category of osteopathic manipulation. They were typically included in the visceral sections of osteopathic principles and practice. The Educational Council on Osteopathic Principles (ECOP) offers no definition of lymphatics as a separate type of osteopathic manipulation. In the ECOP glossary, the only specific mention of lymphatic technique is that of the lymphatic (Miller) pump and the pedal (Dalrymple) pump (1). These techniques are included in this chapter as well as referenced in *Foundations of Osteopathic Medicine* (1).

It is a principle that all osteopathic techniques have some effect on lymphatics. This is accomplished directly, by stimulating flow or removing impediments to flow, or indirectly, by the alleviation of somatic dysfunction and the consequential normalization or balancing (parasympathetic or sympathetic) of the autonomic nervous system. However, certain techniques seem to have a more direct effect on the lymphatic system than others and hence are described in this chapter. Lymph-potentiating techniques are described in other chapters. Examples of techniques with great lymphatic potential of their own are balanced ligamentous tension, or ligamentous articular strain (BLT/LAS); soft tissue; visceral; myofascial release (MFR); and articulatory techniques. These are described in their respective chapters.

Many osteopathic physicians have attempted to affect the lymphatic system. The principle of unimpeded vascular supply has been promoted extensively, and most osteopathic students have heard A.T. Still's rule of the artery quoted; however, Still also stated that he considered the lymphatic system primary in the maintenance of health and, when it is stressed, a major contributor to disease and increased morbidity. He expressed his philosophy with words such as "life and death" when speaking about this system (2).

Philadelphia osteopathic physicians were important to the understanding of the lymphatic system and in developing techniques to affect it. William Galbreath (Philadelphia College of Osteopathic Medicine [PCOM],

1905) developed mandibular drainage, a technique included in this text (3,4). Another PCOM alumnus, J. Gordon Zink, was a prominent lecturer on the myofascial aspects of lymphatic congestion and its treatment. We believe that of the fluid systems, it is the low-pressure lymphatic system that can most easily be impeded and most clinically benefited. We are attempting to use techniques with a strong effect on this system to treat some of our most difficult chronic cases that are complicated by autoimmune and other inflammatory conditions.

Students of osteopathic medicine are typically instructed in the terrible effects of the influenza pandemic of 1918 and 1919. In this respect, many students have been taught the lymphatic (thoracic) pump developed by C. Earl Miller, DO, a graduate of the Chicago College of Osteopathy who practiced just north of Philadelphia. He began using this technique and promoting it to other osteopathic physicians in the mid-1920s. However, Miller's technique was not being used during the influenza epidemic, and it was most likely soft tissue and articulatory techniques that were most commonly used at that time.

A few years ago, Miller's son, himself a doctor of medicine, discussed with us the many cases and techniques that he saw his father use and that he continued to use in his own internal medicine practice. He was kind enough to donate some of his father's equipment to the PCOM archives. What was most interesting to us were the positive effects he said his father's technique had on so many varied conditions. Some were not conditions that have been historically taught as indications for its use. This had a profound effect on us, and we are attempting to develop more research in this field (e.g., Parkinson disease, multiple sclerosis). Bell palsy was the condition that piqued our interest most when considering its clinical value. Miller evidently had extremely rapid positive clinical responses when treating Bell palsy with this technique. It changed our views on the symptoms associated with this process and why stimulation to the chest wall and pulmonary cavity could result in an almost immediate clinical response in a syndrome with most of its symptoms in the facial cranium. We believe that the fluid-stimulating effects can decongest the foramen through which the facial nerve passes, thus alleviating the symptoms.

The clinical effects that can be seen with lymphatic techniques may be secondary to the elimination of somatic dysfunction, whereby related autonomic changes and potential facilitated segments are normalized. This normalization not only has effects on somatic and visceral reflexes, nociception, and vascular tone but also can affect the lymphatic system, which receives autonomic stimulation. The larger lymphatic vessels may even change diameter following sympathetic stimulation (1,5).

Technique Classification

Techniques Removing Restrictions to Lymphatic Flow

Restrictions to lymphatic flow that are related to specific somatic dysfunctions may be removed by techniques from many categories (e.g., BLT/LAS; high volume, low amplitude [HVLA]). This can be thought of as breaking the dam. An example is a first rib dysfunction. Besides causing pain, limited motion, and so on, a first rib dysfunction has the potential to restrict flow through the thoracic inlet. Mobilizing the rib and restoring its normal range of motion and function may remove the restriction to lymphatic flow. Therefore, any technique that is indicated for first rib somatic dysfunction (e.g., MFR, muscle energy technique [MET]) also has the potential to be a lymphatic technique. Another important principle is to remove somatic dysfunctions that are causing secondary autonomic effects (e.g., thoracic dysfunctions causing hypersympathetic tone with consequent lymphatic constriction). In trying to develop a clinical step-by-step treatment protocol, the elimination of a somatic dysfunction that is directly causing a hypersympathetic response (e.g., facilitated segment) may logically be the first step in the treatment. In bypassing this step in the treatment and trying to improve the myofascial status of the thoracic inlet, you will not necessarily affect the etiology of the dysautonomia, and therefore, the "vasoconstrictive" effects will continue to cause restricted lymphatic flow, similar to poor drainage from a clogged drain.

Some other common areas of dysfunction with which this type of technique can be helpful are submandibular restrictions, thoracic inlet restriction secondary to myofascial tension, abdominal diaphragm dysfunction, psoas muscle dysfunction, and dysfunctions affecting the axilla, antecubital fossa, popliteal fossa, and plantar fascia.

Techniques Promoting Lymphatic Flow

Techniques promoting lymphatic flow are generally stimulatory, stroking, oscillatory, or vibratory. Effleurage and pétrissage are common massage variations of this type of technique. Thoracic pump, pedal pump, mandibular drainage, and anterior cervical chain drainage are classical examples of osteopathic techniques that stimulate flow.

This modality has been involved in discussions concerning treatment of patients with a malignancy. Some believe that it is not wise to promote lymphatic flow, while others believe it is indicated because promoting normal flow allows greater clearance of abnormal cells. More research is needed, but we believe that if exercise can be prescribed for specific patients with a malignancy, then lymphatic flow stimulation should also be indicated in those patients.

Technique Styles

The various styles of lymphatic technique belong to their own category of osteopathic manipulative treatment (OMT). Subclassification in this category includes techniques that affect the intrinsic and extrinsic lymphatic pumps.

Intrinsic Lymphatic Pump

These techniques alter autonomic tone or tissue texture in the interstitial spaces. In the interstitium, fluid can accumulate and eventually disrupt normal lymphatic flow. Examples of this style include treatment of facilitated segments in the thoracolumbar region and indirect MFR to the interosseous membrane.

Extrinsic Lymphatic Flow

The extrinsic pump is related to the effects of muscle contraction and motion on the lymphatic system. Therefore, any technique that affects this mechanism is considered an extrinsic style. Examples include abdominal diaphragm or pelvic diaphragm treatment with MFR and MET or treatment of the somatic component of a dysfunction with HVLA (e.g., C3–C5 dysfunction affecting the diaphragm). Any form of exercise or technique affecting muscle activity (e.g., direct pressure, stroking, effleurage) is included in this style.

Indications

Lymphatic congestion and postsurgical edema (e.g., mastectomy)
Mild congestive heart failure
Upper and lower respiratory infections and other areas of infection
Asthma and chronic obstructive pulmonary disease
Pain due to lymphatic congestion and swelling

Contraindications

Absolute Contraindications

1. Necrotizing fasciitis (in area involved)

Relative Contraindications

1. Acute indurated lymph node (do not treat directly)
2. Fracture, dislocation, or osteoporosis if technique style would exacerbate condition
3. Organ friability as seen in spleen with infectious mononucleosis
4. Acute hepatitis
5. Malignancy
6. Bacterial infection with risk of dissemination
7. Chronic infections with risk of reactivation (abscess, chronic osteomyelitis)
8. Diseased organ (treating thyroid in presence of hyperthyroidism)
9. Coagulopathies or patients on anticoagulants
10. Unstable cardiac conditions
11. Moderate to severe congestive heart failure
12. COPD (thoracic pump with activation)

General Considerations and Rules

Lymphatic techniques are similar in scope of principle to the visceral techniques. The physician must consider the patient's health status along with the specific presenting symptoms before deciding to use a particular technique. The area must be stable, and the integument must be able to tolerate the type of pressure, whether probing or frictional. For vibratory or compression techniques, the patient's musculoskeletal status in respect to bone density and motion availability must be relatively normal. If the patient has lymphatic sequelae of autonomic disturbance, the appropriate somatic component must be treated with whichever technique the physician determines is indicated.

These techniques, in addition to affecting lymphatic circulation, may affect the endocrine, autoimmune, and neuromusculoskeletal systems, resulting in increased motion, less pain, and a better overall sense of well-being. The following techniques, as stated previously, are not the only ones affecting the lymphatics. Please see other chapters for ways to enhance lymphatic flow, reduce restriction, or normalize autonomic innervation.

Lymphatic Treatment Protocol (Order)

In developing a treatment protocol for a lymphatic-style treatment, the physician should understand the nature of lymphatic flow from its control mechanisms, anatomical relationships, and the principle with which the lymphatic technique is to be performed (e.g., stimulation vs. removal of impediments). The general historic principle is to treat the most central (proximal) obstruction first. This can be a neurologic control issue (i.e., hypersympathetic reaction causing lymphatic constriction of the larger lumen vessels) or a physical blockage. Also, the physician should be able to discern whether the edema is from other visceral pathology (e.g., congestive heart failure) or a breakdown of the lymphatic system itself. A common problem is to differentiate the cause of unilateral extremity edema. In this case, treating the thoracic inlet first may not be indicated as the obstruction may be more peripheral, such as in the popliteal fossa in a patient with ankle edema.

An example of a treatment protocol is the step-by-step technique implementation for conditions of ear, nose, and throat (ENT), as follows:

1. If present, treat any associated "facilitated" thoracic/costal and/or upper lumbar somatic dysfunction.
2. Release thoracic inlet/outlet myofascial restrictions (i.e., MFR, muscle energy to cervicothoracic junction), and then in stepwise fashion, do/treat the following:

   Anterior cervical arches
   Cervical chain drainage ("milking")
   Submandibular release and suboccipital release
   Mandibular drainage (Galbreath technique)
   Auricular drainage
   Alternating nasal pressure/frontonasal distraction
   Trigeminal stimulation
   Fronto (facial) temporomandibular drainage: effleurage

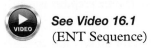 ***See Video 16.1***
(ENT Sequence)

Head and Neck

Anterior Cervical Arches
Hyoid, Cricoid, Thyroid Cartilage Release

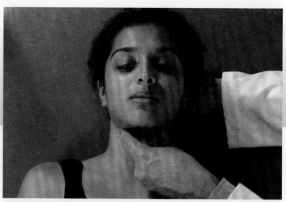

Figure 16.1. Steps 1 to 3, setup.

Indications

Laryngitis
Pharyngitis
Cough
Any dysfunction or lymphatic congestion in the ENT
    region

Technique

1. The patient lies supine, and the physician sits at
   the patient's side, near the head of the table.

2. The physician stabilizes the patient's head by
   placing the cephalad hand beneath the head or by
   gently grasping the forehead.

3. The thumb and index finger of the physician's
   caudad hand form a horseshoe shape (inverted C)
   over the anterior cervical arches **(Fig. 16.1)**.

4. The physician makes alternating contact (*arrows*,
   Figs. 16.2 and 16.3) with the lateral aspects of
   the hyoid bone, thyroid cartilages, then cricoid
   cartilage, which houses the tracheal rings, gently
   pushing them from one side to the other.

5. The physician continues this alternating pressure
   up and down the length of the anterior neck.

6. If there is crepitus between the anterior
   cartilaginous structures and the cervical spine,
   the neck may be slightly flexed or extended
   to eliminate excess friction. (Some crepitus is
   normal.)

7. This technique is continued for 30 seconds to
   2 minutes.

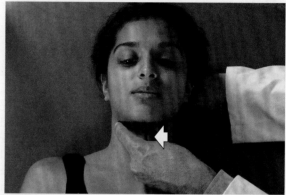

Figure 16.2. Step 4.

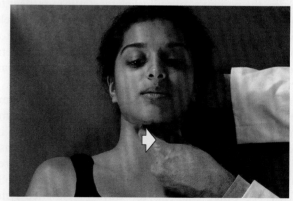

Figure 16.3. Step 4.

Head and Neck

Cervical Chain Drainage Technique

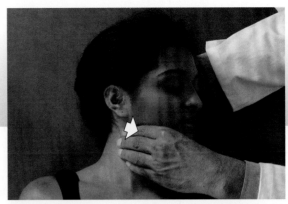

Figure 16.4. Steps 1 to 3, hand placement.

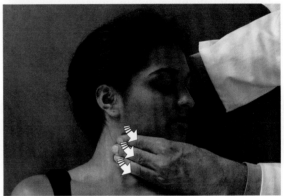

Figure 16.5. Step 4, milking motion.

Indications

This technique is indicated for any dysfunction or lymphatic congestion in the ENT region. Before performing this technique, the physician should treat any dysfunctions centrally (thoracic inlet, first thoracic, first rib, etc.) so that lymphatic flow is not impeded. Note: Some are of the philosophy that the initial contact should begin inferiorly, at the lower end of the chain near the clavicle, and then slowly work upward toward the upper cervical portion and then alternating caudal to cephalad.

Technique

1. The patient lies supine, and the physician sits at the patient's side, near the head of the table.

2. The physician stabilizes the patient's head by placing the cephalad hand beneath the head to elevate it slightly or by gently grasping the forehead.

3. The physician's caudad hand (palmar aspect of the fingers) makes broad contact over the sternocleidomastoid (SCM) muscle near the angle of the mandible (*arrow*, **Fig. 16.4**).

4. From cephalad to caudad, the fingers roll along the muscle in a milking fashion (*arrows*, **Fig. 16.5**). The hand may be moved slightly more caudad along the muscle and repeats the rolling motion, going cephalad to caudad.

5. This same procedure is applied both anterior to and posterior to the SCM muscle to affect both the anterior and posterior lymphatic chains.

6. Caution: Do not perform directly over painful, indurated lymph nodes.

Head and Neck

Submandibular Release

Indications

This technique is indicated for any dysfunction or lymphatic congestion in the ENT region, especially those affecting the tongue, salivary glands, lower teeth, and temporomandibular dysfunctions.

Technique

1. The patient lies supine, and the physician sits at the head of the table.

2. The physician places the index and third fingertips (may include fourth fingers) immediately below the inferior rim of the mandible **(Fig. 16.6)**.

3. The fingers are then directed superiorly into the submandibular fascia to determine whether an ease-bind asymmetry is present (*arrows*, **Fig. 16.7**).

4. The physician then imparts a direct (*arrow*, **Fig. 16.8**) or indirect (*arrow*, **Fig. 16.9**) vectored force until meeting the bind (direct) or ease (indirect) barrier.

5. The force may be applied very gently to moderately.

6. The physician continues until a release is palpated (fascial creep) and follows this creep until it does not recur. This may take 30 seconds to 2 minutes.

7. The physician takes care to avoid too much pressure over any enlarged and painful submandibular lymph nodes.

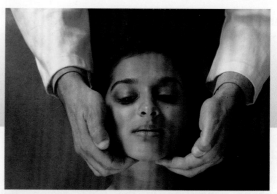

Figure 16.6. Hand and finger position.

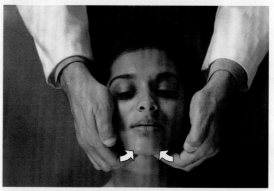

Figure 16.7. Step 3, fingers directed superiorly.

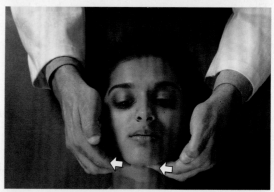

Figure 16.8. Direct.

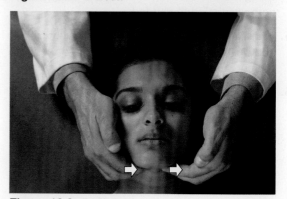

Figure 16.9. Indirect.

Head and Neck

Mandibular Drainage, Galbreath Technique

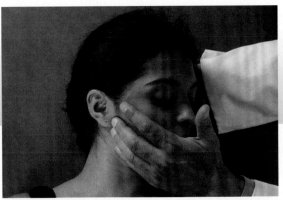

Figure 16.10. Steps 1 to 3, setup and hand placement.

Indications

This technique is indicated for any dysfunction or lymphatic congestion in the ENT or submandibular region, especially dysfunction in the eustachian tubes. Care must be taken in patients with active temporomandibular joint (TMJ) dysfunction (e.g., painful click) with severe loss of mobility and/or locking.

Technique

1. The patient lies supine with the head turned slightly toward the physician, and the physician sits at the patient's side, near the head of the table.

2. The physician stabilizes the patient's head by placing the cephalad hand beneath the head to elevate it slightly.

3. The physician places the caudad hand with the third, fourth, and fifth fingertips along the posterior ramus of the mandible and the hypothenar eminence along the body of the mandible **(Fig. 16.10)**.

4. The patient opens the mouth slightly.

5. The physician's caudad hand presses on the mandible so as to draw it slightly forward (*arrows*, **Fig. 16.11**) at the TMJ and gently toward the midline.

6. This procedure is applied and released in a slow rhythmic fashion for 30 seconds to 2 minutes. It may be repeated on the other side.

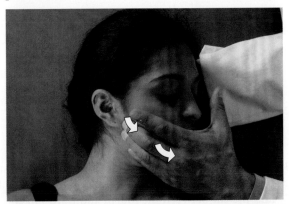

Figure 16.11. Step 5, caudad pressure on mandible.

Head and Neck

Auricular Drainage Technique

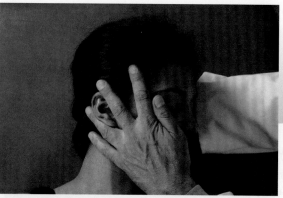

Figure 16.12. Steps 1 to 3, hand placement.

Indications

Any dysfunction or lymphatic congestion in the ear region
Otitis media
Otitis externa

Technique

1. The patient lies supine with the head turned slightly toward the physician, and the physician sits at the patient's side, near the head of the table.

2. The physician stabilizes the patient's head by placing the cephalad hand beneath the head to elevate it slightly.

3. The physician places the caudad hand flat against the side of the head, with fingers pointing cephalad and the ear between the fourth and third fingers **(Fig. 16.12)**.

4. The physician's caudad hand makes clockwise and counterclockwise circular motions (*arrows*, **Figs. 16.13 and 16.14**), moving the skin and fascia over the surface of the skull. There should be no sliding over the skin and no friction.

5. This procedure is applied for 30 seconds to 2 minutes.

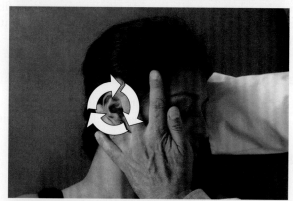

Figure 16.13. Step 4, clockwise.

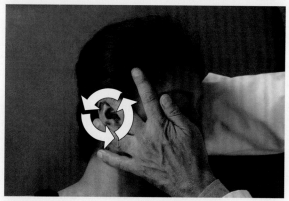

Figure 16.14. Step 4, counterclockwise.

Head and Neck

Alternating Nasal Pressure Technique

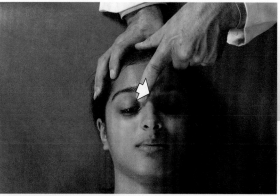

Figure 16.15. Step 4, left.

Indications

This technique is indicated for any dysfunction or lymphatic congestion in the ENT region, especially the ethmoid sinus.

Technique

1. The patient lies supine, and the physician sits at the head of the table.

2. The physician uses an index finger to press on a diagonal (*arrows*, **Figs. 16.15 and 16.16**) into the junction of the nasal and frontal bones, first in one direction and then the other.

3. This procedure is applied for 30 seconds to 2 minutes.

4. Alternative methods based on personal modifications of hand position are acceptable **(Fig. 16.17)**.

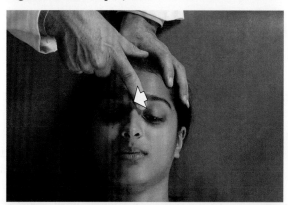

Figure 16.16. Step 4, right.

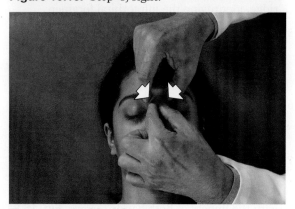

Figure 16.17. Modification.

Head and Neck

Trigeminal Nerve Decongestion/Release Supra-, Infra-, and Mental Foramina Lymphatic Drainage Emphasis

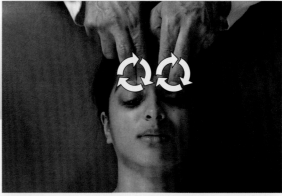

Figure 16.19. Steps 2 and 3, supraorbital foramen.

Indications

This technique is indicated for any dysfunction or lymphatic congestion in the ENT region affecting or exacerbated by inflammation of cranial nerve V **(Fig. 16.18)**.

Technique

1. The patient lies supine, and the physician sits at the head of the table.

2. The physician palpates along the superior orbital ridge, identifying the supraorbital foramen.

3. The physician places the pads of the index and middle finger just inferior to the orbital ridge and produces a circular motion with the fingers of both hands (*arrows*, **Fig. 16.19**).

4. The physician palpates along the inferior orbital ridge, identifying the infraorbital foramen.

5. The physician places the pads of the index and middle fingers just inferior to the infraorbital foramen and produces a circular motion with the fingers of both hands (*arrows*, **Fig. 16.20**).

6. The physician palpates along the mandible, knowing that the three foramina form a straight line, identifying the mandibular foramen.

7. The physician places the pads of the index and middle fingers over the mandibular branch of the trigeminal nerve and produces a circular motion with the fingers of both hands (*arrows*, **Fig. 16.21**).

8. This trigeminal stimulation procedure is applied for 30 seconds to 2 minutes at each of the three locations.

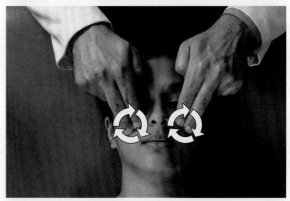

Figure 16.20. Steps 4 and 5, infraorbital foramen.

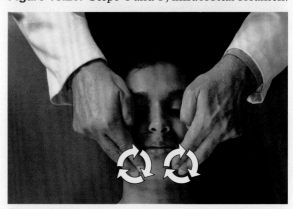

Figure 16.21. Steps 6 and 7, mandibular foramen.

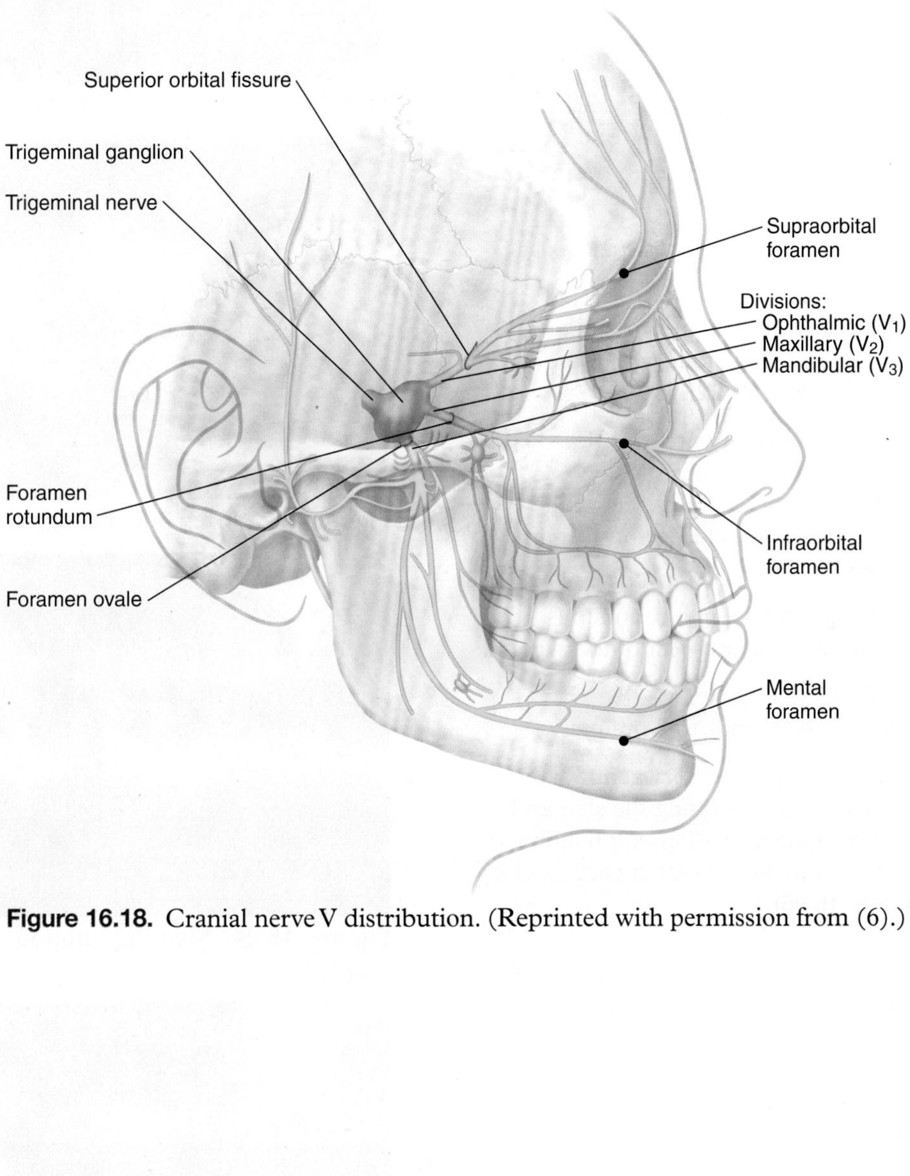

Figure 16.18. Cranial nerve V distribution. (Reprinted with permission from (6).)

Head and Neck

Maxillary Drainage, Effleurage

Indications

This technique is indicated for any dysfunction or lymphatic congestion in the ENT region, especially those affecting the maxillary sinuses.

Technique

1. The patient lies supine, and the physician sits at the head of the table.

2. The physician places the index finger tip pads (may include third fingers) just inferior to the infraorbital foramina **(Fig. 16.22)**.

3. The physician's fingers begin a slow, gentle stroking (effleurage) over the patient's skin immediately parallel to the lateral aspect of the nose until they meet the dental ridge of the gums (*arrows*, **Fig. 16.23**).

4. The fingers continue laterally in a continuous gentle motion toward the alar aspect of the zygoma **(Fig. 16.24)**.

5. This is repeated for 30 seconds to 2 minutes.

6. This may be modified by either very gentle skin rolling over the area or gently lifting the skin and its contiguous subcutaneous tissues and holding at different levels for 20 to 30 seconds at each level in steps 3 and 4 **(Fig. 16.25)**.

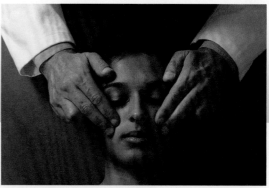

Figure 16.22. Step 2, finger placement.

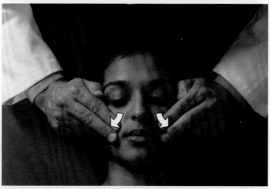

Figure 16.23. Step 3, effleurage.

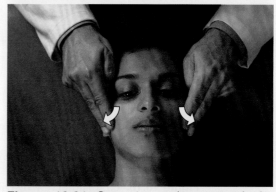

Figure 16.24. Step 4, motion toward the zygoma.

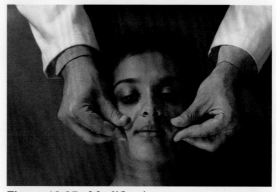

Figure 16.25. Modification.

Head and Neck

Frontal (Facial) Temporomandibular Drainage Lymphatic Emphasis

Indications

This technique is indicated for any dysfunction or lymphatic congestion in the ENT region, especially those affecting the frontal through mandibular regions or in tension headache.

Technique

1. The patient lies supine, and the physician sits at the head of the table.

2. The physician places the index fingertips (may include third fingers) immediately above and medial to the eyebrows **(Fig. 16.26)**.

3. The physician's fingers begin a slow, gentle, stroking (effleurage) laterally that takes them immediately parallel to the supraorbital ridge until they meet the area of the pterion (*arrows*, **Fig. 16.27**).

4. The fingers continue inferiorly in a continuous gentle motion toward the TMJ and inferiorly over the mandible **(Fig. 16.28)**.

5. This is repeated for 30 seconds to 2 minutes.

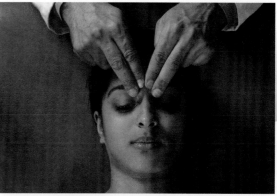

Figure 16.26. Step 2, finger placement.

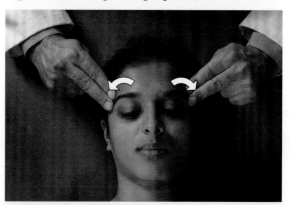

Figure 16.27. Step 3, effleurage.

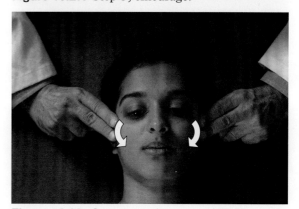

Figure 16.28. Step 4, motion toward TMJ.

Thoracic Region

Thoracic Inlet/Outlet Release
Seated "Steering Wheel" Technique
Myofascial Release/Lymphatic Emphasis

 See Video 16.2

Indications

This technique is indicated for any dysfunction or lymphatic congestion caused or exacerbated by fascial tone asymmetry in the area of the thoracic inlet and outlet.

Contraindications

This technique has no absolute contraindications.

Technique

See Chapter 8 for details.

Thoracic Region

Thoracic Inlet/Outlet Release
Direct Myofascial/Lymphatic Emphasis
Ex: Right Thoracic Outlet, Hypertonicity

Indications

This technique is indicated for any dysfunction or lymphatic congestion caused or exacerbated by fascial tone asymmetry in the area of the thoracic inlet and outlet.

Contraindications

This procedure should not be used if the patient has painful, severely restricted motion of the shoulder (e.g., fibrous adhesive capsulitis, rotator cuff tear).

Technique

1. The patient lies supine with the arm on the dysfunctional side abducted to approximately 90 degrees.

2. The physician stands or sits at the side of the dysfunctional thoracic inlet either caudal or cephalad to the abducted upper extremity **(Fig. 16.29)**. The arm may be supported by the physician's thigh if needed **(Fig. 16.30)**.

3. The physician places the index and third finger pads of the cephalad hand over the area of the thoracic inlet so as to palpate the fascial tone at the insertion of the first rib at the manubrium and the supraclavicular fascia **(Fig. 16.31)**.

4. The physician's caudad hand controls the patient's arm.

5. The physician gently moves the patient's arm through a series of motions (*arrows*, **Fig. 16.32**) to vector a line of tension toward the thoracic inlet. When successful, the physician will palpate the tension at that site.

6. The physician waits for a release (fascial creep) and continues until there is no further improvement in the restrictive barrier. Deep inhalation or other release-enhancing mechanisms can be helpful, as can a vibratory motion produced through the upper extremity with the wrist-controlling hand.

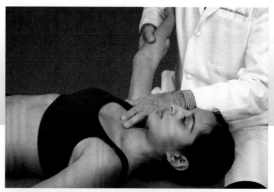

Figure 16.29. Steps 1 and 2, setup.

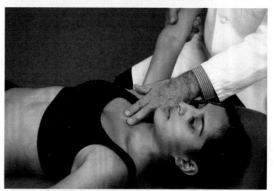

Figure 16.30. Modified supportive position.

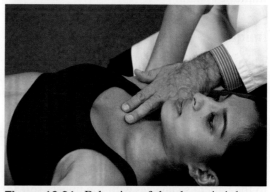

Figure 16.31. Palpation of the thoracic inlet.

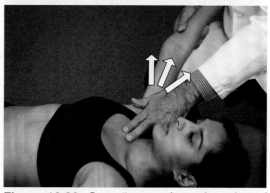

Figure 16.32. Step 5, arm through series of motions.

Thoracic Region

Miller Thoracic (Lymphatic) Pump
Male/Female Patient Variations

 See Video 16.3

Indications

This technique is indicated for infection, fever, lymphatic congestion, rales, and chronic productive cough; also preventive, it may increase titers postvaccination (7–11).

Contraindications

This procedure should not be used if the patient has fractures, osteoporosis, moderate to severe dyspnea, regional incisions, subclavian lines, metastatic cancer, and so on.

Physiologic Goal

The goal is to accentuate negative intrathoracic pressure, increase lymphatic return, loosen mucus plugs via the vibratory component, and potentially stimulate the autoimmune system.

Technique

1. The patient lies supine with the head turned to one side (to avoid breathing or coughing into the face of the physician) and with the hips and knees flexed and the feet flat on the table.

2. The physician stands at the head of the table with one foot in front of the other **(Fig. 16.33)**.

3. The physician places the thenar eminences inferior to the patient's clavicles with the fingers spreading out over the upper rib cage **(Fig. 16.34)**. For female patients, the physician may place the hands more midline over the sternum **(Fig. 16.35)**.

4. The patient is instructed to take a deep breath and exhale fully.

5. During exhalation, the physician increases the pressure on the anterior rib cage, exaggerating the exhalation motion.

6. At end exhalation, the physician imparts a vibratory motion to the rib cage at two compressions per second (*pulsed arrows*, **Fig. 16.36**).

7. Should the patient need to breathe, pressure is relaxed slightly, but the compressions are continued for several minutes.

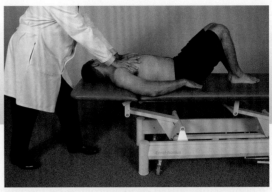
Figure 16.33. Steps 1 and 2, setup.

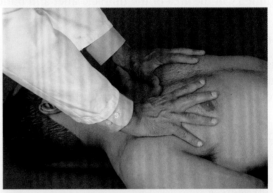
Figure 16.34. Hand position.

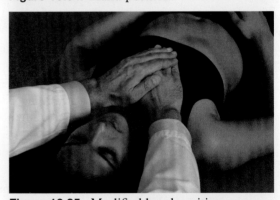
Figure 16.35. Modified hand position.

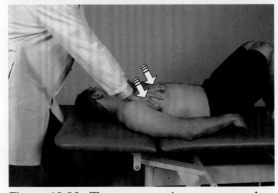
Figure 16.36. Two compressions per second.

Thoracic Region

Miller Thoracic (Lymphatic) Pump Exaggerated Respiration Method Male/Female Patient Variations

 See Video 16.3

Indications

This technique is indicated for infection, fever, lymphatic congestion, rales, and chronic productive cough; it is also preventive.

Contraindications

This procedure should not be used if the patient has a fracture, osteoporosis, moderate to severe dyspnea, regional incision, subclavian line, metastatic cancer, or a similar condition.

Physiologic Goal

The goal is to accentuate negative intrathoracic pressure and increase lymphatic return.

Technique

1. The patient lies supine with the head turned to one side (to avoid breathing or coughing into the face of the physician) and with the hips and knees flexed and the feet flat on the table.

2. The physician stands at the head of the table with one foot in front of the other.

3. The physician places the thenar eminences inferior to the patient's clavicles with the fingers spreading out over the upper rib cage **(Fig. 16.37)**. For female patients, the physician places the hands more midline over the sternum **(Fig. 16.38)**.

4. The patient is instructed to take a deep breath and exhale fully.

5. During exhalation, the physician increases the pressure on the anterior rib cage, exaggerating the exhalation motion (*arrow*, **Fig. 16.39**).

6. During the next inhalation, the physician releases the pressure (*upward arrow*, **Fig. 16.40**) and then reinstates it (*downward arrow*) with the next exhalation.

7. This version of the thoracic pump may be repeated for 5 to 10 respiratory cycles. This may hyperventilate the patient, and light-headedness and dizziness are fairly common.

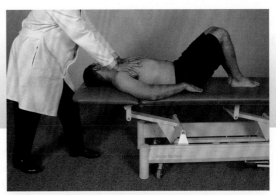
Figure 16.37. Hand position.

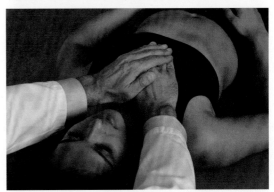
Figure 16.38. Modified hand position.

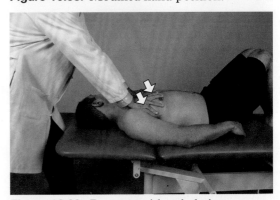
Figure 16.39. Pressure with exhalation.

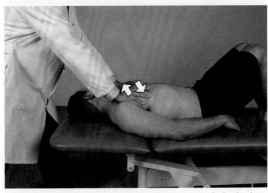
Figure 16.40. Release pressure on inhalation and reinstate it on exhalation.

Thoracic Region

Unilateral Thoracic (Lymphatic) Pump Side Modification Method

 See Video 16.4

1. The patient lies supine, and the physician stands at the side of the table at the level of the patient's rib cage. The patient's hips and knees may be flexed to enhance the effect.

2. The patient's arm is abducted 90 degrees or greater, and the physician exerts traction on the arm with the cephalad hand.

3. The physician places the caudad hand over the lower costal cartilages with the fingers following the intercostal spaces **(Fig. 16.41)**.

4. The patient is instructed to take a deep breath and exhale fully.

5. At end of exhalation, a percussive or vibratory motion (*arrow,* **Fig. 16.42**) is exerted by the physician at two per second.

6. Should the patient feel the need to breathe, pressure is released just enough to permit easy respiration and the vibratory motion continued.

7. This technique is continued for several minutes. It should be repeated, when possible, on the opposite side of the chest.

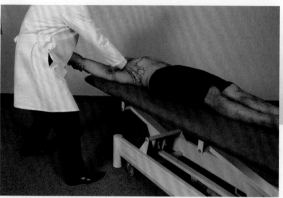

Figure 16.41. Steps 1 to 3, setup and hand placement.

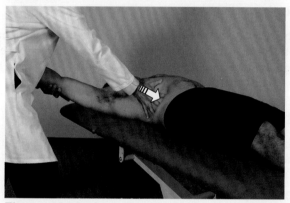

Figure 16.42. Step 5, percussive or vibratory motion.

Thoracic Region

Thoracic (Lymphatic) Pump
Atelectasis Modification Method
Male/Female Patient Variations

 See Video 16.5

Indications

This technique is indicated for atelectasis.

Contraindications

This procedure should not be used if the patient has a fracture, osteoporosis, severe congestion, incision, subclavian line, metastatic cancer, or similar condition.

Physiologic Goal

The goal is to accentuate the negative phase of respiration and clear mucus plugs.

Technique

1. The patient lies supine with the head turned to one side (to avoid breathing or coughing into the face of the physician) and with the hips and knees flexed and feet flat on the table.

2. The physician stands at the head of the table with one foot in front of the other.

3. The physician places the thenar eminences inferior to the patient's clavicles with the fingers spreading out over the upper rib cage (**Fig. 16.43**). For female patients, the physician places the hands more midline over the sternum (**Fig. 16.44**).

4. The patient is instructed to take a deep breath and exhale fully.

5. During exhalation, the physician increases the pressure on the anterior rib cage, exaggerating the exhalation motion.

6. During the next several inhalations, the physician maintains heavy pressure on the chest wall (**Fig. 16.45**).

7. On the last instruction to inhale, the physician suddenly releases the pressure, causing the patient to take a very rapid, deep inhalation, inflating any atelectatic segments that may be present (**Fig. 16.46**).

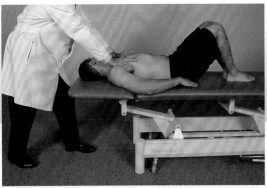

Figure 16.43. Steps 1 to 3, setup and hand placement.

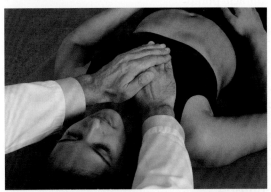

Figure 16.44. Modified hand position.

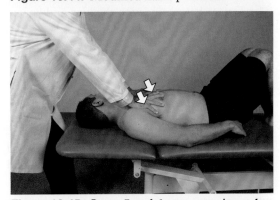

Figure 16.45. Steps 5 and 6, exaggerating exhalation, restricting inhalation.

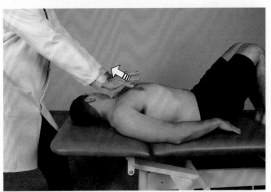

Figure 16.46. Sudden release of pressure.

Thoracic Region

Bilateral Pectoral Traction
Pectoralis Major/Minor, Anterior Deltoid
Myofascial Release/Lymphatic Emphasis

 See Video 16.6

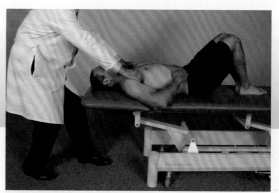

Figure 16.47. Steps 1 to 3, hand position.

Indications

This technique is indicated for lymphatic congestion, upper extremity edema, mild to moderate dyspnea or wheeze, and/or reactive airway or asthma; it facilitates the thoracic pump.

Contraindications

This procedure should not be used if the patient has hypersensitivity to touch at the anterior axillary fold, subclavian line, some pacemakers, metastatic cancer, or similar condition.

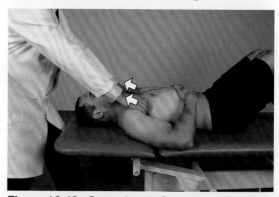

Figure 16.48. Steps 4 to 5, force toward ceiling.

Physiologic Goal

The goal is to increase lymphatic return.

Technique

1. The patient lies supine with the hips and knees flexed and the feet flat on the table.

2. The physician sits or stands at the head of the table with one foot in front of the other.

3. The physician places the finger pads inferior to the patient's clavicles at the anterior axillary fold **(Fig. 16.47)**.

4. The physician slowly and gently leans backward, causing the hands and fingers to move cephalad into the patient's axilla.

5. When the physician's hands and fingers meet a restrictive barrier, a new force is directed upward (*arrows*, **Fig. 16.48**).

6. The patient is instructed to take deep breaths through the mouth, and the physician pulls cephalad with the additional movement caused by the inhalation (*arrow*, **Fig. 16.49**).

7. The patient is next instructed to exhale fully, and the physician resists this movement at the axilla, continuing to pull cephalad and upward (*arrows*, **Fig. 16.50**).

8. Inhalation with cephalad traction and exhalation with resistance to costal depression is continued five to seven times.

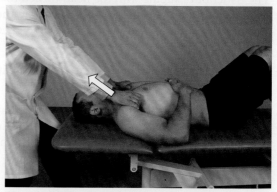

Figure 16.49. Step 6, deep inhalation.

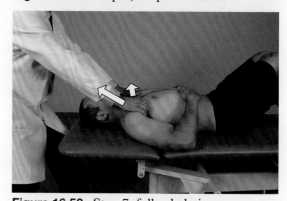

Figure 16.50. Step 7, full exhalation.

Thoracic Region

"Rib Raising" Technique
Bilateral, Upper Thoracic Variation

Indications

This technique is indicated to facilitate lymphatic drainage, improve respiratory excursion of the ribs, and alleviate postoperative paralytic ileus.

Contraindications

Rib and/or sternal fracture
Spinal cord injury and surgery
Malignancy

Technique

1. The patient lies supine, and the physician is seated at the head of the table.

2. The physician slides both hands under the patient's thoracic region.

3. The finger pads of both hands contact the paravertebral tissues over the costotransverse articulation **(Fig. 16.51)**.

4. By leaning down with the elbows, the physician elevates the fingers into the paravertebral tissues (*solid arrows*, **Fig. 16.52**) and then pulls them (*broken arrows*) toward the physician cephalad and lateral.

5. This extends the spine and places a lateral stretch on the paravertebral tissues.

6. This technique may be performed as an intermittent kneading technique or with sustained deep inhibitory pressure for 2 to 5 minutes.

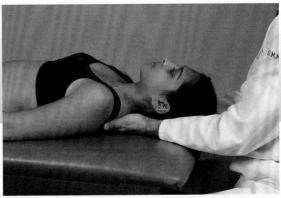

Figure 16.51. Steps 1 to 3, setup and hand placement.

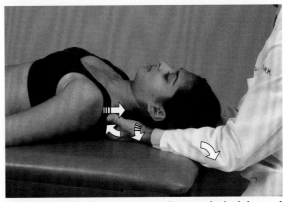

Figure 16.52. Step 4, anterior cephalad lateral force.

Thoracoabdominal Region

Doming the Diaphragm

 See Video 16.7

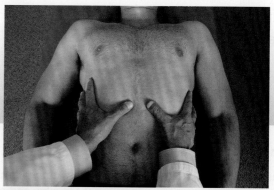

Figure 16.53. Thumb placement.

Indications

This technique is indicated for lymphatic congestion distal to the diaphragm and/or respiration that does not (myofascially) extend fully to the pubic symphysis.

Contraindications

This procedure should not be used if the patient has drainage tubes, intravenous lines, thoracic or abdominal incision, or moderate to severe hiatal hernia or gastro-esophageal reflux symptoms.

Physiologic Goal

The goal is to improve lymphatic and venous return; it may improve immune function.

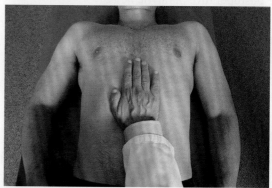

Figure 16.54. Variation of thenar eminence placement.

Technique

1. The patient lies supine with the hips and knees flexed and feet flat on the table.

2. The physician stands to one side at the level of the pelvis, facing cephalad.

3. The physician places the thumbs or thenar eminence just inferior to the patient's lower costal margin and xiphoid process with the thumbs pointing cephalad **(Figs. 16.53 and 16.54)**.

4. The patient is instructed to take a deep breath and exhale. On exhalation, the physician's thumbs follow the diaphragm (*arrows*, **Fig. 16.55**), which permits the thumbs to move posteriorly.

5. The patient is instructed to inhale, and the physician gently resists this motion.

6. The patient is instructed to exhale, and the physician gently follows this motion posteriorly and cephalad (*arrows*, **Fig. 16.56**), as the thumbs are now beneath the costal margin and xiphoid process.

7. The patient inhales as the physician maintains pressure on the upper abdomen and then, on repeated exhalation, encourages further cephalad excursion **(Fig. 16.57)**.

8. This procedure is repeated for three to five respiratory cycles.

This procedure should not be used if the patient has rib or vertebral fracture, spinal cord injury, thoracic surgery, or malignancy in the area to be treated.

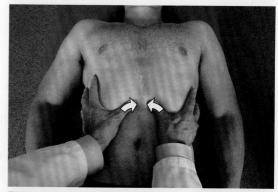

Figure 16.55. Step 4, following exhalation.

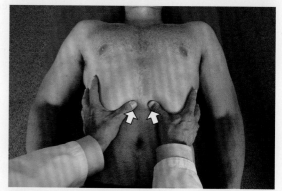

Figure 16.56. Step 6, thumbs beneath costal-xiphoid margin.

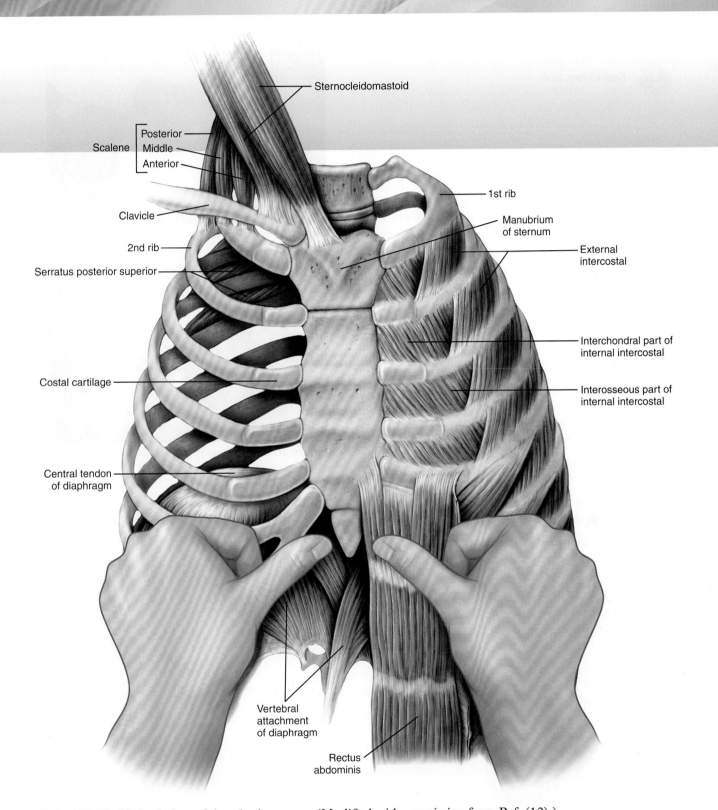

Figure 16.57. Skeletal view of thumb placement. (Modified with permission from Ref. (12).)

Abdominal Region

Mesenteric Release, Small Intestine

 See Video 16.8

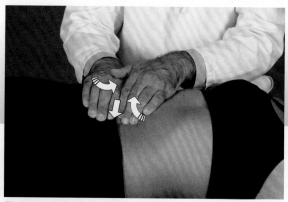

Figure 16.60. Supine position.

Indications

This technique is indicated to enhance lymphatic and venous drainage and alleviate congestion secondary to visceral ptosis.

Contraindications

This procedure should not be used if the patient has an abdominal incision, acute ischemic bowel disease, obstruction, or similar condition.

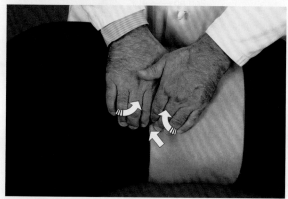

Figure 16.61. Lateral recumbent position.

Technique

The mesentery of the small intestine fans out from its short root to accommodate the length of the jejunum and ileum **(Fig. 16.58)**, and treatment is focused along its length **(Fig. 16.59)**.

1. The patient lies supine **(Fig. 16.60)** or in the left lateral recumbent (sidelying) **(Fig. 16.61)** position.

2. The physician sits on the patient's right side or stands behind the patient.

3. The physician places the hand or hands at the left border of the mesenteric region of the small intestine with the fingers curled slightly.

4. The fingers gently push (*solid arrows*, **Figs. 16.60 and 16.61**) toward the patient's back and then toward the patient's right side (*curved arrows*) until they meet the restrictive tissue barrier.

5. This position is held until the physician palpates a release (20 to 30 seconds), and then the physician follows this movement (fascial creep) to the new barrier and continues until no further improvement is detected.

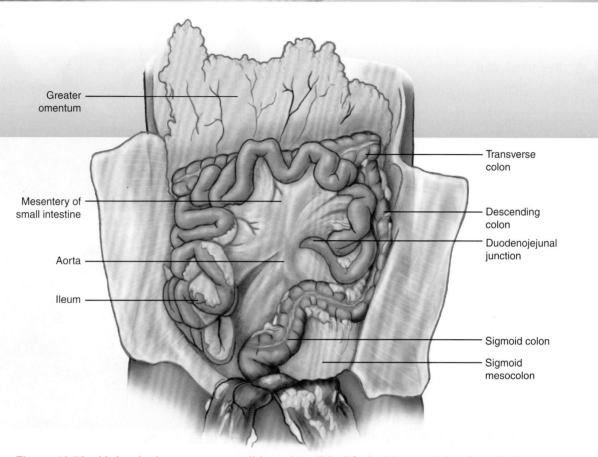

Figure 16.58. Abdominal mesentery, small intestine. (Modified with permission from Ref. (12).)

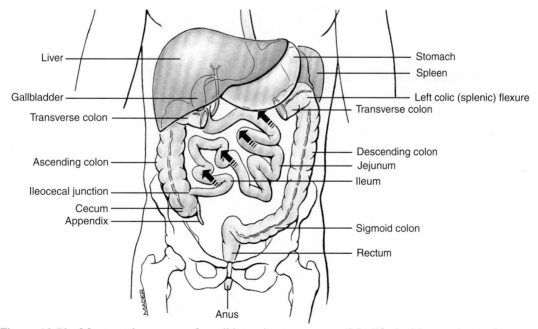

Figure 16.59. Mesenteric vectors of small intestine treatment. (Modified with permission from Ref. (12).)

Abdominal Region

Mesenteric Release, Ascending Colon

 See Video 16.8

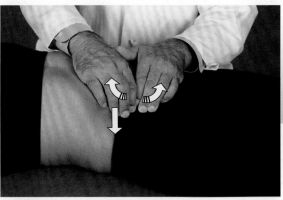

Figure 16.64. Supine position.

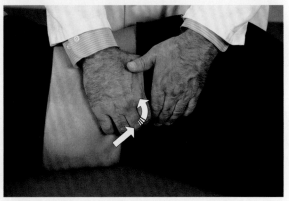

Figure 16.65. Lateral recumbent position.

Indications

This technique is indicated to enhance lymphatic and venous drainage and alleviate congestion secondary to visceral ptosis.

Contraindications

This procedure should not be used if the patient has an abdominal incision, acute ischemic bowel disease, obstruction, or similar condition.

Technique

Treatment is focused along the mesenteric ascending colon attachment **(Figs. 16.62 and 16.63)**.

1. The patient lies supine **(Fig. 16.64)** or in the right lateral recumbent **(Fig. 16.65)** position.

2. The physician sits on the left side or stands behind the patient.

3. The physician places the hand or hands at the right border of the mesenteric region of the ascending colon with the fingers curled slightly.

4. The fingers gently push toward the patient's back (*solid arrows*, **Figs. 16.64 and 16.65**) and then draw toward the patient's left side (*curved arrows*) until they meet the restrictive tissue barrier.

5. This position is held until the physician palpates a release (20 to 30 seconds), and then the physician follows this movement (fascial creep) to the new barrier and continues until no further improvement is detected.

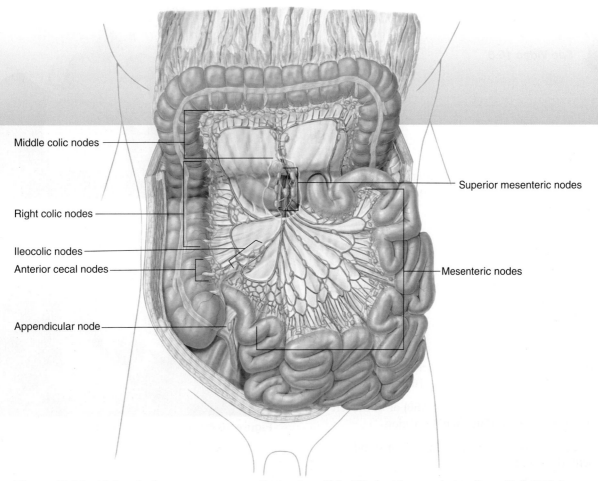

Figure 16.62. Abdominal mesentery, ascending colon. (Modified with permission from Ref. (12).)

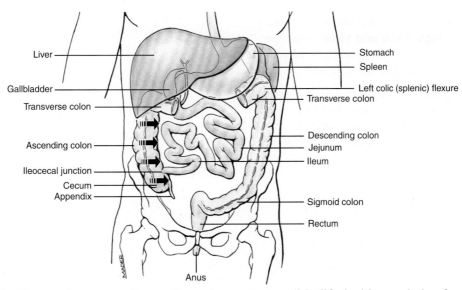

Figure 16.63. Mesenteric vectors of ascending colon treatment. (Modified with permission from Ref. (12).)

Abdominal Region

Mesenteric Release, Descending Colon

 See Video 16.8

Indications

This technique is indicated to enhance lymphatic and venous drainage and to alleviate congestion secondary to visceral ptosis.

Contraindications

This procedure should not be used if the patient has abdominal incisions, acute ischemic bowel disease, obstruction, or similar condition.

Technique

Treatment is focused along the mesenteric descending colon attachment **(Figs. 16.66 and 16.67)**.

1. The patient lies supine **(Fig. 16.68)** or in the left lateral recumbent **(Fig. 16.69)** position.

2. The physician sits on the right side or stands behind the patient.

3. The physician places the hand or hands at the left border of the mesenteric region of the descending colon and sigmoid with the fingers curled slightly.

4. The fingers gently push toward the patient's back (*straight arrows*, **Figs. 16.68 and 16.69**) and then draw toward the patient's right side (*curved arrows*) until meeting the restrictive tissue barrier.

5. This position is held until the physician palpates a release (20 to 30 seconds), and then the physician follows this movement (fascial creep) to the new barrier and continues until no further improvement is detected.

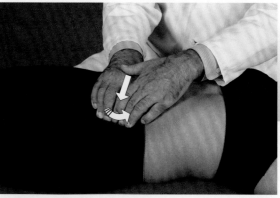

Figure 16.68. Supine position.

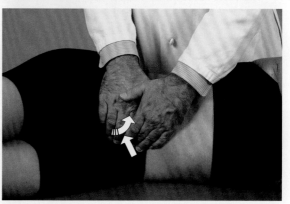

Figure 16.69. Lateral recumbent position.

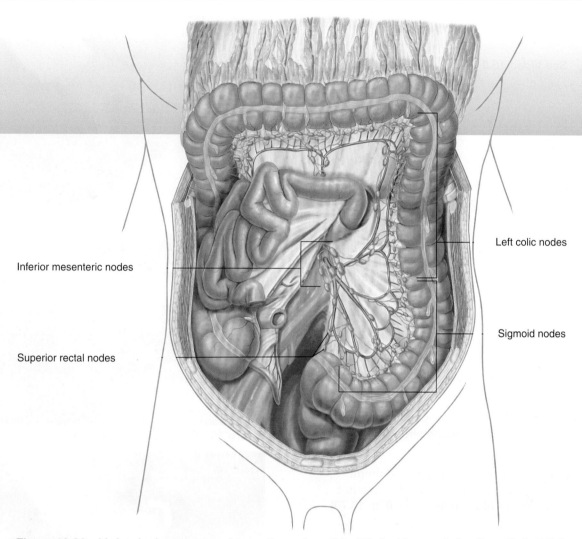

Inferior mesenteric nodes

Superior rectal nodes

Left colic nodes

Sigmoid nodes

Figure 16.66. Abdominal mesentery, descending colon. (Modified with permission from Ref. (12).)

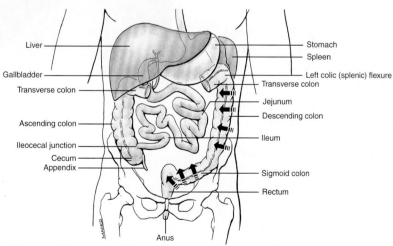

Liver

Gallbladder

Transverse colon

Ascending colon

Ileocecal junction

Cecum

Appendix

Stomach

Spleen

Left colic (splenic) flexure

Transverse colon

Jejunum

Descending colon

Ileum

Sigmoid colon

Rectum

Anus

Figure 16.67. Mesenteric vectors of descending colon treatment. (Modified with permission from Ref. (12).)

Abdominal Region

Presacral Release, Direct/Indirect

 See Video 16.9

Indications

This technique is indicated to enhance lymphatic drainage and relieve venous congestion in the lower abdomen, pelvic region, and lower extremities.

Contraindications

This procedure should not be used if the patient has abdominal incision, acute ischemic bowel disease, obstruction, or similar condition.

Technique

1. The patient lies supine, and the physician stands at either side of the patient.

2. The physician, with the index and third fingers approximated and the thumb abducted, makes a **C** shape.

3. The physician places the fingers and thumb downward in the lower abdominal region just above the ramus of the pubic bone **(Fig. 16.70)**.

4. The physician determines whether an ease-bind asymmetry is present by applying and vectoring forces in multiple directions, including posterior, superior, inferior, clockwise, and counterclockwise (*arrows*, **Fig. 16.71**).

5. The physician, on determining the dysfunctional asymmetry, applies forces in an indirect or direct manner, respectively, until meeting the ease or bind barriers **(Fig. 16.72)**.

6. This position is held until the physician palpates a release (20 to 30 seconds), and then the physician follows this movement (fascial creep) to the new barrier and continues until no further improvement is detected.

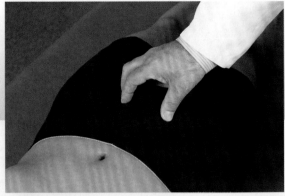
Figure 16.70. Hand placement.

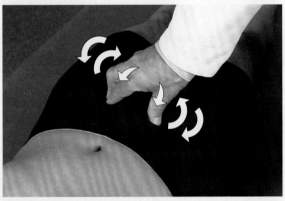
Figure 16.71. Step 4, ease-bind determination.

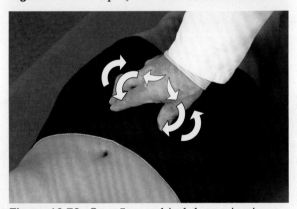
Figure 16.72. Step 5, ease-bind determination.

Abdominal and Pelvic Region

Marian Clark Drainage

 See Video 16.10

Indications

This technique is indicated to improve passive venous and lymphatic drainage from the lower abdomen and pelvis; it also helps to alleviate menstrual cramps.

Technique

1. The patient is in semiprone position on all fours with the contact points being the hands, elbows, and knees **(Fig. 16.73)**.

2. The physician stands at the side of the patient, facing the foot of the table.

3. The physician hooks the pads of the fingers medial to both anterior superior iliac spines **(Fig. 16.74)**.

4. The physician pulls the hands cephalad (*arrow*, **Fig. 16.75**).

5. The physician continues this abdominal traction, and the patient can be instructed to arch the back like a cat.

6. The physician encourages this movement along with a cephalad rocking of the body **(Fig. 16.76)**.

7. This slow rocking movement is repeated for several minutes. The patient may use it as an exercise at home.

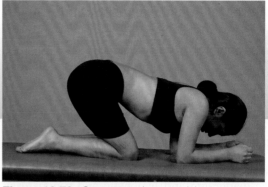

Figure 16.73. Step 1, patient position.

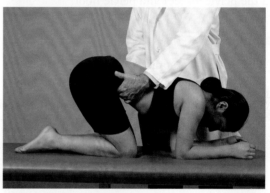

Figure 16.74. Hand position.

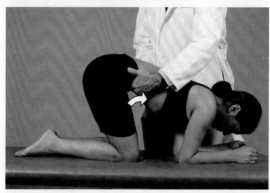

Figure 16.75. Step 4, cephalad direction.

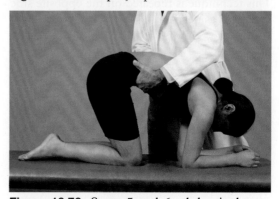

Figure 16.76. Steps 5 and 6, abdominal traction, cephalad rocking.

Pelvic Region

Ischiorectal Fossa Release, Supine

 See Video 16.11

Indications

This technique is indicated to improve motion of the pelvic diaphragm and lymphatic and venous drainage from the pelvic viscera and pelvic floor.

Technique

1. The patient lies supine with the hips and knees flexed.

2. The physician sits at the side of the table opposite the side of the dysfunction to be treated.

3. The physician places the thumb of the hand closest to the table medial to the ischial tuberosity (*arrow*, **Figs. 16.77 and 16.78**) on the dysfunctional side.

4. The physician exerts gentle pressure cephalad (*arrow*, **Fig. 16.78**) into the ischiorectal fossa until resistance is met and then applies a lateral force (*curved arrow*, **Fig. 16.79**).

5. The physician can attempt to feel a fluid ebb and flow with a resultant release or add a release-enhancing mechanism by instructing the patient to inhale and exhale deeply.

6. With each exhalation, the physician exerts increased cephalad pressure on the pelvic diaphragm until no further cephalad and lateral excursion is possible.

7. This technique is repeated on the opposite side of the pelvis as needed.

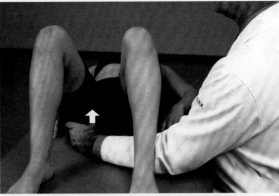

Figure 16.77. Physician and patient positioning.

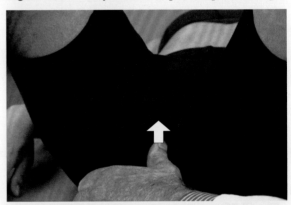

Figure 16.78. Thumb positioning.

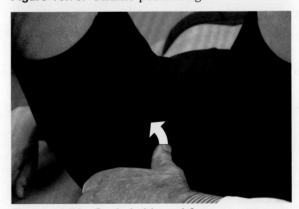

Figure 16.79. Cephalad lateral force.

Pelvic Region

Ischiorectal Fossa Release, Prone

 See Video 16.12

Indications

This technique improves motion of the pelvic diaphragm and venous and lymphatic drainage from the pelvic viscera and pelvic floor.

Technique

1. The patient lies prone, and the physician stands at the side of the table facing the head of the table.

2. The physician places the thumbs medial to the ischial tuberosities on each side **(Fig. 16.80)**.

3. Gentle pressure is exerted cephalad (*arrows*, **Fig. 16.81**) into the ischiorectal fossa until resistance is met, and then a lateral force (*arrows*, **Fig. 16.82**) is applied.

4. The patient is instructed to inhale and exhale deeply.

5. The physician can attempt to feel a fluid ebb and flow with a resultant release or add a release-enhancing mechanism by instructing the patient to inhale and exhale deeply.

6. With each exhalation, the physician exerts increased cephalad pressure on the pelvic diaphragm until no further cephalad and lateral excursion (resistance) is noted.

7. This technique is performed bilaterally as above or directed toward a unilateral restriction. If done for a unilateral restriction, both hands and thumbs are applied as described above, but, after the initial contact and control, only the thumb palpating the restriction applies increased pressure while the opposing hand anchors the pelvis.

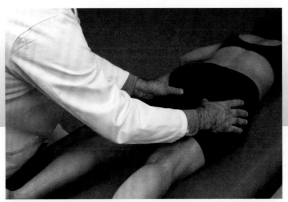

Figure 16.80. Thumb placement.

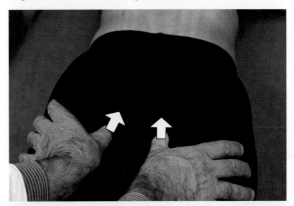

Figure 16.81. Cephalad force.

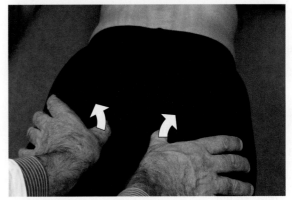

Figure 16.82. Lateral force.

Lower Extremity Region

Pedal Pump (Dalrymple Technique) Supine Method

 See Video 16.13

Indications

This technique is indicated for lymphatic congestion, fever, infection, and inability to use the thoracic pump.

Contraindications

This procedure should not be used if the patient has venous thrombosis; acute ankle sprain; Achilles strain, gastrocnemius strain, or other acute process; and/or painful lower extremity conditions. It should also be avoided in the acute postoperative period in some abdominal surgery patients.

Physiologic Goal

The goal is to accentuate negative intra-abdominal pressure, increase lymphatic return, and increase endothelial nitrous oxide, which may offer anti-inflammatory benefit (13,14).

Technique

1. The patient lies supine, taking care to keep the heels of the feet on the table.

2. The physician stands at the foot of the table with one foot slightly behind the other for balance.

3. The physician places the hands over the dorsal aspect of the patient's feet, and the feet are carefully plantar flexed to their comfortable limit **(Fig. 16.83)**.

4. The physician holds this pressure and begins a quick on-and-off rhythmic pressure (*arrows*, **Fig. 16.84**) at two per second for 1 to 2 minutes.

5. The physician may choose to substitute or add pressure by grasping the plantar surface of the feet at the distal metatarsals **(Fig. 16.85)**. Pressure is then directed cephalad in a similar rhythmic fashion (*arrows*, **Fig. 16.86**) at two per second for 1 to 2 minutes.

6. These rhythmic forces should be parallel to the table, not directed toward the table.

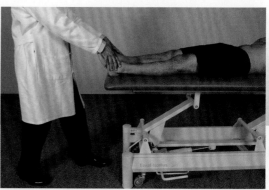

Figure 16.83. Steps 1 to 3, setup, plantar flexion.

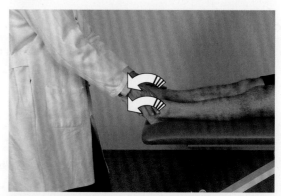

Figure 16.84. Step 4, plantar flexion.

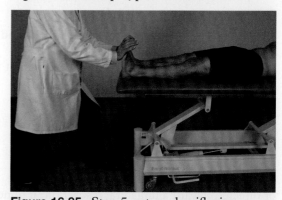

Figure 16.85. Step 5, setup, dorsiflexion.

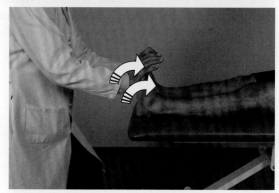

Figure 16.86. Step 5, dorsiflexion.

Lower Extremity Region

Pedal Pump (Dalrymple Technique)
Prone Method

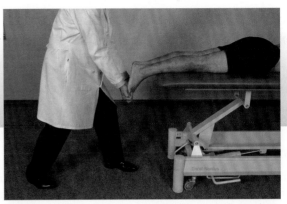

Figure 16.87. Step 1, physician and patient positioning.

Indications

This technique is indicated for lymphatic congestion, fever, infection, and inability to use the thoracic pump.

Contraindications

This procedure should not be used if the patient has venous thrombosis; acute ankle sprain; Achilles strain, gastrocnemius strain, or other acute process; or painful lower extremity conditions. It should also be avoided in the acute postoperative period in some abdominal surgery patients.

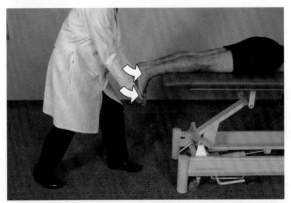

Figure 16.88. Hand and foot positioning.

Physiologic Goal

The goal is to accentuate negative intra-abdominal pressure, increase lymphatic return, and increase endothelial nitrous oxide, which may be of anti-inflammatory benefit.

Technique

1. The patient lies prone with the feet slightly off the table, and the physician stands at the foot of the table with one foot slightly behind the other **(Fig. 16.87)**.

2. The physician grasps the patient's feet at the distal metatarsal region and directs a force (*arrows*, **Fig. 16.88**) to achieve bilateral dorsiflexion.

3. At the comfortable limit of dorsiflexion, the physician begins a rhythmic on-and-off cephalad pressure (*arrows*, **Fig. 16.89**) at one to two per second.

4. This pressure is directed parallel to the length of the table and continued for 1 to 2 minutes.

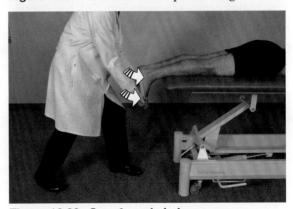

Figure 16.89. Step 3, cephalad pressure.

Lower Extremity Region

Popliteal Fossa Release, Supine
Ex: Left Popliteal Congestion

 See Video 16.14

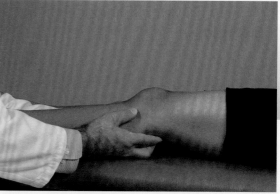

Figure 16.90. Steps 1 to 3, setup and hand placement.

Indications and Physiologic Goal

This technique is indicated to improve lymphatic and venous drainage from the lower extremities (knee, calf, ankle, and foot) and to release any fascial restriction(s) of the popliteal fossa.

Technique

1. The patient lies supine with legs extended on table.

2. The physician, facing the head of the table, sits at the side to be treated.

3. The physician's medial hand reaches around to the medial aspect of the popliteal fossa as the lateral hand grasps the lateral aspect of the popliteal fossa **(Fig. 16.90)**.

4. The physician palpates for any fascial restrictions, including cephalad, caudad, medial, and lateral **(Fig. 16.91)**.

5. The physician engages the tissues with an anterior force through the fingertips while engaging any fascial barriers (e.g., cephalad, caudad, medial, lateral) until resistance is met **(Fig. 16.92)**.

6. The physician can attempt to feel a fluid ebb and flow with a resultant release or add a release-enhancing mechanism by instructing the patient to inhale and exhale deeply. Force is directed into the barrier until no further excursion or relaxation of the tissues is possible.

7. This technique is repeated on the opposite side as needed.

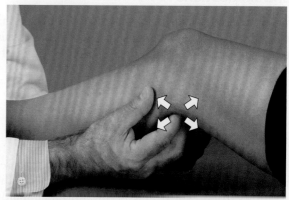

Figure 16.91. Step 4, determining barriers.

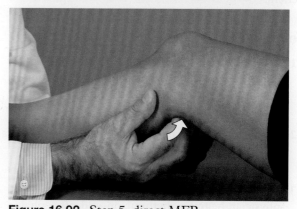

Figure 16.92. Step 5, direct MFR.

Lower Extremity Region

Iliotibial Band (ITB) Effleurage
Ex: Left, ITB Congestion/Inflammation

Indications and Physiologic Goal

Iliotibial band (ITB) syndrome and trochanter bursitis are common painful conditions that can be helped with various styles of OMT (e.g., MFR and soft tissue). Lymphatic drainage of the lateral compartment of the thigh can augment the positive outcome of other styles of treatment by reducing lymphatic congestion in this area and the subsequent decrease in inflammation and other causes of pain (nociception). If myofascial restriction secondary to fibrosis is present, the inelastic qualities may be treated by a gentle "stroking" stretch that is greater and deeper in pressure than effleurage (see Chapter 7).

1. The patient lies in the right lateral recumbent position (affected side down), and the physician stands in front of the patient. If the technique is performed directly on the skin, a skin lotion or powder helps to reduce friction.

2. The webbing between the thumb and index finger of the physician's right hand is placed over the ITB. The physician's left hand is placed over the patient's left greater trochanter to stabilize the pelvis and hip.

3. The physician's right hand is initially placed at the left ITB slightly distal to the trochanter or halfway down the thigh. With a *very* gentle pressure, effleurage stroking from distal to proximal is performed. After a few strokes, the physician's hand moves farther distal and continues the "distal to proximal" stroking up to the trochanter **(Figs. 16.93 to 16.95)**. The physician's hand is minimally placed farther distally with each few strokes, until reaching the terminal/distal ITB. This can be repeated for 1 to 2 minutes.

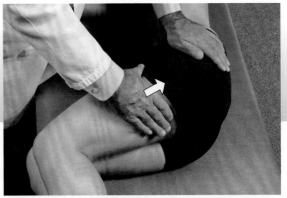

Figure 16.93. Step 3, initial hand placement.

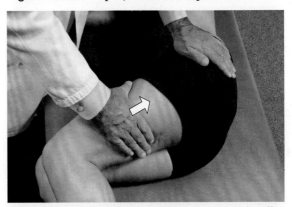

Figure 16.94. Step 3, mid-ITB stroke proximally.

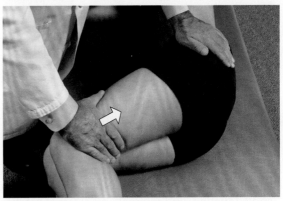

Figure 16.95. Step 3b, distal ITB stroke proximally.

Lower Extremity and Pelvic Region

Hip, Indirect LAS/BLT, Supine

Indications and Physiologic Goal

This technique is indicated to enhance lymphatic drainage and relieve venous congestion in the pelvic region and lower extremities. It is also an excellent technique to treat dysfunctions of the hip joint!

Technique

1. The patient lies supine with the hip and knee flexed on the side to be treated.

2. The physician stands at the side of the table on the side to be treated.

3. The physician places the cephalad thenar eminence on the patient's greater trochanter with the fingers directed posterolaterally and thumb contouring the anterior inguinal region. The initiating force is applied anteromedially (*arrow*, **Fig. 16.96**).

4. The abducted thumb and first two fingers in an inverted C shape of the physician's caudal hand attempt to control the head of the femur anteriorly. This hand applies a force posterolaterally (*arrow*, **Fig. 16.97**).

5. The patient's knee on the dysfunctional side is controlled by the physician's anterior pectoral region or axilla and is placed toward the ease barrier's balance point, determined by moving the hip through flexion and extension, slight abduction and adduction, and internal and external rotation (*arrows*, **Fig. 16.98**).

6. The physician uses the shoulder to apply compression (*arrow*, **Fig. 16.99**) to the patient's knee toward the hip, finding the position of greatest ease with slight hip motions in all three planes. This is the third force to be applied.

7. All three forces are applied simultaneously to find the indirect position of ease. A release-enhancing mechanism may be added by instructing the patient to inhale and exhale deeply. The release is perceived by an increased movement toward the indirect barrier.

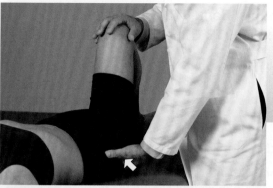

Figure 16.96. Steps 1 to 3, initiating hand placement.

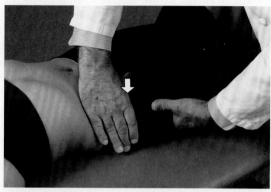

Figure 16.97. Step 4, posterosuperior vectored force.

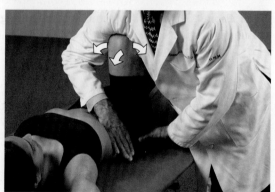

Figure 16.98. Step 5, balancing three forces.

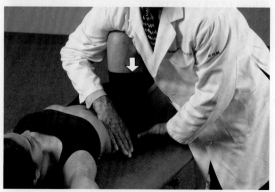

Figure 16.99. Step 6, compression through hip.

Upper Extremity Region

Anterior Axillary Fold Release
Pectoralis Major/Anterior Deltoid Muscles
Ex: Left, Soft Tissue Inhibition Method

Indications

This technique is indicated for lymphatic congestion and upper extremity edema.

Contraindications

This procedure should not be used if the patient has hypersensitivity to touch at the anterior axillary fold, subclavian line, some pacemakers, metastatic cancer, or similar condition.

Physiologic Goal

The goal is to increase lymphatic return.

Technique

1. The patient lies supine, and the physician sits or stands at the side of the patient on the side of the dysfunctional upper extremity.

2. The physician palpates for any increased tone, edema, and bogginess of the tissues **(Fig. 16.100)**.

3. The physician, finding tissue texture changes, places the index and third fingers on the ventral surface of the anterior axillary fold and the thumb in the axilla, palpating the anterior portion from within the axilla **(Figs. 16.101 and 16.102)**.

4. The physician may very slowly and minimally squeeze the anterior axillary fold with the thumb and fingers.

5. This is held for 30 to 60 seconds. It may be repeated on the opposite side as needed.

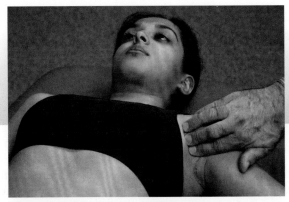

Figure 16.100. Steps 1 to 2, setup.

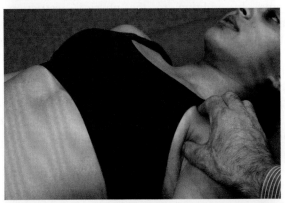

Figure 16.101. Step 3, hand and finger placement.

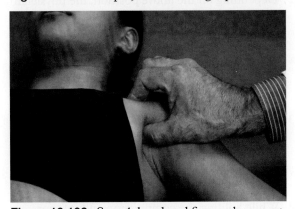

Figure 16.102. Step 4, hand and finger placement.

Upper Extremity Region

Posterior Axillary Fold Release
Pectoralis Major/Anterior Deltoid Muscles
Ex: Right, Soft Tissue Inhibition Method

Indications and Physiologic Goals

This deep, constant pressure technique is indicated for myofascial restrictions that restrict normal lymphatic flow and that can eventually lead to upper extremity edema. In addition to the physical restriction to lymphatic flow that dysfunctional axillary tissues can cause (fibrous changes, hypertonicity), the existence of somatic dysfunction may develop somatosomatic reflexing and eventual somatovisceral reactions that can adversely affect lymphatic and vascular flow through hypersympathetic tone. Eventually, this may lead to further upper extremity edema and/or chest cage lymphatic congestion.

1. The patient lies supine, and the physician sits at the right side of the table or at the right head of the table.

2. Depending on the above position, the physician grasps the patient's posterior axillary fold with either (a) the thumb placed posterior and the index/third fingers anteriorly **(Fig. 16.103)** or (b) grasps the posterior axillary fold with the thumb anteriorly and the index/third fingers posterior **(Fig. 16.104)**.

3. Using the side of table positioning as the example, the physician compresses the thumb and fingers toward each other, "squeezing" the posterior axillary fold and then pulling inferiorly (*white arrows*) to its tension barrier **(Fig. 16.105)**.

4. While holding the compression and inferior (caudal) traction, the patient's arm may be brought to the side, if patient preference dictates **(Fig. 16.106)**.

5. This pressure is held until a release is perceived or for 30 to 60 seconds.

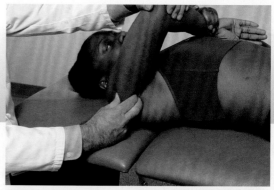

Figure 16.103. Step 2a, head of table positioning.

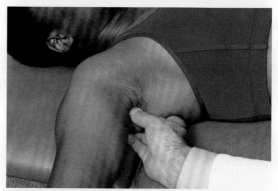

Figure 16.104. Step 2b, side of table positioning.

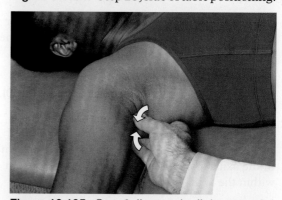

Figure 16.105. Step 3, "squeezing" the posterior axillary fold.

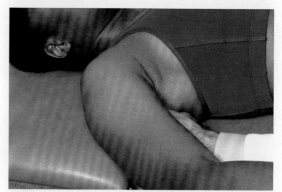

Figure 16.106. Step 4, if preferred, arm brought to the side.

References

1. Chila AG, ed. Foundations of Osteopathic Medicine. 3rd ed. Baltimore, MD: Lippincott Williams & Wilkins, 2011.
2. Still AT. Philosophy of Osteopathy. Kirksville, MO: A.T. Still, 1809.
3. Galbreath WO. Acute otitis media, including its postural and manipulative treatment. J Am Osteopath Assoc 1929:377–379.
4. Pratt-Harrington D. Galbreath technique: a manipulative treatment for otitis media revisited. J Am Osteopath Assoc 2000;100:635–639.
5. Chikly B. Silent Waves: Theory and Practice of Lymph Drainage Therapy. An Osteopathic Lymphatic Technique. 2nd ed. Scottsdale, AZ: IHH, 2004.
6. Agur AMR, Dalley AF. Grant's Atlas of Anatomy. 11th ed. Baltimore, MD: Lippincott Williams & Wilkins, 2005.
7. Knot EM, Tune JD, Stoll ST, et al. Increased lymphatic flow in the thoracic duct during manipulative intervention. J Am Osteopath Assoc 2005;105:593–596.
8. Jackson KM, Steele TG, Dugan EP, et al. Effect of lymphatic and splenic pump techniques on the antibody response to hepatitis B vaccine: A pilot study. J Am Osteopath Assoc 1998;98:155–160.
9. Steele T, Jackson K, Dugan E. The effect of osteopathic manipulative treatment on the antibody response to hepatitis B vaccine. J Am Osteopath Assoc 1996;96(9).
10. Breithaupt T, Harris K, Ellis J, et al. Thoracic lymphatic pumping and the efficacy of influenza vaccination in healthy young and elderly populations. J Am Osteopath Assoc 2001;101(1):21–25.
11. Mesina J, Hampton D, Evans R, et al. Transient basophilia following the applications of lymphatic pump techniques: A pilot study. J Am Osteopath Assoc 1998;98(2).
12. Agur AMR, Dalley AF. Grant's Atlas of Anatomy. 11th ed. Baltimore, MD: Lippincott Williams & Wilkins, 2005.
13. Kuchera M, Daghigh F. Determination of enhanced nitric oxide production using external mechanical stimuli. J Am Osteopath Assoc 2004;104:344 (abstract).
14. Kuchera M. Osteopathic manipulative medicine considerations in patients with chronic pain. J Am Osteopath Assoc 2005;105(Suppl. 4):29–36.

Articulatory and Combined Techniques

17

Technique Principles

This chapter describes articulatory and combined techniques. These techniques are discussed in the same chapter because we believe they tend to have many similarities, using principles from other techniques, especially soft tissue, lymphatic, muscle energy, and high-velocity, low-amplitude (HVLA). The Educational Council on Osteopathic Principles (ECOP) defines the articulatory treatment (ART) modality as "a low-velocity/moderate- to high-amplitude technique where a joint is carried through its full motion with the therapeutic goal of increased freedom range of movement. The activating force is either a springing motion or repetitive concentric movement of the joint through the restrictive barrier" (1). At the Philadelphia College of Osteopathic Medicine (PCOM), we have referred to it simply as *springing technique* and, more recently, have added the term *oscillatory*. It has similarities to both soft tissue and HVLA in that it can affect the myofascial components and articular components, respectively. However, the moderate-to-high amplitude described in the definition does not mean moving through the restrictive barrier at high amplitude. The relationship among the pathologic, physiologic, and anatomic barriers should remain consistent with the principles of HVLA: motion through the restrictive barrier should still be moderated and kept to a minimum. The amplitude is the distance available within the dysfunctional presentation's range.

Combined method (technique) is defined by ECOP as "(a) Treatment strategy where the initial movements are indirect; as the technique is completed, the movements change to direct forces. (b) A manipulative sequence involving two or more osteopathic manipulative treatment systems (e.g., Spencer technique combined with muscle energy technique). (c) A concept described by Paul Kimberly, DO" (1). Kimberly used this term relative to the secondary definition in relating the combination of various forces, including direct, indirect, inherent, gravitational, physician directed, respiratory assist, and others, in treatment (2). Therefore, the techniques in this chapter could well have been classified in other chapters based on the primary focus of each technique.

ART, although primarily affecting the myofascial and articular components of the dysfunction, also significantly affects the circulatory and lymphatic systems. These styles of technique have been part of the recommendations for the osteopathic treatment of the geriatric patient for many years and are relatively safe and well tolerated.

Technique Classification

Direct, Indirect, or Combined

Depending on the ART or combination of methods, all these techniques can be direct, indirect, or both, hence the definition. Articulatory was classically defined as a direct technique, but depending on the physician's preference, the ease and bind barriers may both be met with a gentle springing motion.

Technique Styles

Rhythmic

The physician may choose a rhythmic ART to change the soft tissues or to release an articular restriction. The cadence of the stretch and release in this technique has been described by Nicholas S. Nicholas, DO, FAAO, as "make and break," relating to the on-off pressure applied. This may be slow or moderate and may become "oscillatory."

Mixed

The physician may choose any variation of rhythms, amplitude, or acceleration (velocity) depending on the patient's presentation. Therefore, the patient may be treated with a variety of combined techniques.

Indications

1. Restricted motion in the presence of articular and/or myofascial somatic dysfunction (especially in the frail or elderly)
2. Circulatory and lymphatic congestion

Contraindications

1. Acute moderate to severe strain or sprain
2. Fracture, dislocation, or joint instability in the area affected by the treatment
3. Acute inflammatory joint disease in the area affected by the treatment
4. Metastasis in the area affected by the treatment

General Considerations and Rules

The performance of these techniques can vary with the physician's impression of the severity of the dysfunction and any complicating factors. The techniques range from extremely gentle, with minimal amplitude, to forceful traction. The rhythmic aspects may also vary from slow to fast. In general, compressive forces should be limited in those with osteoporosis, ankylosis, and so on. These techniques have a wide range of application for increasing motion and decreasing edema.

Upper Extremity Region

Shoulder Girdle: *Spencer Technique*

 See Video 17.1

Indications

Adhesive capsulitis
Bursitis
Tenosynovitis
Arthritis

General Considerations

Nicholas S. Nicholas, DO, FAAO, promoted this technique more than any other. Besides publishing one of the early articles extolling its virtue, he spent years lecturing and presenting it to many organizations, especially in athletic medicine. Over his many years in sports medicine and as a consultant to teams, especially as a physician for the Villanova University football team from the 1940s to the 1960s, he had many successful outcomes with this treatment when other treatments had failed. This treatment protocol, when used in conjunction with other osteopathic manipulative techniques to treat the cervical, thoracic, and costal regions, gives the patient an excellent chance of recovery. This technique was, for alliteration purposes, taught as the "seven stages of Spencer" even though there are eight stages. At PCOM, we have taught this technique as having *stages 5A* and *5B* to accommodate the eight stages into seven.

The patient lies in the lateral recumbent position with the shoulder to be treated away from the table. The patient's back is perpendicular to the table, with the lower knee and hip flexed to prevent any forward roll. A pillow is placed under the patient's head to remove any drag on the shoulder from the cervical and shoulder girdle musculature.

Upper Extremity Region

Shoulder Girdle: *Spencer Technique*
Stage 1: Extension

1. The physician stands facing the patient.

2. The physician's cephalad hand bridges the shoulder to lock out any acromioclavicular and scapulothoracic motion. The fingers are on the spine of the scapula, and the thumb is on the anterior surface of the clavicle.

3. The physician's caudad hand grasps the patient's elbow.

4. The patient's shoulder is moved into extension in the horizontal plane to the edge of the restrictive barrier.

5. A slow, gentle springing (*articulatory, make and break*) motion (*arrows,* **Fig. 17.1**) is applied at the end range of motion.

6. *Muscle energy activation:* The patient is instructed to attempt to flex the shoulder (*black arrow,* **Fig. 17.2**) against the physician's resistance (*white arrow*). This contraction is held for 3 to 5 seconds.

7. After a second of relaxation, the shoulder is extended to the new restrictive barrier **(Fig. 17.3)**.

8. Steps 6 and 7 are repeated three to five times and extension is reassessed.

9. Resistance against the attempted extension (*white arrow,* **Fig. 17.4**) (reciprocal inhibition) has been found to be helpful in augmenting the effect.

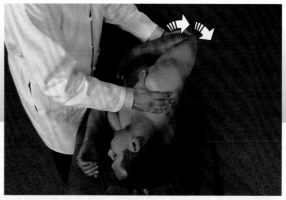
Figure 17.1. Stage 1, steps 1 to 5.

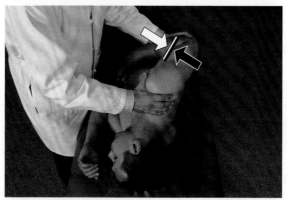
Figure 17.2. Stage 1, step 6.

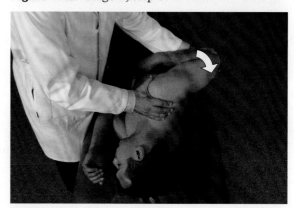
Figure 17.3. Stage 1, step 7.

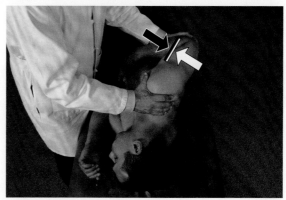
Figure 17.4. Reciprocal inhibition.

Upper Extremity Region

Shoulder Girdle: *Spencer Technique*
Stage 2: Flexion

1. The physician's hands reverse shoulder and arm contact positions. The caudad hand reaches over and behind the patient and bridges the shoulder to lock out acromioclavicular and scapulothoracic motion. The fingers are on the anterior surface of the clavicle, and the heel of the hand is on the spine of the scapula.

2. Using the other hand, the physician takes the patient's shoulder into its flexion motion in the horizontal plane to the edge of its restrictive barrier.

3. A slow, springing (*articulatory, make and break*) motion (*arrows*, **Fig. 17.5**) is applied at the end range of motion.

4. *Muscle energy activation*: The patient is instructed to extend the shoulder (*black arrow*, **Fig. 17.6**) against the physician's resistance (*white arrow*). This contraction is maintained for 3 to 5 seconds.

5. After a second of relaxation, the shoulder is flexed further until a new restrictive barrier is engaged **(Fig. 17.7)**.

6. Steps 4 and 5 are repeated three to five times, and flexion is reassessed.

7. Resistance against the attempted flexion (reciprocal inhibition) has been found to be helpful in augmenting the effect **(Fig. 17.8)**.

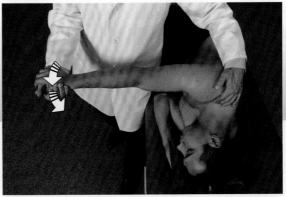

Figure 17.5. Stage 2, steps 1 to 3.

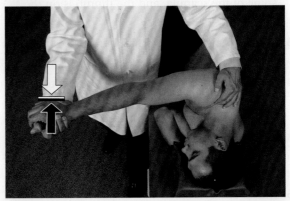

Figure 17.6. Stage 2, step 4.

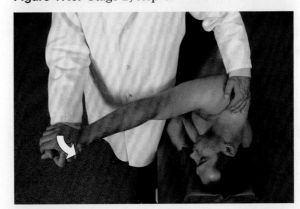

Figure 17.7. Stage 2, step 5.

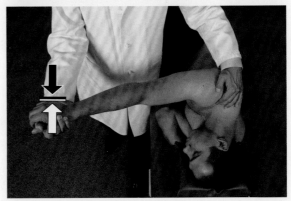

Figure 17.8. Reciprocal inhibition.

Upper Extremity Region

Shoulder Girdle: *Spencer Technique*
Stage 3: Circumduction/Slight Compression

1. The original starting position is resumed with the cephalad hand.

2. The patient's shoulder is abducted to the edge of the restrictive barrier **(Fig. 17.9)**.

3. The patient's arm is moved through full *clockwise* circumduction (small diameter) with slight *compression*. Larger and larger concentric circles are made, increasing the range of motion **(Fig. 17.10)**.

4. Circumduction may be tuned to a particular barrier. The same maneuver is repeated counterclockwise **(Fig. 17.11)**.

5. There is no specific muscle energy activation for this step; however, during fine-tuning of the circumduction, it may be feasible to implement it in a portion of the restricted arc.

6. This is repeated for approximately 15 to 30 seconds in each direction, and circumduction is reassessed.

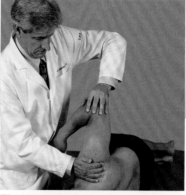

Figure 17.9. Stage 2, steps 1 to 2.

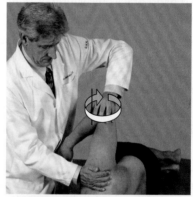

Figure 17.10. Stage 3, step 3.

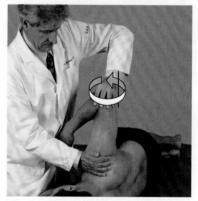

Figure 17.11. Stage 3, step 4.

Upper Extremity Region

Shoulder Girdle: *Spencer Technique*
Stage 4: Circumduction with Traction

1. The patient's shoulder is abducted to the edge of the restrictive barrier with the elbow extended.

2. The physician's caudad hand grasps the patient's wrist and exerts vertical traction. The physician's cephalad hand braces the shoulder as in stage 1 **(Fig. 17.12)**.

3. The patient's arm is moved through full *clockwise* circumduction with synchronous traction. Larger and larger concentric circles are made, increasing the range of motion **(Fig. 17.13)**.

4. The same maneuver is repeated *counterclockwise* **(Fig. 17.14)**.

5. There is no specific muscle energy activation for this step; however, during fine-tuning of the circumduction, it may be feasible to implement it in a portion of the restricted arc.

6. This is repeated for approximately 15 to 30 seconds in each direction, and circumduction is reassessed.

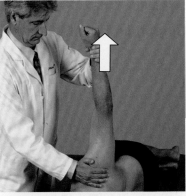

Figure 17.12. Stage 4, steps 1 to 2.

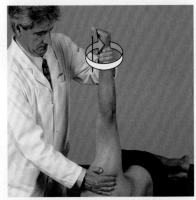

Figure 17.13. Stage 4, step 3.

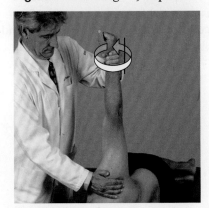

Figure 17.14. Stage 4, step 4.

Upper Extremity Region

Shoulder Girdle: *Spencer Technique*
Stage 5A: *AB*duction

1. The patient's shoulder is abducted to the edge of the restrictive barrier.

2. The physician's cephalad arm is positioned parallel to the surface of the table.

3. The patient is instructed to grasp the physician's forearm with the hand of the arm being treated **(Fig. 17.15)**.

4. The patient's elbow is moved toward the head, abducting the shoulder, until a motion barrier is engaged. Slight internal rotation may be added.

5. A slow, gentle (*articulatory, make and break*) motion (*arrows*, **Fig. 17.16**) is applied at the end range of motion.

6. *Muscle energy activation*: The patient is instructed to adduct the shoulder (*black arrow*, **Fig. 17.17**) against the physician's resistance (*white arrow*). This contraction is held for 3 to 5 seconds.

7. After a second of relaxation, the shoulder is further abducted to a new restrictive barrier **(Fig. 17.18)**.

8. Steps 6 and 7 are repeated three to five times, and abduction is reassessed.

9. Resistance (*white arrow*, **Fig. 17.19**) against the attempted abduction (*black arrow*) (reciprocal inhibition) has been found to be helpful in augmenting the effect.

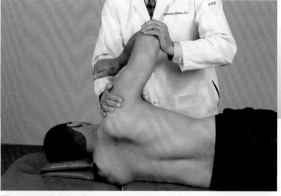

Figure 17.15. Stage 5A, steps 1 to 3.

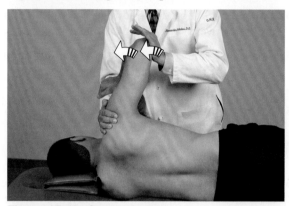

Figure 17.16. Stage 5A, steps 4 to 5.

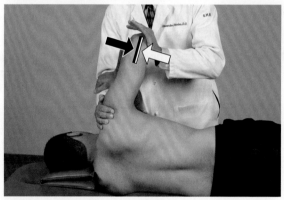

Figure 17.17. Stage 5A, step 6.

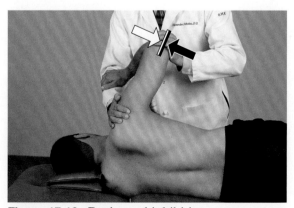

Figure 17.19. Reciprocal inhibition.

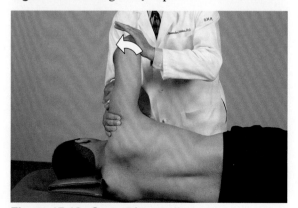

Figure 17.18. Stage 5A, step 7.

Upper Extremity Region

Shoulder Girdle: *Spencer Technique*
Stage 5B: *AD*duction/External Rotation

1. The patient's arm is flexed sufficiently to allow the elbow to pass in front of the chest wall.

2. The physician's forearm is still parallel to the table with the patient's wrist resting against the forearm.

3. The patient's shoulder is adducted to the edge of the restrictive barrier **(Fig. 17.20)**.

4. A slow, gentle (*articulatory, make and break*) motion (*arrow*, **Fig. 17.21**) is applied at the end range of motion.

5. *Muscle energy activation:* The patient lifts the elbow (*black arrow*, **Fig. 17.22**) against the physician's resistance (*white arrow*). This contraction is held for 3 to 5 seconds.

6. After a second of relaxation, the patient's shoulder is further adducted until a new restrictive barrier is engaged **(Fig. 17.23)**.

7. Steps 5 and 6 are repeated three to five times, and adduction is reassessed.

8. Resistance against the attempted adduction using the physician's thumb under the olecranon process (reciprocal inhibition) has been found to be helpful in augmenting the effect **(Fig. 17.24)**.

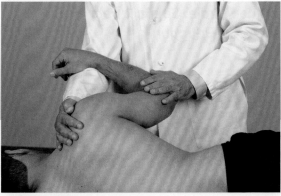

Figure 17.20. Stage 5B, steps 1 to 3.

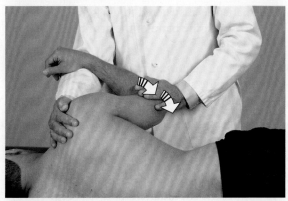

Figure 17.21. Stage 5B, step 4.

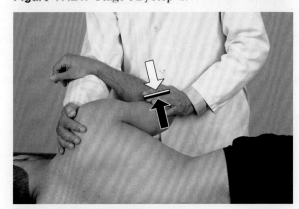

Figure 17.22. Stage 5B, step 5.

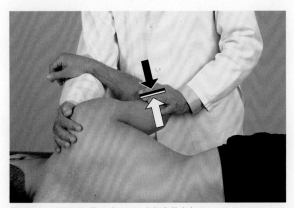

Figure 17.24. Reciprocal inhibition.

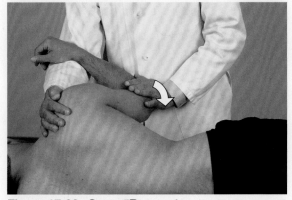

Figure 17.23. Stage 5B, step 6.

Upper Extremity Region

Shoulder Girdle: *Spencer Technique*
Stage 6: Internal Rotation

1. The patient's shoulder is abducted 45 degrees and internally rotated approximately 90 degrees. The dorsum of the patient's hand is placed in the small of the back.

2. The physician's cephalad hand reinforces the anterior portion of the patient's shoulder.

3. The patient's elbow is very gently pulled forward (internal rotation) to the edge of the restrictive barrier **(Fig. 17.25)**. *Do not push the elbow backward*, as this can dislocate an unstable shoulder.

4. A slow, gentle (*articulatory, make and break*) motion (*arrow,* **Fig. 17.26**) is applied at the end range of motion.

5. *Muscle energy activation:* The patient is instructed to pull the elbow backward (*black arrow,* **Fig. 17.27**) against the physician's resistance (*white arrow*). This contraction is held for 3 to 5 seconds.

6. After a second of relaxation, the elbow is carried further forward (*arrow,* **Fig. 17.28**) to the new restrictive barrier.

7. Steps 5 and 6 are repeated three to five times, and internal rotation is reassessed.

8. Resistance against the attempted internal rotation (*arrows*) (reciprocal inhibition) has been found to be helpful in augmenting the effect **(Fig. 17.29)**.

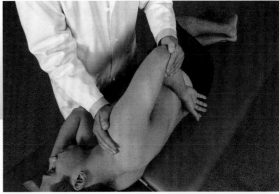

Figure 17.25. Stage 6, steps 1 to 3.

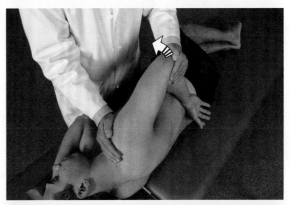

Figure 17.26. Stage 6, step 4.

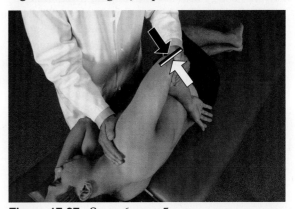

Figure 17.27. Stage 6, step 5.

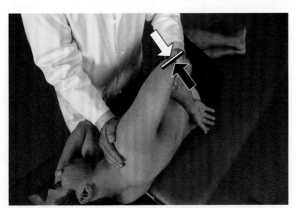

Figure 17.29. Reciprocal inhibition.

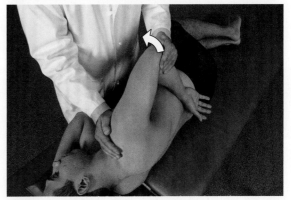

Figure 17.28. Stage 6, step 6.

Upper Extremity Region

Shoulder Girdle: *Spencer Technique*
Stage 7: Distraction in Abduction

1. The physician turns and faces the head of the table.

2. The patient's shoulder is abducted, and the patient's hand and forearm are placed on the physician's shoulder closest to the patient.

3. With fingers interlaced, the physician's hands are positioned just distal to the acromion process **(Fig. 17.30)**.

4. The patient's shoulder is scooped inferiorly (*arrow*, **Fig. 17.31**) creating a translatory motion across the inferior edge of the glenoid fossa. This is done repeatedly in an articulatory fashion.

5. Alternatively, the arm may be pushed straight down into the glenoid fossa and pulled straight out again (*arrows*, **Fig 17.32**) with a pumping motion.

6. *Muscle energy activation*: Scooping traction is placed on the shoulder and maintained. While the traction is maintained (*curved arrow*), the patient is instructed to push the hand straight down on the physician's resisting shoulder (*straight arrows*). This contraction is held for 3 to 5 seconds. After a second of relaxation, further caudad traction is placed on the shoulder until a new restrictive barrier is engaged **(Fig. 17.33)**.

7. Step 6 is repeated three to five times.

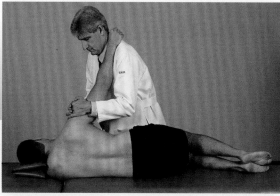

Figure 17.30. Stage 7, steps 1 to 3.

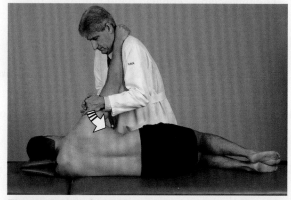

Figure 17.31. Stage 7, step 4.

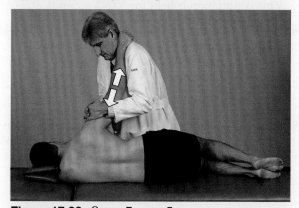

Figure 17.32. Stage 7, step 5.

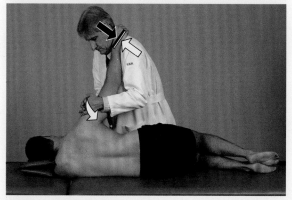

Figure 17.33. Stage 7, step 6.

Upper Extremity Region

Glenohumeral Joint: Glenoid Labrum (Lip) Abduction, Adduction, and Circumduction Ex: Left Shoulder, in 90-Degree Flexion

 See Video 17.2

Indications: Fibrous adhesive capsulitis, tendinitis, tenosynovitis, bursitis, and arthritis

1. The patient lies prone with the left arm/shoulder off the side of the table, and the physician sits facing the patient's affected arm. The patient's hand should not touch the floor, so the table should be elevated or a pillow placed under the patient's chest.

2. The physician's hands encircle the upper (proximal) humerus with the fingers reaching under the axilla until they meet; the thumbs are being placed next to each other, pads down on the humerus, immediately distal to the greater tubercle at the deltoid muscle **(Fig. 17.34)**.

3. The physician engages a slight traction force downward/distal on the arm and then begins to move the shoulder in a "hinge-like" fashion initiating small arcs of abduction **(Fig. 17.35)** and adduction **(Fig. 17.36)**. This and ensuing stages are performed at 10 to 20 full cycles for 15 to 30 seconds each.

4. The patient's arm is then taken back to the neutral starting position, and the humeral head is taken through small clockwise and counterclockwise circular motions (*circular arrows*) in a vertical plane parallel to the long axis of the table for 30 to 60 seconds each **(Fig. 17.37)**.

5. Returning to the neutral position, the physician pushes into the proximal humerus with the thumbs toward the glenoid fossa, adds downward traction, and then draws the arm laterally, followed by an upward, inward, and outward progression, thus forming a motion that would outline a "figure 8" **(Fig. 17.38)**. *Note:* The "8" is seen from a superior view, not a lateral view, distinguishing its motion arc from step 4.

6. The shoulder is then re-examined for functional improvement and pain response. Initially, this technique can be repeated up to three times per week and then titrated to once weekly until function and pain are improved.

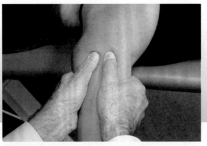

Figure 17.34. Steps 1 and 2.

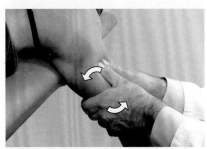

Figure 17.35. Step 3, abduction.

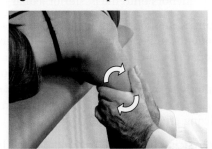

Figure 17.36. Step 3, adduction.

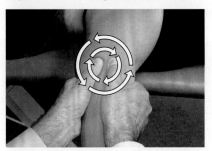

Figure 17.37. Step 4, circumduction.

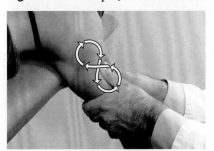

Figure 17.38. Step 5, "the figure 8."

Upper Extremity Region

Shoulder Girdle: Three-Stage Traction
Ex: Left Shoulder Restriction (Capsulitis)

 See Video 17.3

Indications: Improve shoulder range of motion, fibrous adhesive capsulitis, long head of biceps tenosynovitis, short head of biceps, pectoralis minor, and coracobrachialis muscle tendinitis or tendinosis

1. The patient lies supine with the right hand reaching over the chest and grabbing the upper arm to stabilize the glenohumeral joint, and the physician sits at the head of the table.

2. The physician reaches under the patient's left axilla and, with slightly flexed (curled) index and third fingers, anchors onto the posterior axillary fold.

3. The physician's right arm is placed gently onto the patient's upper anterior chest wall to anchor the upper ribs and scapulothoracic articulation. The index and third fingers of this hand curl into the anterior axillary fold while the thumbs of both hands meet over the acromioclavicular joint for a stabilizing effect **(Fig. 17.39)**.

4. The physician begins the treatment by adding a gentle, cephalad-directed traction with both hands and may hold this position for 30 to 60 seconds or use a slow traction "on" and traction "off" (release) "make and break" style **(Fig. 17.40)**.

5. As the patient continues to anchor the left upper arm with the right arm, the physician directs a traction force in a cephalad and lateral direction, making a 60-degree angle from the superior vertical plane. The traction may be performed as in step 4 **(Fig. 17.41)**.

6. The patient's arm is now brought back to the side, and the physician adds a cephalad-directed traction. While the physician holds the traction steady, the patient is instructed to slowly externally rotate **(Fig. 17.42)** and then internally rotate the humerus **(Fig. 17.43)** for 30 to 60 seconds. *Note:* This should not be confused with supination and pronation of the forearm.

7. The shoulder is then re-examined for functional improvement and pain response. Initially, this technique can be repeated up to three times per week and then titrated to once weekly until function and pain are improved.

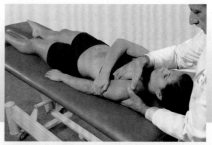
Figure 17.39. Steps 1 to 3.

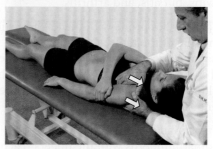
Figure 17.40. Step 4, cephalad traction.

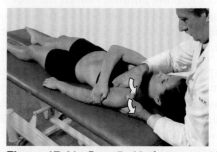
Figure 17.41. Step 5, 60-degree traction.

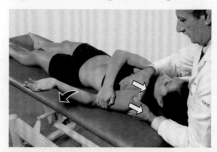
Figure 17.42. Step 6, external rotation.

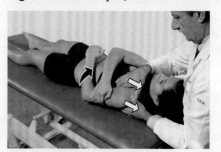
Figure 17.43. Step 6, internal rotation.

Lower Extremity Region

Hip Girdle: *Spencer Technique* Variation
Stage 1: Hip Flexion

1. The patient lies supine, and the physician stands at the side of the table next to the dysfunctional hip.

2. The physician flexes the patient's knee and carries the hip to the flexion-restrictive barrier **(Fig. 17.44)**.

3. A slow, gentle (*articulatory*, *make and break*) motion (*arrows*, **Fig. 17.45**) is applied at the end range of motion.

4. *Muscle energy activation:* The patient pushes (hip extension) the knee into the physician's resistance (*arrows*, **Fig. 17.46**). This contraction is held for 3 to 5 seconds.

5. After a second of relaxation, the hip is carried farther into the new restrictive barrier **(Fig. 17.47)**.

6. Steps 4 and 5 are repeated three to five times, and flexion is reassessed.

7. Resistance against the attempted hip flexion (reciprocal inhibition) has been found to be helpful in augmenting the effect **(Fig. 17.48)**.

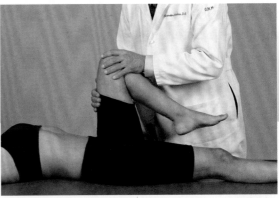

Figure 17.44. Stage 1, steps 1 to 2.

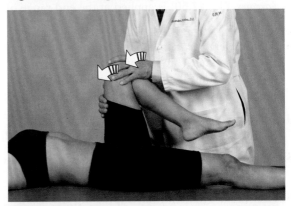

Figure 17.45. Stage 1, step 3.

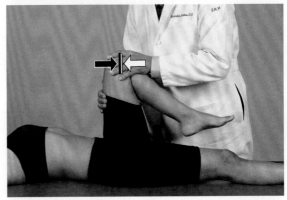

Figure 17.46. Stage 1, step 4.

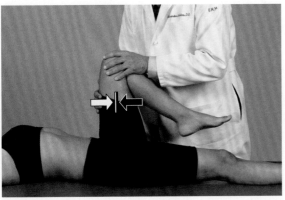

Figure 17.48. Reciprocal inhibition.

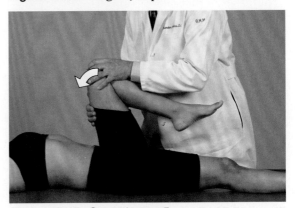

Figure 17.47. Stage 1, step 5.

Lower Extremity Region

Hip Girdle: *Spencer Technique* Variation
Stage 2: Hip Extension

1. The patient's leg is moved off the side of the table and is allowed to descend toward the floor until it meets its extension-restrictive barrier **(Fig. 17.49)**.

2. A slow, gentle (*articulatory, make and break*) motion (*arrows*, **Fig. 17.50**) is applied at the end range of motion.

3. *Muscle energy activation:* The patient is instructed to pull the knee (hip flexion) (*black arrow*, **Fig. 17.51**) into the physician's resistance (*white arrow*). This contraction is held for 3 to 5 seconds.

4. After a second of relaxation, the hip is carried farther into the new restrictive barrier **(Fig. 17.52)**.

5. Steps 3 and 4 are repeated three to five times, and extension is reassessed.

6. Resistance against the attempted hip extension (reciprocal inhibition) has been found to be helpful in augmenting the effect **(Fig. 17.53)**.

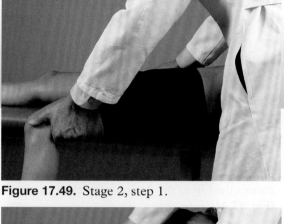

Figure 17.49. Stage 2, step 1.

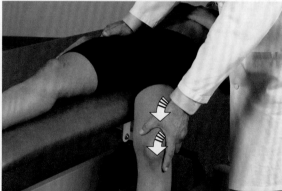

Figure 17.50. Stage 2, step 2.

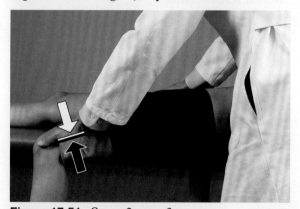

Figure 17.51. Stage 2, step 3.

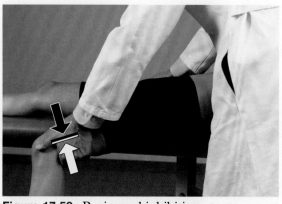

Figure 17.53. Reciprocal inhibition.

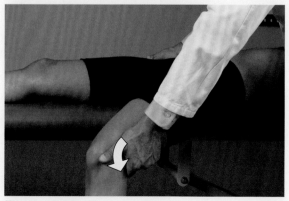

Figure 17.52. Stage 2, step 4.

Lower Extremity Region

Hip Girdle: *Spencer Technique* **Variation**
Stages 3 and 4: Circumduction
Ex: Left Hip, Compression/Traction

1. The physician flexes the patient's hip (with the knee flexed) toward the flexion barrier and adds slight compression (*arrow*, **Fig. 17.54**).

2. The physician circumducts (*arrows*, **Fig. 17.55**) the patient's hip through small and then enlarging circles (clockwise and counterclockwise) for approximately 30 seconds while maintaining compression.

3. The physician extends the patient's knee and grasps the foot and ankle, adding moderate traction (*arrow*, **Fig. 17.56**).

4. Continuing to hold traction, the physician circumducts the patient's hip through small and then increasingly large circles (*arrows*, **Fig. 17.57**) both clockwise and counterclockwise for approximately 15 to 30 seconds.

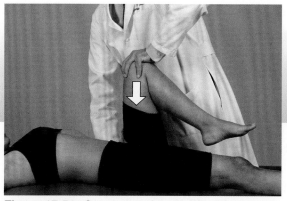

Figure 17.54. Stages 3 and 4, step 1.

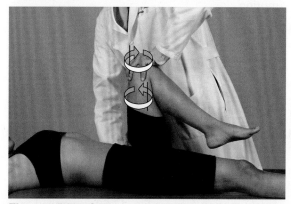

Figure 17.55. Stages 3 and 4, step 2.

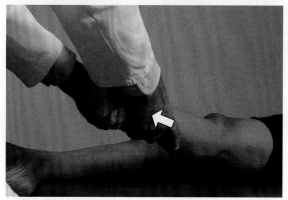

Figure 17.56. Stages 3 and 4, step 3.

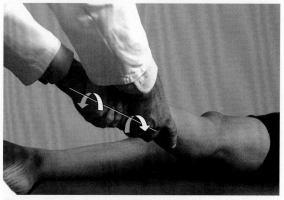

Figure 17.57. Stages 3 and 4, step 4.

Lower Extremity Region

Hip Girdle: *Spencer Technique* Variation
Stages 5 and 6: Internal/External Rotation

1. The physician flexes the patient's hip and knee and internally rotates the hip to its barrier.

2. A slow, gentle (*articulatory, make and break*) motion (*arrows*, **Fig. 17.58**) is applied at the end range of motion.

3. *Muscle energy activation*: The patient is instructed to push the knee (external rotation) (*black arrow*, **Fig. 17.59**) into the physician's resistance (*white arrow*). This contraction is held for 3 to 5 seconds. After a second of relaxation, the hip is carried to the new restrictive barrier.

4. Step 3 is repeated three to five times, and internal rotation is reassessed.

5. The patient is then taken to the external rotation barrier and a slow, gentle (*articulatory, make and break*) motion (*arrows*, **Fig. 17.60**) is applied at the end range of motion.

6. *Muscle energy activation*: The patient is instructed to push the knee (hip internal rotation) into the physician's resistance (*arrows*, **Fig. 17.61**). This contraction is held for 3 to 5 seconds. After a second of relaxation, the hip is carried farther to the new restrictive barrier.

7. Step 6 is repeated three to five times and external rotation is reassessed.

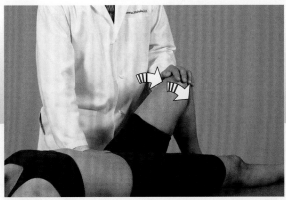

Figure 17.58. Stage 5, steps 1 to 2.

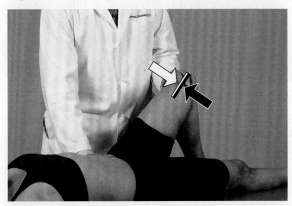

Figure 17.59. Stage 5, step 3.

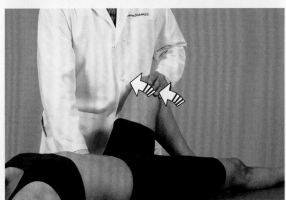

Figure 17.60. Stage 6, step 5.

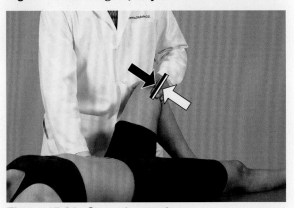

Figure 17.61. Stage 6, step 6.

Lower Extremity Region

Hip Girdle: *Spencer Technique* Variation
Stages 7 and 8: Abduction and Adduction

1. The patient lies supine on the treatment table, and the physician gently takes the patient's straightened leg and abducts it to its restrictive barrier.

2. A slow, gentle (*articulatory, make and break*) motion (*arrows*, **Fig. 17.62**) is applied at the end range of motion.

3. *Muscle energy activation:* The patient is instructed to pull (*black arrow*, **Fig. 17.63**) the knee (hip adduction) into the physician's resistance (*white arrow*). This contraction is held for 3 to 5 seconds. After a second of relaxation, the hip is carried to the new restrictive barrier.

4. Step 3 is repeated three to five times, and abduction is reassessed.

5. The patient is taken to the adduction barrier, and a slow, gentle (*articulatory, make and break*) motion (*arrows*, **Fig. 17.64**) is applied at the end range of motion.

6. *Muscle energy activation:* The patient is instructed to push (*black arrow*, **Fig. 17.65**) the knee (hip abduction) into the physician's resistance (*white arrow*). This contraction is held for 3 to 5 seconds. After a second of relaxation, the hip is carried to the new restrictive barrier.

7. Step 6 is repeated three to five times, and adduction is reassessed.

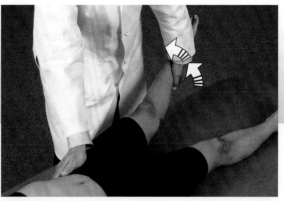

Figure 17.62. Stage 7, steps 1 to 2.

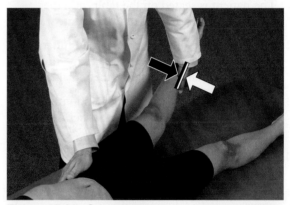

Figure 17.63. Stage 7, step 3.

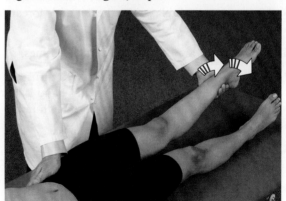

Figure 17.64. Stage 8, step 5.

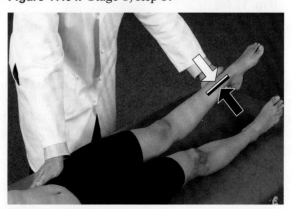

Figure 17.65. Stage 8, step 6.

Upper Extremity Region

Radioulnar Pronation Dysfunction
Long-Lever Supination, Muscle Energy/HVLA
Ex: Right Radial Head, Pronated

 See Video 17.4

Note: This technique affects the long-axis rotational motion of the radius and does not engage the "seesaw" relationship of radial head moving opposite the distal radius.

1. The patient is seated on the table, and the physician stands in front of the patient.

2. The physician holds the patient's dysfunctional arm as if shaking hands and places the thumb of the opposite hand anterior to the radial head.

3. The physician then rotates the hand into supination until the restrictive barrier is engaged **(Fig. 17.66)**.

4. The patient is instructed to attempt to pronate the forearm (*black arrow*, **Fig. 17.67**) while the physician applies an unyielding counterforce (*white arrow*).

5. After a second of relaxation, the patient's forearm is taken into further supination.

6. Steps 4 and 5 are repeated three to five times.

7. If full supination cannot be achieved, a thrust technique may be used. The patient's hand is held in the same fashion with the physician's thumb anterior to the radial head.

8. The elbow is carried into full extension and supination simultaneously.

9. At end extension, a posteriorly directed arc-like thrust is delivered with the thumb into the radius **(Fig. 17.68)**.

10. The physician reassesses the components of the dysfunction (TART).

The long-axis dysfunctions relate to a rotational movement along the length of the radius without anterior and posterior displacement. They are different dysfunctions from the seesaw motions described in the anteroposterior dysfunctions, in which the radial head and styloid process move in opposing directions.

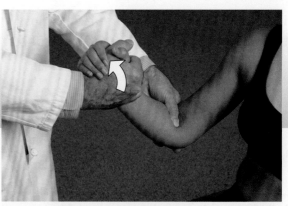

Figure 17.66. Steps 1 to 3.

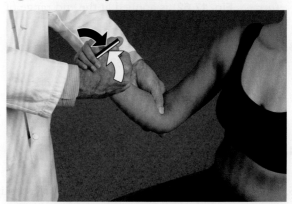

Figure 17.67. Step 4.

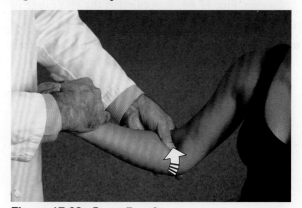

Figure 17.68. Steps 7 to 9.

Upper Extremity Region

Radioulnar Supination Dysfunction
Long-Axis Pronation, Muscle Energy/HVLA
Ex: Right Radial Head, Supinated

 See Video 17.5

Note: This technique affects the long-axis rotational motion of the radius and does not engage the "seesaw" relationship of radial head moving opposite the distal radius.

1. The patient is seated on the table, and the physician stands in front of the patient.

2. The physician holds the patient's dysfunctional arm as if shaking hands and places the thumb of the opposite hand posterior to the radial head giving support.

3. The physician rotates the forearm into pronation (*arrow*, **Fig. 17.69**) until the restrictive barrier is reached.

4. The patient is instructed to attempt to supinate the wrist (*black arrow*, **Fig. 17.70**) while the physician applies an unyielding counterforce (*white arrow*).

5. After a second of relaxation, the patient's forearm is taken into further pronation.

6. Steps 4 and 5 are repeated three to five times.

7. If full pronation cannot be achieved, a thrust technique may be used. The patient's hand is held in the same fashion with the physician's thumb posterior to the radial head.

8. The elbow is carried into full extension and pronation simultaneously.

9. At end extension, an anterior arc-like thrust is delivered with the thumb, which is positioned behind the radial head (**Fig. 17.71**).

10. The physician reassesses the components of the dysfunction (TART).

The long-axis dysfunctions relate to a rotational movement along the length of the radius without anterior and posterior displacement. They are different dysfunctions from the seesaw motions described in the anteroposterior dysfunctions, in which the radial head and styloid process move in opposing directions.

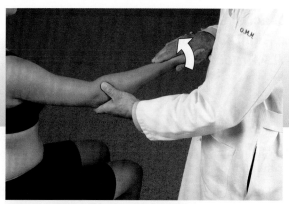

Figure 17.69. Steps 1 to 3.

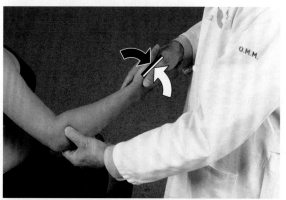

Figure 17.70. Step 4.

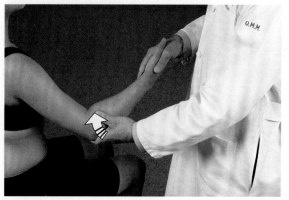

Figure 17.71. Steps 7 to 9.

Pelvic Region

Iliosacral (Innominate) Dysfunction
Ex: Right Anterior Innominate Rotation
HVLA/Traction, Respiratory Assistance

1. The patient lies supine, and the physician stands at the foot of the table.

2. The physician grasps the patient's right ankle and raises the patient's right leg to 45 degrees or more and applies traction on the shaft of the leg (*arrow*, **Fig. 17.72**).

3. This traction is maintained, and the patient is asked to take three to five slow, deep breaths. At the end of each exhalation, traction is increased.

4. At the end of the last breath, the physician delivers an impulse thrust in the direction of the traction (*arrow*, **Fig. 17.73**).

5. The physician reassesses the components of the dysfunction (TART).

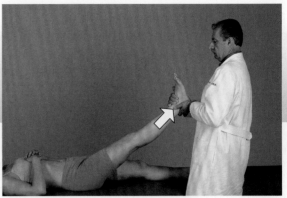

Figure 17.72. Steps 1 to 2.

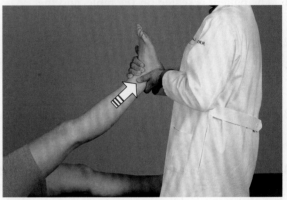

Figure 17.73. Steps 3 to 4.

Cervical Region

C2–C7 Dysfunctions
Ex: C3 NSRRR and SSLRL

1. The patient lies supine, and the physician sits at the head of the table.

2. The physician palpates the articular processes of the segment to be evaluated with the pad of the second or third finger.

3. A translational motion is introduced from left to right (left side bending) and then right to left (right side bending) through the articular processes **(Figs. 17.74 and 17.75)**.

4. At the limit of each translational motion, a rotational springing may be applied in the direction from which the translation emanated (e.g., side bending left, rotation left) **(Fig. 17.76)**.

5. This may be repeated from C2 to C7 for regional improvement or specifically at a local dysfunctional segment.

6. The physician reassesses the components of the dysfunction (TART).

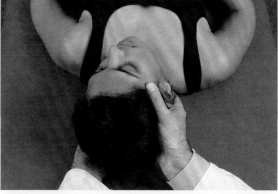

Figure 17.74. Steps 1 to 3, translation to right.

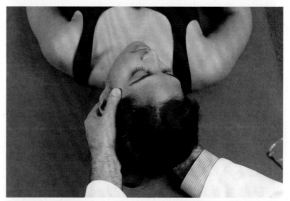

Figure 17.75. Steps 1 to 3, translation to left.

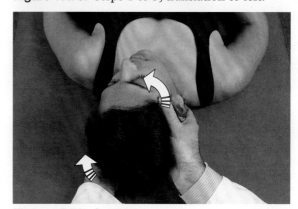

Figure 17.76. Step 4.

Thoracic Region

T1–T4 Dysfunctions
Direct (FSRRR), Type II Method
Ex: T1 ESLRL

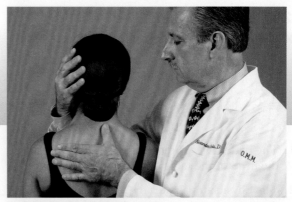

Figure 17.77. Steps 1 to 3.

1. The patient is seated, and the physician either stands behind or sits next to the patient.

2. The physician places the thenar eminence of the posterior hand on the proximal paraspinal thoracic tissues in the dysfunctional area.

3. The physician's other hand reaches in front of the patient and cups the side of the patient's head **(Fig. 17.77)**.

4. As the physician adds a gentle side bending motion of the head toward the physician's side, the thoracic hand applies a springing force perpendicular to the length of the vertebral column **(Fig. 17.78)**.

5. This may be continued throughout the thoracic region or at a local dysfunctional segment as well as can be performed from the other side.

6. The physician reassesses the components of the dysfunction (TART).

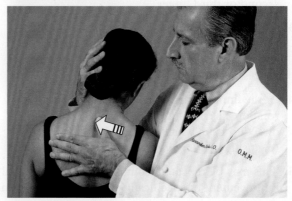

Figure 17.78. Step 4.

References

1. Ward R, exec. ed. Foundations for Osteopathic Medicine. 2nd ed. Philadelphia, PA: Lippincott Williams & Wilkins, 2003.

2. Kimberly P, Funk S, eds. Outline of Osteopathic Manipulative Procedures: The Kimberly Manual. Millennium Edition. Marceline, MO: Walsworth, 2000.

Osteopathic Cranial Manipulative Medicine

Technique Principles

Osteopathic cranial manipulative medicine (OCMM), previously called osteopathy in the cranial field (OCF), as defined by the Educational Council on Osteopathic Principles (ECOP) is a "system of diagnosis and treatment by an osteopathic physician using the primary respiratory mechanism and balanced membranous tension first described by William Garner Sutherland, DO. Osteopathy in the Cranial Field is the title of the reference work by Harold Magoun, Sr., DO" (1). In 2014, ECOP voted to change the name osteopathy in the cranial field to osteopathic cranial manipulative medicine (2).

Sutherland, a student of A. T. Still, began a lifelong study of the cranium, its anatomy and potential biomechanics as they related to health and disease. His interest in the cranium began after first viewing a disarticulated skull when studying in Kirksville, MO (American School of Osteopathy). Although Sutherland is the name most often associated with this form of technique, many others took up his work and continued the study, research, and teaching (3,4). ECOP has defined the primary respiratory mechanism as "a model proposed by William Garner Sutherland, DO to describe the interdependent functions among five body components as follows" (1):

1. The inherent motility of the brain and spinal cord.
2. Fluctuation of the cerebrospinal fluid.
3. Mobility of the intracranial and intraspinal membrane.
4. Articular mobility of the cranial bones.
5. The involuntary mobility of the sacrum between the ilia (pelvic bones) (1).
6. This is considered to be interdependent with the motion at the sphenobasilar synchondrosis.

OCMM has also been called osteopathy in the cranial field (OCF), cranial osteopathy (CO) (1), craniosacral technique (5), and simply cranial technique. It is important that OCMM be used with the aforementioned principles. Other osteopathic techniques can be used on the cranium but are used with their specific principles for treatment effect on somatic dysfunction. For example, counterstrain, soft tissue, myofascial release, and lymphatic techniques can all be used in this region but are not classified as OCMM, OCF, CO, or craniosacral technique. Extensive courses of further study are offered in osteopathic cranial manipulative technique and anatomy, above and beyond the concepts taught in osteopathic medical schools, to prepare physicians to perform this specialty manipulative technique in order to be competent.

Many physicians were reluctant to believe that the cranial bones were capable of movement or that the physician could palpate movement. A number of studies have shown evidence of such motion and suggest that the cranial sutures may not completely ossify (1). A simple example to illustrate that the sutures allow cranial bone mobility is to have one student fix a partner's frontozygomatic sutures bilaterally. This is done by placing one thumb over one frontozygomatic suture and the pad of the index finger of the same hand on the opposite frontozygomatic suture. Then the student gently rocks the zygomatic portion from side to side while the other hand is cradling the head. An audible articular click may occur. The operator, the patient, or both may feel this motion. We have not seen any adverse effects from this maneuver and therefore have confidence in a positive educational outcome.

The reason patients react positively to OCMM is not completely understood, and the underlying cause and effect may be a combination of the stated principles. Some other reasons may include reflex phenomena from connective tissue mechanoreceptors and/or nociceptors or microscopic and macroscopic fluid exchange either peripherally (Traube-Hering-Mayer oscillations) (6) or in the central nervous system. Sutherland, after palpating many patients, felt specific types of motions, and he could not account for these motions based on muscle activity upon reviewing cranial anatomy. Therefore, he began postulating an inherent involuntary mechanism and eventually came to the term *primary respiratory mechanism* (7). ECOP further defines the *primary respiratory mechanism* as:

Primary, because it is directly concerned with the internal tissue respiration of the central nervous system

Respiratory, because it further concerns the physiological function of the interchange of fluids necessary for normal metabolism and biochemistry, not only of the central nervous system but also of all body cells

Mechanism, because all the constituent parts work together as a unit carrying out this fundamental physiology (2)

It is believed that a specific pattern of motion exists and is readily apparent and palpable in each person. This motion pattern is determined by a variety of factors but is thought to be related to the beveling of the sutures and the attachments of the dura. Therefore, to diagnose and treat using OCMM, the physician must know cranial anatomy (e.g., at the pterion, which overlies the middle meningeal artery, the bones overlap as follows: frontal, parietal, sphenoid, and temporal, overlapping alphabetically from inner to outer table).

The internal dural reflections of the falx cerebri, the falx cerebelli, and the tentorium cerebelli are collectively known as the *reciprocal tension membrane* (RTM). The RTM restricts the range of articular motion during normal physiologic movement (1). Distortion in the position or motion of any of the cranial bones may be transmitted to the base and vault through this reciprocal tension membrane. Therefore, restriction of cranial bone motion with distortion of its symmetric motion pattern is termed *cranial somatic dysfunction.*

The biphasic fluctuation of motion that is palpated in the cranial bones has been referred to as the *cranial rhythmic impulse (CRI).* The emphasis in OCMM is placed on the synchronous movement of the cranium with the sacrum (craniosacral mechanism). The physiologic motion between the cranium and sacrum is believed to be around transverse axes with the attachments of the dural tube at the foramen magnum and the second sacral segment. The sacral base (promontory) forms the respiratory axis. This is sometimes called *the core link.* It follows a rhythmic cadence from 8 to 14 cycles per minute (1,4). This impulse may be palpated anywhere in the body, and it is used not only in OCMM but also in balanced ligamentous tension or ligamentous articular strain (BLT/LAS) techniques. Its rate and amplitude may vary in certain disease processes (e.g., fever).

Cranial nomenclature is generally referenced to motion occurring at the sphenobasilar symphysis (SBS) or synchondrosis. The sphenoid articulates with the occiput just below the sella turcica (home to the pituitary gland) at the sphenobasilar synchondrosis. The occiput and the sphenoid rotate in opposite directions.

In sphenobasilar flexion, the basiocciput and basisphenoid move cephalad, while the occipital squama and the wings of the sphenoid move more caudally. These flexion and extension motions are rotational about two transverse axes: one at the level of the foramen magnum and the other through the body of the sphenoid (7). All midline unpaired cranial bones are described as moving in flexion and extension.

Flexion and Extension of the Sphenobasilar Synchondrosis

During flexion of the cranial base **(Fig. 18.1)**, the petrous portions of the temporal bone move cephalad with the SBS driven by the motion of the occiput (8). This produces a flaring outward of the temporal squama called external rotation of the temporal bones. All paired bones move into external rotation synchronous with sphenobasilar flexion. Internal rotation of the paired bones is synchronous with sphenobasilar extension. Therefore, it can be said that in flexion, the skull shortens in the anteroposterior diameter and widens laterally. In extension **(Fig. 18.2)**, the skull lengthens in the anteroposterior diameter and narrows laterally.

Because of the core link between the cranium and the sacrum, the sacrum will synchronously move with the cranium. In SBS flexion, the sacral base moves posterosuperiorly (1), and in SBS extension, the sacrum moves anteroinferiorly. This more recent craniosacral mechanism terminology has caused some confusion because of its difference from the previously used nomenclature for gross sacral motion. In gross sacral biomechanics, a sacral base anterior movement was described as flexion of the sacrum. However, flexion in craniosacral mechanism terminology, is defined as the sacral base moving posteriorly. Some have decided to describe sacral base movements as nodding motions. Thus, forward sacral base movement is called nutation, and backward sacral base movement is called counternutation. No matter which terms one chooses (flexion/extension or nutation/counternutation), the sacral base goes forward in gross flexion and in craniosacral extension. The sacral base moves backward in gross extension and craniosacral flexion.

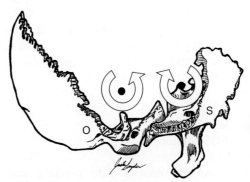

Figure 18.1. Flexion of the sphenobasilar synchondrosis. (O, occipital axis of rotation; S, sphenoidal axis of rotation.)

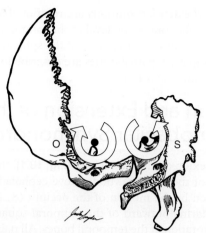

Figure 18.2. Extension of the sphenobasilar synchondrosis. (O, occipital axis of rotation; S, sphenoidal axis of rotation.)

 See Video 18.1
(SBS Flexion/Extension)

See also the video at the American Association of Colleges of Osteopathic Medicine website for a 3-D animation of flexion and extension of the sphenobasilar synchrondrosis (http://www.aacom.org/ome/councils/aacom-councils/ecop/motion-animations/Detail/flexion-and-extension-of-the-sphenobasilar-synchrondrosis).

Craniosacral Mechanism

Dysfunctional patterns of cranial motion have been described as either physiologic or not. Examples of physiologic dysfunctions include torsion, side bending and rotation, and fixed (flexion and extension). Compression, vertical strains (shear), and lateral strains are examples of nonphysiologic dysfunctions. They may be secondary to head trauma, birth trauma, dental procedures, inferior musculoskeletal stress and dysfunction, and postural abnormalities.

Torsion involves rotation of the SBS around an anteroposterior axis. The sphenoid and occiput rotate in opposite directions. Palpation of a *right torsion* feels as if the greater wing of the sphenoid on the right elevates and rotates to the left, while the occipital squama on the right drops into the hands and rotates to the right **(Fig. 18.3)**. It is named for the greater wing that is superior.

 See Video 18.2
(SBS Torsion)

Side bending/rotation is side bending and rotation that occur simultaneously at the SBS. Side bending occurs by rotation around two vertical axes, one through the center of the body of the sphenoid and one

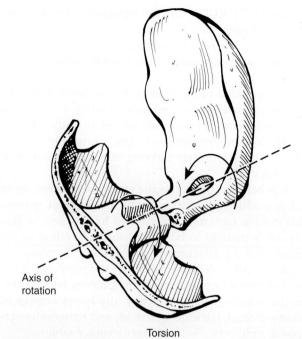

Figure 18.3. Right SBS torsion.

at the foramen magnum. The sphenoid and the occiput rotate in opposite directions about these axes. The rotation component of the dysfunction occurs around an anteroposterior axis, but the sphenoid and the occiput rotate in the same direction. Rotation occurs toward the side of convexity (the inferior side) and is named for such. While palpating a *left side bending rotation*, one notes that the left hand feels a fullness as compared to the right hand (side bending), and one also feels that the left hand is being drawn caudally both at the sphenoid and occiput (rotation) **(Fig. 18.4)**.

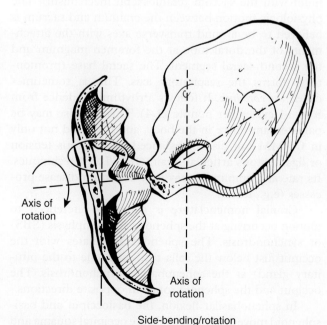

Figure 18.4. Left SBS side bending/rotation.

See Video 18.3
(SBS Side Bending/Rotation)

See also the video at the American Association of Colleges of Osteopathic Medicine website for a 3-D animation of cranial motion that results in a "side bending rotation" somatic dysfunction with axes (http://www.aacom.org/ome/councils/aacom-councils/ecop/motion-animations/Detail/cranial-motion-that-results-in-a-sidebending-rotation-somatic-dysfunction-with-axes).

SBS compression either feels rock hard, like a bowling ball (void of any motion), or the physician begins to feel all of the dysfunctional strain patterns together **(Fig. 18.5)**.

See Video 18.4
(SBS Compression)

Superior/inferior vertical strains involve either flexion at the sphenoid and extension at the occiput (superior) or extension at the sphenoid and flexion at the occiput (inferior). The dysfunction is named by the position of the basisphenoid. During palpation, a superior vertical shear feels as if the greater wings of the sphenoid are drawn too far caudally. In an inferior vertical shear, the sphenoid moves minimally caudad **(Fig. 18.6)**.

See Video 18.5
(SBS Inferior Vertical Strain)

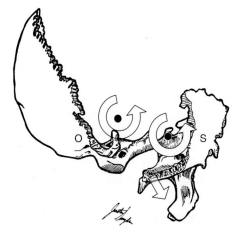

Figure 18.6. SBS inferior vertical strain. (O, occipital axis of rotation; S, sphenoidal axis of rotation.)

See Video 18.6
(SBS Superior Vertical Strain)

Lateral strain involves rotation around two vertical axes, but the rotation occurs in the same direction. This causes a lateral shearing force at the SBS. The dysfunction is named for the position of the basisphenoid, relative to the occiput. During palpation, the lateral strains feel as if the hands are on a parallelogram **(Fig. 18.7)**.

See Video 18.7
(SBS Lateral Strain)

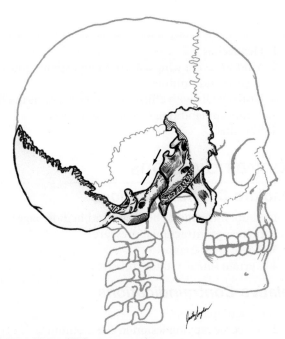

Figure 18.5. SBS compression.

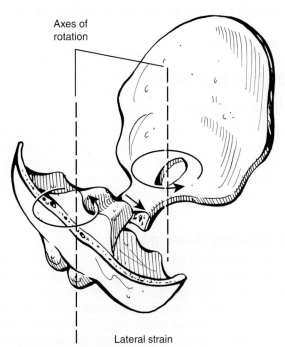

Figure 18.7. SBS lateral strain.

Technique Classification

Direct Technique

In direct OCMM, the dysfunction is moved toward the restrictive barrier (bind, tension). The physician should gently approach the barrier and maintain a light force until a release occurs. If the dysfunction appears to be mostly articular, a direct technique is appropriate. This technique is commonly used on infants and children before full development of the cranial sutures and in very specific dysfunctions in adults (5).

Indirect Technique

In indirect OCMM, the dysfunction is moved away from the restrictive barrier or toward the ease (freedom, loose). The physician attempts to move the dysfunction in the direction of freedom until a balance of tension occurs (balanced membranous tension) (5,7) between the ease and bind. The CRI is monitored, and the inherent forces eventually cause a slight increase toward the ease and then movement back to the original balance position, which is a sign of the release. This technique is most appropriate if the key dysfunction is secondary to a membranous restriction (5).

Exaggeration

Exaggeration method is performed with the physician moving the dysfunction toward the ease, similar to indirect, but when meeting the ease barrier, an activating force is added.

Disengagement

In disengagement, the physician attempts to open or separate the articulation. Depending on how the articulation is felt to be restricted, traction or a compressive force may be added.

Technique Styles

Inherent Force

Use of the body's inherent force through the primary respiratory mechanism is the major method of OCMM. Using the fluctuation of the cerebrospinal fluid, the physician can alter the pressure in one area or another and cause this fluid to change the various barriers. This is most evident in the **V**-spread technique (5).

Respiratory Assistance

As in other techniques, the use of pulmonary respiration can facilitate osteopathic technique. This release-enhancing mechanism will increase movements associated with inhalation and exhalation. For example, it is believed that during inhalation, the SBS tends to move toward flexion, with the paired bones moving more toward external rotation. In exhalation, the unpaired bones move preferentially toward extension and the paired bones into internal rotation. The physician can have the patient breathe in the direction preferred for its related cranial effect and tell the patient to hold the breath at full inhalation or exhalation. This will enhance a release.

Distal Activation

In certain conditions, the physician may prefer to treat the patient's problem from the sacral region or extremities. By applying tension on the sacrum, the physician can guide the mechanism from below and effect the movement of the SBS. In addition, the physician may have the patient actively attempt plantar flexion or dorsiflexion to gain a particular effect on the SBS. Dorsiflexion enhances SBS flexion, while plantar flexion enhances extension (5).

Still Point

In this method, the physician attempts to resist the primary respiratory mechanism that is being monitored through the CRI. This is most commonly called compression of the fourth ventricle (CV4). Success of the CV4 technique relies on inherent forces. In this technique, the physician monitors several cycles of CRI and then permits exhalation motion at the bone being palpated (usually the occipital squama). Then the physician gently resists flexion until a cessation of the cerebral spinal fluid fluctuation is palpated. This is called a *still point*. This position is held for 15 seconds to a few minutes, until the physician appreciates a return of the CRI. This can be applied to the sacrum when contacting the head is contraindicated (e.g., acute head trauma) (5,7).

Indications

1. Headaches
2. Mild to severe whiplash strain and sprain injuries
3. Vertigo and tinnitus
4. Otitis media with effusion and serous otitis media
5. Temporomandibular joint dysfunction
6. Sinusitis

Contraindications

Absolute Contraindications

1. Acute intracranial bleeding and hemorrhage
2. Increased intracranial pressure
3. Acute skull fracture
4. Certain seizure states (relative)

Relative Contraindications

1. Coagulopathies
2. Space-occupying lesion in the cranium

General Considerations and Rules

OCMM may help a number of conditions. Its adverse reactions are few, but the physician should be on alert, as headache, vertigo, tinnitus, nausea, and vomiting can occur, as can some autonomic related effects (e.g., bradycardia). These are mostly seen when students are first learning the technique and do not realize the pressure being imparted into their patient's cranium. This is common, with improper holding technique (location and incorrect pressure) seen at times at the occipitomastoid suture. Headaches, nausea, and vomiting, while not common, are seen occasionally.

Therefore, the physician must take care to contact the patient properly and apply enough but not too much pressure for the appropriate amount of time. The physician should also make sure that the primary respiratory mechanism is present when deciding to end the treatment.

A variation of this technique is using a multiple-hand approach. While one operator is palpating the cranium, another can be on the sacrum or another area of the patient's body. This can potentiate the effect of a treatment.

Cranial Region

Cranial Vault Hold

 See Video 18.8.

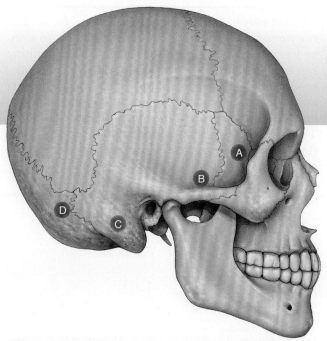

Figure 18.8. Lateral view of skull with dots for finger placement. (Modified with permission from Ref. (2).)

Objectives

The objective is to assess the primary respiratory mechanism as it manifests itself in the cranium and the degree of participation of each bone in the general motion of the cranium.

Technique

1. The patient lies supine, and the physician is seated at the head of the table.
2. The physician establishes a fulcrum by resting both forearms on the table.
3. The physician's hands cradle the patient's head, making full palmar contact on both sides.
4. The physician's index fingers rest on the greater wings of the patient's sphenoid (*A*, **Fig. 18.8**).
5. The physician's middle fingers rest on the zygomatic processes of the patient's temporal bones (*B*, **Fig. 18.8**).
6. The physician's ring fingers rest on the mastoid processes of the patient's temporal bones (*C*, **Fig. 18.8**).
7. The physician's little fingers rest on the squamous portion of the patient's occiput (*D*, **Fig. 18.8**).
8. The physician's thumbs touch or cross each other without touching the patient's cranium (**Figs. 18.9 and 18.10**).
9. The physician palpates the CRI:
   - *Extension/internal rotation*: coronal diameter narrows, anteroposterior diameter increases, and height increases.
   - *Flexion/external rotation*: coronal diameter widens, anteroposterior diameter decreases, and height decreases.
10. The physician notes the amplitude, rate, and regularity of the CRI.
11. The physician notes which bones, if any, have an altered amplitude, rate, and regularity.

The physician may instruct the patient to stop breathing to further distinguish the rhythmic sensations that occur in the CRI. The physician can also have the patient inhale and exhale fully to increase the amplitude of the CRI, which can make it easier to feel.

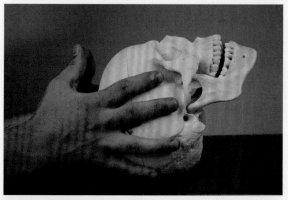

Figure 18.9. Steps 1 to 8.

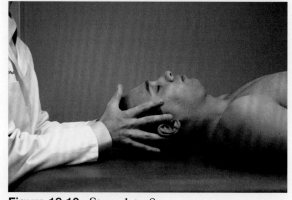

Figure 18.10. Steps 1 to 8.

Cranial Region

Fronto-occipital Hold

 See Video 18.8

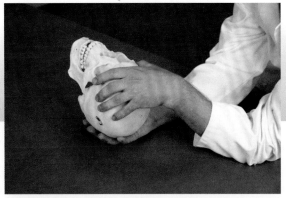

Figure 18.11. Steps 1 to 5.

Objectives

The objectives are to assess the primary respiratory mechanism as it manifests itself in the cranium; to assess the freedom of motion of the cranial base, especially at the SBS; and to assess the frontal bone as it relates to the rest of the CRI.

Technique

1. The patient lies supine, and the physician is seated at the side of the head of the table.

2. The physician places the caudad hand under the patient's occipital squama with the forearm resting on the table establishing a fulcrum.

3. The physician's cephalad hand bridges across the patient's frontal bone, with the elbow resting on the table establishing a fulcrum.

4. The thumb and middle finger of the physician's cephalad hand rest on the greater wings of the patient's sphenoid (if the hand spread is too short, approximate the greater wings).

5. The physician makes full palmar contact with both hands **(Figs. 18.11 to 18.13)**.

6. The physician palpates the CRI:
   - *Extension/internal rotation:* coronal diameter narrows, anteroposterior diameter increases, and height increases.
   - *Flexion/external rotation:* coronal diameter widens, anteroposterior diameter decreases, and height decreases.

7. The physician notes the amplitude, rate, and regularity of the CRI.

8. The physician notes which bones, if any, have an altered amplitude, rate, and regularity.

9. The physician pays particular attention to the SBS, determining whether there is any preferred motion of the sphenoid and the occiput.

The physician may instruct the patient to stop breathing to further distinguish the rhythmic sensations that occur in the CRI. The physician can also have the patient inhale and exhale fully to increase the amplitude of the CRI, which can make it easier to feel.

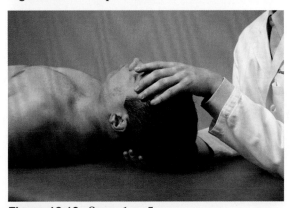

Figure 18.12. Steps 1 to 5.

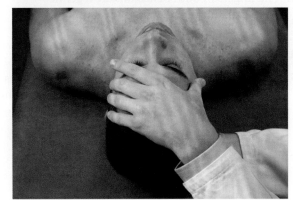

Figure 18.13. Steps 1 to 5.

Cranial Region

Decompression of the Occipital Condyles

 See Video 18.9

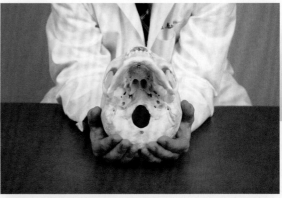

Figure 18.14. Steps 1 and 2.

Objectives

The objective is to balance the reciprocal tension membrane at the hypoglossal canal, permitting normalized function of cranial nerve XII.

Technique

1. The patient lies supine, and the physician is seated at the head of the table with both forearms resting on the table, establishing a fulcrum.

2. The patient's head rests on the physician's palms, and the physician's index and middle fingers (or the middle and ring fingers) approximate the patient's condylar processes (as far caudad on the occiput as the soft tissue and C1 will allow) **(Figs. 18.14 to 18.16)**.

3. The fingers of both hands initiate a gentle cephalad and lateral force at the base of the occiput.

4. The force is maintained until a release is felt.

5. The rate and amplitude of the CRI as it manifests in the basioccipital region are retested to assess the effectiveness of the technique.

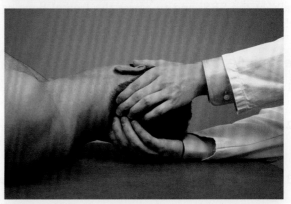

Figure 18.15. Steps 1 and 2.

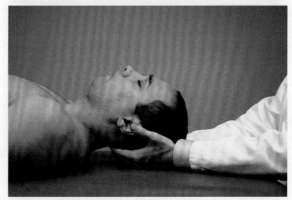

Figure 18.16. Steps 1 and 2.

Cranial Region

Occipitoatlantal Decompression

Objectives

The objective is to treat occipitoatlantal somatic dysfunction that results from rotation of the occiput on its anteroposterior axis, resulting in misalignment of the condyles in the facets of the atlas (8). In general, this technique should be performed after decompression of the occipital condyles.

Technique

1. The patient lies supine, and the physician is seated at the head of the table with both forearms resting on the table, establishing a fulcrum.

2. The physician places the pads of both middle fingers on the posterior aspect of the cranium and slides these fingers down the occiput until the fingers are against the posterior arches of the atlas **(Figs. 18.17 to 18.19)**.

3. The physician applies caudad pressure with both middle fingers to separate the facets from the condylar parts.

4. While the physician maintains this caudad pressure, the patient tucks the chin into the chest, making sure *not* to flex the neck (this is the nodding movement that occurs at the occipitoatlantal joint).

5. This motion carries the occipital condyles posteriorly, tenses the ligaments in the region, and stretches the contracted muscles in the occipital triangle.

6. The physician maintains this position while the patient holds one or more deep inspirations to their limit. This will enhance articular release.

7. The rate and amplitude of the CRI, as it manifests in the basiocciptal region, are retested to assess the effectiveness of the technique. Occipitoatlantal motion testing can also be assessed for normalization.

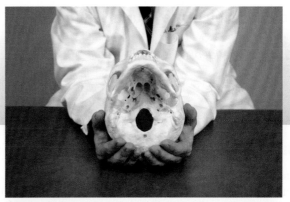

Figure 18.17. Steps 1 and 2.

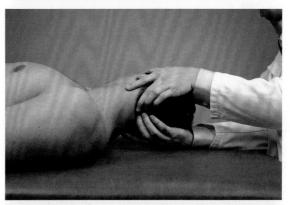

Figure 18.18. Steps 1 and 2.

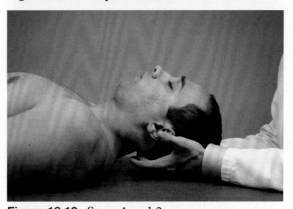

Figure 18.19. Steps 1 and 2.

Cranial Region

Compression of the Fourth Ventricle

 See Video 18.10

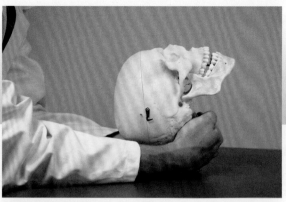

Figure 18.21. Steps 1 to 3.

Objectives

Treatment often starts with compression of CV4 for ill patients. The treatment augments the healing capabilities of the patient, relaxes the patient, and improves the motion of the CRI.

Technique

1. The patient lies supine, and the physician is seated at the head of the table with both forearms resting on the table, establishing a fulcrum.

2. The physician crosses or interlaces the fingers of both hands, cradling the patient's occipital squama.

3. The physician places the thenar eminences posteromedial to the patient's occipitomastoid sutures. *If the thenar eminences are on the mastoid processes of the temporal bones, the compression that follows will bilaterally externally rotate the temporal bones, which may cause extreme untoward reactions* (Figs. 18.20 to 18.23).

4. The physician encourages extension of the patient's occiput by following the occiput as it moves into extension.

5. The physician resists flexion by holding the patient's occiput in extension with bilateral medial forces. *Note:* The occiput is not forced into extension. Rather, it is prevented from moving into flexion. It is as if the physician is taking up the slack created by extension and holding it there.

6. This force is maintained until the amplitude of the CRI decreases, a still point is reached, and/or a sense of release is felt (a sense of softening and warmth in the region of the occiput).

7. As the CRI resumes, the physician slowly releases the force, allowing the CRI to undergo newfound excursion.

8. The rate and amplitude of the CRI are retested to assess the effectiveness of the technique.

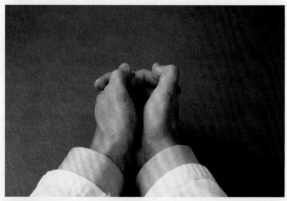

Figure 18.22. Superior view of hand position.

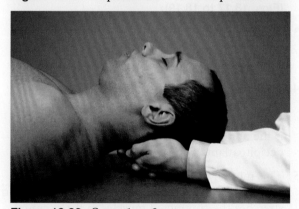

Figure 18.23. Steps 1 to 3.

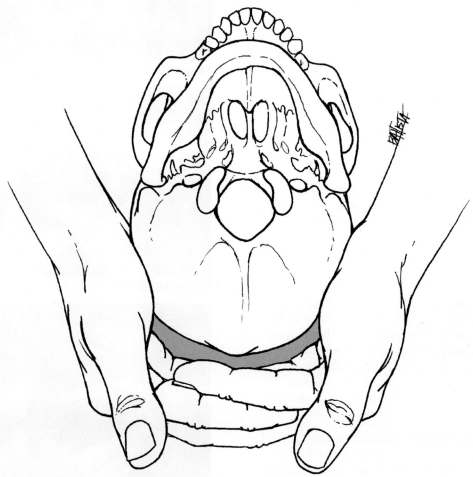

Figure 18.20. Steps 1 to 3.

Cranial Region

Interparietal Sutural Opening (V-Spread)

 See Video 18.11

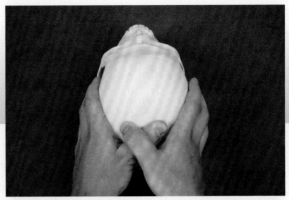

Figure 18.24. Steps 1 to 3.

Objective

The objective is to restore freedom of movement to the sagittal suture, increasing the drainage of the superior sagittal sinus.

Technique

1. The patient lies supine, and the physician is seated at the head of the table with both forearms resting on table, establishing a fulcrum.

2. The physician's thumbs are crossed over the patient's sagittal suture just anterior and superior to lambda.

3. The remainder of the physician's fingers rest on the lateral surfaces of the patient's parietal bones **(Figs. 18.24 to 18.26)**.

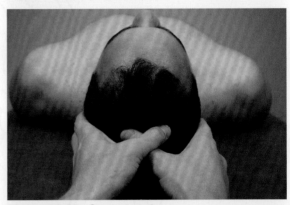

Figure 18.25. Steps 1 to 3.

4. The physician's crossed thumbs gently exert a force, pushing the patient's parietal bones apart at the sagittal suture. The physician's other fingers encourage external rotation of the parietal bones, decompressing the sagittal suture (this may be accompanied by a sensation of softening and warming or an increase in motion and a physical spreading).

5. The physician moves the thumbs anteriorly approximately 1 to 2 cm, and the procedure is repeated. The physician continues to move along the sagittal suture to the bregma. (This technique may be carried even farther forward along the metopic suture.)

6. The rate and amplitude of the CRI, especially at the sagittal suture, are retested to assess the effectiveness of the technique.

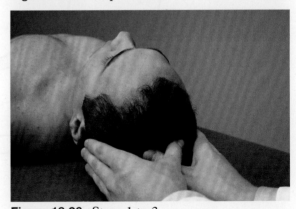

Figure 18.26. Steps 1 to 3.

Cranial Region

Sutural Spread
(Direction of Fluid Technique)

 See Video 18.12

Objective

The objective is to release a restricted cranial suture (e.g., left occipitomastoid suture).

Technique

1. The patient lies supine, and the physician is seated at the head of the table with both elbows resting on the table, establishing a fulcrum.

2. The physician places the index and middle fingers on the two sides of the patient's restricted suture.

3. The physician places one or two fingers of the other hand on the patient's cranium at a point opposite the suture to be released **(Figs. 18.27 to 18.29)**.

4. With the lightest force possible, the physician directs an impulse toward the restricted suture with the hand opposite the suture, initiating a fluid wave. The object is not to physically push fluid through to the opposite side. Instead, the physician is using the fluctuation of the cerebrospinal fluid to release the restriction. The physician uses intention to initiate this wave; this method contracts the fewest muscle fibers and so applies the slightest force.

5. This fluid wave may bounce off the restricted suture and return to the initiating hand, which should receive and redirect the returned wave toward the restricted suture.

6. This back-and-forth action may be repeated for several cycles before the physician feels the suture spread and the wave penetrating the suture does not return to the initiating hand.

7. The rate and amplitude of the CRI at that suture are retested to assess the effectiveness of the technique.

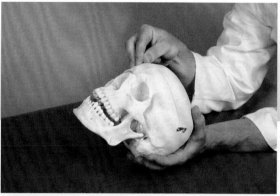
Figure 18.27. Steps 1 to 3.

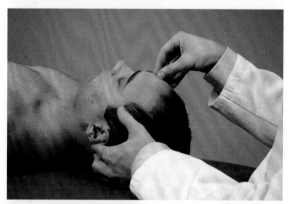
Figure 18.28. Steps 1 to 3.

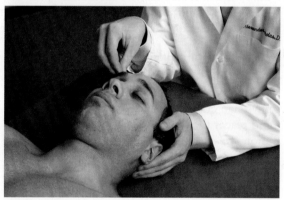
Figure 18.29. Steps 1 to 3.

Cranial Region

Venous Sinus Drainage

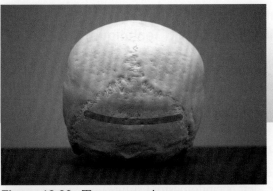

Figure 18.30. Transverse sinus.

Objectives

The objective is to increase intracranial venous drainage by affecting the dural membranes that comprise the sinuses (7). Thoracic outlet, cervical, and occipitoatlantal joint somatic dysfunctions should be treated first to allow drainage from the venous sinuses.

Technique

1. The patient lies supine, and the physician is seated at the head of the table with both elbows resting on the table, establishing a fulcrum.

2. For transverse sinus drainage, the physician places the first and second finger pads of both hands across the superior nuchal line (*blue line*, **Fig. 18.30**) (**Fig. 18.31**).

3. This position is maintained with minimal pressure (the weight of the patient's head should suffice) until a release is felt (apparent softening under the fingers).

4. The physician maintains this pressure until both sides release.

5. For drainage at the confluences of sinuses, the physician cradles the back of the patient's head and places the middle finger of one hand on the inion (*blue dot*, **Fig. 18.32**) (**Fig. 18.33**).

6. Step 4 is repeated until a softening is felt.

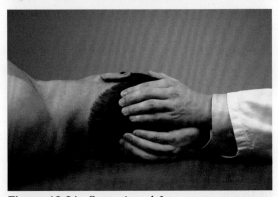

Figure 18.31. Steps 1 and 2.

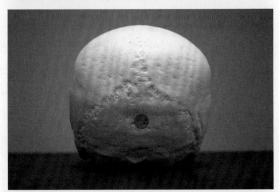

Figure 18.32. Confluence of sinuses.

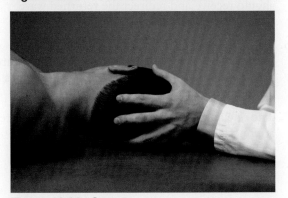

Figure 18.33. Step 5.

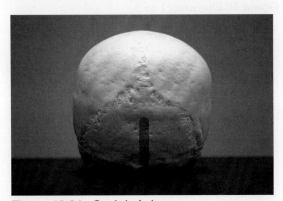

Figure 18.34. Occipital sinus.

7. For occipital sinus drainage, the physician cradles the back of the patient's head and places the second to fourth fingers of both hands in opposition along the midline from the inion to the suboccipital tissues (*blue line*, **Fig. 18.34**) **(Fig. 18.35)**.

8. Step 4 is repeated until a softening is felt.

9. For drainage of the superior sagittal sinus, the physician places two crossed thumbs at lambda and exerts opposing forces with each thumb to disengage the suture.

10. Once local release is felt, the physician moves anteriorly and superiorly along the superior sagittal suture with the crossed thumb forces, noting releases at each location toward bregma (*blue line*, **Fig. 18.36**) **(Fig. 18.37)**.

11. Once at bregma, the physician places the second to fourth fingers of both hands in opposition along the midline on the frontal bone at the location of the metopic suture (*blue line*, **Fig. 18.38**) **(Fig. 18.39)**.

12. The physician continues anteriorly on the frontal bone, disengaging the suture by gently separating each finger on opposing hands.

13. The rate and amplitude of the CRI, especially fluid fluctuations, are retested to assess the effectiveness of the technique.

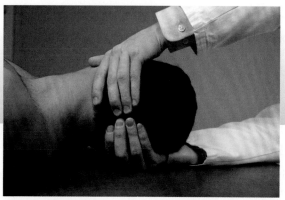

Figure 18.35. Step 7.

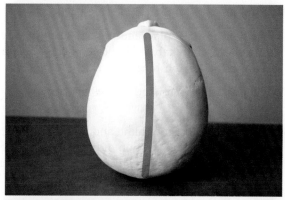

Figure 18.36. Superior sagittal sinus.

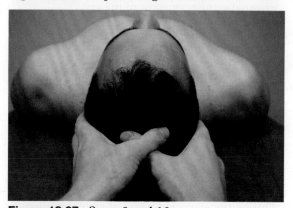

Figure 18.37. Steps 9 and 10.

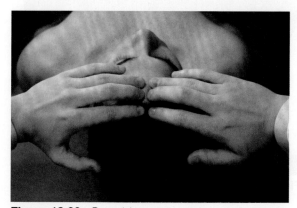

Figure 18.39. Step 11.

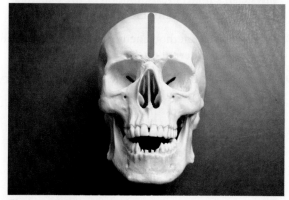

Figure 18.38. Metopic suture.

Cranial Region

Unilateral Temporal Rocking
Ex: Right, External/Internal Rotation

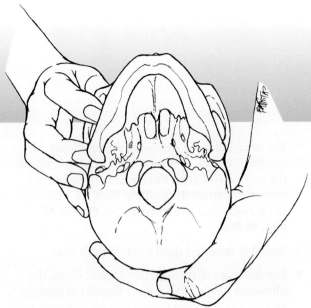

Figure 18.40. Steps 1 to 5, anatomic location of finger placement.

Objective

The objective is to treat a dysfunction in which the temporal bone is held in external/internal rotation.

Technique

1. The patient lies supine, and the physician is seated at the head of the table with both forearms resting on the table, establishing a fulcrum.

2. The physician's left hand cradles the patient's occiput.

3. The physician's right thumb and index finger grasp the zygomatic portion of the patient's right temporal bone, thumb cephalad, and index finger caudad.

4. The physician's right middle finger rests on the external acoustic meatus of the ear.

5. The physician's right ring and little fingers rest on the inferior portion of the patient's mastoid process **(Figs. 18.40 to 18.42)**.

6. During the flexion phase of cranial motion, the physician's ring and little fingers exert medial pressure. This pressure is accompanied by cephalad lifting of the patient's zygomatic arch with the physician's thumb and index fingers, encouraging external rotation of the temporal bone.

7. During the extension phase of cranial motion, the physician's fingers resist motion of the patient's temporal bone toward internal rotation.

8. An alternative method encourages internal rotation and inhibits external rotation.

9. The rate and amplitude of the primary respiratory mechanism, especially at the temporal bone, are retested to assess the effectiveness of the technique.

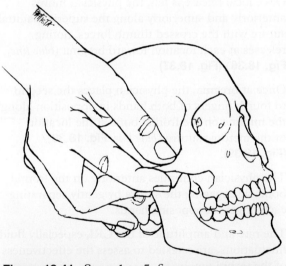

Figure 18.41. Steps 1 to 5, fingers on zygoma.

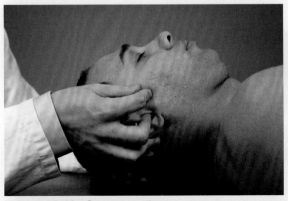

Figure 18.42. Steps 1 to 5.

Cranial Region

Frontal Lift

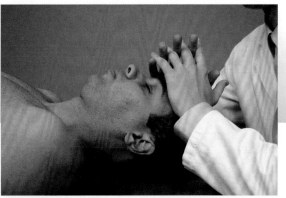

Figure 18.43. Steps 1 to 3, hand placement.

Objective

The objective is to treat dysfunctions of the frontal bones in relation to their sutural or dural connections (i.e., frontoparietal compression, frontonasal compression) (9).

Technique

1. The patient lies supine, and the physician is seated at the head of the table with both forearms resting on the table, establishing a fulcrum.

2. The physician places both hypothenar eminences on the lateral angles of the frontal bones and the thenar eminences of both hands anterior to the lateral aspects of the coronal suture.

3. The physician interlaces the fingers above the metopic suture **(Fig. 18.43)**.

4. The physician's thenar and hypothenar eminences provide a gentle compressive force medially to disengage the frontals from the parietals (*arrows*, **Fig. 18.44**), internally rotating the frontal bones.

5. The physician, while maintaining this medial compressive force, applies a gentle anterior force either on one side or both as needed to disengage the sutural restrictions (*arrows*, **Fig. 18.45**).

6. This position is held until the physician feels the lateral angles of the frontal bones move into external rotation (expansion under the hypothenar eminences).

7. The physician then gently releases the head.

8. The rate and amplitude of the primary respiratory mechanism, especially at the frontal bones, are retested to assess the effectiveness of the technique.

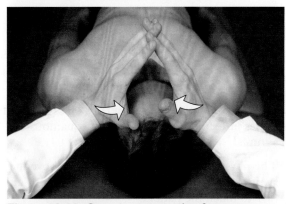

Figure 18.44. Step 4, compressive force.

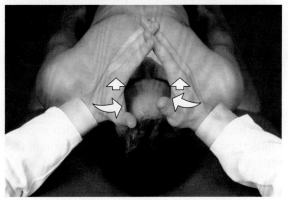

Figure 18.45. Step 5, anterior-guided force.

Cranial Region

Parietal Lift

 See Video 18.13

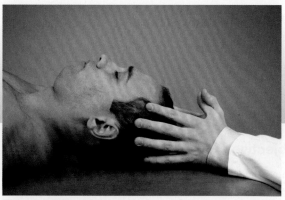

Figure 18.46. Steps 1 to 3.

Objective

The objective is to treat dysfunction of the parietal bones in relation to their sutural or dural connections (i.e., parietotemporal, parietofrontal) (9).

Technique

1. The patient lies supine, and the physician is seated at the head of the table with both forearms resting on the table, establishing a fulcrum.

2. The physician places the fingertips on both parietal bones just superior to the parietal-squamous sutures.

3. The physician crosses the thumbs just above the sagittal suture **(Fig. 18.46)**. *Note:* The thumbs are NOT to touch the patient.

4. The physician presses one thumb against the other (*arrows*, **Fig. 18.47**) (one thumb presses upward, while the other resists it).

5. Pressing one thumb against the other approximates the fingertips. This induces internal rotation of the parietal bones at the parietal-squamous sutures.

6. While maintaining pressure, the physician lifts both hands cephalad until fullness is felt over the fingertips; this fullness is external rotation of the parietal bones (*arrows*, **Fig. 18.48**).

7. The physician gently releases the head.

8. The rate and amplitude of the primary respiratory mechanism, especially at the frontal bones, are retested to assess the effectiveness of the technique.

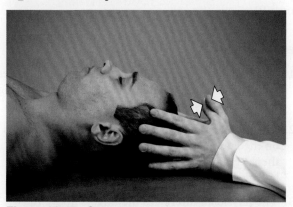

Figure 18.47. Step 4.

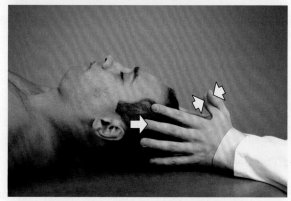

Figure 18.48. Step 6, external rotation of parietals.

Sacral Region

Sacral Hold

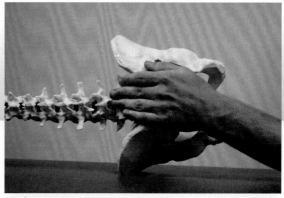

Figure 18.49. Steps 1 to 4.

Objective

The objective is to create free and symmetric motion of the sacrum by palpation of the CRI.

Technique

1. The patient lies supine, and the physician is seated at the side of the table caudad to the sacrum.

2. The patient is instructed to bend the far knee and roll toward the physician.

3. The physician slides the caudad hand between the patient's legs and under the sacrum, and the patient drops his or her weight is on this hand.

4. The physician allows the hand to mold to the shape of the sacrum with the median sacral crest lying between the third and fourth fingers, the fingertips approximating the base, and the palm cradling the apex **(Figs. 18.49 and 18.50)**.

5. The physician presses the elbow down into the table, establishing a fulcrum.

6. The physician palpates the craniosacral mechanism. Sphenobasilar flexion is synchronous with sacral counternutation (sacral base moves posterior). Sphenobasilar extension is synchronous with sacral nutation (sacral base moves anterior).

7. The physician's hand follows these motions, encouraging symmetric and full range of sacral motion.

8. The physician continues to follow and encourage sacral motion until palpation of a release, which is usually accompanied by a sensation of softening and warming of the sacral tissues.

9. The physician retests the quantity and quality of sacral motion to assess the effectiveness of the technique.

The physician can also use the cephalad hand, either sliding it under the patient's lumbar area **(Fig. 18.51)** or laying the forearm across both anterior superior iliac spines. The additional hand placement gives the physician more information about how the sacrum relates to the respective areas.

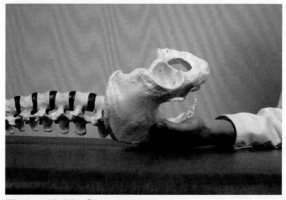

Figure 18.50. Steps 1 to 4.

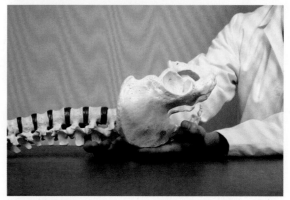

Figure 18.51. Lumbar and sacral contact.

References

1. Ward R, exec. ed. Foundations for Osteopathic Medicine. 2nd ed. Philadelphia, PA: Lippincott Williams & Wilkins, 2003.

2. Educational Council on Osteopathic Principles (ECOP) of the American Association of Colleges of Osteopathic Medicine, Glossary of Osteopathic Terminology, Chevy Chase, Revised October 2014.

3. Arbuckle B. The Selected Writings of Beryl E. Arbuckle. Camp Hill, PA: National Osteopathic Institute and Cerebral Palsy Foundation, 1977.

4. Weaver C. The cranial vertebrae. J Am Osteopath Assoc 1936;35:328–336.

5. Greenman P. Principles of Manual Medicine. 3rd ed. Philadelphia, PA: Lippincott Williams & Wilkins, 2003.

6. Nelson K, Sergueff N, Lipinsky C, et al. Cranial rhythmic impulse related to the Traube-Hering-Mayer oscillation: comparing laser Doppler flowmetry and palpation. J Am Osteopath Assoc 2001;101:163–173.

7. DiGiovanna E, Schiowitz S. An Osteopathic Approach to Diagnosis and Treatment. Philadelphia, PA: Lippincott Williams & Wilkins, 2005.

8. Magoun H. Osteopathy in the Cranial Field. 3rd ed. Boise, ID: Northwest Printing, 1976.

9. Agur AMR, Dalley AF. Grant's Atlas of Anatomy. 11th ed. Baltimore, MD: Lippincott Williams & Wilkins, 2005.

Note: Page numbers in italics denote figures; page numbers followed by t denote tables.